C12

Handbook of
Behavioral Neurobiology

Volume 4
Biological Rhythms

Edited by

Jürgen Aschoff

Max-Planck Institut für Verhaltensphysiologie
Andechs, German Federal Republic

PLENUM PRESS · NEW YORK AND LONDON

Library of Congress Cataloging in Publication Data

Main entry under title:

Biological rhythms.

(Handbook of behavioral neurobiology; v. 4)
Includes index.
1. Biological rhythms. I. Aschoff, Jürgen. II. Series.
QP84.6.B56   591.1'882   80-21037
ISBN 0-306-40585-7

© 1981 Plenum Press, New York
A Division of Plenum Publishing Corporation
227 West 17th Street, New York, N.Y. 10011

Printed in the United States of America

Contributors

JÜRGEN ASCHOFF, *Max-Planck-Institut für Verhaltensphysiologie, Andechs, West Germany*

SUE BINKLEY, *Department of Biology, Temple University, Philadelphia, Pennsylvania*

JOHN BRADY, *Department of Zoology and Applied Entomology, Imperial College of Science and Technology at Silwood Park, Ascot, Berks, England*

CONSTANCE S. CAMPBELL, *Department of Biological Sciences, Northwestern University, Evanston, Illinois*

PETER COLQUHOUN, *Medical Research Council Perceptual and Cognitive Performance Unit, University of Sussex, Brighton, England*

SERGE DAAN, *Zoology Department, Groningen State University, Haren, The Netherlands*

FRED C. DAVIS, *Department of Anatomy and Brain Research Institute, University of California at Los Angeles, School of Medicine, Los Angeles, California*

MICHAEL G. DUBE, *Department of Psychology, University of Florida, Gainesville, Florida*

JAMES THOMAS ENRIGHT, *Scripps Institution of Oceanography, University of California—San Diego, La Jolla, California*

EBERHARD GWINNER, *Max-Planck-Institut für Verhaltensphysiologie, Radolfzell-Möggingen, West Germany*

KLAUS HOFFMANN, *Max-Planck-Institut für Verhaltensphysiologie, Andechs, West Germany*

RONALD J. KONOPKA, *Division of Biology, 216-76, California Institute of Technology, Pasadena, California*

MICHAEL MENAKER, *Department of Biology, University of Oregon, Eugene, Oregon*

MARTIN C. MOORE-EDE, *Department of Physiology, Harvard Medical School, Boston, Massachusetts*

DIETRICH NEUMANN, *Zoologisches Institut der Universität Köln, Köln, West Germany*

TERRY L. PAGE, *Department of Biology, Vanderbilt University, Nashville, Tennessee*

THEODOSIOS PAVLIDIS, *Department of Electrical Engineering and Computer Science, Princeton University, Princeton, New Jersey*

COLIN S. PITTENDRIGH, *Hopkins Marine Station, Stanford University, Pacific Grove, California*

BENJAMIN RUSAK, *Department of Psychology, Dalhousie University, Halifax, Nova Scotia, Canada*

D. S. SAUNDERS, *Department of Zoology, University of Edinburgh, Edinburgh, Scotland*

FRANK M. SULZMAN, *Department of Physiology, Harvard Medical School, Boston, Massachusetts*

FRED W. TUREK, *Department of Biological Sciences, Northwestern University, Evanston, Illinois*

HANS G. WALLRAFF, *Max-Planck-Institut für Verhaltensphysiologie, Seewiesen, West Germany*

WILSE B. WEBB, *Department of Psychology, University of Florida, Gainesville, Florida*

RÜTGER WEVER, *Max-Planck-Institut für Verhaltensphysiologie Andechs, West Germany*

Preface

Interest in biological rhythms has been traced back more than 2,500 years to Archilochus, the Greek poet, who in one of his fragments suggests "$\gamma i\gamma\nu\omega\sigma\varkappa\epsilon\ \delta'o\tilde{i}os\ \dot\rho\upsilon\vartheta\mu\dot os\ \dot\alpha\nu\vartheta\rho\dot\omega\pi o\upsilon s\ \dot\epsilon\chi\epsilon\iota$" (recognize what rhythm governs man) (Aschoff, 1974). Reference can also be made to the French student of medicine J. J. Virey who, in his thesis of 1814, used for the first time the expression "horloge vivante" (living clock) to describe daily rhythms and to D. C. W. Hufeland (1779) who called the 24-hour period the unit of our natural chronology. However, it was not until the 1930s that real progress was made in the analysis of biological rhythms; and Erwin Bünning was encouraged to publish the first, and still not outdated, monograph in the field in 1958. Two years later, in the middle of exciting discoveries, we took a breather at the Cold Spring Harbor Symposium on Biological Clocks. Its survey on rules considered valid at that time, and Pittendrigh's anticipating view on the temporal organization of living systems, made it a milestone on our way from a more formalistic description of biological rhythms to the understanding of their structural and physiological basis.

In the meantime, rhythm research has attracted a steadily increasing number of workers from various disciplines, and the stock of well-documented facts has grown quickly. It therefore seems timely that 20 years after the Cold Spring Harbor Symposium a new effort is made to summarize our knowledge. Volume 4 of the *Handbook of Behavioral Neurobiology* has in its title the term "rhythms," which is broader and less precise than "clocks." Hence, it is possible to include here discussions of rhythmic phenomena that do not necessarily represent time-measuring devices—for example, the short-term rhythms in locomotor activity of animals, the temporal characteristics of sleep, and the ovarian cycle. On the other hand, rhythms of higher frequencies such as the firing of a receptor neurone, heart rate, and respiration are not treated. Instead, emphasis is placed on those rhythms which have evolved in adaptation to temporal programs in the environment, which have become part of the genetic makeup of organisms, and which can be used by organisms as true clocks. Daily (tidal and lunar) and annual rhythms are the main objectives. These have in common that they behave like self-sustaining oscillations and that they can be entrained by periodic factors in the environment; together, they form the special class of the so-called circarhythms.

Circadian rhythms are treated in 14 of the 27 chapters. Discussions include the formal properties of entrainment, surveys on rhythms in behavior of invertebrates and vertebrates, their neural and endocrine control, the genetics and ontogeny of circadian rhythms and their adaptive significance. Two chapters are devoted to human circadian rhythms. In Part III, a discussion of tidal and lunar rhythms is followed by four chapters on annual rhythms, including photoperiodism in insects and vertebrates, and a chapter on human annual rhythms. Although each of the authors follows his own ideas of how to master his task, they all adhere to the same basic concept, including a common terminology (cf. the Glossary). From their chapters, a unified picture emerges of the multioscillatory structure of biological systems and its control by central pacemakers. In essence, then, this volume demonstrates that in behavior and neurobiology temporal organization is of as much relevance as is spatial organization.

The study of the physiological mechanisms underlying circarhythms is a rapidly developing field, and the question of how discrete is the clock from the rest of the body (Pittendrigh, 1976) may soon be answered in the circadian case (M. Suda, O. Hayaishi, and H. Nakagawa, 1979). The overview given in this volume on the present state of the art hopefully will stimulate further research and, hence, become obsolete in some of its parts. However, I think it may also provide a valuable source of information for years to come.

Jürgen Aschoff

References

Aschoff, J. Speech after dinner. In J. Aschoff, F. Ceresa, and F. Halberg (Eds.), *Chronobiological Aspects of Endocrinology. Chronobiologia*, 1974, *1* (Suppl. 1), 483–495.

Bünning, E. *Die Physiologische Uhr*. Berlin: Springer Verlag, 1958.

Chovnik, A. (Ed). *Biological Clocks. Cold Spring Harbor Symposia in Quantitative Biology*, 1961, *25*.

Pittendrigh, C. S. Circadian clocks: What are they? In J. W. Hastings and H. G. Schweiger (Eds.), *The Molecular Basis of Circadian Rhythms* (Dahlem Konferenzen 1975). Berlin: Life Sciences Research Reports, 1976.

Suda, M., Hayaishi, O., and Nakagawa, H. (Eds.). *Biological Rhythms and Their Central Mechanism*. Amsterdam: Elsevier, North Holland, 1979.

Contents

CHAPTER 8

CHAPTER 9

CHAPTER 13

Neural and Endocrine Control of Circadian Rhythms in the Vertebrates 243
Michael Menaker and Sue Binkley

CHAPTER 14

Ontogeny of Circadian Rhythms 257
Fred C. Davis

CHAPTER 21

CHAPTER 22

PART IV RHYTHMS NOT DIRECTLY RELATED TO
ENVIRONMENTAL CYCLES

PART I

Introduction

A Survey on Biological Rhythms

Jürgen Aschoff

The recurrence of any event within a biological system at more-or-less regular intervals can be considered a biological rhythm (Kalmus, 1935). The notion of a *rhythm* is sufficiently vague (i.e., not defined in physical terms) to be useful in listing a wide variety of phenomena that might reflect quite different underlying mechanisms. In the attempt to classify rhythms, restrictive descriptions become necessary that depend on the criteria chosen. Rhythms may be distinguished according to (1) a characteristic such as frequency; (2) the biological system (e.g., a population) in which the rhythm is observed; (3) the kind of process that generates the rhythm; or (4) the function that the rhythm fulfills. Some of these aspects are briefly touched upon in the following paragraphs.

A Spectrum of Rhythms

Biological rhythms extend over many logarithmic units of frequency from one cycle per millisecond to one cycle per several years. They can be observed in single cells, in networks of tissues and organs, in the whole organism, or in populations only. The seven rhythms depicted in Figure 1 are selected to give an impression of the range of frequencies as well as to indicate the various levels of integration at which rhythms manifest themselves. The figure is also useful to introduce the basic question whether a rhythm reflects merely a response to a periodic input coming from outside the biological unit in which it is observed (exogenous rhythm) or whether the rhythm originates from within that unit (endogenous rhythm). In technical terms, exogenous rhythms are analogous to forced oscillations of *passive systems,* that is, systems that can oscillate only under the influence of external periodic perturbations or signals (driving force), and whose oscillations damp out if the input becomes constant. On the other hand, endogenous rhythms are often considered analogous

Jürgen Aschoff   Max-Planck-Institut für Verhaltensphysiologie, D-8131 Andechs, West Germany.

to self-sustaining oscillations of *active systems,* that is, systems whose oscillations continue undamped when the energy supply is kept constant. A less restrictive definition of *endogenous* includes free damped oscillations of passive systems, for which no special term is available in biology, but which may occur frequently in biological systems.

There can be no doubt that rhythms such as the firing rate of a cold receptor in response to a constant thermal stimulus of 33.2°C (Figure 1, a) or the autonomous periodic activity of a pacemaker cell (b) belong to the class of endogenous rhythms. However, rhythms with periods of 24 hr (d) or of one year (f) could be caused by periodic factors in

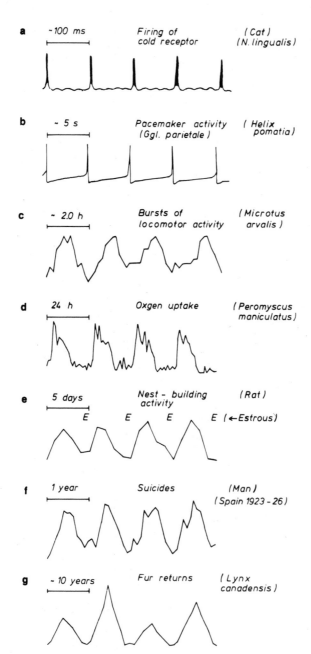

Fig. 1. Biological rhythms. Sources: (a) Hensel and Zotterman, 1951 (background noise from the original record omitted); (b) Courtesy: H. D. Lux, Munich; (c) Daan and Slopsema, 1978; (d) Jameson, Heusner, and Arbogast, 1977; (e) Kinder, 1927; (f) Instituto Nacional de Estadistica, Madrid, 1959; (g) Elton and Nicholson, 1942.

the environment; specially designed experiments are necessary to demonstrate that these rhythms can be also endogenous (see below). The three remaining examples in Figure 1 (c, e, g) pose problems for a variety of reasons. The about 10-year cycle in density of a lynx population (g) is not, as was once assumed, a response to the sunspot cycle but results from a prey–predator interaction (Nicholson, 1955); to classify it as an endogenous rhythm, the definition of the biological "unit" has to comprise both prey and predator (Aschoff, 1959). The 5-day estrous cycle of the rat (e) is most likely an endogenous rhythm like the ovarian cycles of many other species, including man; to justify this classification in its strict sense, it must be demonstrated that the 5-day cycle is not generated by but only coupled to the daily periodic input (cf. Fitzgerald and Zucker, 1976). Finally, for the alternation between activity and rest in intervals of about 2.0 hr (c), the question has to be asked whether it truly represents a "rhythm"; pictures that resemble those of more-or-less regularly recurring bursts in an activity record can be produced on the basis of specific classes of purely stochastic processes (Lehmann, 1976; see also Chapter 19 in this volume). Other rhythm-like phenomena, such as episodic hormone secretion, may fall into the category just mentioned but may as well represent damped oscillations or the outcome of a programmed central neuronal mechanism (Yen, Vandenberg, Tsai, and Parker, 1974).

The Four "Circarhythms"

Within the entire spectrum, rhythms differ extremely with regard to their variability in frequency. This wide difference is indicated in Figure 2 by horizontal bars representing intraindividual (black bars) or interspecific variability (white bars). Most of the rhythms that can be observed in the central nervous system, in the circulatory system, or in respi-

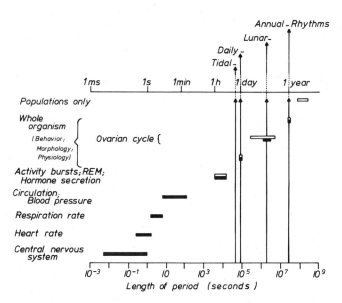

Fig. 2. Spectrum of biological rhythms. White bars (mammals) indicate interspecific variability; black bars (man), intraindividual variability. REM: rapid eye movement. Modified from Hildebrandt (1958) and Aschoff (1959).

ration are characterized by a large intraindividual variability. Other endogenous rhythms, such as the ovarian cycle, show little intraindividual but large interspecific variability. Finally, there are four rhythms (indicated in Figure 2 by vertical lines) that do not vary in frequency under natural conditions because they are synchronized with cycles in the environment. These geophysical cycles are the tides, day and night, the phases of the moon, and the seasons. All four are reflected in the tidal, daily, lunar, and seasonal rhythms of biological systems, and it has been shown in at least a few species that each of these rhythms can persist when isolated from the respective environmental cycle (Aschoff, 1967). Under those artificially constant conditions, the period of the rhythm usually deviates slightly from that of the cycle to which it is normally synchronized; that is, it freeruns with its own "natural" frequency. If such a freerunning rhythm can be shown to persist for many periods without attenuation, the rhythm can be said to belong to the class of systems that are capable of self-sustaining oscillations (endogenous rhythms, in the strict sense of the definition). As a representative example, taken from the domain of daily rhythms, Figure 3 shows records of oxygen consumption in two chaffinches, kept first in light–dark cycles (LD) and thereafter in constant dim illumination. The period τ of the freerunning rhythm is slightly longer than 24 hr in the upper record, and shorter in the lower record (for variability of τ, see Chapter 6).

Since the period of the freerunning rhythm only approximates that of the environmental cycle that it reflects, the prefix *circa* was introduced by Halberg (1959) to characterize daily as *circadian* rhythms and then was later adopted for the three other endogenous rhythms that correspond to cycles in the environment: circatidal, circalunar, and circannual rhythms (Aschoff, 1967). All four circarhythms have common features that are characteristic of self-sustaining oscillations (see Chapter 5). It seems useful to apply the prefix *circa* only to those rhythms that are usually synchronized to environmental cycles and that show their natural frequency (immanent in the system) only under special conditions. As opposed to such a restrictive use of the term, it has been suggested, for example, to call the episodic hormone secretion a *circhoral* rhythm (Dierschke, Bhattacharya, Atkinson, and Knobil, 1970); a consistent application of this usage would lead to designations such as *circasecond* rhythm for heart rate.

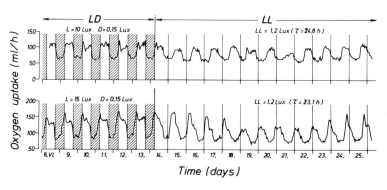

Fig. 3. Rhythms of oxygen uptake in two chaffinches *Fringilla coelebs,* kept for six days in light–dark cycles (LD), thereafter in constant dim illumination (LL). (Unpublished data from Pohl.)

The predominant role of circadian rhythms has been the reason for a subdivision of the spectrum into ultradian rhythms (with periods shorter than circadian) and infradian rhythms (with periods longer than circadian) (Halberg, Engeli, Hamburger, and Hillman, 1965). Typical examples of ultradian rhythms in man are provided by the repetition of phase of rapid eye movements (REM) during sleep in about 90-min intervals (see Chapter 26 in this volume), and by cycles of similar duration that can be observed during wakefulness, for example, in oral activity (Friedman and Fisher, 1967; Oswald, Merrington, and Lewis, 1970) and gross motor activity (Globus, Phoebus, and Boyd, 1973), in performance (Globus, Phoebus, Humphries, and Boyd, 1972; Kripke, 1972; Orr, Hoffman, and Hegge, 1974), in renal excretory activity (Lavie and Kripke, 1977), or in the perception of apparent motions (Lavie, 1976). However, the great variability in frequency, and a progressive elongation of intervals observed in some of these rhythms (Lavie, 1977), render their interpretation difficult. In the rhesus monkey, behavioral ultradian rhythms have been reported with periods of about 45 min (Maxim, Bowden, and Sackett, 1976) and of 90-min duration (Lewis and Kripke, 1977).

Infradian rhythms, apart from those indicated in Figure 2 at the right end of the spectrum, are less well documented. Weekly rhythms observed in animals in the laboratory—for example, in locomotor activity of a centipede (Mead, 1970), in larviposition of a mosquito (Nash and Trewern, 1972), or in enzyme activity of the rat pineal (Vollrath, Kantarjian, and Howe, 1975)—are likely to be due to periodic disturbances and hence belong to the few examples of exogenous rhythms. In the case of man, they may be the result of habits, for example, in food intake of children (Debry, Bleyer, and Reinberg, 1975) or of treatment schedules for patients (Undt, 1976; Brüning, 1978). An explanation becomes more difficult if such a rhythm seems to freerun with a period only approximating 7 days as described for oviposition of the springtail *Folsomia candida* (Chiba, Cutkomp, and Halberg, 1973), but caution in interpreting those data is always warranted (cf. the critical analysis from Richter, 1976). In man, freerunning rhythms with periods of that order have been claimed to be present in the urinary excretion of 17-ketosteroids (Halberg *et al.,* 1965) and of estrone (Exley and Corker, 1966). There are also data that suggest, in the human male, rhythm of about 21 days in testosterone excretion (Kihlström, 1966; Doehring, Kraemer, Keith, and Brodie, 1975) and in body temperature (Empson, 1977). Finally, the many cyclic phenomena should be mentioned that can be observed in medicine and that have given rise to a number of hypotheses, especially in psychiatry (Reiman, 1963; Richter, 1965).

Interaction among Rhythms and Their Teleonomy

Rhythms of different frequencies can be interrelated in various ways (Figure 4). Well known is the modulation of heart rate by respiration. Similarly, many of the ultradian rhythms in the hourly range (e.g., activity bursts, hormone episodes) are modulated in their frequency on a circadian time scale, and the circadian rhythm, in turn, may depend for some of its parameters on a circannual rhythm (see Chapters 6 and 21). Of more interest

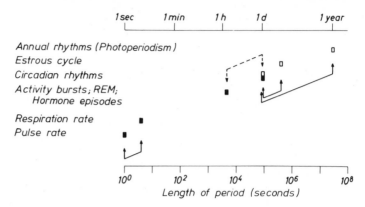

Fig. 4. Demonstrated (———) and suggested (----) interactions (of any kind) between rhythms of different frequencies. Black squares: man; white squares: mammals.

are those observations that suggest a hierarchical order among rhythms, with one rhythm being essential for the proper action of another rhythm. Typical examples are the interaction between the circadian system and the estrous cycle in hamsters (see Chapter 27) and the involvement of circadian rhythms in photoperiodic time measurement (see Chapters 22 and 23 in this volume). In what way ultradian and circadian rhythms may be related to each other still remains to be seen. On the basis of seemingly synchronized hormone episodes in a group of monkeys, a kind of coupling between the two systems has been suggested (Holaday, Martinez, and Natelson, 1977), but the data analysis and conclusions are open to criticism (Kronauer, Moore-Ede, and Menser, 1978). In this context, the question becomes of interest whether the 90-min rhythm (REM) continues from sleep into wakefulness, that is, whether there is a basic rest–activity cycle as suggested by Kleitman (1963).

To illustrate the diversity of functions that can be served by biological rhythms, a few examples should suffice. Within the nervous system, some receptors transfer information by controlled variations of spike frequency (cf. Figure 1, top curve); pulsations, kept in motion by pacemakers, are the basis for the pump functions of heart and lungs; high-frequency rhythms may be useful in stabilizing rhythms of lower frequency. (For a detailed discussion of these problems, cf. Aschoff and Wever, 1962). While these rhythms fulfill important tasks within the organism, the four circarhythms mainly serve in the interplay between the organism and its environment. They have evolved as an adaptation to "niches in time" (Aschoff, 1964) generated by the temporal structure of the environment. By incorporating into its own organization approximate copies of the external temporal programs, an organism acquires time-telling devices, that is, biological clocks (see Chapter 5).

REFERENCES

Aschoff, J. Zeitliche Strukturen biologischer Vorgänge. *Acta Leopoldina,* 1959, *21,* 147–177.
Aschoff, J. Survival value of diurnal rhythms. *Symposia of the Zoological Society of London,* 1964, *13,* 79–98.
Aschoff, J. Adaptive cycles: Their significance for defining environmental hazards. *International Journal of Biometeorology,* 1967, *11,* 255–278.

Aschoff, J., and Wever, R. Biologische Rhythmen und Regelung. In *Probleme der zentralnervösen Regulation*. Bad Oeyenhausener Gespräche V. Berlin-Göttingen-Heidelberg: Springer-Verlag, 1962, pp. 1–15.

Brüning, W. Chronobiologische Untersuchungen über die Sterbehäufigkeit von Kurpatienten im Verlauf von Bäderkuren. Diss. Marburg, 1978.

Chiba, Y., Cutkomp, L. K., and Halberg, F. Circaseptan (7-day) oviposition rhythm and growth of spring tail, *Folsomia candida* (Collembola: isotomidae). *Journal of Interdisciplinary Cycle Research*, 1973, *4*, 59–66.

Daan, S., and Slopsema, S. Short-term rhythms in foraging behaviour of the common vole, *Microtus arvalis*. *Journal of Comparative Physiology*, 1978, *127*, 215–227.

Debry, G., Bleyer, R., and Reinberg, A. Circadian, circannual and other rhythms in spontaneous nutrient and caloric intake of healthy four-year olds. *Diabetes and Metabolism (Paris)*, 1975, *1*, 91–99.

Dierschke, D. J., Bhattacharya, A. N., Atkinson, L. E., and Knobil, E. Circhoral oscillations of plasma LH levels in the ovariectomized rhesus monkey. *Endocrinology*, 1970, *87*, 850–853.

Doehring, C. H., Kraemer, H. C., Keith, H., Brodie, H., and Hamburg, D. A. A cycle of plasma testosterone in the human male. *Journal of Clinical Endocrinology and Metabolism*, 1975, *40*, 492–500.

Elton, C., and Nicholson, M. The ten-year cycle in members of the lynx in Canada. *Journal of Animal Ecology*, 1942, *11*, 215–244.

Empson, J. Periodicity in body temperature in man. *Experientia*, 1977, *33*, 342–343.

Exley, D., and Corker, C. S. The human male cycle of urinary oestrone and 17-oxosteroids. *Journal of Endocrinology*, 1966, *35*, 83–99.

Fitzgerald, K. M., and Zucker, I. Circadian organization of the estrous cycle of the golden hamster. *Proceedings of the National Academy of Sciences USA*, 1976, *73*, 2923–2927.

Friedman, S., and Fisher, C. On the presence of a rhythmic, diurnal, oral instinctual drive cycle in man: A preliminary report. *Journal of the American Psychoanalytic Association*, 1967, *15*, 317–343.

Globus, G. G., Phoebus, E. C., and Boyd, R. Temporal organization of night worker's sleep. *Aerospace Medicine*, 1972, *43*, 266–268.

Globus, G. G., Phoebus, E. C., Humphries, J., Boyd, R., and Sharp, R. Ultradian rhythms in human telemetered gross motor activity. *Aerospace Medicine*, 1973, *44*, 882–887.

Halberg, F. Physiologic 24-hour periodicity: General and procedural considerations with reference to the adrenal cycle. *Zeitschrift für Vitamin-, Hormon- und Fermentforschung*, 1959, *10*, 225–296.

Halberg, F., Engeli, M., Hamburger, C., and Hillman, V. D. Spectral resolution of low-frequency, small-amplitude rhythms in excreted 17-ketosteroids; probably androgen-induced circaseptan desynchronization. *Acta Endocrinologica*, 1965, *103*, 1–54.

Hensel, H., and Zotterman, Y. Quantitative Beziehung zwischen der Entladung einzelner Kältefasern und der Temperatur. *Acta Physiologica Scandinavica*, 1951, *23*, 291–319.

Hildebrandt, G. Grundlagen einer angewandten medizinischen Rhythmusforschung. *Heilkunst*, 1958, *7*, 117–136.

Holaday, J. W., Martinez, H. M., and Natelson, B. H. Synchronized ultradian cortisol rhythms in monkeys: Persistence during corticotropin infusion. *Science*, 1977, *198*, 56–58.

Jameson, E. W., Heusner, A. A., and Arbogast, R. Oxygen consumption of *Scelopourus occidentalis* from three different elevations. *Comparative Biochemical Physiology*, 1977, *56A*, 73–79.

Kalmus, H. Periodizität und Autochronie (= Ideochronie) als zeitregelnde Eigenschaften des Organismus, *Biologia Generalis*, 1935, *11*, 93–114.

Kihlström, J. E. A sex cycle in the male. *Experientia*, 1966, *22*, 630–632.

Kinder, E. H. A study of the nest-building activity of the albino rat. *Journal of Experimental Zoology*, 1927, *47*, 117–161.

Kleitman, N. *Sleep and Wakefulness*. Chicago: University of Chicago Press, 1963.

Kripke, D. F. An ultradian biologic rhythm associated with perceptual deprivation and REM sleep. *Psychosomatic Medicine*, 1972, *34*, 221–234.

Kronauer, R. E., Moore-Ede, M. C., and Menser, M. S. Ultradian cortisol rhythms in monkeys: Synchronized or not synchronized? *Science*, 1978, *202*, 1001–1002.

Lavie, P. Ultradian rhythms in the perception of two apparent motions. *Chronobiologia*, 1976, *3*, 214–218.

Lavie, P. Nonstationarity in human perceptual ultradian rhythms. *Chronobiologia*, 1977, *4*, 38–48.

Lavie, P., and Kripke, D. F. Ultradian rhythms in urine flow in waking subjects. *Nature*, 1977, *269*, 142–143.

Lehmann, U. Stochastic principles in the temporal control of activity behaviour. *International Journal of Chronobiology*, 1976, *4*, 223–266.

Lewis, B. D., and Kripke, D. F. Ultradian rhythms in hand-mouth behavior of the rhesus monkey. *Physiology and Behavior*, 1977, *18*, 283–286.

Maxim, P. E., Bowden, D. M., and Sackett, G. P. Ultradian rhythms of solitary and social behavior in rhesus monkeys. *Physiology and Behavior*, 1976, *17*, 337–344.

Mead, M. Sur l'obtention d'un rythme d'activité de période sept jours chez Scolopendra cingulate (Chilopodes). *Revue du Comportement Animal,* 1970, *4,* 75–76.

Nash, T. A. M., and Trewen, M. A. Hourly distribution of larviposition by *Glossina austeni* Newst and *G. morsitans morsitans* Westw. (Dipt., Glossinidae). *Bulletin of Entomological Research,* 1972, *61,* 693–700.

Nicholson, A. J. An outline of the dynamics of animal populations. *Australian Journal of Zoology,* 1955, *2,* 9–65.

Orr, W. C., Hoffman, H. J., and Hegge, F. W. Ultradian rhythms in extended performance. *Aerospace Medicine,* 1974, *45,* 995–1000.

Oswald, J., Merrington, J., and Lewis, H. Cyclical "on demand" oral intake by adults. *Nature,* 1970, *225,* 959–960.

Reiman, H. A. *Periodic Diseases.* Oxford: Blackwell Scientific Publications, 1963.

Richter, C. P. *Biological Clocks in Medicine and Psychiatry.* Springfield, Ill.: Charles C Thomas, 1965.

Richter, C. P. Artifactual seven-day cycles in spontaneous activity in wild rodents and squirrel monkeys. *Journal of Comparative and Physiological Psychology,* 1976, 572–582.

Undt, W. Wochenperioden der Arbeitsunfallhäufigkeit im Vergleich mit Wochenperioden von Herzmuskelinfarkt, Selbstmord und täglicher Sterbeziffer. In G. Hildebrandt (Ed.), *Biologische Rhythmen und Arbeit.* Wien–New York: Springer-Verlag, 1976, pp. 73–79.

Vollrath, L., Kantarjian, A., and Howe, C. Mammalian pineal gland: 7-day rhythmic activity? *Experientia,* 1975, *31,* 458–460.

Yen, S. S. C., Vandenberg, G., Tsai, C. C., and Parker, D. C. Ultradian fluctuations of gonadotropins. In M. Ferin, F. Halberg, R. M. Richart, and R. L. Vande Wiele (Eds.), *Biorhythms and Human Reproduction.* New York: Wiley, 1974, pp. 203–218.

2

Methodology

James Thomas Enright

Introduction

It would be a pointless exercise to attempt to provide here a summary of the methods that have proved useful for data collection in the study of biological rhythms. Fundamentally different instrumentation is appropriate for monitoring any single biological output, such as locomotor activity, depending on whether the research involves a rodent, a bird, a fish, or an insect. Furthermore, for a given organism, the equipment necessary to monitor, say, body temperature bears little resemblance to that required for monitoring heart rate or urinary output. Hence, a description of the instrumentation and techniques that have been used to measure rhythmic biological variables would constitute an extensive catalog, which would carry with it no assurance that past experience offers an optimal guide for future research. Within the diversity of techniques that have been successful, there appears to be only one useful and almost self-evident guideline: a detailed analysis of a given rhythmic system has rarely if ever been achieved without the development of some sort of automatic or at least semiautomatic data-collecting technique, which greatly reduces the need for human intervention.

Setting aside concerns about data collecting itself, this chapter focuses on general issues of experimental design in rhythm studies: conceptual problems and possible pitfalls. The primary intent is to summarize, for those not thoroughly familiar with the past literature, some of the standard experimental procedures and their limitations, which underlie the conceptual foundation of ongoing research on biological rhythms in many laboratories. For those with experience in this area, the material here may perhaps also be useful as a reminder of the precautions necessary in the rigorous interpretation of experimental results.

James Thomas Enright   Scripps Institution of Oceanography, University of California—San Diego, La Jolla, California 92093.

JAMES THOMAS
ENRIGHT

As a point of departure, it will be useful to consider an idealized experiment addressed to the following questions: (1) Is the organism of interest capable of a self-sustained, free-running rhythm? (2) Is a given environmental factor, when varied in circadian cycles, a zeitgeber for that organism? (3) Does the intensity or "level" of a given environmental factor, when provided continuously, affect the period of the organism's rhythm? and (4) Does the application of a single stimulus of a given sort cause a phase shift of the rhythm? These are four of the most common questions of interest in rhythm research, and while it might seem that little discussion of such elementary issues is warranted, rigorous answers to these questions are not as simple as they may appear. Figure 1 presents schematically an experimental design and the kinds of results that are generally regarded as adequate to fully justify an affirmative answer to all four questions. The format of data presentation in this illustration is based on that usually used for recordings of locomotor activity, and the results shown here might well be those associated with manipulation of light intensity, but the important features of the illustration can be taken as representative of a much more general case, not necessarily involving either locomotor activity or changes in light conditions.

There are several significant features of this diagram that deserve special attention. The initial portion of the figure, illustrating a freerunning rhythm, is a very lengthy record in which the rhythm scans a complete 24-hr day. Why such a long period of observation?

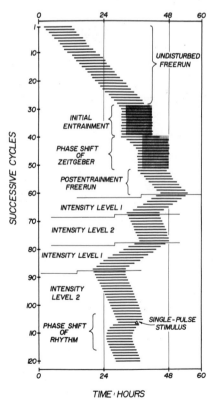

Fig. 1. Hypothetical results from a set of experiments demonstrating a freerunning rhythm, entrainment by a strong zeitgeber, the effect of the "level" of a stimulus (e.g., light intensity) on the period of the rhythm, and a pulse-induced phase shift. Idealized data are presented as an "actogram," a summary format commonly used for recordings of locomotor activity, in which each sequential 24-hr segment of the record is placed beneath that of the preceding day. The black horizontal bars might then correspond, for example, to blocks of perch-hopping activity by a bird, or perhaps to the hours during which body temperature was above some threshold. A vertical sequence of these bars would represent a rhythm with 24-hr period; the "undisturbed freerun" therefore has a period of about 25 hr. See text for detailed interpretation.

Would not the clear demonstration, over even a few cycles, of an apparently stable, non-24-hr period in the biological rhythm represent sufficient evidence for sustained freerun? Such evidence is highly suggestive, but a complete 24-hr scan by the rhythm is required in order to be fully rigorous. Otherwise, it is conceivable that the observed rhythm is subject to some unintended daily environmental cycle, such as laboratory noise or the like, to which it would eventually entrain, with a 24-hr period, and that the several cycles of apparent freerun represent only a gradual phase shift, during the transition before the stable phase relationship with the zeitgeber has been achieved (cf. cycles 40–45 in Figure 1).

Another important requirement, illustrated in the data of this portion of the figure, is that the period of the rhythm be free from long-term oscillatory trends, as it scans the 24-hr day. An organism, in the presence of a weak zeitgeber, may show a rhythm that fully scans the zeitgeber cycle; even though never fully synchronized by that zeitgeber, the rhythm would nevertheless be expected to show oscillatory trends in its cycle-to-cycle period, which reflect periodically changing sensitivity of the organism to the cyclic stimulus (cf. relative coordination, von Holst, 1939). A fully rigorous demonstration of true freerun therefore requires the absence of such oscillatory trends in the cycle-to-cycle period of the rhythm.

The second portion of Figure 1 illustrates entrainment of the rhythm by means of an environmental cycle, and the first and obviously critical feature of this portion of the record in embodied in the fact that the rhythm attains a constant phase relationship with the environmental cycle, following which the rhythm and the zeitgeber have an identical average period. (Note that entrainment does not require that all activity be confined only to one portion of a square-wave environment cycle.) In itself, this phenomenon might seem to be adequate evidence for entrainment, but more is required: it is also essential to demonstrate, as the next portion of the hypothetical record does, that the rhythm follows a phase shift of the zeitgeber. This constitutes a demonstration that the constant phase-relationship between rhythm and zeitgeber is stable, as one expects of true entrainment. Without this precaution, it remains conceivable that the environmental cycle has altered the freerunning period of the rhythm in a completely phase-independent fashion, to an extent that, by coincidence only, led to an approximately 24-hr period in the rhythm. Frequency modulation of that sort, without phase control, should not be mistaken for true entrainment by a zeitgeber.

The final step in rigorous demonstration of entrainment is illustrated in the portion of Figure 1 labeled "postentrainment freerun": the environmental cycle is terminated, and one expects, as illustrated, that the subsequent freerun of the rhythm will begin at a phase determined by that seen during entrainment.[1] Without this precaution, it remains possible that the environmental cycle exerted a strong, exogenous influence on the biological variable monitored, without genuine effect on the underlying timing process. In this latter circumstance, the animal's pacemaker (i.e., the timing center or feedback loop *ordinarily* responsible for rhythmic variation) would have continued to freerun during apparent entrainment, with only its output "masked" by the hypothesized zeitgeber (cf. DeCoursey, 1961, Figure

---

[1]The usual experimental observation resembles that illustrated, with a completely smooth transition of phase between entrainment and subsequent freerun, but this is not a logical necessity. The essential requirement, in demonstrating entrainment, is that freerun, following a given entrainment regime, begin at a *reproducible* phase, relative to that seen in prior entrainment; even large discontinuities of phase at the time of transition are not excluded.

7). In this circumstance, there would be no systematic relationship between the apparent phase of the rhythm during entrainment and the phase at which subsequent freerun begins.

The next portions of Figure 1, which serve to demonstrate that the level of an environmental variable alters freerunning period, require very little commentary. The experimental design, in which stimulus intensity is altered back and forth several times, is not an absolutely essential aspect of the protocol, but it offers two important advantages: each experimental animal serves as its own cross-treatment control, thereby increasing the likelihood of detecting small changes in average period, which might be obscured by interindividual variability in period at any single environmental level; and one thus guards against the risk of being misled by possible monotonic trends or coincidental alterations in freerunning period, which might occur spontaneously, regardless of the manipulated environmental variable.

In the final portion of the record of Figure 1, the single application of a chosen stimulus has produced an enduring modification in the timing of the rhythm, of the sort commonly called a *phase shift*. Following the stimulus, there were several cycles of the rhythm during which the apparent cycle-to-cycle period was shorter than during prior and subsequent freerun. The clarity of the result illustrated here leaves no doubt that the pacemaker that is responsible for the timing of the rhythm has been affected but, as discussed below, the proper description and quantification of this effect are not a simple matter. With this idealized example as background, the balance of this chapter considers several additional complications and possible pitfalls associated with those experimental studies of biological rhythms that are addressed to these same four questions.

COMPLICATIONS FOR INTERPRETATION

THE SEARCH FOR SUSTAINED FREERUNNING RHYTHMS

Confronted with the extensive literature that documents the existence of circadian rhythms in organisms at all phyletic levels, from protozoa to man, an outsider might presume that essentially any healthy animal, when placed under any arbitrarily chosen set of constant conditions, ought to give clear evidence of a persistent freerunning circadian rhythm. That would be very far from the truth, but such a misinterpretation can easily arise because of a bias in the published literature. A persistent rhythm is an "interesting" result; it serves as the basis for further experimentation and may even be considered worthy of publication without further elaboration. The lack of a detectable rhythm, however, is seldom regarded as a basis for a published report. It deserves considerable emphasis here, therefore, that the demonstration of a persistent circadian rhythm requires the judicious—and often very careful—selection of the experimental situation. One of the most important of the environmental variables to be chosen is the intensity of constant light (or darkness) provided. Constant *bright* light frequently inhibits the expression of circadian rhythmicity in organisms at all phyletic levels, and the intensity of light that suppresses rhythmicity is often surprisingly low. For example, few birds remain rhythmic at light intensities greater than about 100 lux, which is appreciably dimmer than ordinary laboratory illumination; and in the pigeon, as an extreme case, rhythmicity has been reproducibly observed only at light intensities of less than 0.5 lux (Miselis and Walcott, 1970). For poikilotherms, the constant temperature provided must also be appropriate, with a loss of rhythmicity often reported at temperatures under 10°C. Even the instrumentation used for data collecting can determine whether or not a freerunning rhythm is detectable, with some registration procedures (e.g., wheel running) being more likely to provide clear evidence of a rhythm than other instrumentation that might seem, in principle, to be measuring a comparable output. Some animals must be provided with a shelter to which they can retire during part of the cycle; others may show a clear rhythm only in the presence of conspecifics. The search for permissive conditions under which a persistent rhythm can be observed in a given organism is often a frustrating exercise with no assurance of success.

Of course, there is a fundamental, logical restriction associated with demonstrating a universal negative, so that no assertion can be justified of the sort, "This species has no freerunning circadian rhythm." The preceding discussion indicates that even a more cautious statement of the sort, "The feeding activity of this animal does not show detectable circadian rhythmicity," must be extensively qualified by specifying the kinds of experimental conditions under which a rhythm was sought.

A further complication in the search for a persistent freerunning rhythm also deserves mention: given a population of individuals, each with a self-sustained rhythm but with interindividual variance in freerunning period, the individuals, acting independently under constant conditions, will progressively move away from mutual synchrony. If the behavior of an entire population (rather than that of the individuals) is then monitored, an initially synchronized group rhythmicity will appear to be progressively damped under constant conditions, eventually reaching a stage indistinguishable from complete arrhythmicity. With a population of animals being monitored continuously, the possibility is clearly evident that progressive damping of the group rhythm could be a population artifact. However, a related problem can arise in other situations where the issue is less transparent.

Consider an assay of rhythmicity that involves sacrificing the individual animals in order to measure, say, the brain level of a given hormone; and assume that predictable temporal differences, of large magnitude, in the typical level of this hormone have been demonstrated in groups of animals kept under a light–dark cycle, as well as during brief freerun. Suppose, now, that a chosen surgical operation is performed on the animals; that a hormone assay is then performed on one group of animals at a given time, several days after surgery, and on another group of animals, say, 12 hr later; and that significant intergroup differences in the hormone levels are no longer detectable. Such a result is open to several possible interpretations. It *may* mean that the surgery has interfered with some fundamental component of the animals' clockworks; but it might also indicate that one has simply induced a wide scatter of phases of the rhythms within each group—perhaps a scatter due to increased variability in freerunning period since surgery, or perhaps a scatter because surgery itself has the capacity to shift the phase of the rhythm by an amount that varies considerably among individuals. The central problem here is that it is difficult, in an experiment based on measurements from groups of individuals, to distinguish between true absence of rhythmicity in the individuals and the presence of an ensemble of ongoing rhythms with widely scattered phases.

In the hypothetical experiment just described, there is an additional complication that pervades essentially all studies of biological rhythms: the need to distinguish between rhythmic variation in the parameter measured and behavior of the pacemaker, which is the underlying cause for the rhythmic variation. In the case described, it is conceivable that the surgery interferes—perhaps permanently or perhaps only transiently—with temporal variation in the hormone measured, without having any lasting effect upon the central timing processes of interest, which normally lead to the observed rhythm. The difficulties associated with distinguishing between an observed rhythm and the pacemaker responsible for that rhythm have widespread ramifications, as is described below, as well as in other sections of this book.

The Demonstration of Entrainment

The full experimental design illustrated in cycles 29 to 60 of Figure 1 serve adequately to demonstrate clear-cut entrainment by a strong zeitgeber, but it is worth reemphasizing the importance of measurement of the subsequent freerunning rhythm. Any environmental factor that exerts a strong direct influence on the biological output being monitored may, when offered with cyclic variation, give superficial evidence suggestive of entrainment, which would represent nothing more than a stimulus–response kind of environmental forcing. Only measurement of subsequent freerun can distinguish between this possibility— that is, an effect on the rhythm only—and true entrainment.

While Figure 1 illustrates complete entrainment such as one would expect from a strong zeitgeber, the situation with weak entraining agents presents a somewhat different picture. The mere fact that entrainment is not obtained when a given environmental cycle is imposed (i.e., the organism fails to achieve the same average period as that of the applied cycle) does not mean that this particular environmental cycle can be disregarded as a *potential* entraining agent. The most sensitive test for the possibility of entrainment requires that the environmental cycle be presented with large-amplitude variation in its "intensity," and that the cycle be presented in a regime, the period of which differs only slightly from that of the unentrained period of the organism's rhythm. A strong zeitgeber like that illustrated in Figure 1 is one that has a broad "range of entrainment," so that even when offered in cycles with a period much different from that seen in freerun, entrainment can occur (Enright, 1965). A weak zeitgeber, however, may be able to entrain the rhythm only when its period is quite close to (but, of course, not identical with) that prevailing in freerun. Even a strong zeitgeber can be converted to a weak one if the amplitude of its oscillation is sufficiently reduced. Simple failure to obtain entrainment in a given experimental situation is therefore an equivocal result; it may mean that the manipulated environmental variable is without effect upon the organism's timing system, or it may simply mean that a potential zeitgeber has been tested at a period value that is outside its range of entrainment. In the latter case, relative coordination (von Holst, 1939) should be expected, but it may not be detectable unless the animal's rhythm is quite regular. As a ramification of this interpretational problem, consider a statement of the sort, "X animals out of N tested were not entrained" by a given environmental cycle. This observation does not provide reliable information about the strength of the zeitgeber cycle; in order properly to quantify such a result, the statement should be supplemented by data on the differences in period between the freerunning rhythms and the intended entraining cycle.

Results of the sort illustrated in the next portions of Figure 1 (cycles 61 to 105) provide clear evidence of induced modification of the freerunning period of the rhythm, but it should be emphasized that a relatively long interval of steady-state period, at each level of the environmental factor, is desirable. In early studies of the effects of environmental temperature on circadian rhythms, when the need for this precaution was not recognized, relatively large changes in period were sometimes reported, based on measurements made over only one to three cycles of the rhythm. Subsequent reinvestigation of these same systems has indicated that a *transition* in temperature can have large transient effects on the monitored rhythm, although the influence of temperature on the steady-state, freerunning period of the pacemaker is quite small. These temporary phenomena following temperature change are of interest in themselves, but because they were confused with true changes in equilibrium period, the remarkable extent to which the circadian systems were able to compensate for differences in temperature was obscured (Bünning, 1973, p. 71).

Measurement of Phase Shift

The response to a single-pulse stimulus, illustrated in the final portion of Figure 1, is an idealized and very clear result, but the interpretation and proper quantification of such experiments deserve further consideration. Problems arise because the issue of fundamental interest in circadian-rhythm studies is usually the effect of the stimulus on the pacemaker that underlies the observed rhythm and not simply the effect on the rhythm itself. As a first precaution, it is therefore necessary to observe the rhythm for several cycles following the stimulus. If one had, for example, at the time of the stimulus illustrated in this case, administered a strong sleeping potion, the animal would have awakened later on the first subsequent cycle (rather than earlier, as illustrated) but might well then, in subsequent cycles, have reverted to a timing essentially unperturbed from prestimulus expectations. In other words, a sleeping potion might affect the observed *rhythm* and not its pacemaker.

In the case illustrated, however, it is clear that the poststimulus rhythm persists in a timing different from the extrapolation of prestimulus trends and that there was thus an effect on the pacemaker. The net result is a rhythm that is phase-shifted, relative to unstimulated expectations. One way of quantifying this result is to measure the extent of the phase difference in the final steady state.

The complication in this method of description is that the stimulus did not immediately induce that full effect; there were several transition cycles of the rhythm, the effects of which cumulated to give the final result. Each of these "transient" cycles might be said to show its own amount of "phase shift," or as an alternative and equally valid description of the result, one might say that there were several cycles during which the "instantaneous period" of the rhythm was shorter than during freerun. The proper interpretation of these transient cycles is more than simply a matter of semantics. One can see directly what the *rhythm* was doing, but what was the state of the pacemaker during this interim? One possible interpretation is that the pacemaker was fully shifted, in the first poststimulus cycle, to a timing or a phase that corresponds to the ultimately achieved steady-state timing. By this interpretation, the transient cycles can be regarded as a reflection of the weak coupling between pacemaker and overt rhythm. A more direct interpretation, however, is that the transient cycles of the observed rhythm may accurately reflect the intervening behavior of the pacemaker, with tight coupling between rhythm and pacemaker.

For those who prefer the first hypothesis, the ultimately achieved phase shift represents a satisfactory summary description of the most interesting aspects of the data. According to the second hypothesis, however, this sort of single descriptive measure is incomplete and would oversimplify the dynamic behavior of the pacemaker. The amount of phase shift (or change in instantaneous period) in each poststimulus cycle would be of interest.

Other instances are described in Chapter 3 of the extent to which hypothesis is a major determinant of what is measured and reported. In the case under consideration here, much of the influence of hypothesis can be avoided by measuring and reporting the result of treatment on each of a sequence of poststimulus days, perhaps as cumulative phase shift of the rhythm, perhaps as a series of values of "instantaneous period." Other researchers can then make their own interpretive decision about what is relevant and significant in the data, rather than having that decision dictated by reporting only one facet of the observed phenomenon.

PLASTICITY OF RHYTHM PROPERTIES

The hypothetical series of experiments summarized in Figure 1 involves an important oversimplification; they incorporate the idealization that the properties of the experimental animal's rhythm under a given set of conditions are highly reproducible. Freerunning period is illustrated as being essentially constant during prolonged freerun as well as after phase shifting; the entrained phase relationship is illustrated as unaltered after the phase shift of the zeitgeber; and the period of the rhythm, at a given level of the constant stimulus, is illustrated as unchanged over repetitive trials. Such idealized behavior permits easy interpretation, but a large body of experimental evidence indicates that this kind of reproducibility is not typical of real experimental animals. Changes in the freerunning period of an organism's rhythm, under a given set of experimental conditions, can occur spontaneously, sometimes in discrete steps and sometimes as a gradual acceleration or deceleration; and changes in freerunning period can also be induced by particular sorts of pretreatment, including both entrainment and phase shift: phenomena known as *aftereffects* (Pittendrigh and Daan, 1976). Any such change in the freerunning period of a rhythm can also be expected, on the basis of elementary theoretical considerations, to be accompanied by changes in the stable phase relationship between the rhythm and any given zeitgeber cycle, as well as by changes in the range of entrainment, so that an environmental cycle that was formerly capable of entraining might lose this ability. Furthermore, changes in the apparent phase relationship between rhythm and zeitgeber commonly occur because of changes in the waveform of a rhythm, even when freerunning period is unaltered. To add even further complexity, nonadditive effects of environmental variables on freerunning period have been documented; for example, temperature may alter the period of a rhythm, when tested at one constant light intensity, and may be without detectable effect at some other light intensity (Enright, 1966).

Biological rhythms are thus complex, nonlinear outputs from pacemaker systems, the properties of which are frequently nonstationary. Careful experimental design, with extensive replication across individuals, can often permit reliable conclusions even in face of this complexity; but even granted the use of the best state of the art in experimental design, most rhythm researchers have learned to be extremely cautious about the extent to which generalization is undertaken.

REFERENCES

Bünning, E. *The Physiological Clock* (rev. 3rd ed.). New York: Springer-Verlag, 1973.

DeCoursey, P. J. Phase control of activity in a rodent. *Cold Spring Harbor Symposia on Quantitative Biology,* 1961, *25,* 49–54.

Enright, J. T. Synchronization and ranges of entrainment. In J. Aschoff (Ed.), *Circadian Clocks.* Amsterdam: North-Holland Publishing Company, 1965.

Enright, J. T. Temperature and the freerunning rhythm of the house finch. *Comparative Biochemistry and Physiology,* 1966, *18,* 463–475.

Miselis, R., and Walcott, C. Locomotor activity in homing pigeons *(Columba livia)*. *Animal Behaviour,* 1970, *18,* 544–551.

Pittendrigh, C. S., and Daan, S. A functional analysis of circadian pacemakers in nocturnal rodents. I. The stability and lability of spontaneous frequency. *Journal of Comparative Physiology,* 1976, *106,* 223–252.

von Holst, E. Die relative Koordination als Phänomen und als Methode Zentralnervöser Functionsanalyse. *Ergebnisse der Physiologie,* 1939, *42,* 228–306.

3

Data Analysis

James Thomas Enright

Introduction

Some General Properties of the Data

The statistical treatment of time-series data has a long history of theoretical development, continuing to the present. A number of modern texts are available on the topic (e.g., Cox and Lewis, 1966; Hannan, 1970; Jenkins and Watts, 1969; Kendall, 1973; Koopmans, 1974; Parzen, 1967; Rosenblatt, 1963), and no attempt will be made here to summarize such general treatments. Instead, the approach here is nonmathematical and pragmatic, with emphasis confined to those techniques and issues of interpretation that have proved to be important for research on biological rhythms whose adaptive significance involves the need for an organism to maintain an appropriate phase relationship with a regularly cyclic environment. The physiological process by which a majority of animals accomplish this objective is an endogenous, entrainable rhythm, usually self-sustaining, in which a single frequency or an extremely narrow range of frequencies dominates the animal's entire physiology and behavior. In such a self-sustaining rhythm, phase is conserved for long intervals, if not indefinitely. These characteristics of biological rhythms create a very special and limited class of problems in data analysis, for which the appropriate and useful techniques are often quite different from those designed for time-series data from other sources.

Another aspect of the data of interest, which distinguishes them from many others, is that the "waveform" of the rhythm is hardly ever a single harmonic oscillation or sine wave. These departures from simple harmonic behavior may occasionally reflect other rhythmic centers with higher frequency (i.e., true harmonic oscillators), but in most cases,

James Thomas Enright Scripps Institution of Oceanography, University of California—San Diego, La Jolla, California 92093.

they probably represent a single data-generating process that is nonsinusoidal in its mechanisms. Furthermore, the properties of a biological rhythm, including period and waveform, often change gradually with time. This plasticity of the data-generating system is also a basic and interesting property, and in most cases, the long-term changes do not reflect other rhythmic centers with very low frequency. These several features of the data of interest cast doubt on the assumption—which is often fruitful in simple physical systems—that an observed time series is optimally treated as the sum of a series of additive sine and cosine components. To interpret biological-rhythm data only in those terms is apt to be a way of "accounting for" the data that obscures mechanisms and phenomena of interest.

DESCRIPTIVE VERSUS INFERENTIAL PROCEDURES

The statistical treatment of any set of observations can be undertaken with either of two very different objectives in mind, the first involving simple description and the second involving inference. In the descriptive uses of statistics, the intent is to *summarize* a particular set of observations in some simple and concise fashion. With the entire data set of interest fully and completely available, no attempt at broader generalization is intended. In contrast, the inferential approach to data involves interest in some general "set" or population of values; the available data are regarded as a sample or subset from this general population. The goal of the analysis is to infer something about the properties of the entire set, on the basis of properties of the sample, and to quantify objectively the degree of confidence that can be placed in this inference. Most of this chapter deals with those kinds of *descriptive* statistics that have proved useful in the study of biological rhythms. A subsequent section then deals, in a less detailed way, with inferential procedures, as applied to rhythm data, and the severe restrictions that limit their usefulness. This may appear to be a misplacement of emphasis, since the broader objective of all science is not simply to describe but to proceed from the particular to the general on the basis of inference. The abbreviated coverage given here to inferential statistics is a result of my conviction that there are seldom any good guidelines, much less firm rules, for quantitatively evaluating how reliable an inference will be, based on statistical analysis of a single time-series record obtained in biological-rhythm studies.

DESCRIPTIVE STATISTICS

OBJECTIVITY IN MEASUREMENT

The usefulness of any summary statistic depends critically on the objectivity of the measurements from which it is derived. The ideal is that any observer, confronted with a given set of phenomena, would report the same unique array of measurement values to be summarized. This ideal, however, may be difficult to achieve; the risk that the observer's biases, originating from hypotheses, will affect his report is a pervasive problem. The only guarantee of objectivity is to have data collection and measurement fully automated, without observer intervention before the final datum is recorded. When such mechanization is unavailable, the use of "blind" observers for data evaluation can be a very useful alternative precaution against subjectivity. If the set of decision-making rules by which a "blind" observer evaluates the record is fully explicit and covers all contingencies, the observer can approximate the function of an automatic measuring device, but there is a residual and often overlooked problem in the context of time-series data. Even the most naive of observers has a tendency to expect approximate repetition within a data sequence, leading to the risk that a "blind" observer will underestimate the true variance of a set of time-series measurements unless each single measurement decision is presented in a completely randomized sequence.

Based on the premise of suitable objectivity in the initial evaluation of the data, the following sections consider several properties of a data series in which a researcher on biological rhythms may be interested, as well as some of the ways of arriving at descriptive, summary statistics.

Determining Phase-Reference Points

For a variety of purposes in rhythm work, it is useful to specify the time point within a complete cycle at which some given event occurs. In fully rigorous usage, *phase* is a concept applicable only to harmonic oscillations, but in research on biological rhythms, the term *phase-reference point*, or sometimes simply *phase*, is loosely used for the time at which a particular event occurs in a cycle that is clearly nonharmonic. Given that the majority of the data of interest have their "energy" concentrated within a narrow frequency band, any useful phase-reference point will in principle represent a stage, in the cycles of that frequency, to which the rhythmic system reproducibly returns. The implicit assumption is that the system passes through a regular sequence of unique "states" in each cycle. The concept of a phase-reference point is therefore of doubtful validity except when applied to an oscillation with constant period, meaning, in the present context, a rhythm that is either in stable freerun or stably entrained. Only in such circumstances is there adequate justification for assuming that the system may pass through a sequence of "states" that are more-or-less equivalent from one cycle to the next.

The choices of phase-reference points that have been made in rhythm studies cover a broad spectrum: the time of attainment of a maximum, or a minimum, or an inflection point in the measured output; the time at which the median of a discrete peak, derived from counts, occurs; the centroid of such a peak; a zero crossing, such as onset of locomotor activity or onset of sleep—the conceivable possibilities are endless. The use that is to be made of a set of phase-reference points will be an important determinant of the optimal choice among these many possibilities.

Phase-Reference Points during Freerun. In some cases, the primary objective in evaluating phase points is to provide a basis for estimating the average period of a free-running rhythm. If this is the only goal in mind, the selection of the most useful reference event can be made by comparing variances of the single-cycle estimates of period resulting from alternative choices of the reference point. Assuming that the period of the rhythm is stable, that phase-reference point which leads to minimum variance of cycle-by-cycle period values will provide the most efficient estimator of overall average period. For example, the variance of single-cycle estimates of period, based on choice of onset of locomotor activity as the reference event, commonly turns out to be smaller than the variance of period estimates based on use of the ends of activity. In experiments in which measurement involves observing large groups of animals, another criterion can be applied: on the basis of replicate experiments, that phase-reference point can be sought which gives minimum intracycle variance in timing among replicate populations (cf. Enright, 1963). Both of these criteria are aimed at finding the most reproducible intracycle reference event within the measurement series, and there is intuitive justification for regarding such reproducibility as a suitable criterion for the approximate equivalence of the "states" of the rhythmic system.

ENTRAINED PHASE RELATIONSHIPS: DESCRIPTION. When a biological rhythm is stably entrained, it may well be of interest to specify the typical time at which a given biological event takes place, with time expressed relative to the entraining cycle. Sometimes the objective may be simply to provide a summary description of a single experiment; in other cases, the objective may be to make cross-individual comparisons under a standard entrainment regime, so as to specify the range of "normal" rhythmic behavior.

A first-order approach to the evaluation of such timing relationships would be to make cycle-by-cycle determinations of the time interval between the biological event of interest and a reference time in the entraining cycle, and then to calculate an average (or perhaps a median) of the values, as well as the variance of the intervals (or perhaps some other measure of dispersion). A similar kind of averaging procedure can also be utilized during stable freerun, in cases in which two separate biological rhythms are monitored in the same individual, with the objective of specifying the average timing relationship between events in the two rhythms.

There are, however, two sorts of problems in the general use of such procedures: (1) the reliable cycle-by-cycle determination of discrete phase-reference points in a data series may be difficult, particularly when the measured variable oscillates in a continuous fashion with a large "noise" component, rather than as a sequence of discrete, on–off events; and (2) the description of a data series in terms of only a single series of once-per-cycle events potentially disregards a great deal of information contained in the full record: the choice of *what* to describe or summarize may well inject an important element of hypothesis into the description. To deal with these kinds of problems, computer-oriented procedures have been developed (Halberg, Tong, and Johnson, 1967), which are referred to as *cosinor analysis,* for which Halberg and his co-workers have found widespread application. The input to the analysis consists of a sequence of measurements, usually made at regular intervals (e.g. readings of body temperature at, say, 3-hr intervals). The analysis seeks that cosine curve which best fits the data series, relying on the criterion of minimum variance of the residuals. Since the period of the cosine curve is dictated by that of the entraining regime, the parameters of the curve to be fitted to the data are its amplitude and its phasing. Once the best-fitting curve has been determined, its phase is commonly expressed in terms of its crest time (corresponding to $0°$), which is designated *acrophase*, relative to some reference time in the entraining cycle (e.g., temperature maximum occurs x hours after onset of lighting).

An extension of the cosinor analysis to data from several indepentent time series also permits calculation of an envelope of "confidence limits" for amplitude and phasing of the overall average best-fitting cosine curve. Considerable caution should be used in evaluating what these confidence limits mean, because they involve assumptions about probability-density distribution that are of uncertain validity; nevertheless, as supplements to a single average of the best-fitting estimates of phase and amplitude, the cosinor ellipses are clearly useful for data summary.

In some situations, cosinor analysis would be decidedly inappropriate. A researcher might, for example, be convinced that the amount of locomotor activity and its broader temporal distribution are irrelevant to an understanding of the animal's clockworks and may decide, on *a priori* grounds, to use, say, activity onset as the phase-reference point for evaluation. Such a choice means, of course, that the summary statistic contains within it a strong element of hypothesis.

The cosinor analysis, in contrast, may appear to be a completely neutral means of summarizing data on phase relationships. In fact, however, the cosine function itself represents an implicit "model" for the data, which affects the nature of the derived summary statistics. Since very few biological rhythms can be adequately described by a single cosine wave, with superimposed random noise, much of the residual variance of the data series around the best-fitting cosine wave may reflect significant features of the waveform that are ignored. As an alternative to a cosine wave, a sawtooth oscillation might, for example, be proposed as a model for the data. The best-fitting sawtooth could then be determined, in terms roughly the equivalent of its phase and amplitude, using a least-squares criterion comparable to that underlying cosinor analysis. With this alternative model, values for peak time and excursion would be derived that would differ somewhat from those derivable by cosinor analysis, and there is no obvious *a priori* basis for preferring one set or another of the estimators. Each would be a partial summary descriptor of the data series; and each is dependent on an implicit model for the waveform underlying the data series.

Since the entire objective of determining phase-reference points is here presumed to be only to summarize an array of data, the impact of hypothesis on the choice of *what* to describe could be reduced by providing summary descriptors of the time within the entraining cycle at which each of several events in the biological rhythm typically occurs. A great deal of information can be conveyed, for example, by reporting the average time at which temperature maximum occurs, with its variance, along with similar data on time of temperature minimum, time of most rapid increase in temperature, time of most rapid decrease, and, say, time at which temperature rises above daily average. This kind of data summary will, of course, involve more detail than a single-value summary, and each researcher must decide for himself about the proper balance between brevity and completeness in the choice of summary descriptors.

ENTRAINED PHASE RELATIONSHIPS: CROSS-TREATMENT COMPARISONS. One of the most important uses in rhythm studies to which determinations of phase-reference points have been put is in the cross-treatment comparison of results, for example, change in timing relationship between animal and zeitgeber, as a function of zeitgeber period. These comparisons are usually designed to be interpretive and to go beyond a simple description of the data, toward testing a prediction or developing a model. The difficulties in selecting the appropriate phase-reference point or points for such comparisons are potentially acute. The problem lies in deciding whether there is cross-treatment equivalence of the reference points being compared, since meaningful comparison depends on the interpretation that the rhythmic system is in each case in a more-or-less equivalent "state."

It is easily conceivable that a rhythm entrained by two different zeitgebers could be fundamentally distorted in different ways by the process of entrainment. If that were to be so, there might not exist *any* time or set of times during the two regimes in which the rhythmic system would be in fully equivalent states. In view of this sort of complication, it is not uncommon (e.g., Enright, 1966) to rationalize the selection of the phase-reference points to be compared on the basis of finding that cross-treatment comparison gives results in conformity with some prior model or expectation. The self-evident interpretational problem involved here is the risk of circular argument, an issue that goes beyond the realm of statistical methods.

DETERMINING AMPLITUDE OF AN OSCILLATION

Some methods of data accumulation do not directly lead to a regular series of quantitative values of the biological output (e.g., actograms based on running-wheel activity). Even when quantitative data are directly available, much of the literature on biological rhythms ignores the amplitude or the range of the measured variable, based on the assumption that it may well be completely unrelated to the central timing process, representing instead only a property of the indicator process that is monitored. Since there is, however, no general consensus on this issue, it seems reasonable, when possible, to seek some summary statistic to characterize "typical" excursion or amplitude of the rhythm. The simplest descriptor would be the average value of the within-cycle peak-to-trough differences. In a noisy record, however, these difference values may have an extremely large variance. Periodogram analysis, which is described in a subsequent section, involves another method of estimating typical peak-to-trough differences, also based on arithmetic averaging, which will have a somewhat smaller variance.

The cosinor analysis, described above, also directly provides an estimate of amplitude, based on the best-fitting cosine function. In addition, a number of other statistics have been proposed that serve to quantify how "rhythmic" a given data series is (e.g., R of Winfree, 1970; and CQ of Halberg, 1964). In an indirect way, these are also indices of the amplitude of a rhythm, the period of which is known. The meaningfulness of any estimate of average amplitude or peak-to-trough differences in a data series depends, of course, on the steady state of the rhythm, and biological rhythms commonly show long-term trends in their excursion. Hence, special care is required in the interpretation of average values calculated over a longer record; the data series should be carefully examined for possible trends that would vitiate the meaning of averages.

ESTIMATING THE PERIOD OF A RHYTHM

The period of a biological rhythm, under nonentraining conditions, is one of its most interesting properties, and a great deal of effort has therefore been devoted to the development of techniques for estimating period from a data series. For some kinds of records, the matter of finding a satisfactory estimator is in fact no problem at all, particularly when many cycles of a stable rhythm are available, in which there are clearly defined zero crossings in each cycle (e.g., onset of activity in some records of locomotor activity.) With the selection of a clear phase-reference point in each cycle, a value for "instantaneous" period can be obtained from each full cycle; if the waveform of the rhythm is also stable over long intervals, then any of several choices of phase-reference point will yield approximately the same estimate of average period, and the most useful phase-reference point would clearly be the one that gives minimum variance of the cycle-by-cycle intervals about the average value of period. It should be noted, however, that an estimate of mean period obtained by simple arithmetic averaging is dependent only on the timing of the first and last phase-reference points in the data series and the number of cycles observed; the detailed internal structure of the time series affects the variance of the estimate but has no influence on the average value. For this reason, the decision about which portion of a given record to evaluate, with its respective starting and ending phase-reference points, may appreciably alter the estimate of mean period; when a relatively short record is available, this choice potentially introduces a serious measure of subjectivity into the summary statistic.

A widely used alternative for estimating average period, given similar kinds of data, is to calculate a least-squares regression line for a sequence of phase-reference points, with the day in the sequence as independent variable and the time of day at which the phase-reference point occurs as the dependent variable. If the rhythm is indeed circadian, the slope of such a regression line (with dimensions of phase advance [−] or delay [+] per day), when added to 24 hr, gives an estimate of average period that is less directly dependent on the timing of the first and last points in the series. For very stable records, with data over many cycles, however, there is seldom an appreciable difference between this estimator and that obtained from direct averaging of the individual, cycle-by-cycle determinations of period.

The evaluation of average period in a data series, in which one cannot reliably recognize a phase-reference point on a cycle-to-cycle basis, is a more difficult problem, and several different analytical procedures are available. The application of the methods to be considered here to circadian-rhythm analysis presumes that the data consist of a long series of observations made at regular intervals of time, with many observations per day. If the original record is a continuous one, it must be reduced to such a series of regular measurements. The first two of the methods to be described here depend on a multiplicative procedure, in which one portion of the record is cross-multiplied with another portion; other methods are also described subsequently, which depend instead on an arithmetic averaging of sequential segments of the data.

The most elementary of the multiplicative procedures is the calculation of an autocorrelation function: the ordinary product–moment correlation coefficient is determined between the original data series, and that same series when it is "lagged" on itself by some fixed number of time units. The first-order serial correlation coefficient involves lagging the data on itself by one time unit (i.e., the interval separating measurements in the original series); the second-order coefficient involves lagging by two time units, and so on. A sequence of these correlation coefficients can then be plotted against the number of lags. For a persistent, stable rhythm in which phase is conserved and in which there is one dominant component present (presumably, for purposes here, a circadian component), this plot of the autocorrelation function is itself an oscillatory sequence, with peaks at lag intervals corresponding to the period of the dominant component; and the troughs, as well as alternate zero-crossings, will also recur at similar, regular intervals. Since this oscillatory autocorrelation function ordinarily shows a much smoother pattern than the original series of observations, with much of the high-frequency "noise" suppressed, one can directly estimate period by taking the average of the intervals between successive recurrences of the same phase-reference point. Unless a very long record is available, so that the autocorrelation can be calculated over a large number of lags, such estimates of average period are apt to have a large variance. Provided, however, that proper procedures are used for determining phase-reference points in the autocorrelation function, the method can serve as an objective and sometimes fully adequate procedure for estimating average period from a noisy record. If, however, the amplitude of oscillations in the autocorrelation function shows progressively greater damping as the number of lags is increased, a cautious interpretation is necessary. Progressive damping suggests that a stable, persistent rhythm may not, in fact, be present in the original data series; at the least, it implies cumulative deviation from perfect periodicity so that the definitional issue of what constitutes a "rhythm" should be carefully considered.

A second multiplicative procedure for estimating period is known as the *power spectrum* (Bingham, Godfrey, and Tukey, 1967). It is a technique initially developed for the physical sciences and rests upon the mathematical principle that any finite sequence of discrete data taken at regular intervals can be fully and completely characterized as discrete values taken at the same intervals from the sum of a finite series of sine and cosine waves, known as the *Fourier components* of the data. The objective of the analysis is to determine certain coefficients that correspond to the amplitudes of these Fourier components. One of several ways of expressing this objective is that the full record of T observations is to be described as

$$\sum_{i=1}^{T} \left(a_i \sin \frac{2\pi i}{T} + b_i \cos \frac{2\pi i}{T} \right)$$

where the values of a_i and b_i are the coefficients of interest, which correspond to the amplitudes of those two components with frequency of i/T. These amplitudes can be interpreted as a measure of the "importance" of each of the array of T values of frequency (or period) into which the series can be decomposed. That period with the greatest amplitudes (expressed as $a_i^2 + b_i^2$, to allow for negative coefficients) can then be taken as a best estimate of the period of the dominant component in the original data series.

Most large computer facilities have program packages available for the complex and tedious calculations involved in determining a power spectrum; the point of departure for the calculations is the autocorrelation function, described above. This kind of analysis has been particularly fruitful for the physical sciences, as well as for the description of certain sorts of biological data, such as electroencephalogram records in which rhythmicity is imprecise and in which phase is not long conserved; but in its elementary form, the method does not prove to be a particularly satisfactory means of estimating period in biological-rhythm studies. The primary reason for these disappointing results is that the estimate of period is a very coarse one; the maximum meaningful resolution attainable is an estimate of power for each of T values of frequency (where T is the total length of the data series), and these components will differ from each other in frequency by steps of $1/T$. Thus, if the total series consists of 10 days of hourly observations, T then being 240, an estimate can be obtained of the power at period values of 240/11, 240/10, and 240/9 hr, that is, 21.82, 24.0, and 26.67 hr. An estimate of maximum power at 24 hr would be expected from a dominant rhythm with a period of any value between about 22.9 and 25.3 hr; ordinarily, in biological-rhythm research, a more refined estimator than this is desired. The fact that the maximum power may be at exactly 24 hr, rather than, say, 24.4 hr, is determined by an arbitrary, *a priori* calculational decision.

An extensive iterative procedure that solves this problem has been devised, but it proves to be very expensive in computer time. The basic idea is to make repeated calculations of the power spectrum on the same data series, each time slightly varying that arbitrary parameter that determines the precise array of period values for which power is estimated. One power spectrum will then, say, give power at periods of 21.82, 24.00, and 26.67

hr; another power spectrum will give power at 21.72, 23.90, and 26.55 hr; and so on. The optimal overall single estimate of period will presumably be that at which maximum power is obtained, but this will, of course, be an estimate without useful confidence limits. An application of this analytical method to a 14-day segment of the recording of locomotor activity is illustrated in Figure 1A. No extensive comparative study has been undertaken in which the success of this procedure is fully evaluated against alternative methods, but one thing seems certain: an iterative search of this sort, based on multiple applications of the power spectrum, should not be taken routinely unless a large budget for computer time is available.

It is, of course, clear that resolving a time series into its Fourier components, as in the power spectrum, involves the implicit assumption that the basic waveform of the rhythm produced by the data-generating process is a simple harmonic function. Any consistent differences between the true waveform and a cosine wave with that period are not recognized as such but are attributed, simply as a matter of definition, to harmonic oscillations of higher frequency. The power spectrum is thus a descriptive method of interpreting a

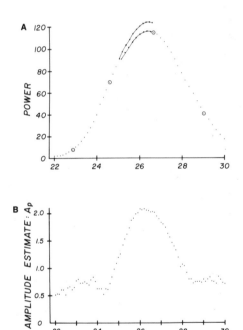

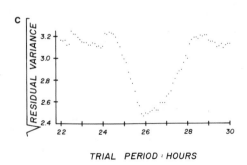

Fig. 1. Results from three kinds of analyses that can be used to estimate the average period from a rather "noisy" 14-day recording of perch-hopping activity of a parakeet under constant conditions (data presented in Table 1 of Enright, 1965a). (A) Power spectrum analyses; the four encircled points represent the results of a single power-spectrum calculation (160 lags); other data points were derived from 22 additional applications of the power spectrum (151–173 lags). The two sets of overlapping points at period values near 26 hr were derived from opposite extremes in lag number. (B) Periodogram analysis of the same data. (C) Modified Lamprecht–Weber analysis of the same data. Note that (A) has 5–7 values per hr, and (B) and (C) have 10 values per hr. Nevertheless, the calculations leading to (A) required more than 6 min of computer time (Burroughs 6700 Computer); and (B) and (C) together required only 14 sec.

time series that is colored by an implied model for the data to be analyzed; the data *can* be so described, but other descriptions can also be formulated, based on other models.

Another method for estimating the period of a dominant component in a time series has been derived from the cosinor procedure for estimating phase and amplitude described above. It has been referred to as *least-squares spectrum analysis* (Halberg, 1964). In the ordinary application of cosinor analysis, the period of the rhythm is presumed to be identical to that of the entraining regime, and the values of phase and amplitude are sought that give the best-fitting cosine wave. If period of a freerunning rhythm is also to be determined, a computerized search procedure can be undertaken in three dimensions, based on minimizing the squared residuals; the three variables of the search would be period, amplitude, and phase. The calculations are somewhat tedious, because optimal phase and amplitude, determined for one value of assumed period, are not generally the optimal phase or amplitude for some different value of assumed period. In principle, however, the analysis should not be as lengthy as multiple applications of the power spectrum; the cosinor analysis assumes that the record consists of a single cosine wave, plus "noise," and the power spectrum procedure insists on a full analysis of that "noise" into its frequency components.

The periodogram represents a calculational procedure for estimating the period of a rhythm that is more economical of computer time than either the power-spectrum or the iterative cosinor procedure, and that is not bound by any implicit assumption about the waveform of the dominant rhythmic component. Instead, the data series itself is used to estimate waveform. The procedure has a long history, going back to Schuster (1898), but its widespread usefulness awaited the availability of modern high-speed computers. The basic method is as follows: the assumption is made that a regular, phase-conservative rhythm is present in the data series, with a period value, P_i; the data are divided into sequential segments of length P_i; these segments are superimposed; and a set of P_i/k average values is calculated for the measured variate, where k is the interval between sequential measurements in the original data series. If there is indeed a single, dominant, persistent, stable rhythm with period P_i underlying the original data series, with superimposed additive "noise," then this sequence of average values will represent an estimate of the average waveform of that rhythm. At the other extreme, if there is no rhythm in the data, the excursion or amplitude of this hypothesized waveform estimate will asymptotically approach zero as the length of the original data series is increased. If this entire procedure is repeated for an extended sequence of assumed values of period for the underlying rhythm, and if a single, dominant oscillatory component in that range is indeed present in the data series, then the value of the assumed period for which the excursion of the hypothetical waveform estimate is maximal will provide an estimator of the period of that rhythm; and the corresponding waveform estimate is then a descriptor of the underlying waveform of that rhythm.

The variance of the average values within such a waveform estimate has been found to permit estimates of period that are more reliable than those obtained from excursion (i.e., range between minimum and maximum). Simple procedures have also been developed for obtaining waveform estimates, and their associated variances, for period values that are noninteger multiples of the basic time unit of observation, k (Enright, 1965b). The periodogram has been calibrated with a variety of artificial inputs; those analyses have led to the recognition of several deficiencies of the procedure, particularly when certain kinds of nonstationarity are present in the data. (Time-series data from biological rhythm experiments often show such nonstationarities, in the form of sudden or gradual changes in period and/or amplitude of the rhythm.) The interested reader should consult Enright (1965b) for a description of some of these problems, as well as for precautions that should be undertaken before a periodogram is interpreted. Binkley, Adler, and Taylor (1973) have developed certain extensions of the periodogram to detect particular kinds of rhythm instability. Binkley (1976) has also undertaken comparisons of the periodogram with the autocorrelation function and the power spectrum as methods for estimating period from records of locomotor activity of birds. Other calibrations of the periodogram, using several different sorts of biological-rhythm data, have been undertaken by Rawson and DeCoursey (1976). In general, the periodogram seems to compare satisfactorily, as a means of estimating the period of a rhythm, with other available methods, even including the calculation of least-squares regression lines through cycle-by-cycle phase-reference points, for cases to which the latter method can be applied. The periodogram involves a great deal more calculation for these latter cases; its advantage lies in its applicability to sets of data that do not permit regression calculations.

Lamprecht and Weber (1970, 1972) have developed still another method of estimating period in biological-rhythm data. The procedure proves to be similar to the periodogram, although Lamprecht and Weber (1970) failed to note the relationship. The initial calculational steps are identical to those of periodogram analysis: the average waveform estimates are obtained for a sequence of assumed values of period. Instead of then examining the excursion or variance within each of these *average* waveform estimates, however, Lamprecht and Weber (1970) proposed fitting each of the estimates of waveform, for trial values of period, to the full original data series, and determining the variance of the residuals. The idea here is that that value of period and the associated waveform, which, when subtracted sequentially from the original data series, leads to minimum residual variance, is the appropriate estimator of period. There has apparently been no published comparison of the Lamprecht–Weber procedure with the periodogram, to which it is so closely related, using artificial or real biological-rhythm data, although Lamprecht and Weber (1970) have compared their method with the autocorrelation function. My limited experience suggests that the Lamprecht–Weber function and the periodogram give quite comparable results, both in terms of reliability of the period estimates and in terms of the breadth and sharpness of the peak (or trough) obtained. An example that illustrates these similarities is shown in Figure 1 B and C. (The extension of the Lamprecht–Weber method used in Figure 1C consisted of the same procedure that is applied in the periodogram for noninteger values of period; see Enright, 1965b.)

Another procedure for estimating period of a biological rhythm has been developed by Blume (1955), referred to as "progressive Fourier analysis"; and still another method has been described by de Prins and Cornélissen (1975), which they called "numerical signal averaging." As its name suggests, progressive Fourier analysis is related to power-spectrum analysis, although it lacks the extensive mathematical and theoretical background of the power spectrum. Numerical signal averaging, on the other hand, is closely related to periodogram analysis. A comparative evaluation of progressive Fourier analysis and numerical signal averaging has been undertaken by Martin and Brinkmann (1977). Their conclusions bear out the preceding comments on the relative merits of Fourier analysis and periodogram procedures: periodogram-related methods are more economical of computer time, often by orders of magnitude, with no loss in reliability or reproducibility of the estimated values of period.

As is indicated by the preceding and by no means exhaustive summary of various methods for obtaining a descriptive estimator for the period of a rhythm from biological time-series, there are many techniques available. Unfortunately, the literature on methods of estimation frequently fails to make any reference to other closely related techniques, much less points out the nature of the relationship. Because new modifications of an older method are seldom compared with previously available methods in terms of their merits and deficiencies, there is no basis for unanimity of opinion about the optimal procedures for any given kind of data. In the absence of unanimity, all I can offer are my own biases, which are in favor of regression-line techniques, (for data that permit this method) and periodogram procedures (for data that do not). A primary advantage of the periodogram is that an empirical calibration of the method is available (Enright, 1965b; Binkley *et al.,* 1973) using various kinds of nonstationarities of the input data, of the sort that commonly arise in observations of biological rhythms. Hence, there is a better basis for understanding the ways in which a periodogram can be *misleading* than is now available for other comparable procedures.

DESCRIPTIVE STATISTICS: AN OVERVIEW

The methods available for descriptively summarizing a set of time-series observations leave a great deal of latitude to the investigator. An obviously important initial requirement is for suitably objective procedures in making the initial measurements. Once this precondition is met, several alternative methods of arriving at summary statistics are then usually available for each aspect of the data to be described. Any summary statistic or set of statistics involves the loss of some of the information present in the original data, and so the choice of exactly what aspects of the data are worth describing and reporting permits (and, in fact, demands) a subjective decision by the researcher about what aspects are "important"; but this represents a general problem in science, not unique to biological-rhythm studies. Even after the decision that a particular element of the data *should* be summarized, the choice of one method rather than another for obtaining the descriptor is apt to involve, at least by implication, a model or hypothesis about the nature of the original data. This, also, is a general problem in descriptive statistics; even when one calculates a mean and a standard deviation, there is commonly the implicit assumption that the Gaussian distribution underlies the data and, hence, that there are a variety of small, additive, random components to the "error" in the observed values. In the selection of appropriate descriptive statistics for summarizing time-series data, the critical problem is that the implicit assumptions may not be obvious to the novice. The unifying theme of the preceding section of this chapter, therefore, has been the exposure of some of these implicit assumptions, so as to show the extent to which hypothesis enters into what is reported, as well as how it is reported.

INFERENTIAL USES OF STATISTICS

THE USE AND ABUSE OF STANDARD INFERENTIAL METHODS

Some of the basic concepts in the inferential use of statistics are (1) that a definable parent population or set of values exists, about which one wishes to generalize; (2) that this generalization will be undertaken on the basis of observations from a small sample or subset from that parent population; and (3) that interesting generalizations necessarily are associated with a certain risk of being mistaken, because of chance alone, and one seeks to obtain an objective, quantitative measure of this risk, usually as a probability. It is, furthermore, a central assumption in most of inferential statistics that the available sample is random (meaning that each element in the general set has an equal a priori probability of entering the sample) and independent (meaning that once a given element in fact enters the sample, this has no effect on the subsequent probability that another given element will enter the sample).

All these matters are usually treated in the introductory pages of standard statistics textbooks; nevertheless, in the ordinary applications of inferential statistics, such issues, which represent the critical foundation for the validity of statistical inference, are routinely ignored. It is a rare publication indeed in which a statistical test is preceded by a careful definition of the general data set of interest, together with an assessment of the assumption that a truly random, independent sample of that set is available for analysis. Biology seems nevertheless to progress, despite such lack of attention to fundamental assumptions, and one may at times wonder how this is possible. As an elementary example, a worker may perform a physiological test on 20 mice from a local breeding colony, divided into two groups of 10, and conclude that treatment A has a different effect on mice than treatment B; and this conclusion is followed by standard statistical symbols (e.g., t test, $p < 0.001$), as though the validity of the conclusion depended on routine application of appropriate inferential statistics, with a probability of less than 1 in 1000 of being mistaken. In fact, if the mice were chosen haphazardly from those in the breeding colony and then assigned randomly (not haphazardly!) to treatment (and how often is even this step ignored?), the set of values about which legitimate statistical inferences can be made consists of the hypothetical array of observations obtainable from these 20 mice, considering all 185,000 permutations of 10 individuals assigned to each treatment. Any conclusion about mice in general, such as stated above, is not based on statistical inference at all but on the implicit (and statistically unjustifiable) assumption that all mice would behave similarly. Such misapplication of statistics commonly leads to correct interpretation only because that latter assumption commonly proves to be not too far from the truth. The use of statistics in a case like this is not, of course, a completely empty gesture; if there had been no significant difference between the two sets of data obtained, no generalization would have been proposed. But even if a "significant" difference is found, it is important to realize that the generalization of interest depends much more on intuition about mice in general than on statistical inference.

It would be unreasonable to insist that research on biological rhythms be based on greater rigor in the use of conventional statistical testing than is usual in other fields of biology. This brief consideration of the sampling theory that underlies statistical inference in general is therefore offered in a spirit of cautionary warning about the cavalier misuses of statistics in all of biology, rather than as defining the minimal standard to be met before any statistical inference is attempted in biological-rhythm research.

If the rhythm data to be analyzed are reduced to a form in which each single number entering the analysis is derived from an evaluation of a separate and independent time series, then the risk involved in using these single values for conventional statistical testing, based on stardard and well-known procedures that are used in other branches of experimental biology, will be no greater than that arising elsewhere. The nature of the single values to be analyzed—whether measures of period, phase, phase shift, or the like—is irrelevant. For example, one could calculate the mean of a set of such single values and derive confidence limits for the mean—incorporating, of course, the additional assumption that the sample averages have a Gaussian distribution. One could test the null hypothesis that one group of these single values belongs to the same general set as another group, obtained under different conditions. One could test the null hypothesis that each of the single values is independent of the value of some other, simultaneously determined variable: standard correlation and regression procedures. Provided that each independent time-series adds only one measurement value or summary descriptor to the analysis (one degree of freedom, in statistical usage), there is nothing special about statistical inference based on data derived initially from a time series. Recognizing that nearly all experimentalists neglect the assumptions of sampling theory that underlie conventional statistics, and that they nevertheless commonly seem to arrive at appropriate conclusions, there is no reason to think that researchers involved in the study of rhythms will be less successful.

RHYTHM-SPECIFIC ISSUES IN INFERENTIAL STATISTICS

The special difficulties of statistical inference based on biological time-series data arise whenever more than one measurement value per animal (or more than one measurement from the same group of animals, for experiments using whole groups) enters the analysis. The distinctive aspect of time-series data lies in the expectation that serial correlation exists: that the measured value obtained at one time is systematically related to the value measured at earlier and later times. Hence, multiple measurements in the observational series involve a special and particularly invidious violation of the assumption that a sample consists of random and independent elements. Casually ignoring this basic problem in the context of time-series data is likely to lead only to disastrous misinterpretations. It is the source of a great many amusing examples of nonsense correlations, such as that between the number of religious ministers and alcohol consumption in New York City.

In dealing with multiple observations taken from a single time series, no statistical inference is possible until one has formulated a fully explicit model for that data-generating process that leads to serial correlation. The statistical dilemma for those involved in biological-rhythm research is that an adequate model is not available; instead, the whole objective of the research is to arrive, eventually, at a plausible functional model for the data-generating process. There is no genuinely satisfactory resolution to this dilemma; the inferential procedures that might be undertaken are either those that involve a trivial and uninteresting model; those that purport to solve the issue of a model by a definitional evasion; or those based on important assumptions that are either patently false or, at best, of uncertain validity.

A trivial model for the data-generating process involves the null hypothesis that the observations constitute a completely random sequence. This hypothesis has an array of explicit consequences; an extensive battery of conventional statistical tests is therefore available to evaluate the adequacy of the model. If the hypothesis of a random sequence *cannot* be rejected for a given data series, the interpretation is quite simple: there is no justification in the available data for making further inquiries or guesses about the nature of the data-generating process. For most biological-rhythm research, however, this model is ordinarily uninteresting and will be rejected out of hand, since it implies not only that there is no rhythm in the data, but that the time at which the measurement was made is an irrelevant consideration.

Granted that the hypothesis of randomness can be rejected, one of the most common of the questions about which a researcher would like to draw inferential conclusions is whether data in a given series show evidence of the existence of a true rhythm. A question of this general form cannot be legitimately answered (Enright, 1965a) except by arbitrary definition: What, exactly, is meant by a *true rhythm?* Once this definitional issue has been resolved in full and complete detail, quantitative predictions can be derived that follow from the definition, and observation can be tested against these expectations. The definition will constitute a complete null hypothesis from which one can proceed, but any inferences will apply only to a "rhythm," as arbitrarily defined in advance.

A more specific question that may be of interest is whether a given set of data includes significant evidence of a "component" with a particular period, P. Again, a definitional issue arises: What exactly is meant by the term *component?* This question can be answered only by arbitrary definition. For example, one possible criterion is that for such a component to be present, a periodogram peak must occur at period $P \pm x$ minutes, a peak that is at least $y\%$ above "background," with *background* defined as the general level of the periodogram for the surrounding 5 hr. Once a "component" has been thus defined, based on a specified technique of data analysis, a clear yes–no answer is obtainable for any single data series; and with data from several animals, one might conclude, for example, that 80% of the animals tested do show this "component." Either conclusion, however, is critically dependent on a definitional decision, about which there is apt to be little unanimity among researchers. When carefully considered, the statistical inferences that might be drawn in cases like this contribute little to the understanding of the physiological systems of interest.

For cases in which a question cannot satisfactorily be resolved by reliance on arbitrary definition, all applications of inferential statistics to a single time-series are plagued with questionable assumptions. For example, there are procedures applicable to power-spectrum analysis for deriving "confidence limits" for the energy in a particular frequency band. The interpretation of these confidence limits in biological-rhythm applications, however, involves not only the questionable implication that decomposition of the data into its Fourier components is a proper way of characterizing the output of the data-generating process, but also the assumption of statistical stationarity of the data-generating system. The sample of data available is assumed to be fully representative not only of the observed behavior of the system but also of its past and its future behavior. It is, however, a familiar observation in biological-rhythm studies that various characteristics of a rhythm—including its average period, its amplitude, and its waveform—can change systematically during an extended interval of measurement. Such violations of the assumption of stationarity vitiate the standard confidence limits derivable from the power spectrum.

As another example, the joint "confidence limits" for phase and amplitude that can be derived from cosinor analyses of multiple records depend explicitly on the assumption that errors involved in estimating the phase and amplitude of the best-fitting cosine wave are associated with an underlying bivariate-normal distribution, an assumption that is untested and that was initially proposed only as a "straw man" (Halberg *et al.*, 1967). In periodogram analysis, a simple statistical test is available to deal with the hypothesis that serial correlation is absent from the data (Enright, 1965b), but this will usually be an uninteresting issue. Any further rigorous statistical test of whether a given peak in the periodogram is a "real" or an artifactual aspect of the data, perhaps due to chance, would depend critically on several assumptions of doubtful validity, although certain precautions for detecting artifacts are available (Enright, 1965b).

Particular concern about the meaning and use of statistical inference in biological-rhythm research arises in cases in which the assumptions underlying the inference are not self-evident in the analysis. A striking and elementary example of this problem arises when evaluating the period of a rhythm and estimating the reliability of the value, given a data series in which cycle-by-cycle determinations of a phase-reference point are available. Two sorts of treatment are available and are in common usage, each having direct foundation in ordinary statistical analysis. One can calculate a mean period and its standard error; or one can calculate the slope and its standard error for a regression line through the array of phase-reference points. Each of these procedures permits the calculation of "confidence limits" on the estimate of average period, following standard procedures. In using one or another of these alternative procedures, the suspicion that something is amiss arises because the two sets of confidence limits, evaluated for any set of data, will differ appreciably from each other. The standard error for the average of cycle-to-cycle values of period is consistently larger than that associated with the slope of a regression line; the longer the data series, the larger the discrepancy. This serious inconsistency arises because of a difference in the interpretation involved in the two analytical techniques about the meaning of the phase-reference-point data, but this difference in assumptions is so subtly hidden that it can easily escape recognition.

In the calculation of an average period, and its standard error, the implicit assumption is that the apparent variability of period length about the average value reflects true cycle-to-cycle variability in the period of the pacemaker underlying the observed rhythm. Any errors involved in estimating phase of the pacemaker are assumed to be small, relative to those in the behavior of the pacemaker itself, so that each cycle in the sequence can be treated as independent of the next. In the calculation of the slope of a regression line through phase-reference points, and the associated confidence limits, the hidden assumption is made that the cycle-to-cycle period of the pacemaker is absolutely invariant and that the departures of the observed phase-reference points from the regression line reflect only unreliable cycle-to-cycle estimation of the true phase of the pacemaker. That is to say, the "error" term of the regression calculation includes possible mistakes in determining corresponding phases of the indicator process, as well as possible cycle-to-cycle random variability in the phase relationship between pacemaker and a rhythmic indicator process; but no variability in period of the pacemaker is allowed for. Pittendrigh and Daan (1976) have demonstrated, for large sets of data on locomotor activity of rodents, that sequential values of period length are not independent of each other (thereby invalidating confidence limits based on the mean value of period), but that the period of the pacemaker apparently has an appreciable intrinsic variability (thereby invalidating confidence limits derived from the regression calculation). Neither set of confidence limits represents properly what the data imply. In addition to this difficulty, there is the general problem involved in the use of such confidence limits for predicting what the organisms can be expected to do at some future time, beyond the observed data series. The rigorous use of any confidence limits to extrapolate from an observed time series demands the further and questionable assumption that no change will occur in properties of the pacemaker.

The emphasis in the preceding section on the fact that so little faith can be placed in the application of rigorous statistical inference to biological-rhythm data, for situations in which the sample includes multiple measurements on the same individual or population of individuals, may well appear to be the counsel of despair. There is, however, an alternative approach to biological-rhythm data that, while it lacks the firm theoretical foundation and mathematical underpinnings of statistical inference, can be very useful. Stripped to its barest essentials, a decision based on statistical testing derives from the question: If the null hypothesis were to be true, what is the probability that this observed result could have arisen by chance alone? Certain kinds of data from biological-rhythm studies, even those consisting of a sequence of measurements from a single individual, are so clear-cut in their implications that a decision can be made comparable to one based on statistical analysis without reliance on statistics at all. Such clear-cut results are those that permit a researcher to assert, "The probability that this phenomenon might arise by chance alone is vanishingly small." The term *probability* in such a statment has no fully objective meaning; it represents a "subjective probability" based on qualitative evaluation, but when used cautiously, such an evaluation is one with which all reasonable observers, even those disposed toward skepticism, would feel forced to agree.

Examples of such clear-cut experimental results are presented in the hypothetical data of Figure 1 in Chapter 2 (p. 12). Consider the case of entrainment illustrated there: the implied null hypothesis is that the observed changes in period of the rhythm, immediately after the environmental cycle had been applied as well as after its phase shift and after its removal, were chance events that would have occurred even in the absence of that imposed environmental cycle. In the face of the data presented, that null hypothesis is highly implausible; the systematic array of coincidences required by the hypothesis seems so unlikely that it can be readily rejected. There is, of course, an implicit, if vague, model for the behavior of the data-generating process also implied in this interpretation; the assumption is that in the absence of extraneous perturbation, the system would continue to behave more or less as it had in the recent past. Since the "more or less" in this model cannot be adequately quantified, the risk of error—that is, the probability level associated with a decision based on this procedure—is unspecified; but we are essentially certain—not quite, perhaps, but nearly so—that the null hypothesis is false. A decision based on such subjective and qualitative evaluations of probability can often be more convincing than a decision based on quantitative assertions about probability, which depend on questionable assumptions.

That the environmental cycle that was applied served to modify the performance of this particular (hypothetical) animal seems well documented by the data presented; but in order to generalize this conclusion to other individuals of that species, one would, of course, demand replication of this kind of result, using other animals in similar experiments.

This description of inference based on subjective probability constitutes a powerful argument in favor of presenting full sets of original data (such as provided by actograms) in publications based on biological-rhythm experiments. Presentation of the original data, or some abstraction closely related to the original data, portraying cycle-by-cycle behavior, can permit the reader to apply his own standards of subjective probability to the implicit null hypotheses. Only then is the skeptical reader able to offer his wholehearted endorsement to an interpretation of the data, untinged by reservations about the validity of assumptions that underlie an inferential statistical test. The proper basis for the application of subjective probability depends, of course, on a set of data so clear-cut that even the confirmed skeptic will feel compelled to agree with the inferences to be drawn. Without full presentation of adequate and appropriate data, this kind of inference would become nothing more than a cavalier and conceivably very biased assertion.

Summary

The unifying theme of the last sections of this chapter is a single, simple message: statistical inference based on time-series data can never provide a fully satisfactory substitute for clear-cut and unequivocal results from a well-designed experiment.

References

Bingham, C., Godfrey, M.D., and Tukey, J. W. Modern techniques of power spectrum estimation. *Institute of Electrical and Electronics Engineers: Transactions on Audio- and Electroacoustics* 1967, *Au 15,* 56–66.

Binkley, S. Computer methods of analysis for biorhythm data. In P. J. DeCoursey (Ed.), *Biological Rhythms in the Marine Environment.* Columbia: University of South Carolina Press, 1976.

Binkley, S., Adler, K., and Taylor, P. H. Two methods for using period length to study rhythmic phenomena. *Journal of Comparative Physiology,* 1973, *83,* 63–71.

Blume, J. Das Auffinden und der mathematische Nachweis der Existenz von Perioden in komplizierten Kurvenschreiben. *Kreislaufforschung,* 1955, *44,* 461–740.

Cox, D. R., and Lewis, P. A. W. *The Statistical Analysis of Series of Events.* London: Methuen Co., 1966.

De Prins, J., and Cornélissen, C. Numerical signal averaging. *Journal of Interdisciplinary Cycle Research,* 1975, *6,* 95–102.

Enright, J. T. The tidal rhythm of activity of a sand-beach amphipod. *Zeitschrift für vergleichende Physiologie,* 1963, *46,* 276–313.

Enright, J. T. Accurate geophysical rhythms and frequency analysis. In J. Aschoff (Ed.), *Circadian Clocks.* Amsterdam: North-Holland, 1965a.

Enright, J. T. The search for rhythmicity in biological time-series. *Journal of Theoretical Biology,* 1965b, *8,* 426–468.

Enright, J. T. Influences of seasonal factors on the activity onset of the house finch. *Ecology,* 1966, *47,* 662–666.

Halberg, F. Organisms as circadian systems: Temporal analysis of their physiologic and pathologic responses, including injury and death. In *Medical Aspects of Stress in the Military Climate.* Washington, D.C.: Walter Reed Army Institute for Research, 1964.

Halberg, F., Tong, Y. L., and Johnson, E. A. Circadian system phase—An aspect of temporal morphology; procedures and illustrative examples. In H. von Mayersbach (Ed.), *The Cellular Aspects of Biorhythms.* Berlin: Springer, 1967.

Hannan, E. J. *Multiple Time Series.* New York: Wiley, 1970.

Jenkins, G. M., and Watts, D. G. *Spectral Analysis and Its Applications.* San Francisco: Holden-Day, 1969.

Kendall, M. G. *Time Series.* London: Griffin, 1973.

Koopmans, L. H. *The Spectral Analysis of Time Series.* New York: Academic, 1974.

Lamprecht, G., and Weber, F. Eine neue Methode zur Bestimmung von Periodenlängen rhythmisch ablaufender physiologischer Prozesse. *Pflügers Archiv. European Journal of Physiology,* 1970, *315,* 262–272.

Lamprecht, G., and Weber, F. Eine neue Methode zur Bestimmung von Periodenlängen II. Das Verfahren der schrittweisen Elimination. *Pflügers Archiv. European Journal of Physiology,* 1972, *336,* 60–71.

Martin, W., and Brinkmann, K. A comparison of the numerical signal averaging of de Prins and Cornélissen and Blume's Pergressive [sic] Fourier Analysis. *Journal of Interdisciplinary Cycle Research,* 1977, *8,* 409–415.

Parzen, E. *Time Series Analysis Papers.* San Francisco: Holden Day, 1967.

Pittendrigh, C. S., and Daan, S. A functional analysis of circadian pacemakers in nocturnal rodents. I. The stability and lability of spontaneous frequency. *Journal of Comparative Physiology*, 1976, *106*, 223–252.

Rawson, K. S., and DeCoursey, P. J. A comparison of the rhythms of mice and crabs from intertidal and terrestrial habitats. In P. J. DeCoursey (Ed.), *Biological Rhythms in the Marine Environment*. Columbia: University of South Carolina Press, 1976.

Rosenblatt, M. *Time Series Analysis*. New York: Wiley, 1963.

Schuster, A. On the investigation of hidden periodicities with application to a supposed 26-day period of meteorological phenomena. *Terrestrial Magnetism*, 1898, *3*, 13–41.

Winfree, A. An integrated view of the resetting of a circadian clock. *Journal of Theoretical Biology*, 1970, *28*, 327–374.

4

Mathematical Models

Theodosios Pavlidis

Introduction

The goal of this chapter is to present certain mathematical models for circadian pacemakers, while keeping the mathematical formalism to a minimum. By necessity, our treatment must be nonrigorous, and the mathematically sophisticated reader is referred to the appropriate literature (e.g., Pavlidis, 1973a). Since most biologists are familiar with the basics of population ecology, we shall use an ecosystem as a paradigm for various concepts of oscillator dynamics. Our first order of business is to clarify the term *model,* since it has been used by different people to mean different things. Basically, a model is a hypothesis about how a physical system works. In general, it must have the following two essential properties: (1) it must summarize the available experimental evidence so that the description of the physical system through the model is more concise than the description through a table of experimental results; and (2) it must predict the behavior of the system under new circumstances. However, it need not say anything about the "deep" structure of the system. Strictly speaking, this structure can never be known. In many cases, it is customary to assume that it coincides with that of a very successful model, but this assumption is not really justified. For example, the acceptance of the heliocentric over the geocentric model in physics is not due to any "real truth" but to the fact that the former gives a more compact description of the planetary system and has far more successful predictions than the latter. It is still theoretically possible that one day somebody will come up with a superior geocentric model. This limitation of models has a certain implication for their value in the search for the circadian pacemaker. It is highly unlikely that they will ever give any direct evidence about the biological structure of the system. On the other hand, they can be helpful in aiding the development of "structural" theories.

THEODOSIOS PAVLIDIS   Department of Electrical Engineering and Computer Science, Princeton University, Princeton, New Jersey 08544. Current address: Bell Laboratories, Murray Hill, New Jersey 07974.

It is a good idea to distinguish between a model and its *instances*. We define the latter term to mean different formulations of a given model that provide both the same degree of "data compaction" and the same set of predictions. It should be emphasized that the common practice in the literature is to refer to such instances as *models,* but this usage tends to confuse the issues involved. Most of the models of the circadian pacemaker can be described quite well in a qualitative fashion, while the instances require explicit mathematical formulations. Therefore, it is appropriate to emphasize models, rather than instances, in a nonmathematical treatise. The reader should not conclude, however, that instances are simple mathematical toys. Quite often, it is impossible to study general models rigorously, and one must resort to *overspecified* formulations that are amenable to precise analysis, either theoretically or by computer simulation, or by a combination of the two methods. Of course, the investigator should always keep in mind what are the essential features of the system he studies.

Basic Concepts from the Theory of Oscillators

We consider an ecosystem consisting of two populations: foxes and rabbits. We assume that we can take an instant census of both species and plot their numbers as shown in Figure 1a. The number of foxes is plotted along the horizontal axis and the number of rabbits along the vertical. The results of the census correspond to a point in the plane. If there is an abundance of rabbits and there are few foxes, then both populations may increase between the two successive censuses (points A and B). When the number of foxes becomes large enough, then the overall rabbit population may decrease, and the next census may correspond to point C. Lack of food will cause a drop in the fox population, but the rabbit population may continue to decline (point D), until there are too few foxes left (point E), when it may start growing again. It takes a while for the foxes to catch up, so that the next census may correspond again to point A. In this way, we have traversed a cycle on the plane. We could have studied the evolution of the populations more closely by taking frequent censuses. Any succession of such points could be joined by a line on the plane. Such lines are called *trajectories* of the system. If they close on themselves (as in the above example), then they are called *periodic trajectories.* There are some closed trajectories that have a privileged position; other trajectories tend toward them, as shown in Figure 1b. They are called *limit cycles.* It may also be possible to plot *zero population growth* (ZPG) curves for either species. In particular, for each size of the rabbit population, we may find the number of foxes needed to keep it constant, and conversely, for each size of the fox population, we may find the number of rabbits necessary for its maintenance. Such curves are shown in Figure 1c. The points where the two of them intersect corresponds to population in equilibrium (neither growing nor declining) and are called *points of equilibrium.* Point X in Figure 1b has this property. Points of equilibrium can be *stable* (Figure 1d) or *unstable* (Figure 1e), if a small change in one or both populations causes the system to return to the equilibrium sizes or to move away from them. The name *singularity* is frequently used for points of equilibrium.

We should emphasize that the presence of periodic trajectories— and in particular, limit cycles—is not necessary for any ecosystem. They can be found only under fairly specific assumptions about the population dynamics (Pavlidis, 1973a). Instead of the fox–rabbit system, one could have studied an autocatalytic enzyme–substrate system. Such systems often exhibit limit cycles (Nicolis and Portnow, 1973). The essential point is that many physical systems that exhibit oscillations involve two quantities, so that the plot of their time course in a plane yields a closed curve. The terms *phase plane* and *state variables* are used, respectively, for the plane where the trajectories are plotted and for the quantities corresponding to the coordinate axes. It is generally true that if a system with two state variables has a limit cycle, then the latter must surround a point of equilibrium (Minorsky, 1962; Pavlidis, 1973a). Very often, this point is unstable. Note that the state variables do not include *parameters* whose values affect the behavior of the system but that are not affected by the system itself. Typical parameters for the ecosystem would be those connected with the climate and, for a chemical system, the ambient temperature.

We may also dispose at this point of a common question: How could evolution produce such a complex system as a limit-cycle oscillator? Actually, the opposite would have been surprising. Limit-cycle oscillations are very common in most regulators used by present-day technology. Since oscillatory behavior is undesirable in such cases, a great deal of design effort is spent toward their elimination or the reduction of their amplitude (Truxal, 1955). Homeostasis is a very complex regulatory systems, and therefore, it is expected to exhibit many modes of oscillations. It remained only for natural selection to choose those with a period that had an adaptive value.

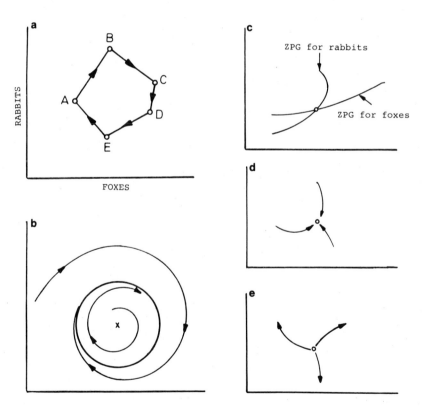

Fig. 1. (a) Illustration of successive censuses of fox and rabbit populations. (b) Plot of trajectories approaching a limit cycle. (c) Segments of zero-population-growth curves. (d), (e) Trajectories near a stable and an unstable equilibrium point.

THEODOSIOS PAVLIDIS

We start our discussion with *Pittendrigh's empirical model,* which was first proposed more than 10 years ago in order to explain certain aspects of the entrainment of the *Drosophila pseudoobscura* eclosion rhythm (see Chapter 3 for a detailed discussion). This model's basic claim is that the 15-min high-light-intensity phase-response curve (PRC) describes the behavior of the system for a combination of such pulses. If we assume that the circadian pacemaker is a limit cycle dynamic system, then the following statements are true. Each point of the limit cycle corresponds to a *phase* or a *subjective circadian time.* The phase-response curve describes a mapping of the limit cycle into itself, since it puts a new phase into correspondence with an old phase.

The empirical model can then be expressed as follows: *The circadian pacemaker is a limit-cycle system and the mapping described by the PRC for 15-min high-intensity-light pulses takes place instantaneously.*

The first assumption is a natural one, since all physical oscillatory systems have limit cycle behavior or can be approximated closely by a system with such behavior. Furthermore, this commonality of limit cycles is to be expected on the basis of physical considerations (Andronov, Vitt, and Khaikin, 1966; Pavlidis, 1973a). The experimental verification of Pittendrigh's empirical model and its expression in terms of limit cycles led to the development of a *topological model* based on an explicit mapping of the limit cycle (Figure 2).

A major observation from the plot of Figure 2 is that the zone of corresponding to circadian times (CT) 4 to 12 has a special meaning. Not only does light (of duration over 15 min) have no effect there, but if the system is exposed to light elsewhere, it is driven in that zone, at least as a first approximation. (We can express the action of light by a parallel from the ecosystem. Light acts like a group of hunters, which, if large enough in number, brings the rabbit population to a very low value almost instantaneously. If there are hardly any rabbits, then the change in the population may be negligible, since the hunters may not be able to find them.) The model can be used to predict the shape of PRCs for light duration longer than 15 min, and it does so successfully (Pavlidis, 1967).

The prediction of the shape of PRCs for shorter light durations is the next problem to be tackled. It is obvious that if a condition of no light leaves the system in the "top" part of the limit cycle and 15-min light pulses drive the system all the way across, then some intermediate values of light intensity and duration should leave the system *within the limit cycle.* (The only alternative is to assume a significant "quantum" action on the part of light: either no effect at all or a very drastic one. In the ecosystem, the gradual effect is simulated by assuming varied numbers of hunters). A number of major predictions result from such an assumption. One is that after a perturbation by weak light, the system will return not

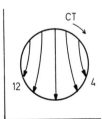

Fig. 2. Mapping of the limit cycle into itself.

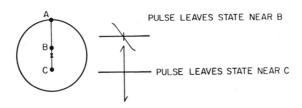

Fig. 3. Illustration of how a slight change in light duration changes the shape of phase-response curve.

immediately to the limit cycle but gradually, in the manner shown in Figure 1b. A second prediction is derived from the fact, mentioned in the previous section, that, in general, a limit cycle surrounds a singularity. The presence of such a point imposes a qualitative change on the shape of the PRCs for light pulses leaving the system above and below the singularity. Those leaving it above would produce PRCs with a zero phase shift at the phase above the singularity; those leaving it below would yield PRCs with a discontinuity. Figure 3 illustrates this phenomenon. A is the "starting" phase; B and C are the points to which weak light pulses bring the system when they are applied at A. The pulse bringing the state to C is slightly stronger than the one bringing it to B.

A computer simulation of an instance of such a model reproduced the weak-light PRCs for the eclosion rhythm, as well as the PRCs of various other organisms (Pavlidis, 1968). In other words, the results were compatible with the hypothesis of a "universal" circadian clock, with the main difference among organisms being sensitivity to light. In the following discussion we refer to this type of model by the term *dynamic,* since it attempts to simulate the dynamics of the circadian pacemaker. We shall discuss some of its instances in the section titled "Instances of the Dynamic Model."

It is possible to apply a light pulse of appropriate strength and timing to bring the state of the system very close to the singularity. If this point is unstable, then the system will return eventually to the limit cycle, but after a rather long time compared with other perturbations. The increase in that time is quite steep, the closer the system is brought to the singularity. Macroscopically, the proximity of the state to the singularity could manifest itself as an arrhythmic behavior, at least temporarily. If the singularity were stable, then such arrhythmic behavior would be permanent, and one would have the following biologically surprising result: "while a strong light stimulus would fail to damp out the oscillation, a weak one (of the same duration) would damp it" (Pavlidis, 1968). Thus the exploration of the interior of the limit cycle seems an interesting but difficult project. The difficulty can be seen from the ecosystem parallel. The hunters must wait till the fox population reaches the right value and then go out and kill a precise number of rabbits, so that both species are on their zero growth curves.

A systematic study of the behavior of circadian pacemakers in the region around the singularity has been carried out by Winfree (1971). For this study, he developed the concept of the *isochrone.* If the state of the system is brought inside the limit cycle, eventually it will return to the original trajectory at some phase. Thus, interior points can be associated with phases. The locus of all points that return to a given phase is called an *isochrone.* All these curves converge on the singularity, so that a typical plot of them in the state space would look like the one shown in Figure 4. For the ecosystem, an isochrone contains all points corresponding to the starting populations of rabbits and foxes, which show peaks (for either

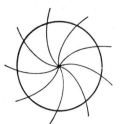

Fig. 4. Plot of isochrones.

species) at the same time. Readers familiar with differential equations should recall that a periodic trajectory inside a limit cycle may be approximated by the equation

$$x(t) = Ae^{at}\sin(wt + \phi)$$

where a and w depend on the coefficients of the differential equation, and A and ϕ depend on the initial conditions. An isochrone is the locus of all points with the same ϕ. For a linear system, the isochrones are straight lines. Winfree (1971) used the property of the singularity as a limit point of the isochrones to determine the characteristics of the stimulus that would bring the system there, and then he proceeded to perform the *critical-pulse experiment*. The eclosion rhythm was indeed damped, and therefore, one of the predictions of the dynamic model was verified. However, there is more to the story. The *Drosophila pseudoobscura* eclosion rhythm can be observed for, at most, nine cycles, and because of the way the experiments had to be performed, there were only two periods available for observing the effects of the critical pulse. Thus, although the existence of a singularity was verified experimentally, not much could be said about its stability. Winfree (1971) proceeded to conduct a *two-pulse experiment,* where the critical pulse was followed by a strong pulse. It turned out that after two days, the state was still near the singularity. Furthermore, if a noncritical weak stimulus was given that left the system inside the limit cycle, there seemed to be no return to it within two days (Winfree, 1975). Thus, the circadian pacemaker behaves as a dynamic system in which the state returns to the limit cycle quite slowly, if at all. Although a simple limit-cycle model could be made to simulate such a behavior by a careful choice of its parameters, this approach is not very desirable. It is difficult to imagine a product of evolution that is highly tuned in this response to a stimulus not encountered under normal environmental conditions. Note that what is surprising is not the existence of a singular point, which had been predicted by the single-oscillator limit-cycle model (Pavlidis, 1968; Taddei-Ferreti and Cordella, 1976), but the slow return to the steady state.

Winfree (1975) has suggested either conservative oscillators or a population of noninteracting oscillators in order to explain this result. Both of these models have disadvantages: It is very difficult to make isoperiodic conservative oscillators (Pavlidis, 1973a) and there are many problems in simulating the phase-shifting and entrainment data by such a model because each trajectory in a nonlinear conservative oscillator has a different period (Pavlidis, 1973a). Furthermore, conservative oscillators are structurally unstable in the sense that they require a very precise choice of parameters (Andronov *et al.,* 1966). Independent oscillators must be extremely precise to simulate freeruns where the period remains constant over a long time. Also they cannot simulate at all a number of other phenomena (see the section titled "Population Phenomena"). It turns out that if we assume that *the circadian clock consists of a population of coupled oscillators,* then it is possible to explain this paradox easily. We shall return to it in the section on population phenomena.

REVIEW OF MODELS DEALING WITH CONTINUOUS LIGHT

The model discussed in the previous section dealt with the response of the system to pulses of light. What happens if light is left on for many days? The models based on the *Drosophila pseudoobscura* eclosion-rhythm PRC predict that the phase of the system will be "frozen" at CT 12. The dynamic model predicts that, depending on the light intensity, a new limit cycle will be followed or the oscillatory behavior will cease, and the system will reach a new singular state. If the oscillations continue they will be, in general, with a different period than under constant darkness (DD). Thus, such models conform to Aschoff's rule (see Chapter 7). If a limit cycle still exists, it will be in a different location in the phase plane, and the same will be true of the singularity. Figure 5 shows such a "shift." Mathematical descriptions of such transformations have been described in detail elsewhere (Pavlidis, 1968, 1973a). The important thing to notice is that the case of pulses can be treated easily under this model.

Indeed, suppose that the system is at A on the DD limit cycle when light is turned on. Under these conditions, the steady state of the system is either the new limit cycle or the new singularity (depending on the light intensity). However, such states are not achieved instantaneously. Instead, the system follows a trajectory starting at A and tending toward the eventual steady state. One such trajectory is shown in Figure 6. If the light is switched off, then the system will be left at point B, inside the DD limit cycle (if the pulse is brief), or at point C, near the "opposite" site of the same cycle (if the pulse is longer), or at point D, outside the DD limit cycle (if the pulse is very long). Thus, we have a reproduction of the phenomena discussed in the previous section.

In the ecosystem, we have represented light by the presence of hunters. The light's intensity is their numbers. Within a certain range of numbers, it is possible for the ecosys-

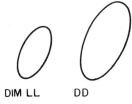

Fig. 5. Illustration of the shift of limit-cycle location under LL.   **DIM LL**   **DD**

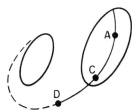

Fig. 6. Effects of pulses under the "continuous" model. Depending on the light duration, the state of the system is at A, C, or D at the end of the light pulse.

tem to survive, but with lower populations in both species, and possibly with a different period.

A few points are worth summarizing here. One is that the "velocity" of the motion of the state along the trajectories under different light intensities is not always the same. However, the change in the period or the phase shifts is due not only to such a change but also to the modification of the *geometry of the motion* under constant light (LL). As a matter of fact, *it is possible to have a situation in which the period is independent of light intensity, but the system exhibits "normal" phase response curves and entrainment as well.* An example of such a model has been described elsewhere (Pavlidis, 1973b). Physically, that particular model is rather unlikely because of the need to choose a certain precise form for its equations, but it demonstrates that a dependence of the period on LL is not a necessary condition for entrainment. In a mathematical sense, the effect of light is to change the velocity *vector* of the system. Under this definition, all PRCs are in a sense also velocity-response curves. However, the latter term is usually reserved to denote the effects on the numerical value of the velocity vector only (Swade, 1969).

Models with light intensity as a parameter would have no problem simulating the PRCs obtained by strong light pulses in rhythms freerunning under dim light. A number of instances of the dynamic model predict that the shape of the two PRCs will be quite similar. Such models also predict the effect of *dark pulses*. Figure 7 shows a plot of the trajectories in the phase plane and the form of the resulting PRC. The latter has been derived on the basis of the isochrones where each trajectory intersects at the end of the dark period.

Entrainment by slowly varying stimuli, like sine waves, is also predicted by the models since they are nonlinear oscillators that can be entrained by their input (Minorsky, 1962; Andronov *et al.*, 1966). It should be emphasized that the mathematical form of all these models is such that light intensity is used as an input. However, when it is held at a constant value, then it can be incorporated into the equations as a parameter. One might then be tempted to use the term *parametric entrainment* for the one caused by slowly varying light stimuli. However, this term has a very specific meaning in the mathematical literature, and it refers to the effects of periodic changes in the coefficients of the equations rather than to changes in a constant term added to them (Andronov *et al.*, 1966).

It is relevant to mention here two recent experiments that concluded that the *Drosophila pseudoobscura* eclosion rhythm is shifted always to CT 12 when transferred from

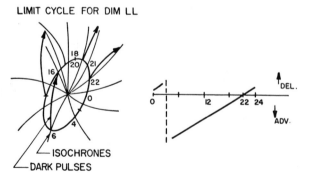

Fig. 7. Effects of dark pulses.

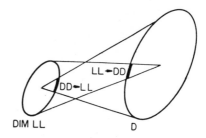

Fig. 8. Phase zones at transfers between LL and DD.

dim LL to DD and to about CT 23 when transferred from DD to dim LL (see Chapter 7). Figure 8 shows a qualitative explanation for these conclusions. Note that a major qualitative prediction is that the zone of phases at the dim-LL-to-DD transfer should be narrower than those observed at the DD-to-dim-LL transfer.

INSTANCES OF THE DYNAMIC MODEL

There have been many specific mathematical models in the literature, some of which merit more attention because of the serious efforts made by their authors to take the experimental evidence into account. One of the first systematic attempts was the model by Wever (1965) described by a second-order differential equation with two quantities: an oscillating variable y and a quantity x, directly dependent on light intensity. The model simulated successfully the PRCs and entrainment of mammals, but it had difficulty in simulating PRCs of large amplitude, like that of the *Drosophila pseudoobscura,* because x acts always in the same manner on y, regardless of the sign of y. Two specific instances of the dynamic model were studied by Pavlidis (1968) and by Pavlidis and Kauzmann (1969). The first was, in essence, the simplest possible mathematical system, which could implement the general model. The second was an implementation in terms of equations of chemical kinetics. That model also suggested a specific mechanism for temperature compensation. A model of a somewhat different type than the above has been proposed by Johnsson and Karlsson (1972). Its major difference is the introduction of a time delay in its equations. This time delay effectively adds another degree of freedom, and it is certainly a realistic assumption for a biological system. On the other hand, it is not clear whether the time delay essentially changes behavior dynamics in the aspects relevant to the simulation of circadian rhythms. The model has been successful in simulating the effects of both continuous and pulsed light as well as rhythm damping by a critical pulse (Engelmann, Karlsson, and Johnsson 1973).

An interesting illustration of the usefulness of mathematical models in biochemical research is offered by the development of the *membrane model* (Njus, Sulzman, and Hastings, 1974; Njus, 1976). There a concrete biochemical mechanism has been suggested for the circadian pacemaker. However, instead of being checked against a long list of experimental data, this model has made use of the dynamic model to check whether the proposed mechanism can create a limit cycle of the proper type.

THEODOSIOS PAVLIDIS

We turn our attention now to a class of phenomena that the previous models have trouble in simulating. We can lump all of them together under the general heading of *freerun period lability*. They include the rhythm-splitting results (see Chapter 5), the spontaneous loss of rhythmicity and then its reappearance (see Chapter 5), the nonmonotonic transients (see Chapter 7), etc. It is possible to modify the simple limit-cycle models to simulate such experiments by allowing random variations of parameters, noise, an increase in the number of state variables involved, etc. All of these factors are feasible in a biological system, but there seems to be another explanation that ties all these things together, namely, that *the circadian pacemaker consists of a population of coupled oscillators*. This assumption is not at all radical in itself, and there is considerable physical evidence in its favor. Multiunit models had been proposed long before the attention of researchers was focused on freerun period liability. For example, they were suggested as a means for achieving low-frequency oscillations out of high-frequency ones (Pavlidis, 1969). Furthermore, they are quite plausible from a biological viewpoint (Vanden Driessche, 1973). Thus, they present a rather natural extension of the single-unit model.

We may point out here another interesting fact. The behavior simulated by the single-unit model (without critical choice of parameters, etc.) involved mostly entrainment and phase shifting. These are essential functions of the circadian pacemaker, and therefore, it is rather unlikely that their study would reveal anything about the structure of the underlying system. Instead, information about the structure of the pacemaker can be elicited best from experiments involving stimuli that are very different than those seen by the organism in its natural environment. Both the long exposures to LL and the critical pulses fall in that category, and both can be explained in terms of populations. It is also beyond doubt that in complex organisms, there is a multiplicity of circadian pacemakers, since phenomena of rhythm dissociation are not uncommon (see Chapters 12 and 17). What is new is the proposition that a given circadian pacemaker may consist of many units, which are coupled in a sufficiently loose manner so that they give rise to overt behavior characteristics of multioscillatory systems.

GENERAL FEATURES OF POPULATIONS OF OSCILLATORS

The most general statement that can be made about populations of interacting oscillators is that there are very few generalizations that can be made about them. The nature of the oscillators themselves, the type of coupling, and, for a given type, the strength of the coupling affect the behavior in a qualitative way. For certain systems the initial conditions are also important. The problem has received considerable attention in the past and has been studied in a variety of contexts. For a review, see Pavlidis (1976). Usually, if all the "units" are close to being identical and the coupling is moderately strong, they tend to synchronize and oscillate together. If the coupling is very strong, then it may alter the dynamics of the system completely and either destroy the oscillatory behavior altogether or produce an oscillation at a frequency quite different than that of the constituent units. For weaker coupling, the behavior may depend on the initial conditions. It should be emphasized that the *similarity between units acts as a "coupling strengthener."* In other words, the same amount of coupling can be moderate, if all units are identical, or weak, if they are different. Not very surprisingly, most of the interesting behavior occurs when the coupling is moderate.

One way to gain some insight into the properties of such systems is to consider an anthropomorphic model of timekeeper interactions. Imagine an island (before the days of radio) in the Arctic (not many environmental clues) where each adult has a poor-quality watch running either too fast or too slow. The watches were mailed to the island by a missionary and were received stopped at random times. Can we ever have a situation where everybody's watch shows more-or-less the same time? One possibility is to have the local chief order an assembly and have everybody synchronize his/her watch. Then, we have a pacemaker, strong or weak, depending on the frequency of such meetings (and on how well the chief is obeyed). Another possibility is to assume a highly egalitarian society where when two people meet they set their watches at some intermediate time. Then, we are faced with a wealth of possibilities, depending on how frequently people meet in comparison to the accuracy of their watches. If they meet quite often, then the answer to our original question is affirmative. It is negative if they meet very infrequently. For intermediate situations, one can envision the effect of initial conditions. We may not be able to reach synchrony, but we may be able to maintain it. There is also the possibility of having a "common time" within each group of islanders but different groups having different times. If for some reason all the watches stop (for example, during a violent storm), then even though each person may restart his/her watch immediately, there may be quite a few days till a common time is established on the island. Such behavior is similar to that observed in the two-pulse experiments conducted by Winfree (1971, 1975). Thus, we have a new possibility for modeling the behavior of the *Drosophila pseudoobscura* eclosion rhythm under weak light pulses.

Let us assume that the main circadian pacemaker consists of two slightly different oscillators with moderate coupling. For appropriate differences in their frequency values, as well as the coupling strength, they will mutually entrain and oscillate at the same frequency but at different phases as shown in Figure 9 (left). The effect of a weak light pulse will be not only to leave them inside their respective limit cycles but also to introduce a significant phase difference among them, as shown in Figure 9 (right). The return to the limit cycle will now be slowed down by the *need of resynchronization.*

This observation is also valid for systems with more than two units. The mathematical

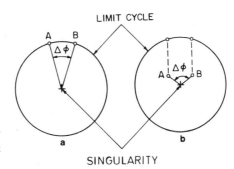

Fig. 9. Illustration of the asynchrony caused by "weak" light pulses in two interacting oscillators of different frequencies.

analysis of such systems, followed by computer simulations (Pavlidis 1969, 1971, 1975, 1976), yields the following results:

1. Even if the units may not synchronize by themselves, they may be brought near synchrony by a zeitgeber and may stay together even after the zeitgeber is removed. However, noise may break their synchrony. When their phases are randomly distributed, they cannot synchronize, but if the distribution is narrowed down, then the coupling strength is enough to pull them together. Thus, the strength of the zeitgeber that may cause synchronization is weaker than that predicted on the assumption of independent oscillators. This can explain the initiation of rhythm by temperature pulses (Zimmerman, 1969).

2. In the absence of a zeitgeber and in the presence of (biological) *noise,* the synchronization is strained. Thus, depending on the individual experiment, synchrony may be lost. Such an event would be more likely if the characteristics of the various units were affected in a different fashion by changes in light intensity. Pittendrigh (1974) has suggested a model of two units, one with period that is an increasing function of light intensity, the other with period that is a decreasing function of light intensity. Such a drastic difference in dependence is not necessarily required. Just having different sensitivity is sufficient to cause a strain in the coupling. The lability of the synchronous state would explain the lability of freeruns (see Chapter 6).

3. In addition to total synchronization, synchronization in groups 180 degrees apart is also a stable state of weakly interacting oscillators (Pavlidis, 1971, 1973a), and this can explain the rhythm-splitting experiments (see Chapter 5).

4. The period of the behavior is a complex function of the periods of the various units. Indeed, suppose that an organism is active whenever the output of at least one unit is above a certain level. Then, a wide distribution of phases may result in many periods of activity and an irregular distribution of the times between, say, starts of activity. In this way, the nonmonotonic transients (Eskin, 1971) are simulated.

Concluding Remarks

The use of a common mechanism to explain both freerun period lability and critical pulse experiments implies an important prediction for the nature of the circadian pacemaker. *Organisms that present significant freerun period lability are also easily brought to an arrhythmic state by critical pulse experiments, and vice versa.* The main obstacle in the verification of this hypothesis lies in the difficulty (if not the impossibility) of achieving significant phase shifts among organisms that have labile freeruns.

There is one more point that requires clarification. It has been mentioned on a number of occasions that the phase response curve of a population of oscillators is qualitatively different than that of individual units and, in particular, that it exhibits greater phase shifts (Wever, 1965; Johnsson and Karlsson, 1972). It turns out that this conclusion depends largely on the way such a phase-response curve is obtained. Theoretically, it is valid only for uncoupled populations. If we compare the average phase of a population before and after a phase shift, then we obtain a phase-response curve that is the average of a set of shifted individual phase-response curves. In general, this curve is a "smoother" curve, with smaller phase shifts. If, on the other hand, we compare the earliest (or a later) phase then bigger phase shifts might be observed.

Temperature effects can be simulated rather easily if a compensating mechanism is assumed. Formally, this idea can be expressed by the statement that the circadian pacemaker never senses the temperature itself but only the difference between some variable y and T, and y follows the variations in T with some delay. Specific biochemical mechanisms for this effect have been postulated elsewhere (Pavlidis and Kauzmann, 1969). The sufficiency of this assumption, at least for the *Drosophila pseudoobscura* data, has been shown in Pavlidis, Zimmerman, and Osborn (1968).

REFERENCES

Andronov, A. A., Vitt, A. A., and Kaikin, S. E. *Theory of Oscillators.* Oxford: Pergamon, 1966.

Engelmann, W., Karlsson, H. G., and Johnsson, A. Phase shifts in the *kalanchoe* petal rhythm caused by light pulses of different durations. *International Journal of Chronobiology,* 1973, *1,* 147–156.

Eskin, A. Some properties of the system controlling the circadian activity rhythm of sparrows. In M. Menaker (Ed.), *Biochronometry.* Washington, D.C.: National Academy of Sciences, 1971, pp. 55–80.

Johnsson, A., and Karlsson, H. G. A feedback model for biological rhythms. I. Mathematical description and properties of the model. *Journal of Theoretical Biology,* 1972, *36,* 153–174.

Karlsson, H. G., and Johnsson, A. A feedback model for biological rhythms. II. Comparisons with experimental results, especially on the petal rhythm of *kalanchoe. Journal of Theoretical Biology,* 1972, *36,* 175–194.

Minorsky, N. *Nonlinear Oscillations.* Princeton, N.J.: Van Nostrand, 1962.

Nicholis, G., and Portnow, J. Chemical oscillations. *Chemical Review,* 1973, *73,* 365–384.

Njus, D. Experimental approaches to membrane models. In J. W. Hastings and H. G. Schweiger (Eds.), *The Molecular Basis of Circadian Rhythms.* Berlin: Dahlem Konferenzen, 1976, pp. 283–294.

Njus, D., Sulzman, F. M., and Hastings, J. W. Membrane model for the circadian clock. *Nature,* 1974, *248,* 116–120.

Pavlidis, T. A mathematical model for the light affected system in the drosophila eclosion rhythm. *Bulletin of Mathematical Biophysiology,* 1967, *29,* 291–310.

Pavlidis. T. Studies on biological clocks: A model for the circadian rhythms of nocturnal organisms. In M. Gerstenhaber (Ed.), *Lectures on mathematics in Life Sciences.* Providence, R.I.: American Mathematical Society, 1968, pp. 88–112.

Pavlidis, T. Populations of interacting oscillators and circadian rhythms. *Journal of Theoretical Biology,* 1969, *22,* 418–436.

Pavlidis, T. Populations of biochemical oscillators as circadian clocks. *Journal of Theoretical Biology,* 1971, *33,* 319–338.

Pavlidis, T. *Biological Oscillators: Their Mathematical Analysis.* New York: Academic Press, 1973a.

Pavlidis. T. The free run period of circadian rhythms and phase response curves. *American Naturalist,* 1973b, *107,* 524–530.

Pavlidis, T. Spatial organization of chemical oscillators via an averaging operator. *Journal of Chemical Physics,* 1975, *63,* 5269–5273.

Pavlidis, T. Spatial and temporal organization of populations of interacting oscillators. In J. W. Hastings and H. G. Schweiger (Eds.), *The Molecular Basis of Circadian Rhythyms.* Berlin: Dahlem Konferenzen, 1976, pp. 131–148.

Pavlidis, T., and Kauzmann, W. Toward a quantitative biochemical model for circadian oscillators. *Archives of Biochemistry and Biophysics,* 1969, *132,* 338–348.

Pavlidis, T., Zimmerman, W. F., and Osborn, J. A mathematical model for the temperature effects on circadian rhythms. *Journal of Theoretical Biology,* 1968, *18,* 210–221.

Pittendrigh, C. S. Circadian organization in cells and the circadian organization of multicellular systems. In F. O. Schmitt and F. C. Worden (Eds.), *Neurosciences Third Study Program.* Cambridge, Mass: MIT Press, 1974.

Swade, R. H. Circadian rhythms in fluctuating light cycles: Toward a new model of entrainment. *Journal of Theoretical Biology,* 1969, *24,* 227–239.

Taddei-Ferreti, C., and Cordella, L. Modulation of *Hydra attenuata* rhythmic activity: Phase response curve. *Journal of Experimental Biology,* 1976, *65,* 737–751.

Truxal, J. G. *Control Systems Synthesis.* New York: McGraw-Hill, 1955.

Vanden Driessche, T. A population of oscillators: A working hypothesis and its compatibility with the experimental evidence. *International Journal of Chronobiology*, 1973, *1*, 253–258.

Wever, R. A mathematical model for circadian rhythms. In J. Aschoff (Ed.), *Circadian Clocks*. Amsterdam: North-Holland, 1965, pp. 44–63.

Winfree, A. T. Corkscrews and singularities in fruitflies: Resetting behavior of the circadian eclosion rhythm. In M. Menaker (Ed.), *Biochronometry*. Washington, D.C.: National Academy of Sciences, 1971, pp. 81–109.

Winfree, A. T. Unclocklike behavior of biological clocks. *Nature*, 1975, *253*, 315–319.

Zimmerman, W. F. On the absence of circadian rhythmicity in *Drosophila pseudoobscura* pupae. *Biological Bulletin*, 1969, *136*, 494–500.

PART II

Daily Rhythms

5

Circadian Systems: General Perspective

COLIN S. PITTENDRIGH

INNATE TEMPORAL PROGRAMS: BIOLOGICAL CLOCKS MEASURING ENVIRONMENTAL TIME

The physical environment of life is characterized by several major periodicities that derive from the motions of the earth and the moon relative to the sun. From its origin some billions of years ago, life has had to cope with pronounced daily and annual cycles of light and temperature. Tidal cycles challenged life as soon as the edge of the sea was invaded; and on land, humidity and other daily cycles were added to the older challenges of light and temperature. These physical periodicities clearly raise challenges—caricatured by the hostility of deserts by day and of high latitudes in winter—that natural selection has had to cope with; on the other hand, the unique stability of these cycles based on celestial mechanics presents a clear opportunity for selection: their predictability makes anticipatory programming a viable strategy. The result has been widespread occurrence in eukaryotic systems of innate temporal programs for metabolism and behavior that are most appropriately undertaken during a restricted fraction of the external cycle of physical change. Feeding behavior in nocturnal rodents is programmed into early hours of the night; the behavior persists at that phase—recurring at intervals close to 24 hr—in animals retained in cueless constant darkness; and mobilization of the enzymes necessary for digestion by the intestine and subsequent metabolic processing in the liver is appropriately programmed to that same (or slightly earlier) time. In plants, photosynthesis can, of course, occur only by day, but that obvious periodicity is not entirely forced exogenously; green cells kept in continuous illumination for weeks continue a circadian periodicity of O_2 evolution reflecting a pro-

---

COLIN S. PITTENDRIGH   Hopkins Marine Station, Stanford University, Pacific Grove, California 93950.

grammed shutdown of the photosystems during the cell's "subjective night" (e.g., Schweiger, Wallraf, and Schweiger, 1964a,b).

Some intertidal isopods (e.g., *Excirolana*; Enright, 1976) feed only during high tides and retreat into the sand when the sea recedes; the intertidal amphipod *Orchestoidea* feeds only on the exposed beach at low tide and retreats below at high water (Benson and Lewis, 1976; McGinnis, 1972; Page, Block, and Pittendrigh, 1980). In both cases, the predictability of the tidal cycle has been exploited by selection: the tidal periodicity of activity and retreat is programmed and persists in a tideless chamber in constant temperature and illumination. In *Orchestoidea,* which feeds on the exposed sand at low tide, activity is further restricted to the hours of darkness at night. Here, then, two periodic programs govern the timing of activity.

Intertidal insects (Neumann, 1976) that undergo metamorphosis in the sea must limit the time of eclosion to low tide, when the pupae are no longer submerged and the freshly emerged adult can fly away. In nature, eclosion does indeed occur only during those nights (every two weeks) that coincide with the lowest neap tides, and in a cueless laboratory environment, it is found that the time of eclosion is again controlled by innate temporal programming; one component of the program has a circadian frequency, other semilunar.

The predictability of even the annual cycles has provided natural selection with the option of innate programming as a viable strategy to ensure seasonally appropriate responses including the anticipation of oncoming opportunities or challenges. The reproductive cycles of several mammals and birds are now known to persist as circannual rhythms in laboratory environments that lack seasonal cues. As Gwinner discusses later (see Chapter 21) the whole gamut of seasonal change in some warblers—including molts, the duration of migratory restlessness, and even change in orientation to navigational cues—is timed by such an innate program.

In all cases—daily, tidal, lunar, and annual—the temporal program is based on undamped biological oscillators whose period (frequency) is an evolved approximation ("*circa-*") to the environmental cycle it copes with and exploits. In all cases where it has been examined (*circa*dian, *circa*tidal, *circa*lunar), the period of the oscillator involved has the remarkable property of temperature compensation: it is stable over a wide range of temperatures (Pittendrigh, 1954, 1974; Sweeney and Hastings, 1960).

The self-sustaining (undamped) feature of the oscillator driving the program is demonstrated by the persistence for years of the circadian rhythm of activity in a rodent. The dependence of the oscillator's motion on metabolic energy is clearly shown by its abrupt arrest with the onset of anoxia in *Drosophila* and its equally prompt resumption even 30 hr later with the return of oxygen and aerobic respiration (Pittendrigh, 1974). The innateness (genetic control) of the oscillation is attested to in many ways, including its susceptibility to change of frequency (period) by laboratory selection (Pittendrigh, 1980b) or chemical mutagenesis (Konopka and Benzer, 1971).

CLOCKLIKE PROPERTIES OF THE "CIRCA-"OSCILLATORS

The pacemakers driving these temporal programs are a distinct subset of biological oscillators characterized by several features that relate to their clocklike function. They are biological clocks for the measurement of environmental time in two conceptually distinct ways: (1) in providing for a proper phasing of the program to the cycle of environmental change, they, in effect, recognize local time; and (2) in assuring an appropriately stable temporal sequence in the program's successive events, they, in effect, measure the lapse of (sidereal) time.

RECOGNITION OF LOCAL TIME: PACEMAKER ENTRAINMENT

The utility of a program intended to match a cycle of environmental change is clearly contingent on its proper phasing to that cycle. This functional prerequisite provides some general explanation of why natural selection has generated programs whose temporal framework is a self-sustaining oscillator rather than an hourglass. Like all such oscillators, the pacemakers driving circadian, circatidal, circalunar, and circannual programs can be entrained by (or can lock onto) an external periodicity whose frequency is reasonably close. In the biological cases that concern us here, the external (environmental) cycle is called a *zeitgeber* or entraining agent. In the circadian case, the 24 hr cycle of light and darkness (LD) is a virtually universal zeitgeber. When entrained by an LD cycle (with period T), the pacemaker's period (τ) is changed from τ to $\tau^* = T$. A mouse that displays a circadian rhythm with $\tau = 23.2$ hr in constant darkness assumes a 24-hr period when exposed to LD 12:12 ($T = 24$). And in the entrained steady state a specific phase-relation (ψ) is established between the pacemaker of the mouse's program and the external light cycle; it is by virtue of its stable entrainment to the LD cycle that the pacemaker can be entrusted with timing, for example, the synthesis of digestive enzymes in anticipation of feeding in the early hours of the night.

An hourglass timer might, in principle, provide the time reference for such a program, but only if initiation of its discharge could be phased—*every day*—to some well-defined external marker of local time. An oscillator has several advantages in this context, including, especially, its provision for complete isolation from a zeitgeber for several cycles: as a freerunning oscillator, it stores information on local time (phase) acquired by prior entrainment (Bünning, 1960). That information is reliable, of course, only if the pacemaker's period (τ) is close approximation to $T = 24$ hr. In the few cases (e.g., *Sarcophaga;* Saunders, 1973) where such isolation from zeitgebers for several days is known to occur, $\bar{\tau}$ is indistinguishably close to 24 hr.

In the majority of cases, $\bar{\tau}$ is in fact only a close approximation (hence *circa*) to the period (T) of the relevant environmental cycles: Why? Why has selection not added the complete precision of $\tau = T$ to the other functional distinctions of "circa-"pacemakers? It could be argued that given the period control ($\tau \rightarrow \tau^* = T$) inherent in entrainment, selection has only demanded that τ be close enough to T to yield to entrainment, but that leaves unexplained a clear statistical trend in $\bar{\tau}$ values. In day-active species $\bar{\tau}$ is generally >24 hr, and <24 hr in night-active species (Aschoff, 1960, 1979). It has been argued (Pittendrigh and Daan, 1976a) that any discrepancy of $\bar{\tau}$ from 24 hr ($= T$) contributes to the day-to-day stabilization of the program's phase (ψ) relative to local time. The phase relation ψ of any oscillator to its zeitgeber is always sensitive to the ratio $\rho = \tau/T$ and especially when $\rho = 1.0$. There is, then, some adaptive advantage to the very *circa* nature of τ in contributing to the reliable recognition of local time. Further, it is seen in a later chapter (see Chapter 7) that the *sign* of τ's difference from T has itself some functional meaning: it contributes to maintaining a particular phase relation between program and light cycle even as photoperiod (or day length) changes throughout the season. In general, the *circa* nature of the period of those biological oscillators that measure environmental time is more than a tolerable approximation to the period of the cycles they match; it has clear utility in stabilizing ψ and hence the reliable recognition of local time.

Measurement of the Lapse of Time: Homeostasis of Pacemaker Period and Angular Velocity

The period (τ) of all those pacemakers that function as clocks measuring environmental time is remarkably stable, even over a wide range of temperatures and other environmental variables (Pittendrigh, 1954, 1974; Pittendrigh and Caldarola, 1973). This general homeostasis of τ, of course, contributes to a stable phase relation between program and light cycle because ψ is sensitive to variation in τ/T and hence in τ. But there is another equally cogent source of selection resulting in the homeostasis of τ. The pacemaker's success in providing a stable temporal framework for the entire program is contingent on maintenance of a stable angular velocity (v) at every phase in its cycle: the sequence of events within the biological program must occur at intervals (fractions of a cycle) as reliably timed as the sequence of external events. In a subsequent chapter (see Chapter 7), it is shown that the detailed time course of the pacemaker throughout its cycle is, in fact, as temperature-compensated as τ itself. The homeostasis of τ could have been effected in other ways not entailing the temperature compensation of angular velocity: acceleration during one fraction of the cycle could be compensated by deceleration elsewhere. But that provision would not produce an oscillator capable of measuring *any fraction* of the cycle with clocklike reliability (Pittendrigh, 1980a,b).

Origin and Diversification of the Pacemaker's Clock Functions

Circadian Programs: Transition from Exogenous Temporal Order to Endogenous Temporal Organization

The stable environmental cycles (day, month, year) that promoted the later evolution of cellular pacemakers with matching periods must have impacted the life of cells from the beginning. In the daily case, for example, the external cycles of light and temperature must have imposed a purely exogenous periodicity on cellular transactions. Moreover, that periodicity was, almost surely, more than just a matter of changing rates in an otherwise stationary steady-state: for a variety of reasons, metabolic pools must have returned to qualitatively different states at different phases in each day's exogenously imposed cycle. That is obvious in the case of photosynthetic autotrophs. Similar effects are expected from temperature cycles, but for different reasons. Metabolic systems are replete with negative feedback loops, many of which have time constants on the order of hours. All such loops are potential oscillators (even if damped) and are therefore prone to lock onto any stable external cycle that can enter the loop. Temperature cycles certainly can: the constituent reactions in metabolic loops are all temperature-dependent. It seems inevitable that any poikilothermic metabolic system enduring longer than a day will be forced into a daily cycle of qualitatively different metabolic states because of this entrainment of feedback oscillations by the temperature cycle acting as exogenous pacemaker. Nothing in this initial temporal order need have been "adaptively," or teleonomically (Pittendrigh, 1958), related to the challenge of external events; it was simply temporal *order* (nonrandomness), not yet information-dependent *organization*. Its essential feature was the predictability of periodic change in *some* aspects of the metabolic system, and its historical role was to set a premium on the coordination in time—by an endogenous pacemaker— of other events in the system in relation to this purely exogenous order. Until more is known about their molecular mechanism, it is idle to speculate further on the detailed origin of the endogenous pacemakers, but their suggested role in providing an arbitrary framework for the temporal organization of eukaryotic life merits further comment. It seems highly unlikely that the success of either DNA replication or mitosis itself depends significantly on environmental conditions at a particular time of day; but the timing of both events is commonly under the control of a circadian pacemaker (e.g., Edmunds, 1971). And as Bruce (1965) noted many years ago, generation times in eukaryotic systems are commonly clustered in the neighborhood of a day. This is two orders of magnitude slower than in most prokaryotes. Why? It could well be that the tempo of eukaryotic life is not so much a necessity imposed by its additional complexity as a consequence of historical commitment to the day outside as a general zeitgeber. Once the environmental cycle becomes "pacemaker" for even part of the system, selection is likely to adjust other rate constants, bringing the period of the entire cell cycle into the range of daily entrainment. Too many circadian rhythms lack any clear relation to either hazard or opportunity in the external day for us to ignore the pacemaker's role as a purely arbitrary clock serving the temporal organization of eukaryotes (Pittendrigh, 1961, 1965). Hufeland (1798) may have been saying this long ago: "Die 24-Stündige Periodik. . . . Sie ist gleichsam die Einheit unserer natürlichen Chronologie."

PACEMAKER PERIOD AND GENERATION TIME

We know of no clear case where an oscillation measuring environmental time has evolved in a system whose "generation time" is shorter than the period of the relevant external cycle. Circannual clocks in animals are known only in individuals (mostly vertebrates) that live longer than one full year. Here the annual cycle of external events is something that the individual organism (not just the population, as such) must cope with, and an innate annual program has potential utility. That is not the case in short-lived species like multivoltine insects, in which response to the annual cycle is a population challenge and must be facultative as far as the individual is concerned. Lunar clocks are similarly unknown in organisms with a generation time of less than a month. And circadian oscillations are known only in cells with generation times (typically) greater than 24 hr.

This restriction of clock periods to individuals living longer than one full cycle (of the clock) is understandable if clock phase cannot be transmitted through the undifferentiated cytoplasm. That is clearly the case in animals where pacemaker function is restricted to highly differentiated cells in the CNS, as in the vertebrate suprachiasmatic nuclei, the eyes of the mollusk *Aplysia,* or the brain of insects. In the moth *Pectinophora*, a phase-settable circadian clock is not differentiated until midway through the 12 days of embryonic development; there is no oscillator to transmit phase or to measure circadian time in the egg itself or in the early embryo (Minis and Pittendrigh, 1968).

The situation in unicellular eukaryotic systems is different. Here, the phase of circadian pacemakers (e.g., those gating cell division itself) can be transmitted from one cell generation to the next (e.g., Edmunds, 1971). The implication that "undifferentiated" eukaryotic cytoplasm is sufficient to sustain pacemaker activity is directly confirmed by the observation that enucleated cell fragments of *Acetabularia* can sustain a circadian rhythm of photosynthesis for up to 30 cycles (Schweiger *et al.,* 1964b). It is tempting, then, to conclude that the apparent absence of circadian pacemakers in prokaryotic cells is not simply attributable to their generation times' being typically less than 24 hr; if prokaryotic cytoplasm could sustain a circadian oscillation at all, it should be transmittable through cytokinesis as it is eukaryotic cytoplasm. The attractive alternative explanation that the complexity of eukaryotic cells is a prerequisite for a circadian clock may well be true but remains uncertain (see Hastings and Schweiger, 1975).

EVOLUTIONARY OPPORTUNISM: DIVERSIFICATION OF PACEMAKER FUNCTIONS

There can be no doubt that the origin of circadian oscillations derives from the benefits of endogenous programming in relation to inevitable exogenous daily change in the life of cells living—typically—longer than 24 hr. That function, primary in the historical sense, remains the principal and most widespread function of circadian pacemakers today. It is, however, not their only function: with its characteristic opportunism, selection has exploited the potential of a temperature-compensated circadian oscillator to perform other clock functions. Two of these, *Zeitgedächtnis* and sun-compass orientation, are limited to animals and clearly dependent on additional complexities of their central nervous system. Another, the photoperiodic time-measurement, is much more widespread but is as clearly secondary (historically) to the pacemaker's primary function of "simple" daily programming.

ZEITGEDÄCHTNIS. Fifty years ago, Beling (1929) showed that honeybees that found an experimental food source at, say 3 P.M. returned to the same food location the following day at essentially the same time. In some sense, they "remembered" 3 P.M with a *Zeitgedächtnis* that was strictly modulo 24 hr and, as Wahl (1932) showed later, was unaffected by temperature within a wide (physiological) range. The bee's *Zeitgedächtnis* is clearly based on a typically temperature-compensated circadian pacemaker that is here being utilized for more than innate programming: it provides a clock reference for the "learning" of significant times of day open to change within the individual's life span. The phenomena of *Zeitgedächtnis*, in the Beling sense, may well be more widespread than the literature still suggests. Formally, identical phenomena are now being reported from vertebrate systems. Suda and Saito (1980) and others found that when rats that normally feed early in the night are forced to eat only in the early morning hours, the anticipatory upsurge in enzymatic activity in the small intestine is shifted from early night to early morning, and it persists at the "learned" phase for several cycles after the animal's return to an *ad libitum* regime. It remains to be seen how much more extensively circadian clocks have been utilized in learned (versus innate) temporal strategies.

SUN-COMPASS ORIENTATION. A great diversity of animals (vertebrate and arthropod) can maintain a constant compass direction throughout the day using the sun's azimuth as compass (see Chapter 16), despite the fact that this directional reference is in constant motion. The time compensation implicit in this behavior involves a circadian pacemaker, as Hoffman (1960) showed in classic experiments many years ago. Birds trained to go in a given compass direction in search of food were isolated from their usual daily zeitgeber for up to 12 days by exposure to constant light. During this time, their activity rhythm was monitored and was found to have a circadian period ($\tau \sim 23.5$ hr, e.g.), which accounted, quantitatively, for the bird's orientation error when challenged, after several days of isolation from its zeitgeber, to find food in the old compass direction. The same circadian oscillator (same τ) that drives the activity–rest cycle can provide time measurement of small fractions of that cycle in compensating for the sun's angular velocity.

THE PHOTOPERIODIC TIME MEASUREMENT. The most common strategy in coping with the annual cycle of environmental change—more common than circannual clocks themselves—involves utilization of day length (or photoperiod) as a reliable marker of phase in the environmental year (see Chapters 22 and 23). A diversity of retreat strategies (hibernation, estivation, "dormancy," diapause) in animals and plants is triggered by the day-length characteristic of the weeks preceding a predictably unfavorable season; and day length similarly initiates reproductive activity in anticipation of that time of year when food or other relevant circumstances will be favorable. This repeated resort of selection to day length as a seasonal cue is undoubtedly explained in part, by its "noise-free" nature as a marker of season; but it has another aspect. In many cases, organisms discriminate day lengths differing by little more than minutes: in some sense, they are—here again, as in sun-compass orientation—measuring time intervals that are a fraction of a day. And again, the time measurement involved is nearly always mediated by circadian oscillations. This particular pacemaker function is now firmly established, not only for plants but for many insects, birds, and mammals, and was predicted many years ago in a now classic paper by Erwin Bünning (1936). How the circadian organization of eukaryotes "measures day length" is a still unclear and major problem in circadian physiology that we return to later.

PACEMAKER VERSUS PROGRAM

UNICELLULAR SYSTEMS

The dinoflagellate *Gonyaulax polyedra* is a unicellular with a circadian temporal program that specifies the time of day when photosynthesis, spontaneous glow, inducible luminescence, and cell division can occur (e.g., Hastings, 1960; Sweeney, 1969). The four "events" occur at markedly different times in the program, which persists as a circadian rhythm as long as the cell population is healthy (Figure 1). The pacemaker driving the program is, as usual, entrainable by light–dark cycles; and single light pulses (e.g., 1-hr duration) cause discrete phase shifts of the freerunning rhythm. The amount and direction (advance, delay) of the phase shift caused by the pulse are characteristic of the phase in the program pulsed by the light. The curve describing the relationship between phase shift ($\Delta\phi_n$) and the phase pulsed (ϕ_n) is a phase-response curve (PRC); it is a useful description of the pacemaker's time course. A pulse given at a phase that delays the photosynthesis rhythm by 2 hr also phase-delays the other three rhythms by 2 hr. The pacemaker of the luminescence, glow, and mitosis rhythms is certainly distinct from (not part of) the photosynthetic machinery itself: the photosynthesis rhythm can be suppressed by N_1-(dichlorophenyl)-N_3-dimethylurea (DCMU) without impact on the rhythmicity of the other three functions (Hastings, 1960). It is as though a "single" pacemaker within the cell were driving all four rhythms, with each rhythm reaching its "maximum" at different phases of the pacemaker's cycle.

Four lines of question emerge from this conceptualization of circadian organization in

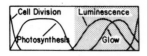

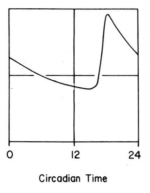

0   12   24

Circadian Time

Fig.1 *Gonyaulax polyedra*. Four different circadian rhythms in this single-celled organism each yield the same phase-response curve: they appear to be driven by a common pacemaker. (Based on the work of Hastings, Sweeney, and co-workers; from Pittendrigh, 1980.)

a single cell: (1) What is the molecular mechanism of the pacemaking oscillation? (2) Is the pacemaker as physically discrete from the rest of the system as it is conceptually? (3) How is the pacemaker coupled to those environmental zeitgebers (light and temperature cycles) that entrain it (and hence the program it drives) to local time? (4) How does the pacemaker exert control over those distinct cellular events it times?

As to molecular mechanism: an increasing body of evidence shows that interference with the rate of protein synthesis on 80S ribosomes (in the cytosol) slows the pacemaker's period; there is other, less extensive evidence that agents impacting membrane properties also change pacemaker period; so does heavy water. However, none of these reassurances that the pacemaker is indeed endogenous provide clear hints about its molecular mechanism: little in the cell can escape the impact of disrupted membrane properties or significant changes in the rate of protein synthesis. (See Hastings and Schweiger, 1975.)

PACEMAKER LOCALIZATION IN MULTICELLULAR SYSTEMS

All the same issues arise in the analysis of multicellular circadian systems. The major goal of understanding the driving oscillation's molecular mechanism remains, of course, as remote as before, but the other three questions are now more tractable. The reason is simple: the larger size of multicellulars makes it possible, using standard surgical and electrolytic lesioning techniques, to address the central issue of pacemaker discreteness. Can the oscillation driving the whole system be physically localized? And if so, how is it coupled to external zeitgebers, on the one hand, and on the other, how is it responsible for a temporal program in the rest of the organism?

When both optic lobes of a cockroach are surgically isolated from the rest of the brain, the animal's circadian rhythm of locomotion is lost; the rhythmicity persists, however, so long as one lobe remains connected to the midbrain (Nishiitsutsuji-Uwo and Pittendrigh, 1968), but that rhythmicity goes when a few cells near the proximal neuropile of the lobe are electrolytically destroyed (Sokolove, 1975; Page 1978). Ablation of the sparrow's pineal (Gaston and Menaker, 1968) similarly leads to circadian arrhythmia, as does electrolytic lesioning of both suprachiasmatic nuclei in rats and hamsters (Moore and Eichler, 1972;

Stephan and Zucker, 1972). The simplest, or most appealing, interpretation in all three cases is that the surgery has either destroyed the pacemaker or severed its access pathway to the rest of the system. That is, of course, not the only possible explanation, and the now strong argument in all three cases rests on other, more crucial observations. In cockroaches, the pacemaker can be phase-shifted by temperature pulses applied to the whole animal; using microthermodes, Page (1980) has shown that localized temperature pulses shift phase only when the thermodes are near the pacemaker site inferred from electrolytic lesioning. In intact rats, Inouye and Kawamura (1979) have recorded circadian rhythmicity of multiple-unit neural activity in many other brain sites as well as in the suprachiasmatic nuclei (SCN). When the SCN is totally isolated by Halasz–Knife surgery, rhythmicity elsewhere in the brain is lost but persists within the isolated SCN: the SCN is evidently an autonomous oscillator, and the rhythms elsewhere are its slaves.

But the clearest evidence of pacemaker localization comes from *in vitro* and transplant techniques. Truman (1972) showed that decapitated pupae of saturnid moths lose circadian timing of their eclosion; that is restored, however, by implantation of a brain into their abdominal hemocoel. Moreover, the time of the host's subsequent emergence is dictated by the phase of the donor's pacemaker in the implanted brain. Zimmerman and Menaker (1979) have reported a virtually identical result for sparrows. As noted, pinealectomy leads to a loss of circadian activity rhythms in sparrows. When the pineal from another bird is implanted into the anterior chamber of the eye of a pinealectomized host, rhythmicity is immediately restored, and moreover, the phase of the donor's rhythm is imposed on the host. The pineal's autonomy as pacemaker is further evidenced by its ability to sustain a rhythm of melatonin secretion *in vitro* (Takahashi, Hamm, and Menaker, 1980) and the ability of pineal cell cultures to sustain a circadian rhythm in the activity of N-acetyl-transferase (Deguchi, 1979). Finally, the eyes of the mollusk *Aplysia* even when excised and cultured *in vitro* maintain an extremely stable and well defined circadian rhythm in the frequency of compound action potentials (Jacklet, 1969).

It is clear that none of these observations attesting to the pacemaker's physical discreteness imply that it is immune to feedback modulation by the rest of the system it drives. In vertebrates, its freerunning period is indeed affected to some extent by circulating levels of testosterone (Daan, Damassa, Pittendrigh, and Smith, 1975; Gwinner, 1974), melatonin (Turek, McMillan, and Menaker, 1976), and estradiol (Morin, Fitzgerald, and Zucker, 1977). Pinealectomy of mice changes the pacemaker's susceptibility to aftereffects (Elliott and Pittendrigh, 1980).

These are, however, minor qualifications to the important conclusion that in metazoan systems, pacemaking activity *can* be localized to anatomically discrete loci; an organ's autonomy (self-sufficiency) as circadian pacemaker is clearly established when it sustains rhythmicity in the isolation of *in vitro* culture, or when in transplantation it carries and imposes circadian phase on a host.

PACEMAKER LOCALIZATION AND ZEITGEBER PATHWAYS

The daily temperature cycle is an effective zeitgeber for circadian pacemakers, especially in poikilothermic and heterothermic animals (e.g., Hoffmann, 1968; Lindberg and Hayden, 1974). There is as yet no evidence that specialized temperature receptors are necessary to mediate its input, and the pervasive effect of temperature change on the whole animal makes no constraint on the pacemaker's localization. That is not always the case with light, however. In two of the five well-studied cases of localization (sparrow pineal and *Aplysia* eye), the pacemaker is actually located within a photoreceptor organ and could be in the receptor cell itself. In two others—crickets (Loher, 1972) and roaches (Nishiit-sutsuji-Uwo and Pittendrigh, 1968)—it lies within the optic lobes in close proximity to the compound eye. And in mammals, it lies close to the chiasm of the primary optic tracts, receiving uninterrupted fibers (RHT) from the retina directly (Moore and Eichler, 1972).

Organized photoreceptors are, however, not essential in many cases of circadian entrainment by light cycles. The *Drosophila* and *Pectinophora* pacemakers can be phase-set by light long before any photoreceptor at the organ level has been differentiated. The pacemaker in a brain explanted into the body cavity of a saturnid moth can be directly set by light. There is an extraocular and extrapineal pathway for light in both sparrows and lizards. Truman (1976) has noted that all the cases of insect extraocular pathways occur in groups that undergo metamorphosis, suggesting that an extraocular pathway is evolved only as needed. That argument, however, leaves the vertebrate cases unexplained. There are effective extraocular pathways for light as circadian zeitgeber in birds, reptiles, and amphibia in spite of the presence of eyes, and indeed, in spite of the ability of those eyes— in both birds and lizards— to mediate entrainment by light. The available facts are both too few and too complex to allow generalization at present, but it is clear from the sparrow and lizard cases that light has several (at least three in the sparrow) input pathways to the circadian system and that different pathways may mediate different effects. In the lizard *Lacerta sicula,* the intact animal obeys Aschoff's rule: its freerunning period shortens in constant light. Blinded animals still entrain (with light reaching the pacemaker by an extraocular route) but their freerunning period is no longer dependent on light intensity (Underwood and Menaker,1976). It may yet prove to be the case that multiple zeitgeber pathways relate to the multiplicity of pacemakers in the system.

Multiple Pacemakers: Mutual Coupling

We now have several demonstrations that metazoan systems do involve a multiplicity of autonomous pacemakers. In cockroaches, circadian oscillators are present in both left and right optic lobes. Each is sufficient to drive the insect's rhythmicity. They maintain synchrony in the intact animal by mutual coupling (Page *et al.,* 1977; Page, 1978). Both eyes of *Aplysia* are autonomous pacemakers; here, the bilateral pair are, at best, only weakly coupled (Hudson and Lickey, 1977), and in nature, their synchrony derives principally from submission to entrainment by a common zeitgeber. In the beetle *Blaps gigas,* each eye is again autonomous, and there is *no* mutual coupling; synchrony in nature depends entirely on access to a common zeitgeber (Koehler and Fleissner, 1978). Bilaterally redundant pacemakers are likely to be the rule and provision for their synchrony variable, depending in part on ecological issues: the tight mutual coupling in roaches (versus desert beetles) may relate to their occasional prolonged isolation from external zeitgebers.

The full range of "splitting" phenomena now known from several vertebrates clearly implies a multiplicity of oscillators in the pacemaking system driving activity rhythms. Hamsters (Figure 2) in constant darkness show a single (though bimodal) band of activity in each circadian cycle. The same is true of the tree shrew *Tupaia.* When hamsters are transferred to constant light (Pittendrigh, 1967, 1974; Pittendrigh and Daan, 1976b) or *Tupaia* to constant darkness (Hoffmann, 1971), the single circadian activity band commonly "splits" into two components that persist at different frequencies—until they again share a common (now different) period, but locked in 180° antiphase to each other. The initial interpretation of this behavior in terms of two mutually coupled oscillators (Pittendrigh, 1974) has now been supported by mathematical demonstrations that mutually coupled pacemakers—whether coupled by discrete (Daan and Berde, 1978) or continuous (Kawato and Suzuki, personal communication, 1979) inputs—do indeed have two alternative steady-state phase relations to each other; one with nearly 0° phase difference and the other with 180° phase difference. A unique case of splitting has been reported from lizards by Underwood (1977). Here, dissociation of daily activity band into two components is induced by a combination of constant light and pinealectomy. The two components move apart as different frequencies and, unlike the hamster and *Tupaia* cases, continue their wholly autonomous freerun for several weeks, failing entirely to recouple in either (0° or 180°) potential steady state: they are clearly being driven by separate oscillators.

It is not yet excluded that the two pacemakers implied by these "splitting" phenomena are simply a bilaterally redundant pair, though it seems unlikely. In the lizard case, they would not be strictly redundant: their freerunning periods are different. In any case, it is more likely that a single pacemaker locus (e.g., SCN) comprises many cells whose synchrony—making them a functional unit—derives from mutual coupling. That proposition yields the simplest explanation for cases such as the hamster in Figure 2, where total

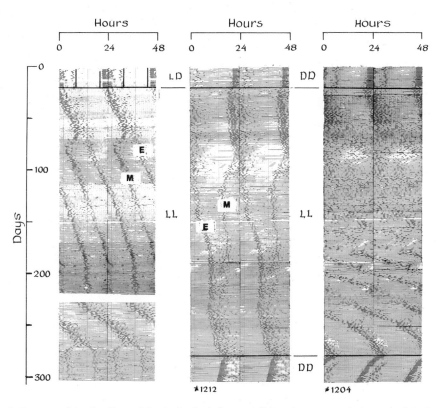

Fig. 2. Response of the circadian activity rhythm in the hamster (*Mesocricetus auratus*) to constant light. In two of the animals (*left and middle*), the rhythm splits into two components (E and M) that freerun with different frequencies until (*left*) they reach 180° antiphase or (*middle*) until the original steady state is regained. The animal at right becomes totally arrhythmic; after more than 100 cycles, a new rhythm "nucleates" out of the arrhythmically distributed activity bursts. (From Pittendrigh, 1974.)

arrhythmia induced by constant light gradually evolves into a clear circadian rhythm by "nucleation" of previously randomly dispersed units of activity. It is as though a population of cellular oscillators with randomly distributed phases gradually locked onto each other by mutual coupling and eventually, as a synchronous unit, imposed a single periodicity of activity on the animal (Pittendrigh, 1974).

Aschoff's (1969) data on the human circadian system attest to a multiplicity of pacemakers in a quite different sense from that implied by splitting: here, entirely different functions (activity–rest and body temperature) have their own pacemaker. In about 16% of the subjects studied, those rhythms shared the same frequency during the early days of isolation from zeitgebers but eventually dissociated and freeran at radically different frequencies. Different pacemakers are clearly implicated; so, too, is their mutual coupling while they are initially synchronous. They then share a common frequency intermediate between those expressed when they uncouple and freerun.

Pacemaker and Slave Oscillations: Hierarchical Entrainment

As previously noted, the sparrow's pineal is sufficiently autonomous as pacemaker so that it not only restores rhythmicity but imposes its own phase on a pinealectomized but otherwise intact bird. However, it is now shown that the sparrow's SCN is also indispensible for its normal circadian rhythmicity: bilateral SCN lesions cause arrhythmia as effectively as pinealectomy (Takahashi and Menaker, 1980). The Inouye and Kawamura (1979) results leave little or no doubt that the SCN is an autonomous pacemaker in rats. Is it so different in sparrows—only an indispensable, nonrhythmic way station mediating the pineal's ultimate control? Or is it also (as in rats) an autonomous oscillator? The latter seems more likely, but if so, the SCN in sparrows is clearly a slave oscillator whose phase is determined by the pineal as system pacemaker.

It is significant in this context that the arrhythmia caused by pinealectomy in sparrows often develops only gradually over many days, as though a remaining slave oscillator were gradually damping or—more likely—several oscillators were gradually losing synchrony in the absence of a central pacemaker to drive them. Certainly, the apparently normal rhythmicity elicited in pinealectomized sparrows by a light–dark cycle is not simply exogenous: the onset of activity phase leads the light when the photoperiod is short (Gaston and Menaker, 1968). The light cycle is merely a zeitgeber, directly entraining residual oscillators left after pinealectomy. Similar results have been reported from insects (Lukat and Weber, 1979; Rence and Loher, 1975; see also Chapter 9), following removal of the presumptive system pacemaker. Roaches made arrhythmic by the removal of both optic lobes become rhythmic when exposed to a temperature cycle. The phase relation of activity rhythm to temperature cycle becomes systematically more negative as the period of the temperature cycle is shortened. The external cycle is again not merely "forcing" a rhythm on the insect; it is directly entraining residual oscillators left after removal of the usual endogenous pacemaker (see Chapter 9).

Pacemaker and Slaves: The Temporal Program

Hierarchical entrainment of multiple slave oscillations may well underlie the temporal structure of metazoan circadian programs. How does a central pacemaker (in the SCN, for example) establish a temporal sequence of events in the daily life of so many different peripheral organs like intestine, liver, and kidney? The possibilities offered by hierarchical entrainment are illustrated by the circadian system that gates emergence behavior in *Drosophila* (Pittendrigh, 1981). It is driven by a temperature-compensated pacemaker (*A*-oscillator, with period τ_A) that is entrainable by light–dark cycles. The gating of emergence is effected by a second oscillator (*B*-oscillator, with period τ_B) that is slave to (entrained by) the pacemaker. The slave is neither temperature-compensated nor directly coupled to light: it maintains a strictly 24-hr period and a reasonably stable phase-relation to the external day only because the pacemaker, itself entrained by the light cycle, in turn entrains the slave. Computer simulations of the system's behavior show (Figure 3) that the phase relation (ψ_{BA}) of slave oscillator (*B*) to pacemaker (*A*) is a function not only of the strength with which the oscillators are coupled (*C*), but also of the slave's freerunning period (τ_B) and its damping coefficient (ϵ_B). (When damped oscillations are taken as slaves, coupling strength (*C*) is without impact on ψ_{BA}.) Variation in τ_B or ϵ (and *C* in the case of undamped

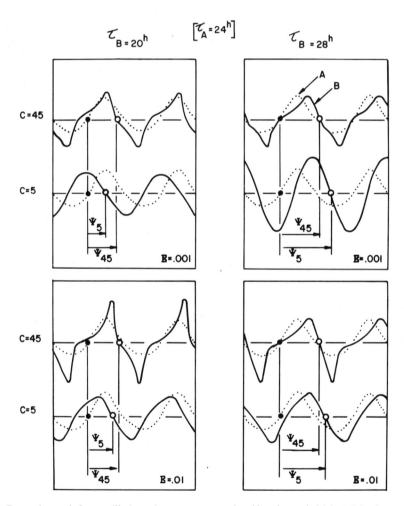

Fig. 3. Pacemaker and slave oscillations. A common pacemaker (dotted curve) driving eight slave oscillators (solid curves) that differ in their freerunning periods (τ_B), damping coefficients (ϵ), and the strength (*C*) with which they are coupled to the pacemaker. The phase relation (ψ) of slave to pacemaker is a function of all three variables. When $\tau_B < \tau_A$, increase of *C* or *E* makes ψ more negative; when $\tau_B > \tau_A$ ψ becomes more positive when *C* or *E* are increased. (From Pittendrigh, 1981.)

slaves) can effect up to 180° change in the phase of slave to pacemaker. That change, moreover, is realizable without change in the pacemaker itself. Genetic variation in τ_B or ϵ provides an opportunity to evolve change in the phase relation of an individual slave to its pacemaker. Laboratory selection exploiting such variation in the *Drosophila* system has yielded two strains ("early" and "late") that differ by 5 hr in the time of day when emergence occurs (Figure 4). The difference is not attributable to the pacemaker whose phase relation to the light cycle (ψ_{AL}) is not measurably different in "early" and "late": what has evolved is ψ_{BA}, the phase relation between the pacemaker and its slave. The temporal sequence of gating signals from the two slaves models the temporal sequence of events in one or more organs driven by the central pacemaker in a circadian system. The significant point is that the temporal program is open to evolutionary adjustment of one component in it without necessary interference with others. Moreover, the slave oscillations in such a hierarchy need not themselves have all the remarkable clocklike properties of the pacemaker; we know of nothing, as yet, in the *Drosophila* case that demands that the slave be self-sustaining; and it is certainly not temperature-compensated. Given its submission to entrainment by the pacemaker, those are dispensable as inherent properties of the slave, although strongly temperature-dependent slaves will make for temperature-inducible lability in the program unless τ_B is set well away from 24 hr. We return here to the general point raised in considering the origin of circadian organization: *any feedback loop in the organism is a potential slave oscillator, and if the circadian pacemaker can make input to the loop, the slave will assume a circadian period and become part of the temporal program*

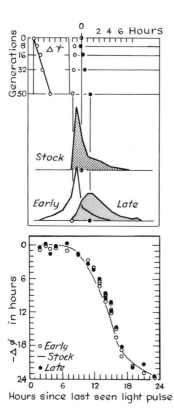

Fig. 4. Laboratory selection of flies emerging earlier and later in eclosion peak has produced two strains that differ genetically in the phase relation of emergence peak to pacemaker. As the lower panel shows, their PRCs have the same phase relation to the light cycle. *Drosophila pseudoobscura* (Pittendrigh, 1967).

that the pacemaker drives. The slave oscillation's phase in that program is open to evolutionary adjustment by change in its intrinsic frequency or damping coefficient.

DISTORTION OF THE TEMPORAL PROGRAM BY EXOTIC LIGHT CYCLES

The hierarchical system exemplified by *Drosophila* has several other features of general interest. The first is its explanation of the transients that characterize the phase-shifting behavior of all multicellular circadian systems so far studied: a light-induced phase shift of the system requires several cycles for completion, although the phase shift of the pacemaker is effected essentially instantaneously. That is now established in the only two cases (*Drosophila*—Pittendrigh, 1974, 1981; hamster—Elliott and Pittendrigh, unpublished, 1980) adequately studied. The system's transients reflect the gradual return of slave oscillations in their steady-state phase relation with the reset pacemaker (Figure 5). The number of cycles required to regain steady state depends on the individual slave's intrinsic period and damping coefficient. When the system comprises many slaves, differing in τ_B and ϵ, the phase shift necessarily entails disruption of the steady-state program as constituent slaves move to new phase at different rates—and some of them even in different "directions" (advance or delay). In Figure 6 a model pacemaker entrains nine slaves whose relative phasing constitutes a simple program. It is reset by a 6-hr advance and then a 6-hr delay. During the several cycles before the new steady state is established, the normal temporal sequence of events is significantly disrupted. This disruption provides a paradigm of the now-familiar physiological disruption entailed by rapid air-transport through several time zones. The stress inherent in that disruption is evidently significant: Aschoff, Saint Paul, and Wever (1971) reported that a weekly 6 hr phase shift reduces the longevity of flies 15%.

As Figure 6 shows, the program created by the nine model slave oscillations is subject to similar disruption when the system is driven by a light cycle with a period (T) different from 24 hr. The steady-state temporal sequence of the nine events changes systematically as T changes. Went (1960) long ago reported that plant growth was optimal in light cycles with $T = 24$ hr; it falls off when T is longer or shorter. A similar impairment of normal function is reflected in the reduced longevity of flies entrained by light cycles longer and shorter than 24 hr (Pittendrigh and Minis, 1972; Saint Paul and Aschoff, 1978). Slave parameters (τ_B and ϵ) have been adjusted by selection to yield a suitable temporal program when $T = 24$ hr; and that program is disrupted when T is changed (see Pittendrigh, 1981).

PHOTOPERIODISM: SEASONAL CHANGE IN THE TEMPORAL PROGRAM

The photoperiodic time measurement is by far the commonest of the "new" functions that selection has found for circadian organization. The commonest class of evidence implicating a circadian element in photoperiodic phenomena comes from experiments utilizing a protocol introduced by Nanda and Hamner in 1959. When an 8-hr light pulse is applied to soybeans, it fails to induce flowering when the duration (T) of the light cycle is 18 hr. However, when T is lengthened by extending the duration of darkness, the incidence of flowering rises and falls as a function of T (modulo 24 hr). That result—found commonly

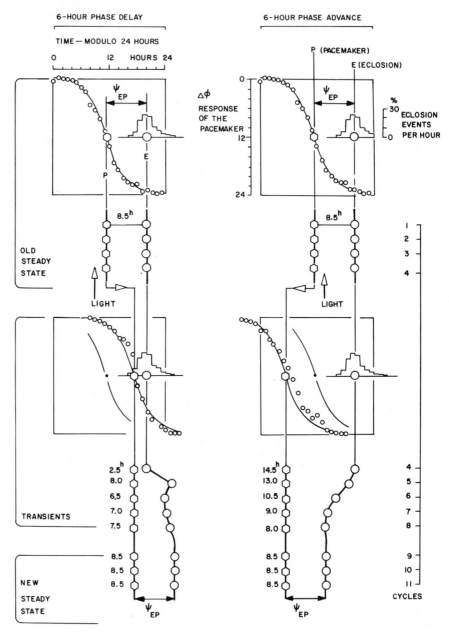

Figure 5. The nature of rhythm transients following a phase shift of its pacemaker, *Drosophila pseudoobscura*. *Right:* The steady-state phase relation (ψ_{EP}) Of pacemaker (P), as measured by its PRC phase (hexagon as phase-reference point) and eclosion peak (E), whose median (open circle) is taken as phase-reference point. Four successive cycles of a steady state (with ψ_{EP} = 8.5 hr) are shown. A light pulse falling at circadian time 20.5 on Day 4 causes an instantaneous 6-hr phase advance of the pacemaker, changing ψ_{EP} to ψ_{EP} = 14.5 hr. Another four cycles (Days 4–7) are required before steady state is regained with ψ_{EP} = 8.5 hr. *Left:* Comparable history of a 6-hr phase delay.

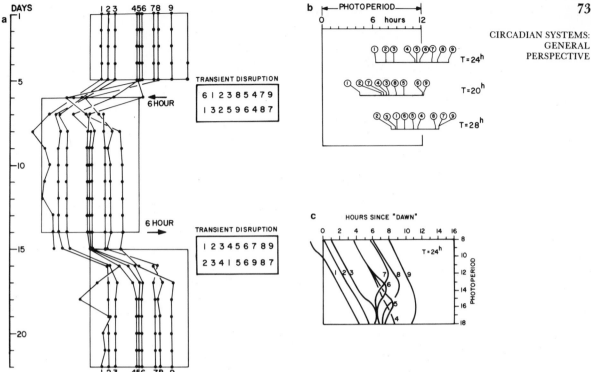

Fig. 6. A model circadian program. Nine events in the organism are timed by nine separate slave oscillations coupled to a common pacemaker. The slaves differ on their freerunning periods, their damping coefficients, and the strength with which they are coupled to the pacemaker; they consequently reach their maxima at different times in the circadian cycle. (a) Five days of steady-state entrainment in LD 12:12 are followed by an abrupt 6-hr phase advance of the light cycle and hence the pacemaker. The temporal structure of the program is significantly disrupted as the nine slaves regain steady state at different rates. The same is true (but with less disruption) during the slaves' transients following a delay. (b) The program is again disrupted when the period (T) of the light cycle is 20 or 28 hr rather than 24 hr. (c) The program is subject to seasonal change as photoperiod is lengthened in the 24-hr day. (From Pittendrigh, 1981.)

in insects, birds and mammals, as well as in plants—leaves no doubt that circadian organization plays some causal role in the photoperiodic induction studied. However, neither the Nanda–Hamner protocol nor any other experimental design that tests and confirms the basic proposition yields any unequivocal evidence on how the circadian system recognizes change in photoperiod.

Bünning's classic paper of 1936, which introduced the basic proposition, went further and suggested how the time measurement was effected. Some phases of the daily cycle are illuminated in the entrained steady state realized by long photoperiods, but not in those by short photoperiods. Bünning proposed that the crucial issue was simply whether or not some *specific phase* in the circadian cycle coincided—or did not—with light. In this class of model, later characterized as "external coincidence" (Pittendrigh, 1972), a photochemical event initiates a reaction sequence that culminates in photoperiodic induction, and the substrate of the photochemical reaction is present only during a limited phase of the circadian cycle.

A quite different class of model ("internal coincidence") focuses on changing phase-relationships among constituent oscillations within the circadian system itself (Pittendrigh, 1960). The central proposition is that the state of the system (the temporal sequence of constituent events) is changed by change in photoperiod: "on one side of the critical photoperiod phase-relations among constituent oscillator elements allow a particular reaction sequence to proceed; on the other side of that (photo) period widely different (phase) relations keep this metabolic pathway closed" (Pittendrigh, 1960). Tyschenko (1966) has published a specific variation on this theme of "internal coincidence" in which separate oscillations in the system are differentially coupled to dawn and dusk as discrete entraining signals. It is, however, unclear that this complication of the original model is necessary. Figure 6 plots the phase relation of the nine slave oscillations (differing in τ_B and ϵ) in the model "temporal program" to a common pacemaker (and hence to themselves) for various photoperiods in a 24-hr day. Their phases change differentially as day length changes; the temporal program is clearly subject to seasonal change: two of the slaves (i.e., numbers 5 and 8 in Figure 6c) separated by several hours on a short day become synchronous (as to phase) on longer days. Again, the impact of change in photoperiod on the mutual phasing of slaves is mimicked by change in T, the length of the light cycle itself. Thus, distortion of the innate temporal program "internal coincidence") provides an adequate explanation of the typical Nanda–Hamner result (Figure 7), and in so doing it also sheds light on the possible meaning of the simple "circadian surface" found in Beck's (1962) *Ostrinia* data by Pittendrigh (1966), as well as the "entended circadian surfaces" he predicted (Pittendrigh, 1972) and Saunders (1972, 1973, 1974) subsequently found in the photoperiodic responses of *Sarcophaga* and *Nasonia* (Figure 7). The "amplitude" of the Nanda–Hamner (or "resonance") curves changes with photoperiod: the curve for each photoperiod is a different transect along the extended circadian surface. Thus, the existence of the extended surface depends on the interaction of pulse length (photoperiod) and cycle length (T) in determining the phase relations among constituent oscillations in the system (Figure 8).

The phase relation (ψ_{BA}) of slave to pacemaker in *Drosophila* is not only open to change by selection but strongly temperature-dependent (Pittendrigh, 1981). If that is generally the case, the amplitude (height) and detailed topography of extended circadian surfaces should also be open to change by selection and temperature. "Critical day length" (i.e., photoperiod inducing a response in 50% of the individuals tested) has been changed by natural selection in latitudinal races of several insect species (Danilevskii, 1965) and by artificial selection in the moth *Pectinophora* (Pittendrigh and Minis, 1972). It is also commonly temperature-dependent in insects (see Danilevskii, 1965, and Saunders, 1976, for review). It is a striking feature of many of these cases that the photoperiodic response curve is not simply displaced on its x-axis (photoperiod length); the change in "critical day length" is effected by depression of the entire curve (Figure 7). Saunders (1976) offers an attractive explanation of this temperature dependence in the response based on an additional "photoperiodic counter"; it certainly cannot be explained as a time measurement executed by a circadian pacemaker itself which is temperature-compensated. On the other hand, it is fully accommodated by the present approach to photoperiodic effects as change in the mutual phase-relations among slave oscillations in the circadian program as such. Temperature-induced changes in the period and/or damping coefficient of different slaves can readily change their mutual timing; and with the amplitude of the surface changed by temperature, we expect not only depression of the entire photoperiodic response curve (as against shift on its axis), but also the depression of Nanda–Hamner transects along the surface that Saunders (1973) has found to be the case; Figure 9 illustrates, not with a model but the concrete example of early and late strains in *Drosophila,* how temperature can radically impact the mutual timing of two slave oscillators. At 25°C, the slave oscillation(s) in early phase *leads* those of late by 3.7 hr, and at 10°C, early phase *lags* late by 1.1 hr.

It is clear that at least part of a circadian temporal program based on a multiplicity of slaves to a common pacemaker can respond, with significant change in internal timing, to seasonal change in day length, and this approach to the photoperiodic phenomena has yet to be fully explored. (So, too, have the related possibilities provided by "complex pacemakers"; see Pittendrigh and Daan, 1976b.) It is equally clear, however, that were the entire population of slave oscillators to respond so differentially to change in photoperiod (and temperature!), the whole strategy would provide an unacceptably labile "program." However, as Figure 6 shows, many combinations of period (τ_B) and damping coefficient (ϵ) can be selected to produce slaves (e.g., numbers 1,2, and 4 in Figure 6c) that maintain an essentially constant phase-relation to each other through a wide range of photoperiods. The troublesome task for natural selection may not have been to find some aspect of cir-

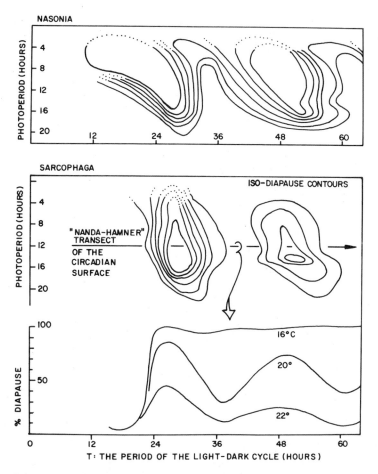

Fig. 7. Extended circadian surfaces for the photoperiodic control of diapause in two insects (*Nasonia vitripennis* and *Sarcophaga argyrostoma*). The percentage of diapause induced by a light–dark cycle is a function of photoperiod duration (ordinate) and cycle length, or *T* (abscissa). Lines connect all the light cycles that induce a given percentage of diapause: they are contours on a circadian surface that peaks modulo τ. The standard "Nanda–Hamner" protocol (see text) is a transect across the surface: the amplitude of the surface is evidently temperature-dependent. (From Pittendrigh, 1981; based on data summarized in Saunders, 1976.)

cadian organization that provides a clue to season; it may well have been to stabilize the bulk of the program throughout the year.

CONVERGENCE: UNITY IN THE DIVERSITY OF CIRCADIAN SYSTEMS

The physiology of circadian systems embraces an unusual diversity of phenomena. There is little, if anything, in common in the concrete detail of underlying mechanisms in flies and mammals other than a general neural substrate for the system pacemaker. Insect photoperiodism involves a midbrain oscillator, prothoracic gland tropic hormone, ecdysone, etc. In mammals, it involves the SCN, pineal, gonads, etc. In mollusks, the repertoire of constituent components is surely different—even if entirely unknown at present.

Nevertheless, there is some underlying unity in the diverse circadian systems of insect, vertebrate, and mollusk. What they appear to share is temporal organization at all levels (cell, tissue, organ) based on the general properties of interacting oscillators; their similar-

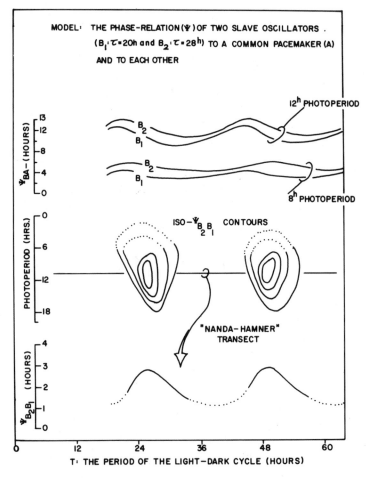

Fig. 8. A model circadian surface. Two slave oscillators, with different freerunning periods, are coupled to a common pacemaker. Their mutual phase-relation ($\psi_{B_2B_1}$) changes with photoperiod and the length (T) of light-dark cycles. Iso-($\psi_{B_2B_1}$) contours form a circadian surface. (From Pittendrigh, 1981.)

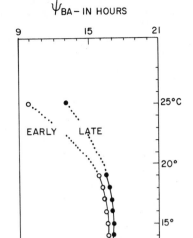

Fig. 9. The temperature dependence of the phase relation between two slave oscillators coupled to a common pacemaker. *Early* and *late* strains of *Drosophila pseudoobscura*. The two strains were created by selection at 20°C. *Late*, which phase-lags *early* at that temperature, phase-leads at lower temperatures. (From Pittendrigh, 1981.)

ities are entirely convergent and concern the formal structure of the organization. The functional integrity of a "unit pacemaker" is surely based on the mutual coupling of constituent cells; mutual coupling is also involved when the pacemaking system comprises more than one functional unit, as in bilaterally redundant pairs or the separate pacemakers for activity and body temperature in man. The potentials inherent in hierarchical entrainment are as surely exploited, to a greater or less extent, in the pacemaker's timing of events in peripheral organs.

It is obvious that progress in understanding any one circadian system (e.g., in a mouse) demands elucidation of the concrete neuroendocrine mechanisms in that particular organism. It is, nevertheless, just as sure, if less obvious, that no amount of neuroendocrine detail will suffice in understanding the system without reference to its multioscillator matrix. The potentialities for temporal organization inherent in the couplings of a multioscillator system have only begun to be explored, and their further elaboration is likely to provide guideposts for more traditional approaches in clarifying how circadian systems are put together.

REFERENCES

Aschoff, J. Exogenous and endogenous components in circadian rhythms. *Cold Spring Harbor Symposia in Quantitative Biology*, 1960, *25*, 11–28.

Aschoff, J. Desynchronization and resynchronization of human circadian rhythms. *Aerospace Medicine*, 1969, *40*, 844–849.

Aschoff, J. Circadian rhythms: Influences of internal and external factors on the period measured in constant conditions. *Zeitschrift Tierpsychologie*, 1979, *49*, 225–249.

Aschoff, J., Saint Paul, U., and Wever, R. Die Lebensdauer von Fliegen inter dem Einfluss von Zeit-verschiebungen. *Naturwissenschaft*, 1971, *58*, 574.

Bech, S. D. Photoperiodic induction of diapause in an insect. *Biological Bulletin,* 1962, *122,* 1–12.

Beling, I. Uber das Zeitgedachtnis der Bienen. *Zeitschrift für vergleichende Physiologie,* 1929, *9,* 259–338.

Benson, J. A., and Lewis, R. D. An analysis of the activity rhythm of the sand beach amphipod, *Talorchestia guoyana. Journal of Comparative Physiology,* 1976, *105,* 339–352.

Bruce, V. G. Cell division rhythms and the circadian clock. In J. Aschoff (Ed.), *Circadian Clocks.* Amsterdam: North-Holland Publ. Company, 1965, pp. 125–138.

Bünning, E. Die endonome Tagesperiodik als Grundlage der photoperiodischen Reaktion. *Berichte deutsches Botanisches Gesellschaft,* 1936, *54,* 590–607.

Bünning, E. Biological clocks. *Cold Spring Harbor Symposia in Quantitative Biology,* 1960, *25,* 1–10.

Daan, S., and Berde, C. Two coupled oscillators: simulations of the circadian pacemaker in mammalian activity rhythms. *Journal of Theoretical Biology,* 1978, *70,* 297–313.

Daan, S., and Pittendrigh, C. S. A functional analysis of circadian pacemakers in nocturnal rodents. II. The variability of phase response curves. *Journal of Comparative Physiology,* 1976a *106,* 252–266.

Daan, S., and Pittendrigh, C. S. A functional analysis of circadian pacemakers in nocturnal rodents. III. Heavy water and constant light: Homeostasis of frequency? *Journal of Comparative Physiology,* 1976b, *106,* 267–290.

Daan, S., Damassa, D., Pittendrigh, C. S., and Smith, E. An effect of castration and testosterone replacement on a circadian pacemaker in mice *(Mus musculus). Proceedings of the National Academy of Sciences, USA,* 1975, *72,* 3744–3747.

Danilevskii, A. S. *Photoperiodism and Seasonal Development of Insects.* Edinburgh and London: Oliver and Boyd, 1965.

Deuguchi, T. Circadian rhythm of serotonin *N*-acetyltransferase activity in organ culture of chicken pineal gland. *Science,* 1979, *203,* 1245–1247.

Edmunds, L. N. Persistent circadian rhythm of cell division in *Euglena:* Some theoretical considerations and the problem of intercellular communication. In M. Menaker (Ed.), *Biochronometry.* Washington, D.C.: National Academy of Sciences, 1971, pp. 594–611.

Enright, J. T. Resetting a tidal clock: a phase-response curve for *Excirolana.* In P. J. DeCoursey (Ed.), *Biological Rhythms in the Marine Environment.* Columbia: University of South Carolina Press, 1976, pp. 103–114.

Gaston, S., and Menaker, M. Pineal function: The biological clock in the sparrow? *Science,* 1968, *160,* 1125–1127.

Gwinner, E. Testosterone induces "splitting" of circadian locomotor activity rhythms in birds. *Science,* 1974, *185,* 172.

Hastings, J. W. Biochemical aspects of rhythms: Phase shifting by chemicals. In *Cold Spring Harbor Symposia on Quantitative Biology,* 1960, *25,* 131–143.

Hastings, J. W., and Schweiger, H. G. The molecular basis of circadian rhythms. *Dahlem Workshop Report,* 1975.

Hoffmann, K. Experimental manipulation of the orientational clock in birds. *Cold Spring Harbor Symposia in Quantitative Biology,* 1960, *25,* 370–388.

Hoffmann, K. Temperaturcyclen als Zeitgeber der circadianen Periodik. *Verhandlungen der Deutschen Zoologischen Gesellschaft.* Innsbruck, 1968, pp. 265–274.

Hoffmann, K. Splitting of the circadian rhythm as a function of light intensity. In Michael Menaker (Ed.), *Biochronometry.* Washington, D.C.: National Academy of Sciences, 1971, pp. 134–150.

Hudson, D., and Lickey, M. Weak negative coupling between the circadian pacemakers of the eyes of *Aplysia. Neuroscience Abstracts,* 1977, *3,* 179.

Hufeland, C. W. *Makrobiotik oder die Kunst das menschliche Leben zu verlängern.* Berlin: G. Reimer, 1823.

Inouye, S. T., and Kawamura, H. Persistence of circadian rhythmicity in a mammalian hypothalamic "island" containing the suprachiasmatic nuclei, 1980. *Proceedings of the Natural Academy of Sciences, USA,* 1979, *76,* 5962–5966.

Jacklet, J. W. Circadian rhythm of optic nerve impulses recorded in darkness from isolated eye of *Aplysia. Science,* 1969, *164,* 562–563.

Koehler, W. K., and Fleissner, G. Internal desynchronization of bilaterally organized circadian oscillators in the visual system of insects. *Nature* (London), 1978, *274,* 708–710.

Konopka, R., and Benzer, S. Clock mutants of *Drosophila melanogaster. Proceedings of the National Academy of Sciences, USA,* 1971, *68,* 2112–2116.

Lickey, M. E., Block, G. D. Hudson, D. J., and Smith, J. T. Circadian oscillators and photoreceptors in the gastropod, *Aplysia. Photochemistry and Photobiology,* 1976, *23,* 253–273.

Lindberg, R. G., and Hayden, P. Thermoperiodic entrainment of arousal from torpor in the little pocket mouse, *Perognathus longimembris. Chronobiologia,* 1974, *1,* 356–361.

Loher, W. Circadian control of stridulation in the cricket, *Teleogryllus commodus* Walker. *Journal of Comparative Physiology*, 1972, *79*, 173–190.

Lukat, R., and Wever, F. The structure of locomotor activity in bilobectomized cockroaches *(Blaberus fuscus)*. *Experientia*, 1979, 35, 38–39.

McGinnis, J. W. A tidal rhythm in the terrestrial sand beach amphipod *Orchestoidea corniculata*. Unpublished student research report, Hopkins Marine Station, Stanford University, 1972.

Minis, D. H., and Pittendrigh, C. S. Circadian oscillation controlling hatching: Its ontogeny during embryogenesis of a moth. *Science* (Washington), 1968, *159*, 534–536.

Moore, R.Y., and Eichler, V. B. Loss of a circadian adrenal corticosterone rhythm following suprachiasmatic lesions in the rate. *Brain Research*, 1972, *42*, 201–206.

Morin, L. P., Fitzgerald, K. M. and Zucker, I. Estradiol shortens period of hamster circadian rhythms. *Science*, 1977, *196*, 305–307.

Nanda, K. K., and Hamner, K. C. Photoperiodic cycles of different lenghts in relation to flowering in *Biloxi* soybean. *Planta*, 1959, *53*, 45–52.

Neumann, D. Entrainment of a semi-lunar rhythm. In P. J. deCoursey (Ed.), *Biological Rhythms in the Marine Environment*. Columbia: University of South Carolina Press, 1976, pp. 115–128.

Nishiitsutsuji-Uwo, J., and Pittendrigh, C. S. Central nervous system control of circadian rhythmicity in the cockroach. III. The optic lobes, locus of the driving oscillation? *Zeitschrift für vergleichende Physiologie*, 1968, *58*, 14–46.

Page, T. L. Interactions between bilaterally paired components of the cockroach circadian system. *Journal of Comparative Physiology*, 1978, *124*, 225–236.

Page, T. L., Caldarola, D. C., and Pittendrigh, C. S. Mutual entrainment of bilaterally distributed circadian pacemakers. *Proceedings of the National Academy of Sciences, USA*, 1977, *74*, 1277–1281.

Page, T. L. Block, G. G., and Pittendrigh, C. S. Unpublished observations, 1980.

Pittendrigh, C. S. On temperature independence in the clock system controlling emergency time in *Drosophila*. *Proceedings of the National Academy of Sciences, USA*, 1954, *40*, 1018–1029.

Pittendrigh, C. S. Adaptation, natural selection and behavior. In A. Roe and C. G. Simpson (Eds.), *Behavior and Evolution*. New Haven, Conn.: Yale University Press, 1958, pp. 390–416.

Pittendrigh, C. S. Circadian rhythms and circadian organization of living systems. *Cold Spring Harbor Symposia on Quantitative Biology*, 1960, *25*, 159–182.

Pittendrigh, C. S. On temporal organization in living systems. *Harvey Lectures*, 1961, *56*, 93–125.

Pittendrigh, C. S. Biological clocks: The functions, ancient and modern, of circadian oscillations. *"Science in the Sixties," Proceedings of the 1965 Couldcroft Symposium*, Air Force Office of Scientific Research, 1965, pp. 96–111.

Pittendrigh, C. S. The circadian oscillation in *Drosophila pseudoobscura* pupae: A model for the photoperiodic clock. *Zeitschrift für Pflanzenphysiologie*, 1966, *54*, 275–307.

Pittendrigh, C. S. Circadian rhythms, space research and manned space light. In *Life Sciences and Space Research*. Vol. 5. Amsterdam: North-Holland Publ. Company, 1967, pp. 122–134.

Pittendrigh, C. S. Circadian surfaces and the diversity of possible roles of circadian organization in photoperiodic induction. *Proceedings of the National Academy of Sciences, USA*, 1972, *69*, 2734–2737.

Pittendrigh, C. S. Circadian oscillations in cells and the circadian organization of multicellular systems. In F. O. Schmitt and F. G. Worden (Eds.), *The Neurosciences: Third Study Program*. Cambridge, Mass.: MIT Press, 1974, pp. 437–458.

Pittendrigh, C. S. Functional aspects of circadian pacemakers. In M. Suda, O. Hayaishi, and H. Nakagawa (Eds.), *Biological Rhythms, Their Central Mechanism*. New York: Elsevier Press, 1980.

Pittendrigh, C. S. Circadian organization and the photoperiodic phenomena. In B. K. Follett (Ed.), *Biological Clocks in Reproductive Cycles*. Bristol: John Wright, 1981.

Pittendrigh, C. S., and Caldarola, P. C. General homeostasis of the frequency of circadian oscillations. *Proceedings of the National Academy of Sciences, USA*, 1973, *70*, 2697–2701.

Pittendrigh, C. S., and Daan, S. A functional analysis of circadian pacemakers in nocturnal rodents. I. Stability and lability of spontaneous frequency. *Journal of Comparative Physiology*, 1976a, *106*, 233–252.

Pittendrigh, C. S., and Daan, S. A functional analysis of circadian pacemakers in nocturnal rodents. IV. Entrainment: Pacemaker as clock. *Journal of Comparative Physiology*, 1976b, *106*, 291–331.

Pittendrigh, C. S., and Daan, S. A functional analysis of circadian pacemakers in nocturnal rodents. V. Pacemaker structure: A clock for all seasons. *Journal of Comparative Physiology*, 1976c, *106*, 333–355.

Pittendrigh, C. S., and Minis D. H. Circadian systems: Longevity as a function of circadian resonance in *Drosophila pseudoobscurra*. *Proceedings of the National Academy of Sciences, USA*, 1972, *69*, 1537–1539.

Rence, B., and Loher, W. Arrythmically singing circkets: Thermoperiodic re-entrainment after bilobectomy. *Science*, 1975, *190*, 385–387.

Saint Paul, U., and Aschoff, J. Longevity among blowflies (*Phormia terranovae* R. D.) kept in non-24 hour light–dark cycles. *Journal of Comparative Physiology*, 1978, *127*, 191–195.

Saunders, D. S. The temperature-compensated photoperiodic clock "programming" development and pupal diapause in the flesh-fly *Sarcophaga argyrostoma*. *Journal of Insect Physiology*, 1971, *17*, 801–812.

Saunders, D. S. Circadian control of larval growth rate in *Sarcophaga argyrostoma*. *Proceedings of the National Academy of Sciences, USA*, 1972, *69*, 2738–2740.

Saunders, D. S. The photoperiodic clock in the flesh-fly, *Sarcophaga argyrostoma*. *Journal of Insect Physiology*, 1973, *19*, 1941–1954.

Saunders, D. S. Evidence for "dawn" and "dusk" oscillators in the *Nasonia* photoperiodic clock. *Journal of Insect Physiology*, 1974, *20*, 77–88.

Saunders, D. S. *Insect Clocks*. London: Pergamon Press, 1976, pp. 1–279.

Schweiger, E., Wallraff, H. G. and Schweiger, H.-G. Endogenous circadian rhythm in cytoplasm of *Acetabularia:* Influence of the nucleus. *Science* 1964a, *146*, 657–659.

Schweiger, E., Wallraff, H. G. and Schweiger, H.-G. Über tagesperiodische Schwankungen der Sauerstoffbilanz kernhaltiger und kernloser *Acetabularia mediterranea*. *Zeitschrift für Naturforschung*, 1964b, *19*, 499–505.

Sokolove, P. G. Localization of the cockroach optic lobe circadian pacemaker with microlesions. *Brain Research*, 1975, *87*, 13–21.

Stephan, F. K., and Zucker, I. Circadian rhythms in drinking behavior and locomotory activity of rats are eliminated by hypothalamic lesions. *Proceedings of the National Academy of Sciences, USA*, 1972, *69*, 1583–1586.

Suda, M., and Saito, M. Coordinative regulation of feeding behavior and metabolism by a circadian timing system. In M. Suda, O. Hayaishi, and H. Nakagawa (Eds.), *Biological Rhythms, Their Central Mechanism*. New York: Elsevier Press, 1980.

Sweeney, B. M. *Rhythmic Phenomena in Plants*. New York: Academic Press, 1969.

Sweeney, B., and Hastings, J. W. Effects of temperature upon diurnal rhythms. *Cold Spring Harbor Symposia on Quantitative Biology*, 1960, *25*, 87–104.

Takahashi, J., and Menaker, M. Brain mechanisms in avian circadian systems. In M. Suda, O. Hayaishi, and H. Nakagawa (Eds.), *Biological Rhythms, Their Central Mechanism*. New York: Elsevier Press, 1980.

Takahashi, J., Hamm, H. and Menaker, M. Circadian rhythms of melatonin release from individual superfused chicken pineal glands *in vitro*. *Proceedings of the National Academy of Sciences, USA*, 1980 *77*, 2319–2322.

Truman, J. W. Physiology of insect rhythms. II. The silk moth brain as the location of the biological clock controlling eclosion. *Journal of Comparative Physiology*, 1972, *81*, 99–114.

Truman, J. W. Extraretinal photoreception in insects. *Photochemistry and Photobiology*, 1976, *23*, 215–225.

Turek, F. McMillan J. P. and Menaker, M. Melatonin: Effects on the circadian locomotor rhythm of sparrows. *Science*, 1976, *194*, 1441–1443.

Tyschenko, V. P. Two-oscillatory model of the physiological mechanism of insect photoperiodic reaction. *Zhurnal Obshcei Biologii*, 1966, *33*, 21–31.

Underwood, H. Circadian organization in lizards: The role of the pineal organ, *Science*, 1977, *195*, 587–589.

Underwood, H., and Menaker, M. Extraretinal photoreception in lizards. *Photochemistry and Photobiology*, 1976, *23*, 227–243.

Wahl, O. Neue untersuchungen über das Zeitgedachtnis der Bienen. *Zeitschrift für vergleichende Physiologie*, 1932, *16*, 529–589.

Went, F. Photo-and Thermoperiodic effects in plant growth. *Cold Spring Harbor Symposia in Quantitative Biology*, 1960, *25*, 221–230.

Zimmerman, N. H., and Menaker, M. The pineal gland: A pacemaker within the circadian system of the house sparrow. *Proceedings of the National Academy of Sciences, USA*, 1979, *76*, 999–1003.

6

Freerunning and Entrained Circadian Rhythms

JÜRGEN ASCHOFF

INTRODUCTION

Circadian rhythms "freerun" in constant conditions like self-sustaining oscillations, and they can be synchronized (entrained) by periodic factors in the environment, the zeitgebers. The period τ of the freerunning rhythm depends on the species, on the individual and its physiological state, on environmental conditions, and on the experimental history. Under conditions of entrainment, the rhythm keeps a distinct phase-relationship to the zeitgeber. The record of locomotor activity of a pig-tailed macaque, *Macaca nemestrina,* reproduced in Figure 1, illustrates a few of the major principles. When exposed to a light–dark cycle (LD), the monkey is active during L, with onset of activity occurring shortly before light-on; in constant conditions (LL), the period is shorter than 24 hr and, on the average, somewhat shorter in 0.03 lux than in 0.1 lux; there is day-to-day variability of intervals between the onsets of activity around the mean τ that in itself changes slightly over time (especially in 0.03 lux); reentrainment by the zeitgeber after Day 78 is accomplished by a series of delay transients. A more detailed discussion of those phenomena follows below.

FREERUNNING RHYTHMS

DEPENDENCE OF FREQUENCY ON EXTERNAL AND INTERNAL FACTORS

LIGHT. In most species, τ of a freerunning rhythm depends on the intensity of illumination. In many diurnal species, τ shortens with an increase in light intensity, and it

JÜRGEN ASCHOFF   Max-Planck-Institut für Verhaltensphysiologie, Andechs, West Germany.

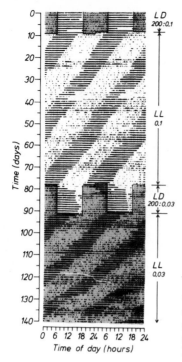

Fig. 1. Circadian rhythm of locomotor activity (black marks) in a pig-tailed macaque, *Macaca nemestrina*, alternatively kept in light–dark cycles (LD) and in conditions of constant dim illumination (LL). Intensity of illumination (in lux) given at the right margin. Original record duplicated once. (From Aschoff, 1979a. Reprinted with permission of Paul Parey Verlag, Berlin.)

lengthens in nocturnal species. In general, this rule is supported by data from fishes, reptiles, and birds. Mammals behave differently in so far as the majority of diurnal species also lengthens τ when light intensity increases. Most of the data available from vertebrates are summarized in Figure 2. For arthropods, no consistent rule emerges from the data published so far (cf. Figure 15 in Aschoff, 1979a).

At higher intensities of illumination, locomotor activity often becomes arrhythmic, and other rhythms damp out. The intensity at which this occurs may be quite low, as in some insects (Pittendrigh, 1960); it seems to be higher in diurnal than in nocturnal species, and higher in mammals than in birds (see Figure 2). One has to be careful in interpreting the disappearance of a rhythm as a "stopping" of the circadian pacemaker as opposed to an "uncoupling" of the overt rhythm or a desynchronization among a multiplicity of oscillators.

Circadian periods measured in continuous darkness (τ_{DD}) scatter within a range from 22 hr to more than 26 hr. In mammals, τ_{DD} tends to be above 24 hr in diurnal species ($\bar{\tau}_{DD} = 24.24 \pm 0.52$ hr; 11 species) and below 24 hr in nocturnal species ($\bar{\tau}_{DD} = 23.85 \pm 0.56$ hr; 26 species); six diurnal avian species have a mean $\bar{\tau}_{DD}$ of 24.82 $\pm$ 1.01 h (Aschoff, 1979a). In arthropods, τ_{DD} values below 24 hr prevail. As has been outlined by Pittendrigh and Daan (1976b), the species-specific differences in τ_{DD}, together with the species-specific responses of τ to light, may reflect parts of a "strategy of entrainment" for diurnal and nocturnal species.

TEMPERATURE. A near independence of τ from ambient temperature was first clearly demonstrated for the rhythm of emergence in *Drosophila pseudoobscura* by Pittendrigh (1954). However, most of the lower organisms, plants, and poikilothermic animals studied later on show a slight dependence of τ on temperature, with Q_{10} values either above or below 1.0 (see the review article of Sweeney and Hastings, 1960). More recently, similar dependencies have been described for birds and mammals. A survey of all data available suggests that with an increase in ambient temperature, τ shortens in most diurnal and lengthens in nocturnal species (see Figure 23 in Aschoff, 1979a). The dependence of τ on temperature is less than that on light intensity and certainly far below any dependence that could be expected from metabolic effects of temperature. Models to explain this unique feature of circadian systems are usually based on mechanisms of compensation (e.g., Brinkmann, 1971). The phenomenon of temperature compensation has been discussed by Pittendrigh and Calderola (1973) as the special case of a general homeostatic conservation of frequency of circadian oscillations.

VARIOUS EXPERIMENTAL CONDITIONS. If in a continuously illuminated cage a dark nestbox is provided where the animal can hide, τ differs from that measured in the empty cage (Saint Paul, 1973). The reason is that by alternating between shelter and cage, the animal itself produces an LD cycle that influences τ via the response curve (see Chapter 7) of the circadian system. Similar effects can be observed when the animal is allowed to turn lights on and off by itself. Usually, such self-selected LD cycles result in lengthening of τ as shown for birds, monkeys, and man (for references, see Aschoff, 1979a). Other observations suggest that τ of an activity rhythm is longer if measured in animals with access to a running wheel, as compared with those whose activity is recorded in spring-suspended cages, and that animals living together in a group may have rhythms with a shorter τ than animals kept singly (see Figures 11 and 12 in Aschoff, 1979a).

INTERNAL FACTORS. There is increasing evidence that hormones influence freerunning rhythms. In mice, castration results in a lengthening of τ, and testosterone replacement in a shortening (Daan, Damassa, Pittendrigh, and Smith, 1975). Similarly, τ gets shorter in female hamsters after implantation of estradiol (Morin, Fitzgerald, and Zucker, 1977), and in the house sparrow, *Passer domesticus*, after implantation of melatonin (Turek,

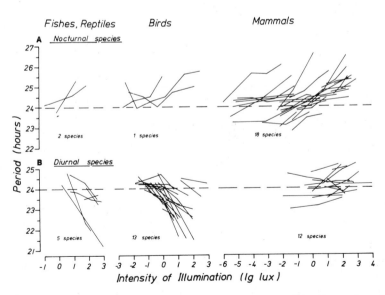

Fig. 2. Dependence of circadian period on intensity of illumination in constant light. (For species and reference sources, see Aschoff, 1979a.)

McMillan, and Menaker, 1976). In view of these observations, seasonal changes in τ are likely to reflect changes in the endocrine system (Aschoff, 1960). Observations made in several avian species indicate that τ is shorter in spring than in fall (Pohl, 1974; Gwinner, 1975).

Differences in τ between the sexes, suggested by data obtained from chaffinches, *Fringilla coelebs* (Aschoff, 1979a), and cockroaches (Page and Block, 1980) could not be found in either the house sparrow (Eskin, 1971) or the pocket mouse, *Perognathus longimembris* (Lindberg, Gambino, and Hayden, 1971). With increasing age, a shortening of τ has been described for three species of rodents (Pittendrigh and Daan, 1974), but no age effects on τ were seen in the blowfly, *Phormia terraenovae* (Saint Paul and Aschoff, unpublished) or in cockroaches (Page and Block, 1980).

VARIABILITY OF FREQUENCY

STABILITY AND PRECISION. Freerunning rhythms are rarely perfectly stable, and they often show long-lasting changes in τ (see Figure 3 in Aschoff, 1979a). As a measure of such lability, Pittendrigh and Daan (1976a) have made use of the standard deviation of several τ estimates, computed from 10-day intervals within one long activity record. It turns out that lability increases the more the mean τ deviates from 24 hr. This rule applies to intra- and interindividual differences in lability, as well as to differences among species (see Table 2 in Pittendrigh and Daan, 1976b).

Whereas *stability* (the converse of the just-defined *lability*) is related to long-term trends in frequency, the standard deviation of consecutive intervals of the rhythm around their mean τ can be considered the converse of *precision*. As exemplified in Figure 3A, precision reaches maximal values (= least SD) as τ comes close to 24 hr. In these experiments, τ has been computed from onsets of activity. It should be noted that usually precision (P) of end of activity is less than that of onset, and that the ratio $P_{end} : P_{onset}$ is positively correlated with τ (Aschoff, Gerecke, Kureck, Pohl, Rieger, Saint Paul, and Wever, 1971a).

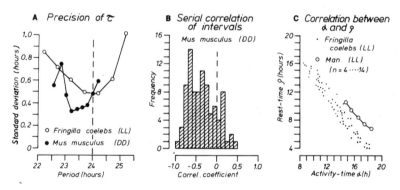

Fig. 3. Properties of freerunning activity rhythms. (A) standard deviation of τ as a function of mean τ (○ after Aschoff *et al.*, 1971a; ● after Daan and Aschoff, unpublished). (B) Serial correlation between consecutive onset intervals (after Pittendrigh and Daan, 1976a). (C) Correlation between activity time and rest time (after Aschoff *et al.*, 1971a).

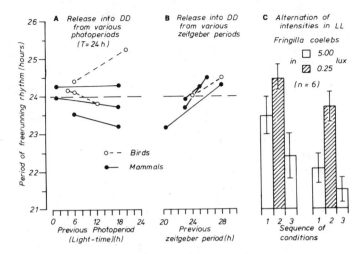

Fig. 4. Aftereffects. (A) and (B) Circadian periods measured in DD after prior entrainment to LD zeitgebers with either various photoperiods or various T values. (C) Period in LL before and after exposure to dimmer LL in two groups of chaffinches. (For species and reference sources, see Figures 5, 6, and 7 in Aschoff, 1979a.)

The day-to-day variability of a rhythm as described by precision is composed of noise in the pacemaker and noise in the coupling between pacemaker and overt rhythm. The second type of noise results in a negative serial correlation between consecutive intervals in the overt rhythm (Figure 3B).

There is a further interdependence that can be observed in records of locomotor activity in which several hours of more-or-less uninterrupted activity (activity time α) can clearly be separated from "sleep" (rest time ρ). Often, the correlation coefficient between α and its following ρ is negative, resulting in a stabilizing of the period τ (Aschoff *et al.*, 1971a). Negative correlations between mean values of α and ρ are shown in Figure 3C. These findings are in conflict with theories based on the assumption that sleep is a "restoring" process and hence should be positively correlated with the duration of prior wakefulness.

HISTORY DEPENDENCE. As was first noticed by Pittendrigh (1960), entrainment to zeitgebers with different properties can result in differences in the τ values measured afterward in constant conditions. Two types of such aftereffects can be distinguished: the period may be influenced (1) by the LD ratio (photoperiod) of the entraining zeitgeber and (2) by the zeitgeber period. From the data summarized in Figure 4, no consistency can be seen in the dependence of various species on long or short photoperiods (Figure 4A). Contrary to this, there is a strong positive correlation between τ and the period T of the zeitgeber to which the rhythm had been entrained previously (Figure 4B).

Another class of aftereffects results from phase shifts produced either by entrainment interposed between two freeruns or by a single stimulus, such as a light pulse applied in constant conditions. Often, advance shifts result in a shortening, and delay shifts in a lengthening of τ. (For reference, see Aschoff, 1979a; Pittendrigh and Daan, 1976a). Finally, there can be aftereffects on τ, measured in relatively bright light, from previous exposure to DD or to a lower intensity of illumination in LL. The latter case is illustrated in Figure 4C.

ENTRAINED RHYTHMS

DIVERSITY OF ZEITGEBERS

Next to a light–dark cycle, a cycle of lower and higher temperatures can be a powerful zeitgeber, at least for lower organisms and poikilothermic animals. In lizards, a cycle with a range of only 0.9°C suffices to entrain the activity rhythms of about one-third of the animals tested (Hoffman, 1969). Homeothermic animals are less easily entrained by temperature. Eskin (1971) had to use cycles with ranges of more than 30°C to get entrainment in the house sparrow; for the pig-tailed macaque, a range of only 16° can be enough (see Figure 15 in Aschoff, 1979b). In the attempt to demonstrate a zeitgeber, care has to be taken to seperate effects on the rhythm that imply phase control via the pacemaker from "masking effects" (Aschoff, 1960) that reflect mere actions on the overt rhythm, such as enhancement or suppression of activity (see Figure 10). Masking, in the first place, obscures the behavior of the pacemaker but may eventually influence the phase of the pacemaker via more indirect pathways (feedback mechanisms?) (Aschoff, 1978b, 1979b).

In contrast to light and temperature, information on the entraining capability of other factors is scarce. A more-or-less convincing documentation is available, for example, for air pressure (Hayden and Lindberg, 1969), timing of meals (Sulzman, Fuller, and Moore-Ede, 1977), and species-specific song (Gwinner, 1966; Menaker and Eskin, 1966). The third example points to the possible importance of social zeitgebers in general, due to which mutual entrainment can occur among animals kept together in constant conditions. Certainly, mutual entrainment also plays its role under natural conditions, as has been shown for the cave-dwelling insectivorous bat *Hipposideros speoris* (Marimuthu, Subbaraj, and Chandrashekaran, 1978) as well as for the members of a beaver family, *Castor canadensis,* all exhibiting the same freerunning rhythm when living under ice (Bovet and Oertli, 1974).

In view of the multioscillatory structure of the circadian system (see Chapters 5, 12, and 17), it seems likely that various rhythms measured in one organism differ in their entrainability by zeitgebers. One of the consequences is "partial entrainment," that is, a situation where, in the presence of a zeitgeber, parts of the circadian system start to freerun while others remain entrained (Aschoff, 1978b; cf. Fig. 13 in Chapter 17).

ENTRAINABILITY AND PHASE RELATIONSHIPS

THE PHASE-ANGLE DIFFERENCE. In the steady state of entrainment, the phase-angle difference ψ between rhythm and zeitgeber depends (1) on properties of the zeitgeber and (2) on the responsiveness of the circadian system to the entraining signals of the zeitgeber. Together, these factors constitute what may be called the strength of a zeitgeber (Aschoff, 1960). Given a certain strength, the major determinant for ψ is the ratio between the period τ of the circadian rhythm (when freerunning) and the period T of the zeitgeber. The essential rule describing this relationship is illustrated in Figure 5. Figure 5A demonstrates the dependence of ψ on τ: when entrained by the same zeitgeber, a relatively fast rhythm leads the zeitgeber in phase (ψ positive), and a relatively slow rhythm lags in phase (ψ negative). As shown in Figure 5B, the converse occurs when a rhythm of medium frequency becomes entrained by a zeitgeber of either higher frequency (ψ negative) or of lower frequency (ψ positive).

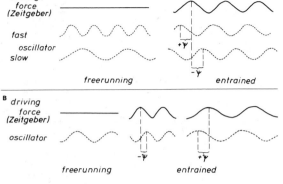

Fig. 5. (A) Entrainment of two oscillations (fast and slow) by the same zeitgeber. (B) Entrainment of an oscillation by zeitgebers of high or low frequency. ψ: phase-angle difference between oscillation and zeitgeber. (From Aschoff: Circadian rhythms: General features and endocrinological aspects. In D. Krieger [Ed.], *Endocrine Rhythm*, © 1979, Raven Press, New York. Reprinted with permission of the publisher.)

Dependence on τ and T. Examples of the dependence of ψ on τ are given in Figure 6, based on experiments with lizards and chaffinches. All animals were first kept in constant conditions to measure their τ. Thereafter, the lizards were entrained by temperature cycles, the birds by LD cycles. In both species, the ψ values become smaller as τ increases. To illustrate the dependence of ψ on T, Figure 7 presents activity records of three canaries, *Serinus canaria;* their rhythms were first freerunning in LL and then entrained by LD cycles with periods of 22, 24, and 26 hr, respectively. When measured between onset of activity and light-on, ψ is zero in $T = 22$ hr (masking?), slightly positive in $T = 24$ hr, and positive by about 2.5 hr in $T = 26$ hr. The figure further demonstrates that a change in photoperiod (reduction of light time from 50% to 25% of the cycle) results in an increase of the ψ values in $T = 24$ hr and 26 hr. This indicates that an LD cycle with only 25% L is a less strong zeitgeber than one with 50% L. Presumably, masking effects obscure the decrease in ψ that should be observed in $T = 22$ hr.

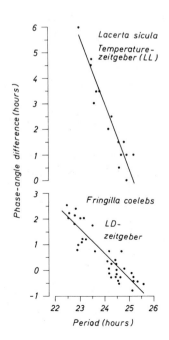

Fig. 6. Dependence of the phase-angle difference during entrainment on the circadian period measured in constant conditions. Data for lizards (above) from Hoffmann (1969), for chaffinches (below) from Aschoff and Wever (1966).

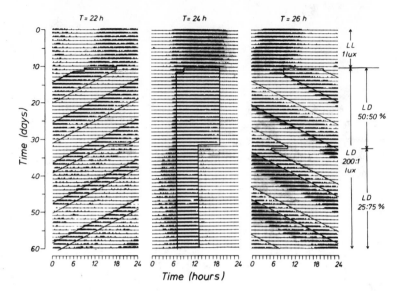

Fig. 7. Activity rhythms of three canaries, *Serinus canaria,* kept for 10 days in constant dim illumination (LL), thereafter in LD cycles with 50% L, followed by cycles with 25% L. *T:* zeitgeber period. White area: 200 lux; shaded area: 1 lux. (From Aschoff *et al.,* 1979.)

Dependence on Photoperiod. Dependencies of ψ on the LD ratio are summarized in Figure 8 for insects; in some species, the phase angle seems to stay parallel to light-off (A), in others parallel to light-on (C), and in a third group (B), the phase angle keeps a close relationship to the middle of light time. These examples are useful in discussing briefly which parts of an LD cycle, in principle, may provide the entraining signals. Light-off as the main (or only) phase determining signal seems to be suggested by the patterns presented in Figure 8A, and light-on by the patterns presented in Figure 8C. To explain the patterns in Figure 8B, one might assume that both steps in light intensity have equal weight in determining the phase of the rhythm. Such considerations could be valid on the assumption that only discrete signals affect the rhythm via what is called *nonparametric entrainment.* The picture becomes more complex if one takes into account the possibility of *parametric entrainment,* that is, a more-or-less continuous action of the zeitgeber (e.g., light intensity in the case of LD) on the angular velocity of the circadian oscillator. A detailed discussion of these problems follows in Chapter 7.

RANGES OF ENTRAINMENT AND LOSS OF ENTRAINMENT. Self-sustaining oscillations can be entrained to periods that deviate from their own "natural" period within certain limits only. These limiting frequencies encompass the "range of entrainment" (Klotter, 1960). The size of this range increases with the strength of the zeitgeber as defined above (page 86), and it also depends on the "degree of persistence" (Klotter, 1960) of self-sustainment in the circadian system. From a survey on ranges of entrainment obtained from 19 species (Aschoff and Pohl, 1978), two major conclusions can be drawn: (1) ranges are relatively small (up to 10 hr) in vertebrates, they are larger for insects (about 20 hr), and they reach extreme values in plants and unicellular organisms; (2) the larger the range of entrainment, the smaller is the change in ψ for 1-hr change in zeitgeber period. These generalizations are illustrated in Figure 9. Secondary ranges of entrainment (of smaller

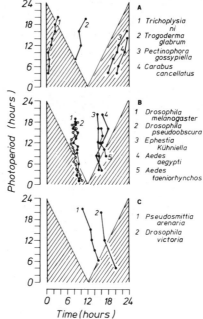

Fig. 8. Phase angles of various insect rhythms entrained by LD zeitgebers with different LD ratios. Shaded area: dark time. (Various sources from the literature.)

size) occur around T values that are close to multiples or submultiples of τ (entrainment by demultiplication).

There are difficulties in measuring precisely a range of entrainment. It often occurs that toward the limits of the range, entrainment becomes unstable, resulting in periodic fluctuations of τ ("relative entrainment"; Wever, 1972). Furthermore, various overt rhythms measured in one organism can have different ranges of entrainment (Aschoff, 1978a), a phenomenon complementary to that of "partial entrainment" (see page 86). Some data, finally, suggest that the circadian system as it is "stretched" or "compressed" by long or short zeitgeber periods, respectively, may lose its capability to produce self-sustaining

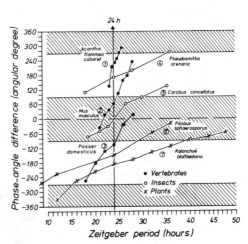

Fig. 9. Dependence of the phase-angle difference (expressed in degree; one full zeitgeber period = 360°) on the zeitgeber period. Shaded area: dark time. (For reference sources, see Aschoff and Pohl, 1978.)

oscillations. This phenomenon would result in extremely large or even "unlimited" ranges of entrainment.

Outside the range of entrainment, a circadian rhythm freeruns with a period close to that measured in constant conditions. Its frequency, however, is modulated by the signals of the zeitgeber through which it crosses, a phenomenon called *relative coordination*. An example is provided in Figure 10 by the activity record of a chaffinch that was initially entrained by a zeitgeber composed of two 1-hr light pulses. Reduction of the pulses to 30 min and, later on, to 15 min resulted in a loss of entrainment; the frequency of the then freerunning rhythm was slowed down and advanced twice during each zeitgeber period. The relative coordination shown in the last section of the record (where only one 15-min pulse is left) is a transformed image of the phase-response curve. In addition, Figure 10 provides good examples of "masking" by the light pulses. Loss of entrainment may also occur in the field, for example, in beavers living under ice (Bovet and Oertli, 1974), or under conditions of natural daylight at high latitudes in midsummer, as described for the woodmouse, *Apodemus flavicollis* (Erkinaro, 1969), and the brook trout, *Salvelinus fontinalis* (Eriksson, 1972).

PHASE SHIFT OF THE ZEITGEBER

After a sudden shift of zeitgeber, it usually takes a series of transient cycles for the rhythm to regain its original phase relationship to the zeitgeber. If the phase of the zeitgeber is shifted by not more than about 6–9 hr, a delay of the zeitgeber is followed by delay transients of the rhythm, and an advance by advance transients. After a shift of the zeitgeber

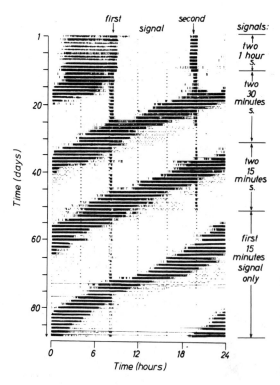

Fig. 10. Activity rhythm of a chaffinch, *Fringilla coelebs*, in skeleton LD cycles with stepwise reduction of the L pulses (signals). Signals indicated by the positive masking effects on activity. (From Enright: Synchronization and ranges of entrainment. In J. Aschoff [Ed.], *Circadian Clocks,* © 1965, North Holland Publishing Co., Amsterdam. Reprinted with permission of the publisher.)

for 9 or more hours, the rhythm may become reentrained through transients that go in a direction opposite to that of the zeitgeber. In those cases, the major determinant is given by the period measured in constant conditions: rhythms with a short τ tend to undergo advance transients; rhythms with a long τ, delay transients (Hoffmann, 1969).

The time needed for reentrainment is negatively correlated with the strength of the zeitgeber (see page 86) and to some extent is positively correlated with the amount of zeitgeber shift. (For examples of these interdependencies, see Aschoff *et al.*, 1975.) In most of the species tested, the duration of reentrainment also depends on the direction of the shift. In diurnal birds, reentrainment after an advance shift takes about half as long as after a delay shift. In contrast, nocturnal mammals become reentrained faster after a delay than after an advance shift (see Figure 5 in Aschoff, 1978c). The sign of this "asymmetry effect" seems to depend on whether the "prevailing" τ of a species is longer or shorter than 24 hr (Aschoff *et al.*, 1975).

It should be noted that rates of reentrainment differ among various overt rhythms measured in the same organism. As a consequence, the temporal order normally represented by the circadian system is disturbed during reentrainment. Frequent repetitions of such disorders can be harmful to the organism, as has been shown in the blowfly; the life expectancy of flies shifted weekly by 6 hr is 25% shorter than that of unshifted control flies (Aschoff *et al.*, 1971b).

One further complication has to be mentioned. In contrast to the "normal" shift, where all overt rhythms follow the shifted zeitgeber in the same direction, it can happen that the system splits into two components, one of which becomes reentrained by advance transients, the other one by delay transients (see Chapter 17, Figure 16). Cases of such a "reentrainment by partition" have especially been observed in man, either after eastbound flights across nine time zones or after advance shifts of artificial zeitgebers in an isolation unit (see Figure 9 in Aschoff, 1978c).

CONCLUDING REMARKS

The message of the survey given in the foregoing paragraphs emphasizes, first of all, the usefulness of treating circadian rhythms as oscillators in a technical sense. A thorough application to circadian rhythms of rules derived from the science of oscillations has substantially increased our understanding of the circadian system. This system, with its genetically fixed constituents (see Chapters 10 and 14), is characterized by a kind of "rigidity," which renders its frequency and other properties partially independent of internal as well as external influences. On the other hand, the system has to be sensitive to external stimuli, and this sensitivity must be phase-dependent, because otherwise entrainment could not occur (see Chapter 7). There is also flexibility in the system, at least within certain limits, as especially demonstrated by the range of entrainment (see page 88). It seems, in addition, that some of the properties of the system can undergo long-lasting or even permanent changes (like changing gears), illustrated by the phenomenon of aftereffects (see page 85). Finally, it must be reemphasized that the circadian system, although often behaving like *one* oscillator, most likely consists of a multiplicity of oscillators that are coupled to each other with variable strength, that differ in their power to produce self-sustaining oscillations, and that may partly be organized in a hierarchical order (see Chapters 5, 12, and

17). Hence, the existence of "master oscillators" (pacemakers) that control the multioscillator system is to be expected (see Chapters 5, 9, and 13). By mutual coupling, control through pacemakers and, what is equally important, by the entraining signals of zeitgebers, a precise temporal order is produced that characterizes the healthy organism (see Chapters 12 and 17).

REFERENCES

Aschoff, J. Exogenous and endogenous components in circadian rhythms. *Cold Spring Harbor Symposia on Quantitative Biology,* 1960, *25,* 11–28.

Aschoff, J. Circadian rhythms within and outside their ranges of entrainment. In I. Assenmacher and D. Farner (Eds.), *Environmental Endocrinology.* Berlin–Heidelberg–New York: Springer-Verlag, 1978a.

Aschoff, J. Features of circadian rhythms relevant for the design of shift schedules. *Ergonomics,* 1978b *39,* 739–754.

Aschoff, J. Problems of re-entrainment of circadian rhythms: Asymmetry effect, dissociation and partition. In I. Assenmacher and D. Farner (Eds.), *Environmental Endocrinology.* Berlin–Heidelberg–New York: Springer-Verlag, 1978c.

Aschoff, J. Circadian rhythms: Influences of internal and external factors on the period measured in constant conditions. *Zeitschrift für Tierpsychologie,* 1979a, *49,* 225–249.

Aschoff, J. Circadian rhythms: General features and endocrinological aspects. In D. Krieger (Ed.), *Endocrine Rhythms.* New York: Raven Press, 1979b.

Aschoff, J., and Pohl, H. Phase relations between a circadian rhythm and its zeitgeber within the range of entrainment. *Naturwissenschaften,* 1978, *65,* 80–84.

Aschoff, J., and Wever, R. Circadian period and phase-angle difference in chaffinches (*Fringilla coelebs* L.). *Comparative Biochemical Physiology,* 1966, *18,* 397–404.

Aschoff, J., Gerecke, U., Kureck, A., Pohl, H., Rieger, P., Saint Paul, U. von, and Wever, R. Interdependent parameters of circadian activity rhythms in birds and man. In M. Menaker (Ed.), *Biochronometry.* Washington, D.C.: National Academy of Sciences, 1971a.

Aschoff, J., Saint Paul, U. von, and Wever, R. Die Lebensdauer von Fliegen unter dem Einfluss von Zeitverschiebungen. *Naturwissenschaften,* 1971b, *58,* 574.

Aschoff, J., Hoffman, K., Pohl, H., and Wever, R. Re-entrainment of circadian rhythms after phase shifts of the zeitgeber. *Chronobiologia,* 1975, *2,* 23–78.

Aschoff, J., Berthold, P., Gwinner, E., Pohl, H., and Saint Paul, U. von. Biological clocks in birds. *Proceedings of the 17th International Congress of Ornithology,* Berlin, 1979.

Bovet, J., and Oertli, E. F. Free-running circadian activity rhythms in free-living beaver *(Castor canadensis). Journal of Comparative Physiology,* 1974, *92,* 1–10.

Brinkmann, K. Metabolic control of temperature compensation in the circadian rhythm of *Euglena gracilis.* In M. Menaker (Ed.), *Biochronometry.* Washington, D.C.: National Academy of Sciences, 1971.

Daan, S., Damassa, D., Pittendrigh, C.S., and Smith, E. R. An effect of castration and testosterone replacement on a circadian pacemaker in mice *(Mus musculus). Proceedings of the National Academy of Sciences,* 1975, *72,* 3744–3747.

Enright, J. T. Synchronization and ranges of entrainment. In J. Aschoff (Ed.), *Circadian Clocks.* Amsterdam: North-Holland Publishers, 1965.

Eriksson, L. O. Free-running circadian rhythm hos bäckröding (*Salvelinus fontinalis* Mitchell) under naturliga ljusförhållanden. *Fauno och Flora,* 1972, *67,* 233–234.

Erkinaro, E. Der Verlauf desynchronisierter, circadianer Periodik einer Waldmaus *(Apodemus flavicollis)* in Nordfinnland. *Zeitschrift für vergleichende Physiologie,* 1969, *64,* 407–410.

Eskin, A. Some properties of the system controlling the circadian activity rhythm of sparrows. In M. Menaker (Ed.), *Biochronometry.* Washington, D.C.: National Academy of Sciences, 1971.

Gwinner, E. Entrainment of a circadian rhythm in birds by species-specific song cycles (Aves, Fringillidae: *Carduelis spinus, Serinus serinus). Experientia,* 1966, *22,* 765.

Gwinner, E. Effects of season and external testosterone on the freerunning circadian activity rhythm of European starlings *(Sturnus vulgaris). Journal of Comparative Physiology,* 1975, *103,* 314–328.

Hayden, P., and Lindberg, R. G. Circadian rhythm in mammalian body temperature entrained by cyclic pressure changes. *Science,* 1969, *164,* 1288–1289.

Hoffmann, K. Zum Einfluss der Zeitgeberstärke auf die Phasenlage der synchronisierten circadianen Periodik. *Zeitschrift für vergleichende Physiologie*, 1969, *62*, 93–110.

Klotter, K. General properties of oscillating rhythms. *Cold Spring Harbor Symposia on Quantitative Biology*, 1960, *25*, 185–187.

Lindberg, R. G., Gambino, J. J., and Hayden, P. Circadian periodicity of resistance to ionizing radiation in the pocket mouse. In M. Menaker (Ed.), *Biochronometry*. Washington, D.C.: National Academy of Sciences, 1971.

Marimuthu, G., Subbaraj, R., and Chandrashekaran, M. K. Social synchronization of the activity rhythm in a cave-dwelling insectivorous bat. *Naturwissenschaften*, 1978, *65*, 6000.

Menaker, M., and Eskin, A. Entrainment of circadian rhythms by sound in *Passer domesticus. Science*, 1966, *154*, 1579–1581.

Morin, L. P., Fitzgerald, K. M., and Zucker, I. Estradiol shortens the period of hamster circadian rhythms. *Science*, 1977, *196*, 305–306.

Page, T. L., and Block, G. D. Circadian rhythmicity in the cockroach: Effects of age, sex, and prior light history. *Journal of Insect Physiology*, 1980.

Pittendrigh, C. S. On temperature independence in the clock controlling emergence time in *Drosophila. Proceedings of the National Academy of Sciences*, 1954, *40*, 1018–1029.

Pittendrigh, C. S. Circadian rhythms and the circadian organization of living systems. *Cold Spring Harbor Symposia on Quantitative Biology*, 1960, *25*, 159–184.

Pittendrigh, C. S., and Calderola, P. C. General homeostasis of the frequency of circadian oscillations. *Proceedings of the National Academy of Sciences*, 1973, *70*, 2697–2701.

Pittendrigh, C. S., and Daan, S. Circadian oscillations in rodents: A systematic increase of their frequency with age. *Science*, 1974, *186*, 548–550.

Pittendrigh, C. S., and Daan, S. A functional analysis of circadian pacemakers in nocturnal rodents. I. The stability and lability of spontaneous frequency. *Journal of Comparative Physiology*, 1976a, *106*, 223–252.

Pittendrigh, C. S., and Daan, S. A functional analysis of circadian pacemaker in nocturnal rodents. IV. Entrainment: Pacemaker as clock. *Journal of Comparative Physiology*, 1976b, *106*, 291–331.

Pohl, H. Interaction of effects of light, temperature and season on the circadian period of *Carduelis flammea. Naturwissenschaften*, 1974 *9*, 406.

Saint Paul, U. von. Die Aktivitätsperiodik bei Vögeln mit und ohne dunklem Schlafkasten. *Journal für Ornithologie*, 1973, *114*, 429–442.

Sulzman, F. M., Fuller, C. A., and Moore-Ede, M. C. Feeding time synchronizes primate circadian rhythms. *Physiology and Behaviour*, 1977, *18*, 775–779.

Sweeney, B. M., and Hastings, J. W. Effects of temperature upon diurnal rhythms. *Cold Spring Harbor Symposia on Quantitative Biology*, 1960, *25*, 87–104.

Turek, F. W., McMillan, J. P., and Menaker, M. Melatonin: Effects on the circadian locomotor rhythm of sparrows. *Science*, 1976, *194*, 1441–1443.

Wever, R. Virtual synchronization towards the limits of the range of entrainment. *Journal of Theoretical Biology*, 1972, *36*, 119–132.

Additional recommended readings:

Aschoff, J. (Ed.). *Circadian Clocks*. Amsterdam: North-Holland Publishing Company, 1965.

Hastings, J. W., and Schweiger, H. G. (Eds.). *The Molecular Basis of Circadian Rhythms*. Berlin: Dahlem Konferenzen, 1975.

7

Circadian Systems: Entrainment

COLIN S. PITTENDRIGH

INTRODUCTION

The circadian rhythmicity of eukaroytic organisms is dictated by an innate program that specifies the time course through the day of many aspects of metabolism and behavior. The programmed sequence of events in each cycle of the rhythm has been evolved to parallel the sequence of predictable change (physical and biological) in the course of the day-outside: it constitutes an appropriate day-within. It is a characteristic, almost defining, feature of these circadian programs that their time course is stabilized with almost clocklike precision to parallel the stable time course of the environmental day. There is equally clear functional significance to the program's being driven by a self-sustaining oscillator; thus, the program is subject to entrainment by one or more of the external cycles whose period it closely approximates. It is this entrainability that provides for proper phasing of the program to the sequence of external changes that it has been evolved to cope with and exploit.

ENTRAINMENT: GENERAL FEATURES

Figure 1 illustrates two aspects of the entrainment of oscillating systems in general. One oscillator (o) whose freerunning period is τ can couple to and be entrained by another (z), sometimes called the *zeitgeber*, with a different but similar period (T). In the entrained steady-state o's period is changed from τ to τ^* which is equal to T, and a unique phase relation ($\psi_{o,z}$) is established between the entrained oscillator (o) and its zeitgeber (z). The freerunning period (τ) of circadian oscillators is close to but usually different from 24 hr; they entrain to one or more of several (zeitgebers) in the external environment, all of which have a period (T) that is dictated by the earth's rotation and is, therefore, precisely 24 hr.

COLIN S. PITTENDRIGH   Hopkins Marine Station, Stanford University, Pacific Grove, California 93950.

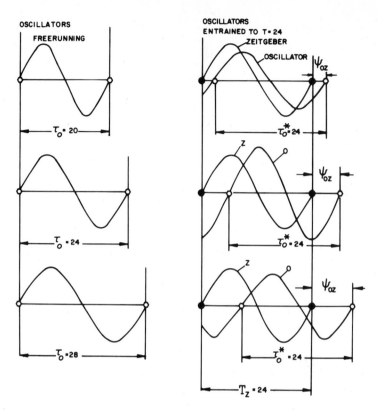

Fig. 1. Three oscillators with different freerunning periods (τ_o) are entrained by a common zeitgeber with period τ_z. When entrained $\tau_o \rightarrow \tau_o^* = \tau_z$; ψ_{oz} is larger, the longer τ_o.

The rhythms of mouse and bird activity shown in Figure 2, which are circadian ($\tau = 23.7$ hr and $\tau = 24.5$ hr, respectively) when freerunning in an aperiodic environment, become *daily* (with $\tau \rightarrow \tau^* = 24$ hr) when they entrain to a natural light–dark cycle. In steady state, the bird's activity is programmed into the day and that of the mouse into the night.

The daily temperature cycle (Hoffmann, 1968; Zimmerman, Pittendrigh, and Pavlidis, 1968; Lindberg and Hayden, 1974) in nature is an effective zeitgeber for many circadian rhythms, especially in poikilotherms, but the light–dark (LD) cycle generated by the earth's rotation is by far the most universal and important entraining agent. This is not surprising: sunrise and sunset are the most well-defined and noise-free environmental markers of local time. The remainder of this chapter focuses on entrainment by LD cycles: How does the daily alternation of ~½ cycle of light and ~½ cycle of darkness entrain the pacemaking oscillation that is responsible for a circadian rhythm?

DISCRETE VERSUS CONTINUOUS ENTRAINMENT MECHANISMS

Whatever the details of mechanism may be, the effect of the daily light-pulse (photoperiod) is to change the period (τ) of the circadian oscillator (or "pacemaker") by an amount equal to $\tau - T$, where T is 24 hr. In Figure 2, the daily photoperiod lengthens τ of the mouse by 0.3 hr and shortens τ of the bird by 0.5 hr. In asking how the $\Delta\tau$ is affected by the zeitgeber, it is convenient to distinguish two broadly defined categories of entrainment mechanism based on experience with other oscillating systems (Bruce, 1960). In the first case, the zeitgeber's input to the oscillator is *continuous* through a large part—even all—of the cycle and exerts control by a continuous change in the oscillation's angular velocity, accelerating at some phases and decelerating at others. In the second case, the zeitgeber's impact is brief, causing an abrupt *discrete* phase-shift of the oscillator, either advancing or delaying it by an amount equal to $\tau - T$.

The circadian oscillator timing eclosion in *Drosophila* is susceptible to entrainment by either mechanism: it can be entrained to a low-amplitude sine wave of light intensity (continuous entrainment) or to a train of very brief pulses (discrete entrainment). It is, then, an open question whether the action of a "natural" photoperiod (e.g., a 12-hr "pulse") is continuous, discrete, or a mixture of both.

The phenomena of "skeleton" photoperiods (Pittendrigh and Minis, 1964) suggest that it is a mixture. The *Drosophila* system (τ = 24 hr) will entrain to light cycles of T = 24 whether the duration of the light pulses is as short as a minute (or less) or as long as 18 hr. Every effective photoperiod within that range must generate a net $\Delta\tau$ of zero ($\tau - T$). For that $\Delta\tau$ requirement to be met, the phase of the oscillator, relative to the photoperiod, must change as the photoperiod changes; thus ψ_{RL}, the phase relation (ψ) of rhythm (R) to light cycle (L), is slightly but significantly dependent on photoperiod. Figure 3 illustrates this dependence and shows that light cycles involving two brief pulses separated by t hours (with $t < 11$ hr) lead to entrained steady states in which ψ_{RL} is the same as that generated by single pulses (photoperiods) of t hours. The two brief pulses constitute a "skeleton" (PPs) of the corresponding "complete" (PPc) photoperiod. It is as though the net effect of the complete photoperiod is the sum of two of the discrete effects associated with its beginning and end. However, the remarkable simulation of PPc by PPs is poorer when PPs exceeds ~11 hr and fails outright when t, duration of the photoperiod, exceeds

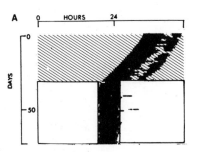

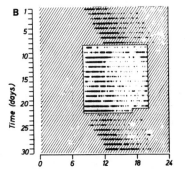

Fig. 2. (A) A deermouse *(Peromyscus leucopus)* freeruns in constant darkness for about 30 days, with τ = 23.7 hr, then is entrained by an LD cycle (18:6). It is night-active. (B) A bird *(Fringilla coelebs)* freeruns in very dim LL (0.5 lux) for 8 days with τ = 24.5 hr, then is entrained by an LD cycle (12:12). It is day-active.

~14 hr (Figure 3). Evidently, there is some small continuing action of light in the middle of the long photoperiod, and its effect is significant and detectable only when the photoperiod duration approaches or exceeds $\tau/2$. In attempting to clarify this complexity, we begin with an analysis of the discrete effects of brief pulses.

The Phase-Response Curves (PRCs) of Circadian Pacemakers

The hamster in Figure 4 (Pittendrigh, 1980a) was allowed to freerun in DD, and every few weeks was exposed to a 15-min light pulse given at successively different phases

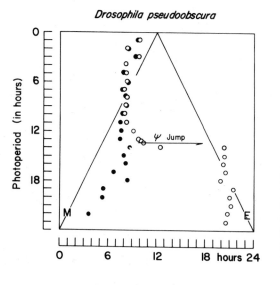

Fig. 3. Entrainment by "complete" and "skeleton" photoperiods of the pupal eclosion rhythm in *Drosophila pseudoobscura*. Plotted points (solid, complete photoperiods; open, skeleton photoperiods) indicate the phase of the eclosion peak for several photoperiods. See text concerning ψ jump. M = morning; E = evening. (Based on Pittendrigh and Minis, 1964.)

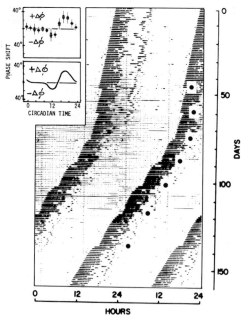

Fig. 4. Derivation of the phase-response curve (PRC) for the circadian pacemaker of the hamster, *Mesocricetus auratus*. The animal freeruns in constant darkness; it receives a succession of single 15-min light pulses (black dots) given at different phases of the activity cycle. The phase shift (delays following the first two pulses; advances later) caused by each pulse is plotted as function of the phase pulsed to yield the PRC. (From Pittendrigh, 1980.)

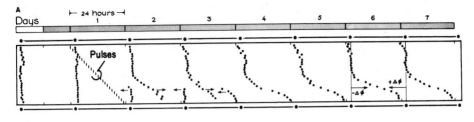

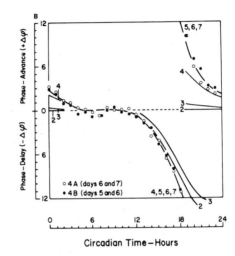

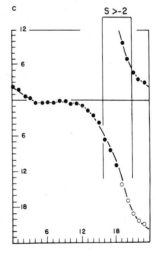

Fig. 5. Derivation of a PRC for the pacemaker of the *Drosophila pseudoobscura* eclosion rhythm. (A) Time course of the rhythm in 24 experimental populations (and 1 control) is given as a series of points marking the midpoint of the eclosion peak. Each population, otherwise freerunning in darkness, receives a single 15-min light pulse ($\sim$100 lux), shown as a short black bar; the light pulse is given at a different phase of the rhythm in each population. Following several transient days, a steady-state phase shift is realized by each population. (B) The PRC plots the phase shift ($\Delta\phi$) as a function of the phase (ϕ) pulsed. Different curves are given for the shifts measured on successive days after the pulse. The advance transients go more slowly than the delays. All phase shifts are in steady state by Day 5 after the pulse. (C) The PRC can be given as all delays yielding a monotonic curve. The slope(s) of the PRC is more negative than -2 between ct 15.7 and ct 20.6

of the rhythm. Each pulse caused a phase shift ($\Delta\phi$), either delaying ($-\Delta\phi$) or advancing ($+\Delta\phi$) the rhythm. When the magnitude and sign of the $\Delta\phi$ caused by the pulse is plotted as a function of the phase (ϕ) of the cycle pulsed, we obtain a phase-response curve (PRC).

Figure 5 illustrates the derivation of another PRC, for the *Drosophila pseudoobscura* eclosion rhythm (Pittendrigh, 1960). Twenty-five separate pupal populations were synchronized by prior exposure to LD 12:12 and released into a DD freerun. One population

COLIN S.
PITTENDRIGH

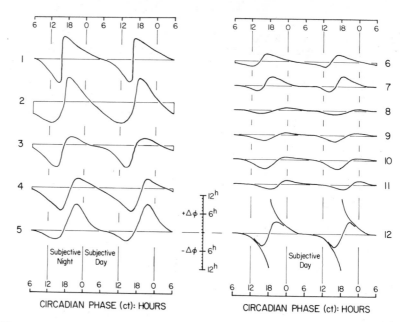

Fig. 6. Phase-response curves for light pulses from a diversity of organisms, unicellular, plant, insect, and vertebrate. Based on data from various sources. (1) *Sarcophaga* (fly); pulse = 3^h, 100 lux; (2) *Coleus* (green plant); pulse = 4^h, 13,000 lux; (3) *Leucophaea* (cockroach); pulse = 6^h, 50,000 lux; (4) *Euglena* (unicellular); pulse = 4^h, 1,000 lux; (5) *Gonyaulax* (unicellular); pulse = 3^h, ? intensity; (6) *Anopheles* (mosquito); pulse = 1^h, 70 lux; (7) *Mesocricetus* (hamster); pulse = 0.25^h, 100 lux; (8) *Peromyscus leucopus* (deer mouse); pulse = 0.25^h, 100 lux; (9) *Peromyscus maniculatus* (deer mouse); pulse = 0.25^h, 100 lux; (10) *Mus musculus* (house mouse); pulse = 0.25^h, 100 lux; (11) *Taphozous* (bat); pulse = 0.25^h, 100 lux; and (12) *Drosophila pseudoobscura* (fruitfly); pulse = 0.25^h (Type 0 PRC) and 1 millisecond (Type 1 PRC).

served as control, and each of the others received a 15-min pulse at a different phase of the cycle. The steady-state phase shift caused by the pulse was measured on the fifth, sixth, and seventh days after the pulse was administered. The PRC again plots the dependence of the phase shift ($\Delta\phi_n$) on the phase (ϕ_n) pulsed. The phase (ϕ or ct) of the oscillation is described in terms of circadian time (ct). The full cycle of the rhythm is taken to be 24 circadian hours; 1 circadian hour is $\tau/24$ hr of real (sidereal) time. In *Drosophila* ct 0 is that phase of the cycle that occurs when dawn would have occurred in the first DD day following release from LD 12:12. The half cycle from ct 0–ct 12 is the "subjective day" (SD) in the oscillatory program; and ct 12–ct 0 is the "subjective night" (SN). The hamster's activity onset in DD following LD 12:12 begins immediately after the last seen L/D transition and is taken as a well-defined marker of the beginning of the subjective night; hence, it defines ct 12 for that species.

Figure 6 gives PRCs for a diversity of other circadian pacemakers; unicellulars, plants, invertebrates, and vertebrates. The curves for the rodents, and for *Drosophila* responding to "weak" (millisecond) pulses, appear qualitatively different from that of *D. pseudoobscura* responding to "strong" (0.25-hr) pulses, but in fact, they are not. Winfree (1970) distinguished two groups of PRCs based on the slope of the associated phase-transition curve (PTC), which plots *new* phase (caused by the pulse) as a function of old phase (when the pulse was given); Figure 7 compares the PRCs and PTCs of *D. pseudoobscura* and *D. melanogaster* based on the same (0.25-hr) pulses. The *D. melanogaster* curve is like that of *D. pseudoobscura* responding to weaker (millisecond) pulses; its PTC has an average slope of 1.0, and its PRC is therefore referred to as Type 1. The *D. pseudoobscura* PTC has average slope zero, and its PRC is accordingly referred to as Type 0.

There are clear differences in detail, but all the PRCs in Figure 6 have the same basic pattern: (1) the subjective day (ct 0–ct 12) is characterized by small responses to light; (2) the subjective night by major responses to light; (3) phase delays characterize the end of the SD and early SN; (4) and are followed by phase advances in the late SN and early SD.

The rodent curves—given on an expanded scale in Figure 8—suggest an interesting relationship between PRC shape and τ: the shorter τ, the greater the ratio D/A, where D is the area under the delay and A the area under the advance part of the PRC. This trend among species is also found within the species: in individuals with shorter τ, D/A is greater than in conspecifics with longer τ (Daan and Pittendrigh, 1976a). It is also found within the individual (Figure 9). When τ is shortened—as an aftereffect caused by previous entrainment—the D/A ratio is increased (see also Daan and Pittendrigh, 1976a). This interdependence of τ and PRC shape remains to be explained: it is not a necessary or even a general feature of self-sustaining oscillations (Pavlidis, 1973). Daan and Pittendrigh (1976a) and Pittendrigh and Daan (1976a) noted, however, that it is functionally useful in contributing to the stabilization of ψ, the phase relationship between pacemaker and light cycle.

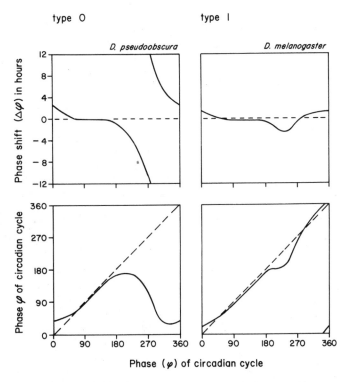

Fig. 7. Type 0 and Type 1 phase-response curves and their associated phase-transition curves: *D. pseudoobscura*, 15-min (100-lux) pulses, Type 0; *D. melanogaster*, 15-min (100-lux) pulses, Type 1. The phase-response curve plots the $\Delta\phi$ characteristic of each ϕ pulsed; the phase transition curve plots the new phase ($\phi\cdot$) to which the pacemaker is reset when pulsed at a given phase (ϕ).

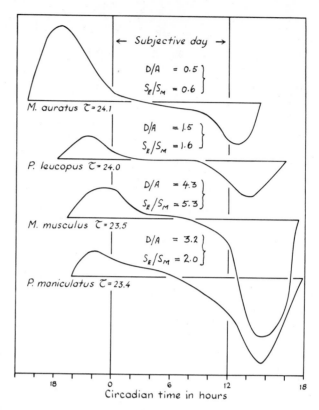

Fig. 8. PRCs based on 15-min (100-lux) light pulses for four rodent species with different $\bar{\tau}$. D (area under delay part of curve); A (area under advance part). S_M average slope of morning (advance) curve; S_E average slope of evening (delay) curve. (From Pittendrigh and Daan, 1976b.)

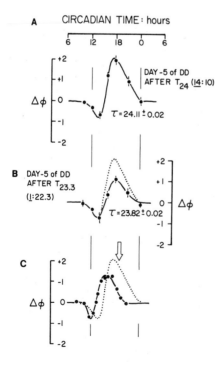

Fig. 9. The hamster *(Mesocricetus auratus)* PRC. (A) After release from LD 14:10 ($T = 24$ hr). (B) After release from LD 1:22.3 ($T = 23.3$ hr), with the 14:10 PRC (dotted) for comparison. After $T = 23$, τ shortens (aftereffect) and D/A increases. (C) A single light pulse (open arrow) at ct 19 causes a phase advance that requires several cycles to be expressed by the rhythm. On the first day after the pulse, the pacemaker has already phase-advanced, however, as measurement of its PRC shows. The initial phase-shift is expressed principally by the advance section of the PRC. (Dotted curve is the unshifted control.) (J. Elliott and C. S. Pittendrigh, unpublished observations.)

The PRCs in Figure 6 are all based on steady-state phase shifts, many of which (especially the phase advances) require many transient cycles to develop (see Figure 5). It has been shown for the *Drosophila* system that these rhythm transients do not reflect the phase-shifting behavior of the pacemaking oscillation that drives the rhythm. Figure 10 summarizes relevant evidence on this point. When a "first" pulse falls at ct 20.5, it causes a 6-hr phase advance of the rhythm, which requires 4 cycles to be expressed. The pacemaker, however, resets essentially instantaneously, as is shown by experiments that utilize a series of "second" (or "tester") pulses to track its time course in achieving the 6-hr phase advance. When the pacemaker's PRC is advanced a full 6 hr as an instantaneous response to the first pulse, it accurately predicts the $\Delta\phi$ responses that "tester" pulses generate at successively later hours after the "first" pulse. The transients of the directly observed rhythm (as distinct from its pacemaker) reflect the motion of a second (slave) oscillation gradually regaining a steady-state phase relation to its reset pacemaker. (Pittendrigh, 1981).

The rapid resetting behavior of the *D. pseudoobscura* pacemaker is illustrated by Figure 11, based on Pavlidis's (1973) mathematical model, in which there are two state variables (R and S). The figure shows the steady-state freerun of the pacemaker as a phase-plane portrait: it is a limit cycle. Following strong light pulses, the oscillator is immediately reset to a different phase on the limit cycle where $R = 0$; it then resumes its steady state motion. Strong pulses occurring before ct 18.5 cause delays; after that phase, they cause advances. Weaker pulses reduce R but leave the system inside the limit cycle on a different *isochron*, thus causing smaller phase shifts. Weak pulses yield a Type 1 PRC; strong pulses yield a Type 0 PRC.

The essentially instantaneous phase-shift caused by strong, brief pulses makes the PRC a useful tool in analyzing several features of discrete entrainment.

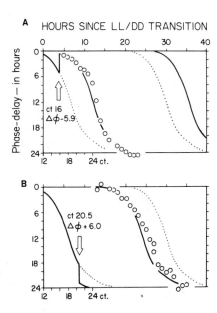

Fig. 10. The "instantaneous" nature of the *D. pseudoobscura*'s pacemaker phase-shifts. (A) A "first" pulse (open arrow) is given at ct 16; second "tester" pulses are used to track the time course of the pacemaker after the first pulse. It is well predicted by the assumption (solid curve) of an instantaneous 6-hr delay of the PRC. (B) The same protocol shows that a pulse at ct 20.5 causes an instantaneous 6-hr advance. (Based on Pittendrigh, 1980.)

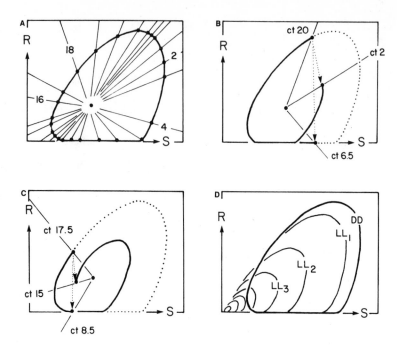

Fig. 11. Phase-plane portraits of the time course of the *D. pseudoobscura* pacemaker. Computed from Pavlidis's (1973) equations, which involve two state variables, R and S: the state of the (periodic) system at any time is defined by the values of R and S. (A) The steady state in constant darkness (DD); the lines radiating from the "center" (singularity) of the limit cycle are isochrons: the intersection of each isochron with the limit cycle defines a phase or circadian time ct. When displaced from its limit cycle (e.g., top right), the system moves on the phase plane, passing through successive isochrons at the same rate as it does on the limit cycle, to which it eventually returns. (B) Light pulses given at ct 20 cause phase advances. The stronger pulse drives the system to $R = 0$, causing a major phase advance. The weaker signal displaces the system to the isochron of ct 2, causing a smaller phase advance. (C) Light pulses at ct 17.5 cause phase delays, setting the system back to earlier isochrons. (D) The dynamics of the system change in constant light (LL); successively higher intensities (1,2, 3, . . .) displace the singularity of the system to smaller values of both R and S, and the associated limit cycle becomes smaller, until at a high enough intensity it vanishes to a singularity. On release into DD from a high intensity, its DD motion begins (no matter what the final LL phase) from an isochron close to ct 12.

Discrete Entrainment of the Pacemaker by Exotic Light Cycles

The Phase Relation, ψ, of Pacemaker and Zeitgeber in Entrained Steady States

When a circadian pacemaker, such as *Drosophila*'s (Figure 12), entrains to cycles of brief (e.g., 15-min) light pulses and T is not equal to τ, the action of the pulse in each cycle is to cause a phase shift ($\Delta\phi$) given by

$$\Delta\phi = \tau - T \tag{1}$$

Thus when $\tau = 24$ hr and $T = 27$ hr, the pulse causes a 3-hr delay ($\Delta\phi = -3$); and when $T = 21$, a 3-hr advance ($\Delta\phi = +3$). Given knowledge of τ and the resetting behavior of the pacemaker illustrated in Figure 10, we can use the PRC (for 15-min pulses) to predict (1) the phase of the pacemaking oscillation that coincides with the light pulse in each cycle and (2) the time course of the pacemaker after each pulse. Figure 12 analyzes the $T = 27$ and $T = 21$ cases. For example, when $T = 27$, the light pulse falls at ct 14.3, causing $\Delta\phi = -3$: the pacemaker immediately resets to ct 11.3, resumes its steady-state motion, and 27 hr later reaches ct 14.3. These predictions are tested by measuring the succession of $\Delta\phi$ responses elicited by "tester" pulses administered at successively later times to pupal populations released into DD from $T = 27$. The observed responses are fully predicted by assuming that (1) the last entraining pulse did indeed fall at ct 14.3 and (2) following its "instantaneous" $\Delta\phi$ of 3 hr, the pacemaker resumed steady-state motion from ct 11.3. Comparable predictions and their test are also given for the $T = 21$ case.

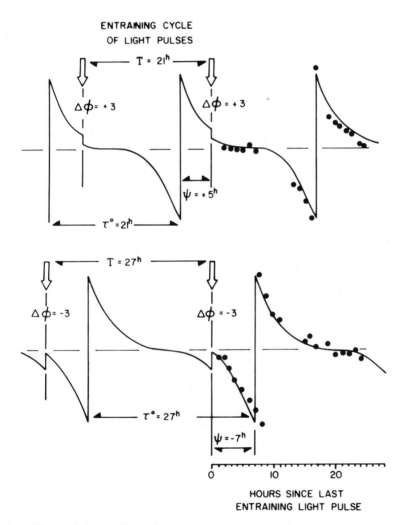

Fig. 12. *Drosophila pseudoobscura*. The steady states created by light cycles (15-min pulses) with $T = 21$ and $T = 27$ hr. In T21, the pulse falls at ct 23.4, causing a 3-hr advance in each cycle; in T27, it falls at ct 14.3, causing a 3-hr delay. The predicted phase-relation of pacemaker to light cycle is tested by measuring the phase of the PRC after release from entrainment. (Based on Pittendrigh, 1967a.)

COLIN S.
PITTENDRIGH

It is clear that the PRC for a given light pulse can be used not only to predict the precise phase-relation of the pacemaker to cycles of such pulses for any value of T within the "limits of entrainment"; it can also be used to predict what those limits are. An analytical study by Ottesen (1965) showed that a stably entrained steady state can be achieved only when the necessary $\Delta\phi$ (defined by $-T$) is obtained at a phase on the PRC where its slope(s) lies between 0 and -2. Using PRCs like the hamster's (Figure 8), where the negative slope never exceeds -2, the shortest and longest light cycles to which the pacemaker will entrain are given by

$$T_{max} = \tau + (-\Delta\phi_{max}) \tag{2}$$
$$T_{min} = \tau + (+\Delta\phi_{max}) \tag{3}$$

However, in some cases, such as $D.$ $pseudoobscura$ (Figure 5), the slope of the PRC exceeds -2 in the middle of the subjective night, and the large $\Delta\phi$ values elicited by single pulses cannot be utilized to entrain the pacemaker. The maximum "usable" $\Delta\phi$ values occur at pacemaker phases just before S becomes, then exceeds, -2 (Figure 5). This analytical result explains why, in $D.$ $pseudoobscura$, the limits of frequency-following entrainment, using 15-min pulses, are $T = 28.5$ and $T = 18.5$, not $T = 36$ and $T = 12$, as was originally proposed (Pittendrigh, 1965); all $\Delta\phi$ values in the PRC greater than $+5.5$ and -4.5 fall where S exceeds -2 (see Ottesen, Daan, and Pittendrigh, 1980).

FREQUENCY DEMULTIPLICATION

The common expression "limits of entrainment" suggests that entrainment fails altogether when the zeitgeber's period (T) gets too far away from τ. That is not the case when the PRC is Type 0 as in $D.$ $pseudoobscura$. T values of 18.5 hr and 28.5 hr are only the limits of simple *frequency following*: within that range the entrained pacemaker follows the frequency of its zeitgeber, and the light pulse falls at the same circadian phase *in each successive cycle*. Beyond those T values, entrainment still occurs, but the frequency of the pacemaker is half that of the zeitgeber: the light pulse falls at the same circadian phase *in every second cycle*. This is called *frequency demultiplication* and is a property of self-sustaining oscillators in general. Figure 3 in Wever (1960) illustrates how such an oscillator may entrain to several whole multiples of its zeitgeber's frequency.

When for example, the interval (T) between light pulses is 12 hr, the pacemaker entrains by frequency demultiplication and assumes a period of 24 hr. This leads to the phenomena of "skeleton photoperiods" as a special case of frequency demultiplication.

ENTRAINMENT BY "SKELETON" PHOTOPERIODS

The formal simplicity of discrete entrainment, involving abrupt phase shifts of the pacemaker, makes it possible to compute nearly all the phenomena associated with "skeleton" photoperiods (PPs). All that is needed is information on the pacemaker's period and its PRC for the pulses that constitute the skeleton. The entrained steady state is reached when

$$\Delta\phi_1 + \Delta\phi_2 = \tau - T \qquad (4)$$

where $\Delta\phi_1$ and $\Delta\phi_2$ are the successive phase shifts caused by the two pulses defining the skeleton photoperiod. Figure 13 shows the time course of the *D. pseudoobscura* pacemaker reaching steady state after exposure to 24-hr zeitgeber cycles with skeleton photoperiods of 8 and 16 hr. It is clear that any skeleton zeitgeber is open to two "interpretations": the cycle that defines an 8-hr skeleton photoperiod also defines one of 16 hr. As Figure 13A shows, no matter which interval is seen first (8 hr or 16 hr), the phase relation (ψ_{PL}) of the pacemaker (P) to the light (L) cycle that develops is characteristic of the shorter (8-hr) complete photoperiod. This is true in *D. pseudoobscura* (Figure 14a) for all skeleton regimes where one of the two dark intervals is greater than 13.7 hr: no matter what the initial conditions between pacemaker and zeitgeber, when the steady state is reached the subjective night of the pacemaker lies in the larger of the two intervals. There is, as it were, a "minimum tolerable night" (MTN) length of 10.3; when that interval is less, the pacemaker is forced into a ψ jump, after which its subjective night is in the longer dark period. The cause of the ψ jump is clear from Figure 13: when the subjective night is placed in the 8-hr interval, the phase shift at the end of the 16-hr interval causes so great a phase delay that the next pulse (8 hr later) again causes a delay. Steady state demands a succession of

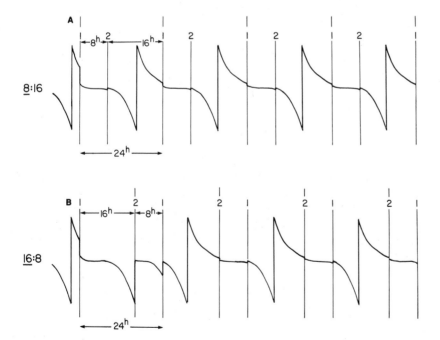

Fig. 13. *Drosophila pseudoobscura*. Entrainment by skeleton photoperiods; two 15-min pulses per 24 hr. Entrainment to LD 8:16 and16:8, with the first pulse falling at ct 21. In both cases, in the eventual steady state the subjective night of the PRC falls in the longer (16-hr) interval. See text. (Based on Pittendrigh and Minis, 1964.)

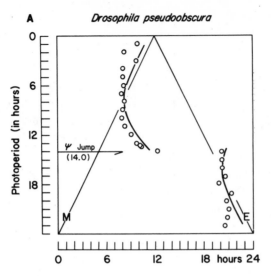

A   *Drosophila pseudoobscura*

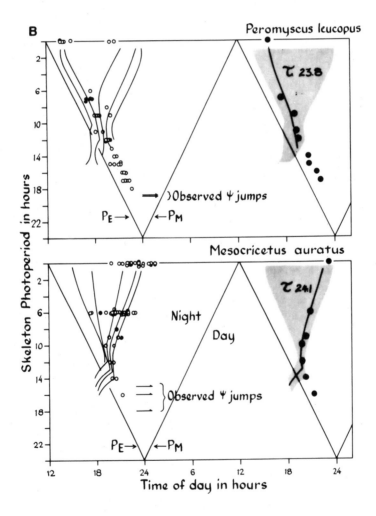

Fig. 14. Entrainment by "skeleton photoperiods"; two brief pulses per cycle of 24 hr. The phase relation of rhythm to light cycle changes with the photoperiod (interval between the pulses) and observed phases (open circles in the case of *Drosophila*, large solid circles in the rodents *Peromyscus* and *Mesocricetus*) are well predicted (solid curves) from the observed $\bar{\tau}$ and PRC of each species. (*Drosophila* redrawn from Pittendrigh and Minis, 1964; *Peromyscus* and *Mesocricetus* from Pittendrigh and Daan, 1976b.)

$+\Delta\phi$ and $-\Delta\phi$ responses, and that succession is not possible when the interval embracing the subjective night becomes less than ~ 10 hr. The length of the minimum tolerable night depends, of course, on both τ and PRC shape: it is different in hamsters and deermice (Figure 14) than in *Drosophila*.

Figures 13 and 14 show that the entrained steady states of *Drosophila*, hamster, and deermouse exposed to a full range of skeleton photoperiods can be computed with acceptable precision from knowledge of their different τs and PRC shapes. The minimum tolerable night of *Drosophila* is also accurately predicted, but both rodents tolerate shorter nights than the model of discrete entrainment predicts (Pittendrigh and Daan, 1976b). We return to this subject later.

There is a narrow range of skeleton photoperiods ($10.3 < 13.7$) in *D. pseudoobscura*, where the two dark intervals are close to $\tau/2$, and within which two different steady states are possible for any zeitgeber (Ottesen *et al.*, 1980; Pittendrigh, 1966). This range of "bistability" is readily computed from the model of entrainment summarized by equation (4). Which of the alternative steady states is realized depends on (1) the pacemaker phase hit by the first pulse and (2) the duration of the first dark interval in the zeitgeber cycle. As Figure 15 illustrates for the case of PPs 11:13 and 13:11, the model's predictions are well matched by observation.

The phenomena of bistability are of interest primarily in elucidating experiments with exotic light cycles designed to clarify the relationship between circadian pacemakers and the photoperiodic time-measurement (see Chapter 22; and Pittendrigh and Minis, 1971). Other aspects of discrete entrainment by two-pulse zeitgebers have general relevance because many nocturnal animals, like the rodents in Figure 14, are indeed entrained by the

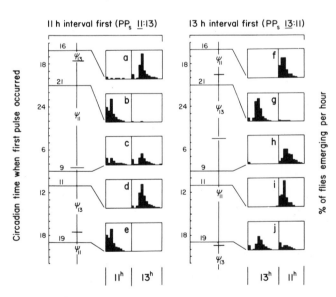

Fig. 15. *Drosophila pseudoobscura*. The "bistability" phenomena; entrainment to skelton photoperiods (PPs) of 11:13 and 13:11. Two steady states are possible for each skeleton photoperiod, depending on the phase of the pacemaker illuminated by the first pulse in the entraining cycle. In one of them (ψ_{11}), the eclosion peak falls in the 11-hr interval; in the other (ψ_{13}), it falls in the 13-hr interval. The model of entrainment summarized by equation (4) predicts (line to the left of each panel of data) which steady state (ψ_{13} or ψ_{11}) will be realized as a function of the phase (ct) of the first pulse. (Pittendrigh and Ottesen, unpublished data.)

interaction of two light pulses each day. The animals retreat to darkness after sunrise and emerge just before sundown. For them, the issue of a minimum tolerable night is real: the mechanism outlined here suggests their MTN is much longer than the short nights they experience at high latitudes; and the behavior reported in Figure 14 indicates they have a way of escaping the ψ jump. We return in a later section to how such nocturnal species escape the ψ jump on long days. Diurnal species escape it by a different mechanism involving the continuing action of light throughout the "complete" photoperiods to which they are inevitably exposed.

Entrainment by "Complete" Photoperiods

The action of continuous illumination (LL) on circadian systems provides some indirect evidence on the probable effect of the light that continues throughout the "complete," as distinct from "skeleton," photoperiod. One widespread effect of LL (Figure 16), reviewed in detail in Chapter 6, is change in the period ($\Delta\tau$) of the freerunning rhythm. Daan and Pittendrigh (1976b) have explored, by computer simulation, the suggestion that PRC shape provides a basis for predicting LL effects. The hypothesis is (1) that a simple linear transformation of the pacemaker's PRC yields a velocity-response curve (VRC); (2) that continuous light changes (relative to that in DD) the angular velocity (v) of the pacemaker at every phase of its cycle; (3) that the Δv at each phase has the same sign as the $\Delta\phi$ caused by a brief pulse at that phase; (4) that the magnitude of Δv is proportional to that

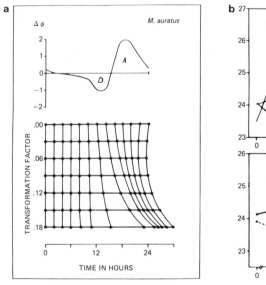

Fig. 16. The "velocity-response curve" (VRC) approach to interpreting the action of continuous illumination (LL) on circadian pacemakers. (a) The hamster *(Mesocricetus)* PRC is used to compute the relative acceleration or deceleration by light (of several intensities) of 12 fractions of the cycle; the net effect is to lengthen τ. (b) The VRC approach uses the known PRCs of three rodents to predict (top) the slopes of τ as a function of intensity in the three species; M.m. = *Mus musculus*, P.l. = *Peromyscus leucopus*, M.a. = *Mesocricetus auratus*. Observation (bottom) matches this prediction. (Based on Daan and Pittendrigh, 1976a.)

of the corresponding $\Delta\phi$; and (5) that Δv, like $\Delta\phi$, is intensity-dependent. Thus, in LL the pacemaker is slowed $(-\Delta v)$ in the late subjective day and early night when pulses elicit $-\Delta\phi$ responses; and it is speeded up $(+\Delta v)$ in the late subjective night and early day. The net change in angular velocity causes the observed change in τ (Figure 16). Clearly, the change in τ will depend on the shape of the pacemaker's PRC (hence, VRC): as the ratio (D/A) of the areas under the delay (D) and advance (A) sections of the PRC increases, the effect of LL will be to lengthen τ proportionally. The utility of this approach (Daan and Pittendrigh, 1976b) to the action of continuing light rests, at present, on its success in explaining the relative coordination of some pacemakers (Swade, 1969) to low-amplitude sine waves of light intensity and in predicting (Daan and Pittendrigh, 1976b) the different effects of LL (various intensities) on the freerunning period of several species of nocturnal rodents (Figure 16). The larger D/A in the PRC, the greater is the $\Delta\tau$ caused by LL; and the steeper is the slope of the τ (intensity) curve. Computer simulations using this VRC model of LL action show that D/A has to be very small indeed if LL is to shorten τ as it does in some diurnal species (birds).

The VRC approach to LL action also has potential bearing on another common effect of LL: at relatively high intensities, rhythmicity is lost entirely. The cause of this arrhythmia is not always clear and may well be different in, for example, multicellulars and unicellulars. Nevertheless, all LL arrhythmias so far studied share a common characteristic: when the system is transferred to darkness, rhythmicity is promptly restored, and its phase, relative to the preceding LL/DD transition, implies that the dark motion began from a phase (ct 12 or close to it) at the beginning of the subjective night. This finding has been taken to imply that the preceding LL stopped the pacemaker at ct 12 (Johnsson and Karlsson, 1972; Pittendrigh, 1966): its complete arrest explains the LL arrhythmia; and its arrest at ct 12 explains why, when permissive conditions (DD) return, it renews its motion from that phase. As Figure 17 shows, continuing illumination need last for only about one-half cycle ($\sim\tau/2$ hr), or less, for this effect to be detected. Following entrainment by 24-hr LD cycles involving any photoperiods longer than 10 or 11 hr, the pacemaker's motion in darkness always begins from ct 12 (Pittendrigh, 1960, 1966).

The two common effects of LL ($\Delta\tau$ and arrhythmia) are evidently part of a continuum: (1) Δv effects at lower intensities cause a change of τ; and (2) at higher intensities, the $-\Delta v$ effects at the beginning of the subjective night can be large enough to cause total arrest ($v = 0$) near ct 12.

This continuum is exemplified by *Drosophila*, where the facts involve further complexities (Pittendrigh and Daan, 1980). High LL intensities cause arrhythmia, and transfer to DD reinitiates a rhythm whose phase projects to ct 12 at the beginning of the dark freerun. The rhythm persists, however, at low intensities with τ longer than in DD. Transfer of the persisting low-intensity LL rhythm to DD now resets the phase of the pacemaker to $\sim$ct 12, *no matter when* (at what phase) in the persisting LL rhythm *the step into darkness occurred*. Clearly, the observation that DD freeruns following prolonged light always begin from $\sim$ct 12 does *not*, of itself, imply that the pacemaker was necessarily *stopped* at that phase (Figure 18).

Figure 11 uses phase-plane portraits of the *D. pseudoobscura* pacemaker (Pavlidis's model) to explain this result. The oscillation persists at low light intensities, but its amplitude is reduced and the limit cycle is displaced on the phase plane; both effects increase as the light intensity is increased. The LL limit cycle eventually lies entirely outside that for

COLIN S.
PITTENDRIGH

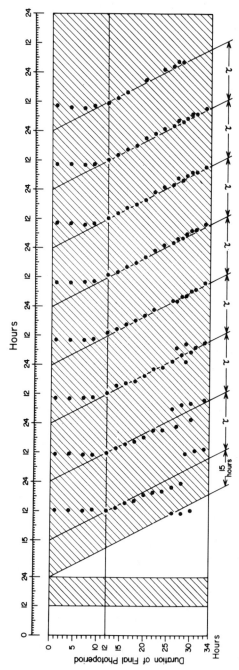

Fig. 17. Light lasting longer than ∼10 hr sets the pacemaker to ct 12. *Drosophila pseudoobscura* eclosion rhythm. Thirty-four populations entrained by the same LD 12:12 cycle, all see the beginning of a final photoperiod at the same time, which is that of previous "dawns." Each population, however, sees a different final photoperiod before entering DD. The phase of all the subsequent DD freeruns following photoperiods longer than ∼10 hr is given by $n\tau + 15$ hr, indicating that the freerun began from ct 12. The plotted points are midpoints of eclosion peaks, which fall at ct 3 in this strain at 20° C. (From Pittendrigh, 1960.)

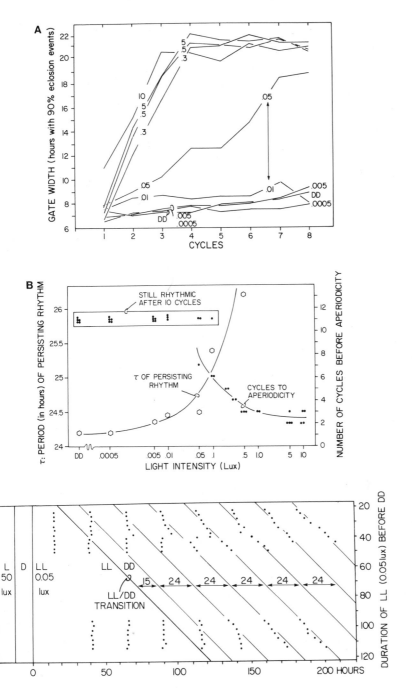

Fig. 18. The effect of low-intensity LL on the *D. pseudoobscura* eclosion rhythm. (A) The approach to arrhythmicity at different light intensities is shown as the increase of the "daily" eclosion peak's width in successive cycles of a freerun in LL. At very low intensities (0.0005 and 0.005 lux), the width of the daily peak increases no faster than it does in DD. At higher intensities (>0.01 lux) rhythmicity is reached rapidly. (B) One curve summarizes the rate at which rhythmicity is lost as a function of intensity; the other shows the dependence of τ (in what periodicity persists) as a function of intensity. (C) In continuous low-intensity light (0.05 lux), the rhythm persists for many cycles. When the system is transferred from 0.05 lux to DD, the phase of the subsequent steady state indicates that the pacemaker was reset to ct 12 no matter at what phase in the LL rhythm the light was turned out. (Pittendrigh and Daan, unpublished observations.)

DD. In this case, when the light is turned out, the DD trajectory always begins on or near the isochron of ct 12, no matter when in the LL cycle the step into darkness occurred. At high enough intensities, the amplitude of the LL cycle is reduced to zero: the oscillator is indeed stopped. But whether stopped in LL or not, the DD motion begins from (or close to) the isochron of ct 12, which is the beginning of the subjective night.

There is clear functional significance to the action of high-intensity light in long, complete photoperiods: by leaving the pacemaker on or near the ct 12 isochron, it avoids the ψ jump that occurs in entrainment by the corresponding two-pulse skeleton photoperiod. In *D. pseudoobscura*, when the dark interval of the skeleton regime that embraces the subjective night gets shorter than 10.3 hr, the evening pulse falls, at times, later than ct 12 and causes such large delays that the morning pulse again causes a delay. It is because long, complete photoperiods never leave the pacemaker at a phase later than ct 12 that night lengths as short as 6 hr can be tolerated without the morning light again causing a delay.

Entrainment by complete photoperiods clearly involves additional (continuous) effects of light not present in the entrainment of nocturnal forms by skeleton regimes. There is nevertheless some similarity in that the entrained steady state derives from the *interaction of morning advances and evening delays*. In the one case (nocturnal), these derive nearly exclusively from abrupt discrete phase-shifts. In the other (diurnal), the abrupt phase-advance due to the onset of light is supplemented by further advance as light causes $+\Delta v$; that is then succeeded by $-\Delta v$ (a delay), which never lets the pacemaker get beyond ct 12.

THE STABILITY OF ENTRAINED STEADY STATES

SKELETON PHOTOPERIODS

A stable phase-relation between the pacemaker and its zeitgeber (light cycle) is a clear prerequisite if the preprogrammed biological change is to be appropriately timed to changes outside. Figure 19 illustrates some of the issues involved by plotting the phase relation (ψ_{oz})

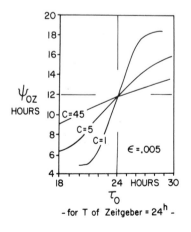

Fig. 19. The phase relation (ψ_{oz}) between an oscillator (o) and its zeitgeber (z) is a function not only of the oscillator's period (τ_o) relative to that of its zeitgeber (T_z) but also the strength of the coupling (c) between them. ψ_{oz} is maximally sensitive to τ_o variation when the coupling is weak and τ_o is close to T_z.

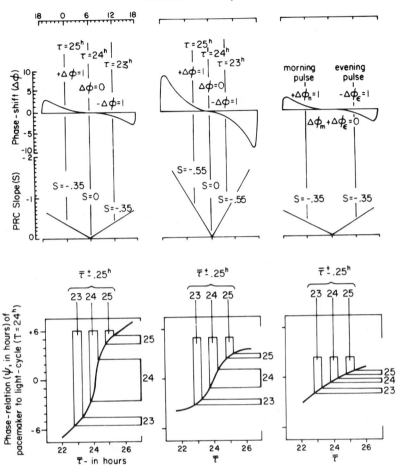

Fig. 20. The phase relation of a circadian pacemaker to its zeitgeber as a function of τ, PRC shape, and the number of entraining signals per cycle. See text. (From Pittendrigh, 1980.)

between a self-sustaining oscillator (o) and its zeitgeber (z). ψ_{oz} is affected by variation in both τ_o and the strength of the coupling (c) between oscillator and zeitgeber. ψ_{oz} becomes more negative as τ_o lengthens; an increase of C makes ψ more negative when $\tau_o < T_z$, but makes it more positive when $\tau_o > T_z$. In general ψ_{oz} is more labile when C is weak and extremely labile when $\tau_o \simeq T_z$. Thus, when τ_o and T_z are the same (e.g., 24 hr), a small ($\pm$ 15-min) range of ψ_o variation is amplified into a 5-hr range of ψ_{BA} variation. A stable phase-relation between oscillator and zeitgeber is the harder to maintain when their average periods are the same.

The same effect is seen when we analyze a circadian pacemaker's entrainment in terms of its period (τ), PRC, and a light cycle with period T (Figure 20). The upper panel gives the PRC itself and its slope (s) as a function of ϕ. The lower panel plots the steady-state phase relation (ψ_{PL}) of pacemaker to light cycle ($T = 24$ hr: 1 brief pulse/cycle) for a range of τ values. ψ_{PL} becomes more negative as τ increases; and the dependence of ψ_{PL} on τ is maximal when $\tau \simeq T$. The underlying issue is the slope of the PRC: the further τ gets from T, the greater the phase shift (advance or delay) necessary for entrainment; and as the necessary $\Delta\phi$ itself increases, so does the slope (s) of the PRC. Thus, the instability (variation) of ψ_{PL} caused by the day-to-day instability of τ around its mean ($\bar{\tau}$) is maximal when $\bar{\tau} = T$ and $s = $ zero; it is progressively smaller the further $\bar{\tau}$ gets from T, and s becomes larger (Pittendrigh, 1980b).

The remarkable homeostasis of the period of circadian pacemakers, including its well-known temperature compensation, is surely significant in this context: without such stabilization of the pacemaker's freerunning period, its phase in the entrained steady state would be unacceptably unstable. It also seems likely that the maximization of ψ instability when $\bar{\tau} = T$ has been one source of natural selection for *circadian,* rather than 24-hr, values of $\bar{\tau}$. This view, that $\bar{\tau} \neq T$ is a *strategy*—not a tolerated approximation—is encouraged by the finding in three laboratories that the standard deviation on $\bar{\tau}$ (a measure of its day-to-day instability) is steadily reduced as $\bar{\tau}$ approaches T (Aschoff, Gerecke, Kureck, Pohl, Rieger, Saint Paul, and Wever, 1971; Kramm, 1980; Pittendrigh and Daan, 1976b). It is as though the intensity of selection for τ's homeostasis is relaxed as the strategy of setting $\bar{\tau}$ away from T is pursued.

The apparent covariation of PRC shape and τ (within the individual animal) noted earlier may also contribute to the day-to-day stabilization of ψ_{PL} (Daan and Pittendrigh, 1976a), but the greatest contribution comes from the interaction of the two phase shifts each day (morning and evening) that are entailed by the long photoperiods in nature. Figure 20 (right) considers the same model pacemaker as before, but now entrained by a 24-hr zeitgeber with two pulses (12 hr apart) in each cycle. The addition of the second pulse amounts to an increase in coupling strength. Thus, the dependence of ψ_{PL} on τ is much smaller, and again the slope of the PRC is the issue: both signals (morning and evening) necessarily fall at PRC phases where s is greater than before. Moreover, the variation is shared by the two pulses (Pittendrigh, 1980).

An entirely different aspect of ψ instability is raised by the "ψ-jump" phenomenon associated with discrete entrainment involving morning and evening light pulses. When the *Drosophila* pacemaker (p. 107) entrains to a two-pulse zeitgeber cycle, no steady state can be realized in which the pacemaker's subjective night lies between two pulses less than 10.3 hr apart; that is the "minimum tolerable night" (MTN). When the night interval becomes shorter, the pacemaker "phase-jumps," and in the new steady state, its subjective night falls within the longer interpulse interval. The MTN can be reduced by two modifications of the pacemaker, both of which are found in nocturnal rodents and presumably contribute to their avoiding seasonal enforcement of a ψ jump. One is to reduce the amplitude of the whole PRC: the discrete entrainment mechanism predicts that, given their PRCs, both hamsters and deermice *(Peromyscus leucopus)* will tolerate shorter night lengths than *Drosophila*, and indeed, they do (Figures 3 and 14). The second pacemaker modification that reduces MTN is to shorten τ: for a given PRC shape, the shorter τ, the shorter the MTN. Pittendrigh and Daan (1976a and b) found that as day length increased (even in skeleton photoperiodic regimes) the period (τ) of these nocturnal rodents shortened as an "aftereffect" of the long photoperiod; as summer proceeds, then, τ is shortened by experience of lengthening photoperiods, and the minimum tolerable night is accordingly shortened.

The long light pulse ("complete photoperiod") experienced each day by diurnal species has a major impact on the stability of entrained steady states. First, it entirely eliminates the potential hazard of a seasonal ψ jump. Second, by assuring that pacemaker motion begins each night from the same (ct 12) phase (or isochron), day-to-day instability of ψ is reduced.

SEASONAL CHANGE IN THE EXTERNAL DAY: τ AND PRC SHAPE

Two-pulse zeitgebers clearly enhance the day-to-day stability of ψ_{PL} but raise other problems associated with seasonal change not only in day length (photoperiod) but in the whole pattern of associated environmental change. The issues involved are introduced by the case of nocturnal rodents where two-pulse (discrete) entrainment is the mechanism involved. Figure 21 (left) assumes that the animal has a symmetric PRC and $\tau = 24$ hr. As spring advances to summer, the interval between morning (M) and evening (E) pulses increases, and the two pacemaker phases (ϕ_M and ϕ_E) pulsed by light each day are necessarily different. Even the reset phases (ϕ'_M and ϕ'_E), to which the pacemaker promptly resets, are different as day length increases. Yet, the available evidence supports the intuitive assumption that for a night-active species, the program's "onset" should maintain a nearly constant phase relation to the onset of darkness (sundown), and that of a day-active species to sunup. The mechanism of discrete entrainment demands that the net daily phase shift ($\Delta\phi_M + \Delta\phi_E$) caused by morning and evening light remain constant through the year and equal to $\tau - 24$ hr. Some seasonal displacement of a nocturnal pacemaker relative to evening light is therefore inevitable as day length increases, but it can be minimized by increasing the slope (S_E) of the PRC at the beginning of the subjective night (where $\Delta\phi_E$ occurs) and reducing its slope (S_M) at the end of the subjective night (where $\Delta\phi_M$ occurs). Thus, any seasonal increment in $|\Delta\phi|$ demanded by increasing day length reduces the seasonal change in ϕ_E and (as the increasing slope of the PRC approaches -1) more nearly returns the pacemaker to a constant ϕ'_E. The coincidence of sundown and a fixed program phase is thereby conserved; it is the coincidence of sunup with a fixed program phase that is sacrificed. It is clear (Figure 21) that as $-\Delta\phi_E$ becomes larger, in the early subjective night, so does the slope of the PRC; it follows that as τ is shortened and the $-\Delta\phi_E$ necessary for entrainment increases, the evening light pulse falls on the PRC where the slope (S_E) is steeper and seasonal variation in ϕ_E and ϕ'_E are accordingly further reduced.

The discrete entrainment mechanism is such, then, that to conserve a constant phase relation between the evening pulse and program onset, a night-active species needs an asymmetric PRC with $S_E > S_M$; and that the shorter τ is, the better the conservation of ψ_{PL} will be. Nocturnal rodents are indeed characterized by short τs and asymmetric PRCs with $S_E > S_M$ (hence $D > A$); see Figure 8. As noted earlier (p. 110), there is an empirical regularity correlating PRC shape with the $\Delta\tau$ caused by constant light (LL): as D/A (hence S_E/S_M) increases, so does the $\Delta\tau$ caused by LL. The section of Aschoff's rule concerning night-active species states that their period is usually less than 24 hr and that constant light lengthens it more than it does in day-active species. These features ($\tau < 24$ hr;

Circadian Phase (ϕ or ct)

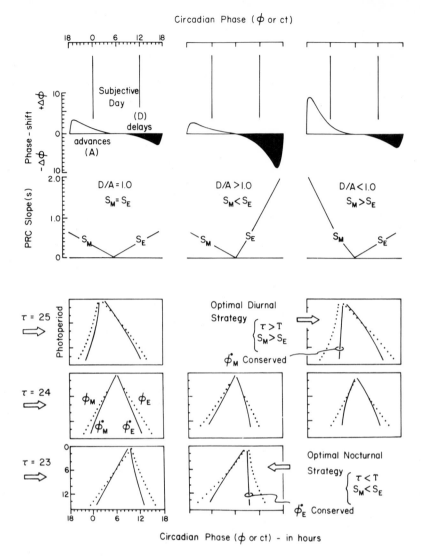

Circadian Phase (ϕ or ct) - in hours

Fig. 21. Optimum pacemaker properties (τ and PRC shape) for nocturnal and diurnal species. See text. In the lower panels, the dotted curves plot the circadian phases (ϕ_M and ϕ_E, respectively) illuminated by morning and evening light pulses; the solid curves plot the phases (ϕ'_M and ϕ'_E) to which the pacemaker is immediately reset. ϕ'_E is invariant with change in photoperiod when $\tau < T$ and $S_E > S_M$. (From Pittendrigh 1980.)

$\tau_{LL} \gg \tau_{DD}$) are, then, what one expects when nocturnal species adopt the optimal strategy ($\tau < 24$ hr; $S_E > S_M$, hence D/A large), given the discrete entrainment mechanism. The rule is evidently reflecting widespread adoption of that strategy in nocturnal animals (Pittendrigh, 1981; Pittendrigh and Daan, 1976b).

Were day-active species also entrained by a discrete two-pulse mechanism, the other half of Aschoff's rule would have a similar functional significance. The optimum strategy would be $\tau > 24$ hr and $S_M > S_E$ (hence D/A reduced); constant light would not lengthen τ of such pacemakers as much as it does in night-active species (D/A large), and in extreme cases ($D \gg A$), it would shorten it. However, entrainment in nature involves other complications, the most obvious of which is that day-active species are *not* entrained by discrete morning and evening pulses. The complete photoperiod they see in its entirety will ensure a nearly constant program phase (ct 12) at sundown (unless PRC amplitude and slope are very much reduced in the early subjective night); to maintain constant phase (ϕ_M') at the beginning of the day, the initial $\Delta\phi$ response at dawn must be large, again suggesting $S_M > S_E$ as an optimal PRC shape. In any case, it is unlikely that the correlation between the statistical trends in Aschoff's rule and the optimal pacemaker parameters suggested by the discrete entrainment mechanism is wholly coincidental.

Seasonal Change in the External Day: Complex Pacemakers

Constant phasing of an innate program's "onset" to dawn or dusk is surely part of the challenge of seasonal change in the pattern of the external day. But there are other issues exemplified by the case of *Salmo trutta* (Figure 22) in very high latitudes. The trout's activity is markedly bimodal, one peak tracking dawn through the year and the other sunset. Their phase relation is so reduced in midwinter that activity is effectively unimodal and diurnal, and in midsummer unimodal and nocturnal (Eriksson, 1973).

An "eocrepuscular" distribution of activity is also common in many diurnal insects, where one activity peak follows dawn and the other anticipates dusk. Much the same is true of at least some nocturnal species: the nightly activity of hamsters and mice (Figure 24) is in fact bimodal, with one peak following sundown and the other anticipating sunup. Part of the seasonal change in pattern may well be exogenously controlled, but not all: when released to freerun in darkness, hamsters in the laboratory retain, at least initially, the activity pattern dictated by the prior photoperiod (Pittendrigh and Daan, 1976a). The innate contribution to the daily activity pattern is clearly not a single or inflexible program needing only to be phased properly as day length changes.

Several features of the system in vertebrates suggest a flexibility of circadian programs

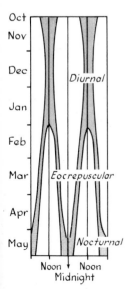

Fig. 22. The annual cycle of change in the daily activity pattern of young trout *Salmo trutta* (redrawn from Eriksson, 1973). The wide band of diurnal activity seen in the winter splits into two components in the spring as the photoperiod lengthens. One component follows sunrise; the other follows sunset. They re-fuse into a single nocturnal band in midsummer, when the Arctic photoperiod increases toward 24 hr. (From Pittendrigh and Daan, 1976b.)

that derives from a two-oscillator structure of the pacemaker itself (Pittendrigh, 1974; Pittendrigh and Daan, 1976b). The remarkable history-dependence of the pacemaker's freerunning period, as well as the phase angle between the two components in each night's activity, both elude explanation in terms of a single oscillator. But both are readily explained if the pacemaker comprises two mutually coupled oscillators, one of which (E) is the primary responder to evening light and the other (M) to morning light (Figure 23). E and M may have different freerunning periods (τ_E and τ_M) but, when coupled, share some intermediate period (τ_{EM}). τ_{EM} is malleable, changing as the phase relation (ψ_{EM}) of the constituent oscillators changes with, for example, change in photoperiods. E times the first component in nightly activity and M the second. The most direct evidence of such pacemaker complexity comes from the phenomena of "splitting" (Pittendrigh, 1960, 1967b, 1974), when the mutual coupling transiently fails, and the E and M components freerun with different frequencies in the same animal (Figure 24) until they reach 180° antiphase to each other; they then lock on to each other, and the mutually coupled system shares a common frequency that is higher than it was before the split occurred. Daan and Berde (1978) and Kawato and Suzuki (personal communication, 1980) have shown that a pair of oscillators mutually coupled by either a discrete (Daan–Berde) or a continuous (Kawato–Suzuki) mechanism do indeed have two alternative steady-state phase relations to each other, and they differ by 180°. Daan and Berde showed that such a "complex pacemaker" has all the special properties, including the history dependence of τ, found in the circadian pacemakers of higher animals.

What remains to be explored in further theoretical development of the model are the details of the complex pacemaker's PRC: Is the interaction of E and M such that, as τ_{EM} varies, PRC shape (e.g., D/A) also changes? Recent observations from two laboratories (Elliott and Pittendrigh, unpublished, 1980; Takahashi and Menaker, personal communication, 1980) show that the hamster pacemaker behaves in a way that is somewhat different from *D. pseudoobscura*'s and is, on the other hand, what one expects of a complex pacemaker. A single light pulse given at ct 19 phase-advances the rhythm. The two-pulse type of experiment described earlier (p. 103) for *Drosophila* shows that, as in the fly case,

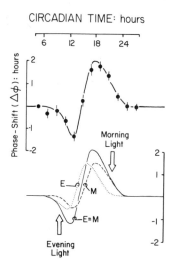

Fig. 23. The PRC of a complex pacemaker (e.g., hamster *Mesocricetus auratus*) is thought to reflect the interaction of two mutually coupled pacemakers. One of them (E) is the principal responder to light seen in the evening; the other (M) is the principal responder to morning light. See also Figure 9.

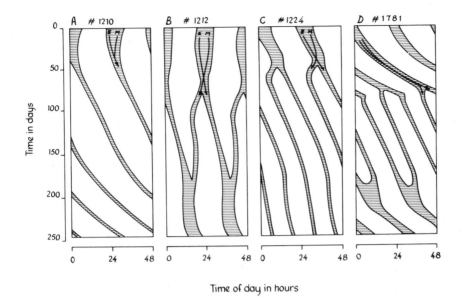

Fig. 24. The "splitting" of hamster *(Mesocricetus)* circadian activity rhythms into three distinct components under constant light. The two components (*E* and *M*) are nearly synchronous in DD; in LL, they move apart at different frequencies and usually reentrain to each other with a 180° phase difference. They are thought to be controlled by two separate but mutually coupled pacemakers; τ of the coupled system is shorter when the split develops. Sometimes the split system spontaneously reverts to the alternative steady state with larger τ. (From Pittendrigh and Daan, 1976c.)

the pacemaker's shift is immediately detectable in the first cycle following the pulse. In the hamster, however, it is only the advance part of the PRC that is shifted in the first day (see Figure 9C); it is as though only the morning (*M*) oscillator was immediately advanced and the evening (*E*) oscillator will require several other cycles before it regains a steady-state phase relation (ψ_{EM}) with its coupled partner.

System Entrainment versus Pacemaker Entrainment

So far we have considered the entrainment of a circadian system entirely in terms of its pacemaker; it is the primary oscillator ("simple" or "complex") responding directly to the external zeitgeber, and its phase relation to the outside world is the principal determinant of phase in the rest of the system it drives. There is, however, more to it, as the eclosion rhythm of *Drosophila pseudoobscura* shows.

The phase relation of pacemaker to light cycle (ψ_{PL}) is temperature-compensated, as one expects given the temperature compensation of τ; but the phase relation of the eclosion peak itself to the light cycle (ψ_{EL}) is not (Figure 25). Thus the phase relation (ψ_{EP}) of eclosion to pacemaker is not fixed: it is markedly temperature-dependent and it also changes (Figure 25) as photoperiod changes in a 24-hr day. It is also, informatively, dependent on the value of T, the period of the zeitgeber cycle. The phase of pacemaker to light (ψ_{PL}) has been shown (p. 105) to be as predicted by the discrete entrainment model when T is made longer ($T = 27$ hr) or shorter ($T = 21$ hr) than τ. When the pacemaker's period is

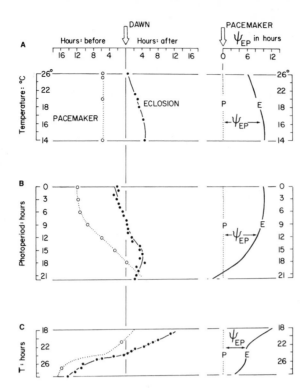

Fig. 25. The phase relation (ψ_{EP}) between eclosion peak (E) and its pacemaker (P) is labile in *D. pseudoobscura*. (A) It is markedly temperature-dependent, becoming more negative at lower temperatures. (B) It changes with photoperiod length in a 24-hr LD cycle; it becomes more positive as photoperiod lengthens. (C) It becomes more negative as the pacemaker's period shortens because of entrainment by an external LD cycle (period T). (Pittendrigh, unpublished.)

systematically varied by entrainment within the range $T = 18-28$ hr, the phase relation (ψ_{EP}) of eclosion peak to pacemaker becomes systematically greater the shorter the pacemaker's period. All these and other features of system entrainment in *Drosophila* have been shown (Pittendrigh, 1981) to derive from the involvement of a second oscillator, slave to the pacemaker, that is directly responsible for rhythm timing. The temperature dependence of slave parameters (its period and its damping coefficient) are responsible for the temperature dependence of rhythm phase.

The principal significance of this distinction between pacemaker and system entrainment lies, currently, in its bearing on photoperiodic phenomena, which has been outlined in Chapter 5.

PERSPECTIVE

The entrainment of circadian systems in nature is surely a more complex phenomenon than the present discussion suggests. In poikilotherms, the temperature cycle certainly plays at least a supplementary role as zeitgeber. How it interacts with the light cycle remains to be adequately explored, and there is ample evidence that this interaction is important in the "photoperiodic" phenomena, many of which are at least in part "thermoperiodic" (e.g., see Danilevskii, 1965; Saunders, 1973). Nor has space been given to complexities of entrainment by light that derive from the gradual (twilight) changes at dawn and sunset (see, e.g., Wever, 1967). For simplicity, the zeitgeber's period (T) has been taken as free of variance, and attention has been focused on the instability of τ; but when, as in animals, programmed behavior patterns dictate when the light is seen, instabilities of τ are translated to day-to-day instability of T.

The discrete mechanism worked out initially for *Drosophila* entrainment by two-pulse zeitgebers in the laboratory does seem to explain the major features of entrainment in nocturnal animals. For day-active species, it provides, at best, a starting point in defining some relevant questions: How does the light (no longer a discrete pulse) in the earlier and later "halves" of the day successively speed up and slow down the pacemaker to change τ to τ^* = T? Much remains to be clarified in the entrainment of diurnal organisms in which it is (significantly?) difficult to get PRCs for pulses as well defined as those in nocturnal species.

Nevertheless, development of the discrete mechanism has led to some empirical regularities in pacemaker properties that promise, on one hand, to provide functional (adaptive) significance not only to the general circadian period of the pacemaker but also to the statistical trends summarized as Aschoff's rule. And on the other hand, they provide strong suggestions about the structure of the pacemaker in higher animals. The susceptibility of τ to an "aftereffect" caused by photoperiod, and the covariance of τ and PRC shape seem especially significant. They not only contribute functionally to conserving pacemaker phase through the cycle of seasonal change; they strongly suggest that the pacemaker is a "complex" of two mutually coupled oscillators on whose interaction the covariance of τ and PRC shape depends.

REFERENCES

Aschoff, J., Gerecke, U., Kureck, A., Pohl, H., Rieger, P., Saint Paul, U. von, and Wever, R., Interdependent parameters of circadian activity rhythms in birds and man. In M. Menaker (Ed.), *Biochronometry*. Washington, D.C.: National Academy of Sciences, 1971, pp. 3–24.

Bruce, V. G. Environmental entrainment of circadian rhythms. *Cold Spring Harbor Symposia in Quantitative Biology*, 1960, 25, 29–48.

Daan, S., and Berde, C. Two coupled oscillators: Simulations of the circadian pacemaker in mammalian activity rhythms. *Journal of Theoretical Biology*, 1978, 70, 297–313.

Daan, S., and Pittendrigh, C. S. A functional analysis of circadian pacemakers in nocturnal rodents. II. The variability of phase response curves. *Journal of Comparative Physiology*, 1976a, 106, 252–266.

Daan, S., and Pittendrigh, C. S. A functional analysis of circadian pacemakers in nocturnal rodents. III. Heavy water and constant light: Homeostasis of frequency? *Journal of Comparative Physiology*, 1976b, 106, 267–290.

Danilevskii, A. A. *Photoperiodism and Seasonal Development of Insects*. Edinburgh and London: Oliver and Boyd, 1965.

Eriksson, L. O. Spring inversion of the diel rhythm of locomotor activity in young sea-going trout (*Salmo trutta trutta* L.) and Atlantic salmon (*Salmo salar* L.). *Aquilo. Ser Zoologica*, 1973, 14, 69–79.

Hoffmann, K. Temperaturcyclen als zeitgeber der circadiane periodik. *Verhandlungen der Deutschen Zoologischen Gesellschaft*, Innsbruck, 1968, 265–275.

Johnsson, A., and Karlsson, H. G. The *Drosophila* eclosion rhythm, the transformation method and the fixed point theorem. *Report*, Lund Institute of Technology, 1972, 51 pp.

Kramm, K. Why circadian rhythms? *American Naturalist*, 1980, in press.

Lindberg, R. G., and Hayden, P. Thermoperiodic entrainment of arousal from torpor in the little pocket mouse, *Perognathus longimembris*. *Chronobiologia*, 1974, 1, 356–361.

Ottesen, E. O. Analytical studies on a model for the entrainment of circadian systems. Bachelor's thesis, 1965, Princeton University.

Ottesen, E. O., Daan, S., and Pittendrigh, C. S. The entrainment of circadian pacemakers: Stable and unstable steady states. Manuscript in preparation, 1980.

Pavlidis, T. *Biological Oscillators: Their Mathematical Analysis.* New York and London: Academic Press, 1973.

Pittendrigh, C. S. Circadian rhythms and the circadian organization of living systems. *Cold Spring Harbor Symposia in Quantitative Biology,* 1960, *25,* 159–184.

Pittendrigh, C. S. On the mechanism of the entrainment of a circadian rhythm by light cycles. In J. Aschoff (Ed.), *Circadian Clocks.* Amsterdam: North-Holland Publishing Co., 1965, pp. 277–297.

Pittendrigh, C. S. The circadian oscillation in *Drosophila pseudoobscura* pupae: A model for the photoperiod clock. *Zeitschrift für Pflanzenphysiologie,* 1966, *54,* 275–307.

Pittendrigh, C. S. Circadian Systems. I. The driving oscillation and its assay in *Drosophila pseudoobscura.* *Proceedings of the National Academy of Sciences, USA,* 1967a, *58*(4), 1762–1767.

Pittendrigh, C. S. Circadian rhythms, space research and manned space flight. In *Life Sciences and Space Research.* Vol. 5. Amsterdam: North-Holland Publ. Press, 1967b, pp. 122–134.

Pittendrigh, C. S. Circadian oscillations in cells and the circadian organization of multicellular systems. In F. O. Schmitt and F. G. Worden (Eds.), *The Neurosciences: Third Study Program.* Cambridge, Mass.: MIT Press, 1974, pp. 437–458.

Pittendrigh, C. S. Some functional aspects of circadian pacemakers. In M. Suda, O. Hayaishi, and H. Nakagawa (Eds.), *Biological Rhythms and Their Central Mechanism.* New York: Elsevier Press, 1980, pp. 3–12.

Pittendrigh, C. S. Circadian organization and the photoperiodic phenomena. In B. K. Follett (Ed.), *Biological Clocks in Reproductive Cycles.* Bristol: John Wright, 1981.

Pittendrigh, C. S., and Daan, S. A functional analysis of circadian pacemakers in nocturnal rodents. I. stability and lability of spontaneous frequency. *Journal of Comparative Physiology,* 1976a, *106,* 233–252.

Pittendrigh, C. S., and Daan, S. A functional analysis of circadian pacemakers in nocturnal rodents. IV. Entrainment: Pacemaker as clock. *Journal of Comparative Physiology,* 1976b, *106,* 291–331.

Pittendrigh, C. S., and Daan, S. A functional analysis of circadian pacemakers in nocturnal rodents. V. Pacemaker structure: A clock for all seasons. *Journal of Comparative Physiology,* 1976c, *106,* 333–355.

Pittendrigh, C. S., and Daan, S. Response of the *Drosophila pseudoobscura* circadian pacemaker to low intensity continuous illumination. Manuscript in preparation, 1980.

Pittendrigh, C. S., and Minis, D. H. The entrainment of circadian oscillations by light and their role as photoperiod clocks. *American Naturalist,* 1964, *98,* 261–294.

Pittendrigh, C. S., and Minis, D. H. The photoperiodic time-measurement in *Pectinorphora gossypiella* and its relation to the circadian system in that species. In M. Menaker (Ed.), *Biochronometry.* Washington, D.C.: National Academy of Sciences, 1971, pp. 212–250.

Saunders, D. S. Thermoperiodic control of diapause in an insect: Theory of internal coincidence. *Science* (Washington), 1973, 358–360.

Swade, R. H. Circadian rhythms in fluctuating light cycles: Toward a new model of entrainment. *Journal of Theoretical Biology,* 1969, *24,* 227–239.

Wever, R. Possibilities of phase control, demonstrated by an electronic mode. *Cold Spring Harbor Symposia in Quantitative Biology,* 1960, *25,* 197–207.

Wever, R. Zum Einfluss der Dämmerung auf die circadiane Periodik. *Zeitschrift für vergleichende Physiologie,* 1967, *55,* 255–277.

Winfree, A. T. The temporal morphology of a biological clock. In M. Gerstenhaber (Ed.), *Lectures on Mathematics in the Life Sciences.* Vol. 2. Providence, R.I.: American Mathematical Society, 1970.

Zimmerman, W., Pittendrigh, C. S., and Pavlidis, T. Temperature compensation of the circadian oscillation in *Drosophila pseudoobscura* and its entrainment by temperature cycles. *Journal of Insect Physiology,* 1968, *14*(5), 669–684.

8

Behavioral Rhythms in Invertebrates

JOHN BRADY

INTRODUCTION

Two divergent approaches have been followed in research on the rhythmicity of behavior. One has been followed by physiologists, who have measured behavior simply as an easy means of inferring the phase of the underlying driving oscillator. The other has been followed by experimental behaviorists, who have found themselves inconvenienced by diel changes in the responsiveness of their subjects. The former have had much interest in circadian processes, but little in the integration of behavior; the latter have had much interest in behavior, but little in the nature of circadian control.

Only rarely has behavior been put in a circadian perspective, or have circadian rhythms been put in a behavioral one. This chapter attempts to do both while cataloging the more important types of behavioral rhythm that have been found in invertebrates. There is rather little to be learned about the circadian control of invertebrate rhythms in the behavioral literature, and the circadian literature deals mainly with only two forms of behavior—locomotor activity in actographs and eclosion (emergence) in populations of insects (a highly atypical form of daily behavior).

Inevitably, this chapter concentrates on insects, for it is on them that much the most work has been done: Saunders (1976) gave 700 references to insect clocks, where Palmer (1973) gave less than 200 for all tidal rhythms, although it is on marine invertebrates that most of the relevant work has been done. If the insects are excluded, probably less than 50 papers exist on invertebrate behavioral circadian rhythms.

Note: The references provided below are not intended to be comprehensive; they either

JOHN BRADY   Department of Zoology and Applied Entomology, Imperial College of Science and Technology at Silwood Park, Ascot, Berks, SL5 7DE, England.

indicate the most important relevant work, or are the most recent papers, from which earlier related studies can best be traced (literature review completed November 1978).

LOCOMOTOR ACTIVITY RHYTHMS

Because of the ease of recording it (see Brady, 1974, p. 6), by far the most commonly studied form of behavioral rhythm is in locomotor activity—generally walking, running, swimming, or flight. Apart from its ease of measurement, such behavior has two important advantages for the investigation of circadian physiology. First, it can be studied in individuals, so that everything that occurs pertains to the temporal organization of one animal and does not arise by population effects, such as may occur in gated emergence rhythms (see p. 133), and must occur in field observations based on trapping. Second, it can reasonably be assumed that changes in locomotor activity reflect fairly fundamental circadian changes taking place in the CNS.

A survey of the more recent or more important studies of locomotor rhythms throughout the invertebrate phyla is given in Table I. The fact that a wide range of activities falls under the general heading of "locomotor activity" is evident and implies the perhaps obvious fact that whatever its central nervous causation, different animals perform their locomotor activity rhythmically for different adaptive purposes.

In nature, such activity is mostly performed as a response to direct external stimulation: to falling light intensity (e.g., Buck, 1937; Tychsen and Fletcher, 1971), rising temperature (e.g., Hawking, Gammage, and Worms, 1965), odors (e.g., Bartell and Shorey, 1969), visual movement (e.g., Brady, 1972b), and so on. In the laboratory, on the other hand, in conditions that provide such stimuli at invariant intensity (i.e., in constant light [or dark], temperature, smell, visual field, etc.), any locomotor activity that is performed must occur either as a result of internal "motivational" changes in the thresholds for these particular stimuli or as a result of central nervous excitation or disinhibition releasing so-called spontaneous activity.

These motivational changes arise from a number of physiological inputs, of which the most important are sex-hormone levels, food or water deprivation, and circadian (or tidal) rhythmicity. They tend to act independently on three distinct time scales in small invertebrates, namely, life span, days, and 24 hr. They inevitably interact, however, so that circadian patterns of locomotor activity are much affected by hunger, for example, and locomotor responses to food vary markedly according to circadian time.

Thus, in the tsetse fly, two clear components are detectable in "spontaneous" flight activity measured in rocking-cage actographs in LD 12:12 (Figure 1A). On the one hand, there is a biphasic circadian rhythm (which freeruns in DD; Brady, 1972a), and on the other, there is a marked increase in the level of activity over a 4-day period of food deprivation, from 8 flight bursts during the first 24 hr after a blood meal to 31 flight bursts during the 4th day. The level of spontaneous activity is thus modulated by two internal physiological inputs: the circadian clock and hunger. In addition, however, the diel *pattern* of the activity changes during the course of the 4 days' starvation, with the evening peak increasing 8-fold while the morning and midday activity levels only double. Furthermore, high and low temperatures alter the diel pattern in yet other ways (Brady and Crump, 1978). Hunger and temperature thus modulate the circadian clock-induced changes and

Table I. Examples of Circadian (C) and Tidal (T) Rhythms of Locomotor or Related
Activities in Various Invertebrate Phyla—with the Most Recent, Key References

Genus (class/order)	Rhythm type	Author
Protista		
Hantzschia (Diatom.)	Vertical migration in mud (T and C)	Palmer and Round, 1967
Euglena (Flagell.)	Motility and phototaxis (C)	Brinkmann, 1971
Coelenterata		
Cavernularia (sea pen)	Expansion of fans (C)	Mori, 1960
Metridium (anemone)	Expansion/contraction (C)	Batham and Pantin, 1950
Nematoda		
Edesonfilaria (Filaria)	Presence in peripheral blood of host (C)	Hawking *et al.*, 1965
Platyhelminthes		
Convoluta (Turbellaria)	Vertical migration in mud (T)	Martin, 1907
Annelida		
Lumbricus (Oligochaeta)	Speed of movement (C)	Bennett and Reinschmidt, 1965
Mollusca		
Limax (Gastropoda)	Locomotion (C)	Sokolove, Beiswanger, Prior, and Gelperin, 1977
Bembicium (Gastropoda)	Locomotion (T)	Zann, 1973
Mytilus (Lamellibranch.)	Opening and filtration (T)	Rao, 1954
Aplysia (Nudibranch.)	Locomotion (C)	Lickey *et al.*, 1976
Echinodermata		
Thyone (Holothuroidea)	Locomotion and feeding (C)	Stier, 1933
Arthropoda: Crustacea		
Talitrus (Amphipoda)	Walking/foraging (C)	Bregazzi and Naylor, 1972
Excirolana (Isopoda)	Swimming (C/T)	Enright, 1976
Peltidiadae (Copepoda)	Vertical migration in plankton (C/T)	Enright and Hamner, 1967
Uca (Decapoda)	Walking (T)	Palmer (1973)
Arthropoda: Myriapoda		
Callipus (Diplopoda)	Walking (C., cavernicole)	Gilhodes, 1974
Arthropoda: "Arachnida"		
Bdella (Acari)	Running (C and T)	Treherne, Foster, Evans, and Ruscoe, 1977
Ornithodoros (Acari)	Postfeeding drop-off (C)	Doube, 1975
Leiobunum (Opiliones)	Walking (C)	Fowler and Goodnight, 1974
Buthotus (Scorpiones)	Walking (C)	Cloudsley-Thompson, 1973
Arthropoda: Insecta		
Periplaneta (Dictyopt.)	Running (C)	Roberts, 1974
Teleogryllus (Orthopt.)	Running and singing (C)	Sokolove, 1975
Oncopeltus (Hemipt.)	Migratory flights (C)	Caldwell and Rankin, 1974
Anopheles (Dipt. Nemat.)	Flight and mating (C)	Jones and Gubbins, 1978
Glossina (Dipt. Cyclor.)	Flight, etc. (C)	Brady, 1975
Apis (Hymenopt.)	Flight and feeding (C)	Spangler, 1973
Epiphyas (Lepidopt.)	Flight and mating (C)	Bartell and Shorey, 1969

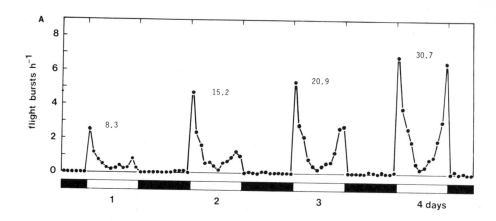

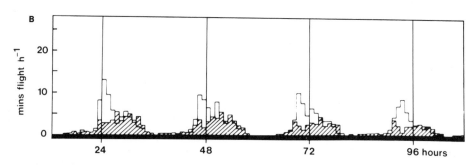

Fig. 1. (A) Rhythm of spontaneous flight activity in male tsetse flies *(Glossina morsitans)* in LD 12:12, expressed as mean number of spontaneous flights per hour per fly ($n = 23$ flies) (activity occurs exclusively in bursts of < 1 min). Figures above curves: mean number of flight bursts per 24 hr. Abscissa: days since last blood meal. Note differential increase in evening peak with increasing level of activity. (B) Freerunning rhythm of flight activity in female *Anopheles gambiae* in DD, expressed as mean minutes of flight per hour per mosquito. Open columns: 29 virgin females. Cross-hatched columns: 25 inseminated females. Abscissa: hours since start of DD. Note loss of early peak after insemination. (Used with permission from Jones and Gubbins, 1978.)

alter the effect of the clock's input differentially according to the overall activity level (Brady and Crump, 1978).

Jones and Gubbins (1978), who performed a more thorough investigation of this phenomenon in female *Anopheles gambiae,* found that insemination, feeding, and oviposition caused marked changes, not only in the total amount of flight performed per day, but also in its 24-hr pattern, both in LD 12:12 and in DD (Figure 1B). More spectacularly, in ants, permanent loss of locomotor rhythmicity occurs as a result of mating (McCluskey and Carter, 1969). Similar irreversible changes occur in the phasing of activity in silkmoths as a result of earlier developmental influences: male *Antheraea pernyi* reared at 25°C are active for the last 2 hr of the scotophase of LD 16:8, but if reared at 12°C and tested as adults at 25°C, they are then active for much of the scotophase (Truman, 1973).

Such differential changes in circadian behavioral pattern as a consequence of internal physiological inputs seem to have been little studied but are presumably common. Circadian pattern changes caused by external, environmental inputs, on the other hand, are well known (Aschoff, 1960). Changing the day length in LD cycles, for example, frequently changes circadian patterns (Schnabel, 1968; Tsutsumi, 1973; Tychsen, 1978), and

Aschoff's rule (see Saunders, 1976, p. 10) may be considered a form of such effects. More relevant are the differential effects of light intensity on behavioral *pattern*. Thus, the oviposition rhythm of *Drosophila melanogaster* changes from a biphasic pattern with equal early and late photophase peaks at 5 lux to a single late photophase peak at 60 lux (Allemand, 1977). Since this oviposition is mostly diurnal, it seems unlikely that the change in its pattern can be due to simple photoinhibition (though the further bias toward ovipositing exclusively in the early scotophase at 28 klux may well be). A still more striking change is shown in Figure 2; not only did Lohmann's cockroaches have different freerunning periods in DD and 5-lux LL (thus following Aschoff's rule), but the whole pattern of their activity was radically different.

Similar but apparently less dramatic pattern changes occur in response to different constant temperatures. Thus, in LD 12:12, caterpillars of the arctiid moth *Halisidota argentata* tend to be nocturnal at 10°C but diurnal at 5°C (Edwards, 1964); and the flight response to female sex pheromone by male *Argyrotaenia velutinana* moths in LD 16:8 peaks several hours earlier at 16°C than it does at 24°C (Cardé, Comeau, Baker, and Roelofs, 1975). The interaction of temperature *cycles* and photoperiod with locomotor patterns is, of course, more complicated (e.g., Dreisig, 1978), especially in nature (e.g., Buck, 1937; Batiste, Olson, and Berlowitz, 1973; Dreisig, 1975). In tidal isopods, 2 hr of water turbulence converts the swimming rhythm from having a single peak to having two persistent peaks 12 hr apart; at first sight, this looks as striking a change as the cockroach's (Figure 2), but it is presumably due to the evocation of an inherent tidal rhythm (Enright, 1976).

All these changes in the daily distribution of locomotor activity indicate that the circadian control of behavior must be highly complex. It not only involves the much-studied phase shifting of activity peaks to zeitgeber changes but also controls radical changes in 24-hr *pattern*. Moreover, such pattern changes are both dramatically qualitative, as in Figure 2, and differentially quantitative, as in the different effects of insemination and oviposition in *Anopheles gambiae* (Jones and Gubbins, 1978) or in the correlation between pattern

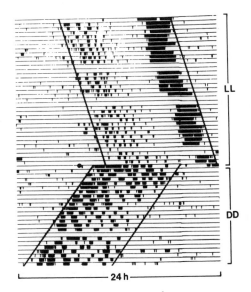

Fig. 2. Freerunning circadian locomotor rhythm of a male cockroach *(Leucophaea maderae)* in LL (5 lux) and DD. (Used with permission from Lohmann, 1967.) Note marked change of daily pattern between LL and DD.

change and total activity level in tsetse flies (Brady and Crump, 1978; as implied in Figure 1A above). Whether these effects indicate that the underlying circadian clock system oscillates differently under different physiological circumstances, or that there is a complex differential coupling between the clock and the behavior-controlling centers, is far from clear (see p. 140).

FEEDING RHYTHMS

One adaptive function that locomotion serves is feeding, and it is no surprise to find that in an active species like the cockroach, feeding is cophasic with locomotion, though feeding occupies only a small part of the span of peak locomotion (Lipton and Sutherland, 1970). In most insects that fly, on the other hand, feeding is incompatible with flight, so that the two behaviors must alternate during the activity peak or else must occur at different phases. Thus, in *Oncopeltus fasciatus,* which is a migratory lygaeid bug, the peak tendency for flights lasting more than 10 min is in midphotophase (in LD 16:8), whereas peak feeding occurs early and late in the photophase (Caldwell and Rankin, 1974). Likewise, peak flight activity in *Anopheles gambiae* occurs early in the scotophase (both in LD and at the equivalent time in DD; Jones and Gubbins, 1978), whereas peak biting activity in the field is after midnight (Haddow and Ssenkubuge, 1962; biting rhythmicity has yet to be measured in the laboratory, however). On the other hand, the tsetse fly shows a biphasic rhythm in proboscis-probing responsiveness that is broadly parallel with its rhythm of flight activity (Brady, 1975; Figure 4B and G below).

For more primitive animals, feeding *is* locomotion. That would seem to be true for some planktonic filter-feeders, for instance. For any sessile animal, the only form of locomotion is passing the environment past or through it as it feeds and respires. The rhythm of water pumping and filtration by the bivalve *Mytilus edulis* falls into this category, being measurable in constant conditions as a tidal rhythm in the rate of clearance of colloidal graphite from the water (Rao, 1954). Similarly in other bivalves, there are persistent tidal rhythms of shell opening (Morton, 1970). Such rhythms in mollusks generally also show clear circadian components, just as tidal locomotor rhythms in Crustacea usually do (see Palmer, 1973, p. 383; also Table I above).

MATING RHYTHMS

A greater tendency to mate at particular times of day is apparently as fundamental a behavioral rhythm as are circadian changes in locomotor activity—fungi, algae, and protozoa all exhibit mating rhythms. For example, *Paramecium aurelia* shows a temperature-compensated circadian rhythm in its frequency of cellular agglutination and pairing (Karakashian, 1965).

Aside from *Paramecium* and the insects, the only other invertebrate mating rhythms that seem to have been investigated are in marine species with lunar or semilunar monthly rhythms—for example, the annelid palolo worm (Hauenschild, Fischer, and Hofmann, 1968). In insects, however, circadian mating rhythms are well known and have been extensively studied in the laboratory. Mating swarms (especially in nematocerous Diptera—Wright, Kappus, and Venard, 1966), pheromones (especially in moths—Shorey and Gaston, 1965), singing (especially in Orthoptera—Dumortier, 1972), and luminescent displays (in fireflies and glowworms—Dreisig, 1978) fall into this general category. Bates (1941) seems to have been the first to discover the persistence of such rhythms in constant conditions, demonstrating that *Anopheles superpictus* swarm at about 24-hr intervals in constant dim light. Later work has revealed that in some species, the peaks of swarming coincide with a sharp increase in the males' responsiveness to the female flight tone, because of the males' erecting their antennal fibrillae (sound-sensitive hairs) for only an hour or so around the dusk peak of locomotor activity (Charlwood and Jones, 1979). Rather similarly, male Queensland fruitflies *(Dacus tryoni)*, in constant conditions, show a dusk-centered, broad, but steep-sided peak in responsiveness to females (Tychsen, 1978); in nature, this peak is restricted to about 30 min at dusk by the males' sensitivity to a critical low light intensity (10 lux) (Tychsen and Fletcher, 1971). The precision of such mating "gates" in nature must often act as species-isolating mechanisms.

The most extensively studied insect mating rhythms concern sex pheromones. There are at least three major rhythmic components of this behavior. First, the "attracted" sex usually has a locomotor rhythm with peak activity coinciding with peak mating (Bartell and Shorey, 1969; Fatzinger, 1973). Second, the female's (or male's) "calling" behavior—usually involving perching (i.e., reduced locomotion) and exposure of the pheromone gland—occurs more-or-less exclusively at certain times of day, usually peaking in the center of the opposite sex's locomotor phase (Bartell and Shorey, 1969; Traynier, 1970; Hammack and Burkholder, 1976). Third, the motile attracted sex has a peak of responsiveness to the pheromone that overlaps the calling peak (Traynier, 1970; Cardé *et al.,* 1975). The calling sex also appears to be most receptive to the other's copulatory attempts at these times (Vick, Drummond, and Coffelt, 1973). All these components of the behavior have been shown to freerun in constant conditions, though not all in any one species. The circadian control of pheromone-mediated mating behavior thus evidently involves complex interactions of antagonistic and allied responses in both sexes, one sex showing increased locomotion when the other shows less, and both showing increased responsiveness to stimuli from the other.

Several insects employ acoustic displays to bring the sexes together (e.g., crickets, cicadas, mosquitoes, and fruitflies). The rhythmic control of such stridulation has been investigated in crickets and grasshoppers and has been shown to be endogenously timed (Sokolove, 1975; Dumortier, 1972). The phase of peak stridulation usually lasts several hours and overlaps extensively between related species (Dumortier, 1972), so that the characteristics of the song rather than its phase setting must be the species-isolating mechanism (cf. the situation in Diptera, above). Orthoptera, unlike mosquitoes, cannot sing and locomote simultaneously, and in *Teleogryllus commodus,* the two behaviors are performed roughly 180° out of phase, both in LD and when freerunning in DD (Sokolove, 1975). However, under some circumstances these activities may occupy the same circadian phase, and in *Eugaster guyoni,* they peak at roughly the same times of day except in individuals that are singing particularly intensely, when locomotion is suppressed (Nielsen, 1974). In *Teleogryllus,* both rhythms, and also the rhythm of spermatophore production, freerun at identical frequencies and respond identically to surgical interference with the CNS—clearly implying control from a single driving oscillator system (Sokolove, 1975; Sokolove and Loher, 1975).

One of the earliest pieces of true circadian research (30 years before that term was invented) was Buck's (1937) investigation of the flashing rhythm in *Photinus pyralis* fireflies. He found that flashing could be induced at any time by a change from light to darkness, but that for at least 4 days in constant dim light, sharp circadian peaks of flashing occurred, phased to the change to LL. This work has since been greatly extended in a study of the neurophysiological control of the similar rhythm in *Luciola lusitanica* by Bagnoli and her colleagues (1976). No other circadian rhythms (with the possible exception of those in *Aplysia*—Lickey, Block, Hudson, and Smith, 1976; see Chapter 9) have been investigated in such elegant neurophysiological detail. Dreisig (1978) has studied the environmental control of the comparable, but physiologically quite different, rhythm in the glowworm, *Lampyris noctiluca*.

RHYTHMS IN REPRODUCTIVE BEHAVIOR

Just as mating is commonly under circadian control, so is the subsequent female behavior concerned with the release of offspring. Thus, the oviposition rhythm of bollworms (Minis, 1965), grasshoppers (Loher and Chandrashekaran, 1970), and mosquitoes (Gillett, Corbet, and Haddow, 1961), and the larviposition rhythm of tsetse flies (Phelps and Jackson, 1971) are all clearly circadian. No doubt the diel oviposition rhythms of other species, such as *Drosophila melanogaster* (Allemand, 1977) and spider mites (*Tetranychus urticae*—Polcik, Nowosielski, and Naegele, 1965) will also prove to be so. One should perhaps be cautious in assuming circadian control of such behavior, however, since the oviposition rhythm of the bug *Oncopeltus fasciatus,* although retained for five generations in LL, is apparently not temperature-compensated: the female's frequency of oviposition is directly related to the rate of egg development (Rankin, Caldwell, and Dingle, 1972). On the other hand, this may merely imply that the vitellogenic cycle is temperature-dependent (as it must be) and that the circadian control of the oviposition behavior breaks down in constant light (as would be expected).

Most research seems to have been on insects, though related lunar monthly rhythms in marine invertebrates are known (e.g., in the isopod crustacean *Excirolana chiltoni*—Klapow, 1972; and in the flatworm *Convoluta roscoffensis*—Keeble, 1910). Presumably, these are controlled also with regard to circadian (or tidal) time on the days when the release of offspring occurs. Certainly the equivalent lunar monthly eclosion rhythms of the marine midge *Clunio marinus* are (Neumann, 1976).

Sometimes peak locomotor activity is associated with peak oviposition, implying that the former subserves the latter (adaptively). Thus, in *Anopheles gambiae,* peak oviposition occurs just after dusk (Haddow and Ssenkubuge, 1962), and the major flight peak at dusk is greatly enhanced in females prevented from ovipositing (Jones and Gubbins, 1978). The same might also appear to be true in *Oncopeltus*, which both flies and oviposits most around noon, but this seems not to be so, since long flights occur in young, migratory females, and oviposition occurs only in mature, postmigratory females (Caldwell and Rankin, 1974). No actograph studies have been made of this species, however, so that the precise circadian flight–oviposition relationship in mature females is unknown.

There is a whole class of circadian rhythms that involve events that occur only once in the life of each individual (e.g., adult eclosion and egg hatch). These appear as "rhythms," therefore, only in mixed-age populations, but they are nevertheless timed by a circadian clock in each individual, which performs its act only at certain times of day, that is, when its circadian "gate" is open (a concept adopted by Pittendrigh, 1966). Thus, *Drosophila pseudoobscura* pupate at all times of day in LD 12:12 but emerge as adults only between dawn and noon (a "gating" rhythm that freeruns at about 24-hr intervals in DD). If an individual then misses a given day's emergence gate, it must wait 24 hr for the next one, or 48 hr for the one after that.

The phenomenology of gating adult eclosion in *Drosophila* has been by far the most extensively investigated (Pittendrigh, 1966; Pittendrigh and Skopik, 1970), but circadian gating has also been demonstrated in the eclosion of silkmoths (Truman, 1971), bollworms (Minis, 1965), tsetse flies (Phelps and Jackson, 1971), blackflies (Hunter, 1977), and marine midges (Neumann, 1976). Although in *Drosophila* and silkmoths it is indeed eclosion of the adult that is gated, that is not always so. In mosquitoes, it is pupation that is gated, with adult eclosion simply following at a fixed, unentrainable, temperature-dependent interval thereafter (Nayar, 1967; Jones and Reiter, 1975). Although larval ecdyses may not themselves be gated, the circadian oscillator that controls the pupation or adult eclosion gate may be already running in the larvae, since in *Drosophila* it is entrainable right back in the first larval instar (Zimmerman and Ives, 1971). The circadian gating of egg-hatching seems to have been studied only in bollworms (Minis and Pittendrigh, 1968) and mosquitoes (Nayar, Samarawickrema, and Sauerman, 1973) but may well be common.

The concept of gating has been applied mostly to once-in-a-lifetime events such as eclosion or hatching, which are primarily thought of as developmental steps. However, they in fact all concern distinct, "one-off" behavior patterns and are more properly thought of as *gated behavior* rather than gated development, since the morphogenetic component is always complete hours or days before the hatching or eclosion behavior commences. Thus, in silkmoths, Truman (1976) has shown that when the cephalic neurosecretion that controls eclosion (see chapter 9) is injected into fully developed pupae (pharate adults), it elicits eclosion behavior within about 2½ hr—at any time of day. The specific behavioral program involved in eclosion is wired into the ventral nerve cord (Truman, 1978) and is switched on by this eclosion hormone, whose secretion from the brain is gated by a circadian clock.

No other once-in-a-lifetime behaviors have been investigated in such detail, but the same principles must generally apply, since it is essentially the behavior that is gated, not the development, and the behavior inevitably involves discrete, never-to-be-repeated programs. The control of gated behavioral "rhythms" is therefore qualitatively different from the control of the more typical kind of ongoing, daily-repeated behaviors considered in the previous sections (see p. 139). There are forms of such daily-repeated behavior, however, whose control in effect involves gating.

Insemination in those species whose females copulate only once is a striking case. Female *Anopheles gambiae*, for example, can mate only during the hour or so after dusk, because that is when they are most active and when the males are sensitive to their flight tone (see p. 131). Furthermore, once mated, their major early scotophase activity peak is lost (Figure 1B). This behavior is thus functionally gated: if a female is not inseminated at dusk on one day, she must wait 24 hr till the next dusk.

In the same class of gated behavior is the postfeeding drop-off "rhythms" of larval ticks. These may take days to engorge and must leave the host to molt. They improve their chances of finding a host for the next instar, however, by dropping off when the host is in its nest. Since this latter event is regulated by the host's own circadian activity pattern, the tick adjusts its dropping off accordingly—by gating it to the appropriate phase of the host's rhythm (Doube, 1975).

In a different phenomenological sense, oviposition may also be gated, since it generally occurs at a particular circadian phase but can only do so if eggs are available. This is evidently the case in some tropical mosquitoes, such as *Anopheles funestus,* which oviposits in the early part of its locomotor phase (as in *A. gambiae*; see p. 132) and does so every other day if the mean temperature is above 25.5°C but only every third day if the temperature is less than 24.5°C (Gillies, 1953), the difference being due to the fact that the gonotrophic cycle takes more than 40 hr at the lower temperature. A quite different condition occurs in *Oncopeltus fasciatus,* however. In this species, ovariectomized females show an "oviposition" behavior rhythm that is indistinguishable from that of intact controls (in LD—Rankin *et al.,* 1972; cf. p.132).

Rhythms in Orientation Behavior

Circadian changes in the intensity of orientational responses, especially to light, have been reported in many animals, including photosynthetic Protista (*Euglena gracilis*—Feldman and Bruce, 1972; Brinkmann, 1971; *Hantzschia virgata*—Palmer and Round, 1967), photosynthetic flatworms (*Convoluta roscoffensis*—Martin, 1907), crustacea (*Daphnia magna*—Ringelberg and Servaas, 1971; *Uca pugnax*—Palmer, 1964), and insects (*Drosophila*—Dürrwächter, 1957; waterboatmen—Rensing, 1965; grain weevils—Birukow, 1964). The *Hantzschia* rhythm is in vertical migration in tidal sand and is interesting from the oscillator control viewpoint because in LL the upward, positive phototaxis occurs only during the subjective circadian photophases that would coincide with low tide—both circatidal and circadian control of behavior is thus involved.

Such phototactic rhythms may indeed be due to circadian changes in photopositive responsiveness, but strictly speaking, none of the responses reported have been shown to be due to oriented photo*taxes* rather than *kineses,* and all evidently contain strong kinetic components associated with the locomotor activity rhythm, so that the apparent orientation rhythms may arise more from a circadian change in the level of locomotor activity than from a change in photoresponsiveness *per se* (for taxes versus kineses, see, e.g., Wigglesworth, 1972, p. 315). Thus, the "phototactic" (? = photokinetic) rhythms of Feldman's *Euglena,* Rensing's waterboatmen, and Birukow's weevils are all closely in phase with their locomotor activity rhythms, and though not yet measured, the same seems likely to be true of the other species. The best indication for a real photopositivity rhythm is in *Daphnia,* in which Ringelberg and Servaas (1971) showed a circadian change in the light intensity threshold for upward (i.e., directed) swimming.

This general criticism cannot apply to those cases where there is a rhythmic change in orientation *angle,* that is, a quantitative change in a directed orientation (taxis). Thus pondskaters have been claimed to show a daily (presumably circadian) cycle in their angle of orientation to gravity (Birukow, 1960). Similarly, dung beetles may rhythmically change their angle of orientation to a light (Birukow, 1960; a sun-compass reaction—see the following section below). These observations still await confirmation, but if correct would indicate that the orientation rhythms exactly parallel the animal's circadian locomotor rhythm in each case and that the orientation response itself must change rhythmically (the parallelism is highly interesting in a different context, also—see p. 139).

A rather different kind of tactic rhythm has been found in wood crickets. When placed in the center of a 30-cm-diameter white cylindrical arena, they walk toward broad vertical black stripes on the walls, with a frequency varying across the 24 hr (LD 12:12) from about 20% to 90% of trials (Campan, Lacoste, and Morvan, 1975). This rhythm bears no obvious relationship with locomotor level (measured as running speed), however, except for a tendency to be roughly 180° out of phase with it.

Time Sense

Several invertebrates exhibit the specific kind of orientational rhythm associated with successful sun-compass orientation, that is, menotactic orientation in which a constant angle is maintained with respect to the sun or the moon (see Wigglesworth, 1972, p. 320). If the journey involved is brief, no significant directional error is incurred, but since the sun moves by a mean of 15° azimuth per hour (azimuth = compass direction to horizon vertically below sun), journeys of more than an hour or so would be inaccurate if not corrected for the sun's movement. Bees, pondskaters, sandhoppers, crabs, and many migratory vertebrates can all do this (see Walraff, this volume; Brady, 1979).

In sandhoppers, correction for the sun's movement takes the following form. They live in the supralittoral zone, in which they remain buried during the day, but from which they emerge to forage inland during the night. When disturbed, or at the end of foraging, they escape homeward by moon-compass orientation in a course at 90° to the local coastline. The direction is time-compensated to an accuracy of about ±20° (Enright, 1972), which is presumably good enough for the purpose. More accurate time compensation occurs in honeybees, which can both find a food source along a learned sun-compass direction without previous experience of it (Gould, 1975) and indicate against gravity by their waggle dances on the comb the correct sun-compass direction of such food. Moreover, "marathon dancers" can indicate the direction of a new nest site at any time of day *or night* for hours at a time, without leaving the darkness of the hive, to an accuracy of about ±2° (von Frisch, 1967, p. 351).

That this ability is due to the animal's underlying circadian control of behavior is indicated by its close temporal link with the locomotor rhythm, at least in bees (Beier and Lindauer, 1970; Spangler, 1973). The essential circadian component in sun-compass orientation is the ability to "know" the time of day continuously, without reference to external time cues—hence the phrase "continuously consulted clocks" used to identify the phenomenon. The central nervous system can evidently read the time with considerable accuracy (in bees to about ±8 min) at any point in its circadian cycle, so that the behavior involved in the associated orientation is continuously coupled to the circadian oscillator system (a point of major interest for circadian behavioral control; see p. 139).

Rhythmicity in Learning

The earliest report of rhythmicity in invertebrate learning seems to be Arbit's finding (1957) that earthworms trained with electroshock reinforcement needed a mean of 45 trials to learn the correct turn in a T-maze during the morning, but only 32 trials to learn the same task at night (cf. the parallel change in locomotion and light-withdrawal reflex in the following section). The next study seems to have been Sukumar's (1975) on shock-avoidance learning in male grasshoppers, which when trained at four different times of day showed peak performance at 0800 hr local time; it is curious that no such rhythmicity was detectable in females, however.

Insects and most other invertebrates (except cephalopods) are generally poor learners. Bees (and other higher Hymenoptera), on the other hand, have highly developed learning abilities, and while rhythmicity in learning has not been demonstrated in them, they nevertheless exhibit what may be thought of as learned phase-settings. In the wild, they learn the time of day to visit flowers that make their nectar available only at specific times (von Frisch, 1967, p. 253). Furthermore, they can be trained to visit artificial food sources at up to nine different times per day and will even remember to come to the correct scent at the correct time, if trained to two scents at different times (Koltermann, 1974).

Rhythmic Changes in Responsiveness

For rhythms to occur in behavior (that is, in feeding, mating, oviposition, etc.), there must be rhythmic changes in the thresholds of the responses involved. Only rarely, however, have either sensory (i.e., receptor) or behavioral thresholds been studied in relation to circadian rhythms. One behavioral example, already noted (p. 134), is the circadian change in light intensity threshold of the upward swimming response in *Daphnia* (Ringelberg and Servaas, 1971). Another is in the pheromone concentration threshold of the sex responses of male moths (Payne, Shorey, and Gaston, 1970; Figure 3A below). A third is in the sucrose concentration threshold of the proboscis extension reflex in blowflies (Hall, 1980).

These seem to be the only cases where behavioral thresholds have been measured across circadian time with full experimental rigor, that is, by testing at different times of day a series of stimulus intensities on a group of individuals, and measuring the intensity necessary to elicit a 50% response. However, circadian behavioral observations on groups of animals are assumed to have the same neural implication when the population fluctuates across the day in its responsiveness (i.e., as the proportion responding) to a periodically presented, standard stimulus. This occurs, for example, in the responsiveness of tsetse flies to moving stripes (Brady, 1972b; Figure 4C below); the responsiveness of male *Dacus* fruitflies to females (Tychsen, 1978); and the responsiveness of blowflies to sugar (Hall, 1980). More commonly, behavioral rhythms are measured with the stimulus (food, oviposition site, mate, etc.) continuously present, in which case there may be no rhythm in responsiveness itself, but merely an adventitious rhythm in stimulation frequency or intensity due to the animals' own movements, which inevitably change in amount because of the locomotor rhythm.

Rhythms in responsiveness can arise, in principle, in three ways: (1) peripherally, from changes in receptor sensitivity; (2) centrally, from changes in CNS integrative thresholds; or (3) from a combination of the two. The first occurs widely in arthropod eyes. Thus, the ommatidial screening pigments migrate distally and proximally with a circadian rhythm in the superposition compound eyes of beetles (Jahn and Wulff, 1943) and crabs (Aréchiga, Huberman, and Naylor, 1974), affecting their light-evoked retinal responses (electroretinogram—Aréchiga and Fuentes, 1970) and their optomotor visual acuity (Meyer-Rochow and Horridge, 1975). By different physiological mechanisms, similar peripheral sensitivity changes also occur in the simple eyes of king crabs (Behrens, 1974), scorpions (Fleissner, 1977), and spiders (Blest, 1978).

Although this kind of peripheral rhythm may thus be widespread in visual systems, the only nonvisual example so far reported is that of the rhythm in some male mosquitoes' antennal sensitivity to the female flight tone (p. 131). No comparable receptor sensitivity rhythms have been detected in the three other behavioral rhythms that have been examined from this point of view. The first of these cases concerns male moths' responsiveness to female sex pheromone. In *Trichoplusia ni,* there is a clear circadian change in the behavioral threshold, but no such change in the electroantennogram (Figure 3A), a situation also true for male saturniids (Riddiford, 1974). The second case concerns the proboscis extension reflex of blowflies responding to tarsal stimulation with sugar. Again, a clear circadian rhythm is apparent in the behavioral responsiveness (this time, whether measured as the sugar concentration threshold of the response or as the proportion of flies responding), but no circadian change occurs in the level of afferent signals from the tarsal chemoreceptors (Figure 3B; this rhythm, moreover, freeruns for at least two cycles in LL—Hall, 1980). The third, less convincing case concerns the response of tsetse flies to slowly moving visual stimuli. Here again, a clear circadian rhythm in behavioral responsiveness occurs (Figure 4C), but the indirect, psychophysical evidence implies that this is not due to changes in the eyes' sensitivity (Brady, 1975).

In these last three examples, therefore, the strong implication is that the rhythms in behavioral responsiveness are due not to peripheral rhythms in receptor sensitivity, but to rhythms in the central nervous integration of the relevant afferent signals.

OVERALL CIRCADIAN ORGANIZATION OF BEHAVIOR

It is apparently characteristic of circadian behavioral rhythms that in any one species, many behaviors are closely cophasic. The most detailed study has been of the tsetse fly (Figure 4), but cophasic parallel rhythms of the same general kind occur in earthworms (learning ability, locomotion, and light-withdrawal response—Arbit, 1957; Bennett and Reinschmidt, 1965); waterboatmen (locomotion and phototaxis [= kinesis?]—Rensing, 1965); pondskaters (locomotion and geotactic angle—Birukow, 1960); mosquitoes (flight, mating, and oviposition—Jones and Gubbins, 1978; Haddow and Ssenkubuge, 1962); moths (pheromone responsiveness and flight—Bartell and Shorey, 1969); and also vertebrates (birds—Ollason and Slater, 1973; and man—Aschoff, Giedke, Poppel, and Wever, 1972).

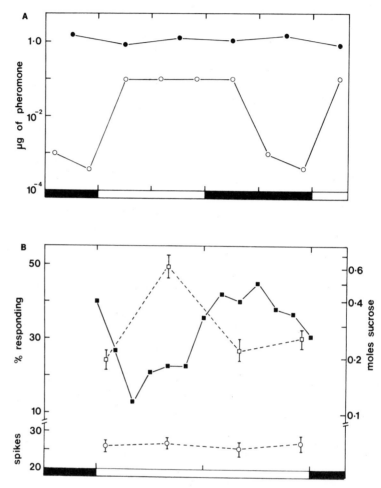

Fig. 3. Comparison of behavioral and receptor threshold changes with circadian time in two insects (in LD 12:12 as on abscissae). (A) Change in responsiveness of male moths *(Trichoplusia ni)* to synthetic female sex pheromone. Solid circles: dose required to elicit detectable electrical response from the antennae (electroantennogram) (n = 7–10 males). Open circles: dose required to elicit a behavioral response in 50% of males. Last two points of both curves plotted twice. (Compiled from Payne *et al.,* 1970.) (B) Change in responsiveness of male blowflies *(Protophormia terraenovae)* to sucrose stimulation of the tarsi. Solid squares and left ordinate: percentage of flies (n = 83) extending their proboscis to stimulation of the tarsi with 1.0 M sucrose. Open squares and right ordinate: concentration of sucrose necessary to elicit the proboscis extension response in 50% of flies (n = 181) (= sucrose threshold; note log scale). Circles: spikes generated by one tarsal chemoreceptor hair in the first half second of stimulation with 0.3 M sucrose (17 flies, with two hairs each tested at each time). Bars: ±SE. Abscissa: LD 12:12 with only part of scotophase shown. (Compiled from Hall, 1980.)

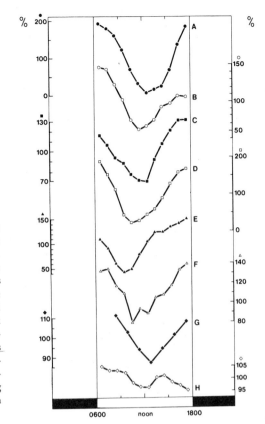

Fig. 4. Parallel behavioral rhythmicity in the tsetse fly *(Glossina morsitans)*. Ordinate units: percentages of the respective mean response levels. (A) The number of flies coming to bite a bait ox in the field (Zimbabwe). (B) Percentage of flies flying spontaneously in actographs (cf. Figure 1A). (C) Percentage of flies taking off to visual stimulation with a large, slowly moving black stripe. (D) Percentage of flies taking off to stimulation with human odor. (E) Percentage of flies resting on well-lit surfaces. (F) Defecation frequency. (G) Percentage of flies probing an artificial feeding surface. (H) Percentage of flies flying toward the visual stimulus used in (C). (Used with permission from Brady, 1975.)

The coincidence of some of these rhythms may be due to the direct and indirect effects of the locomotor rhythm (see pp. 134 and 136), but in many cases, the behaviors involve different sensorimotor systems, as in the earthworm, pondskater, and tsetse fly examples. It therefore appears probable that parallel behavioral circadian rhythmicity is a general phenomenon, and that much of each species's behavior is coupled to its circadian clock system in a manner that modulates many of its different responses in phase across the day. That, in turn, implies unitary circadian control of threshold levels, and since the evidence suggests central rather than peripheral control in many cases (p. 137), a simple hypothesis for the whole system would be that the differing response rhythms all derive from a daily cycle in central excitability, that is, in the signal-passing thresholds of some integrative zone in the CNS (Brady, 1975).

However, any such hypothesis must accommodate at least the following points:

1. Unlike the circadian gating of once-in-a-lifetime behavioral acts (p. 133), circadian control of ongoing, daily behavioral rhythms must be exerted right around the clock. This is evident from the kind of locomotor rhythms that are clearly continuously modulated (e.g., tsetse fly—Brady, 1975) and from the fact that bees, sandhoppers, and other sun-compass-orienting species can "read" circadian time continuously (p. 135).

2. Again, unlike the control of gated "rhythms," the control of ongoing behavior must be exerted in a probabilistic, nonrigid manner; the phase of peak locomotor activity, for

example, is not exclusively filled with locomotion, and conversely, some locomotion usually occurs during the phase of rest. To be adaptive, behavior must allow the animal to adjust to the exigencies of the moment (e.g., arrival of food, mate, predator), so the circadian control of it cannot be all-or-none in the way that, say, eclosion behavior is, once it is switched on (p. 133).

3. Circadian changes in behavior occur around mean levels that change from day to day as a consequence of other physiological inputs, such as "hunger" (p. 126).

4. Circadian changes in responsiveness commonly involve central processing of sensory information rather than peripheral modulation of sensory sensitivity (p. 137).

5. In each individual, circadian changes in many different sensorimotor systems occur in phase (p. 139).

6. Circadian changes often occur in peripheral, receptor sensitivity (p. 137).

7. By no means all behaviors in an animal change in phase across the day, and some, particularly those that are mutually exclusive, are conspicuously out of phase (pp. 130, 131).

8. Phase slippage occurs across circadian time, with differential changes occurring in daily patterns as a result of other inputs and with whole phases sometimes dropping out of the day's pattern (pp. 126, 128).

Whereas the idea of circadian central excitability changes can account for the first five points reasonably well and may be stretched to accommodate point 6 and the part of point 7 that concerns 180° out-of-phase rhythms (Brady, 1975), it seems to explain partially out-of-phase rhythms and the phenomenon covered in point 8 less well.

No satisfactory model for the overall circadian control of all behavior has yet been proposed, but two points are reasonably clear. First, although hormones certainly do affect behavior (for invertebrates, see Riddiford, 1974; Aréchiga et al., 1974), simple circadian changes in hormonal titer would seem too crude and unadaptable a system to control the subtle daily changes that actually occur in behavior (see also Brady, 1974, pp. 57, 69). Second, circadian changes in the excitability of integrative centers in the CNS must be involved to some degree, for that is how behavior arises. Just how the circadian oscillator system is coupled to such centers in a way that allows for continual changes in circadian pattern (point 8) is as yet far from clear, however. Possibly the different brain centers that integrate different behavioral outputs are *each* capable of circadian oscillation within themselves and together comprise a central nervous multioscillator system (Brady, 1979) whose component oscillators are normally maintained either in phase (for cophasic behaviors) or at constant phase angles to each other (for out-of-phase behaviors). Differential excitability in these centers would then cause the circadian pattern of behavior to change.

References

Allemand, R. Influence de l'intensité d'éclairement sur l'expression du rythme journalier d'oviposition de *Drosophila melanogaster* en conditions lumineuses LD 12:12. *Compte Rendu Hebdomadaire des Séances de l'Académie des Sciences. Paris.* 1977, Ser. D, *284*, 1553–1556.

Arbit, J. Diurnal cycles and learning in earthworms. *Science,* 1957, *126*, 654–655.

Aréchiga, H., and Fuentes, B. Correlative changes between retinal shielding pigments position and electroretinogram in crayfish. *The Physiologist,* 1970, *13*, 137.

Aréchiga, H., Huberman, A., and Naylor, E. Hormonal modulation of circadian neural activity in *Carcinus maenas* (L.). *Proceedings of the Royal Society of London,* 1974, *B. 187*, 229–313.

Aschoff, J. Exogenous and endogenous components in circadian rhythms. In *Biological Clocks—Cold Spring Harbor Symposia on Quantitative Biology*, 1960, *25*, 11–28.

Aschoff, J., Giedke, H., Poppel, E., and Wever, R. The influence of sleep-interruption and sleep-deprivation on circadian rhythms in human performance. In W. P. Colquhoun (Ed.), *Aspects of Human Efficiency Diurnal Rhythm and Loss of Sleep*. London: English Universities Press, 1972, pp. 135–150.

Bagnoli, P., Brunelli, N., Magni, F., and Musumeci, D. Neural mechanisms underlying spontaneous flashing and its modulation in the firefly *Luciola lusitanica*. *Journal of Comparative Physiology*, 1976, *108*, 133–156.

Bartell, R. J., and Shorey, H. H. A quantitative bioassay for the sex pheromone of *Epiphyas postvittana* (Lepidoptera) and factors limiting male responsiveness. *Journal of Insect Physiology*, 1969, *15*, 33–40.

Bates, M. Laboratory observations on the sexual behavior of anopheline mosquitoes. *Journal of Experimental Zoology*, 1941, *86*, 153–173.

Batham, E. J., and Pantin, C. F. A. Phases of activity in the sea-anemone *Metridium senile* L. and their relation to external stimuli. *Journal of Experimental Biology*, 1950, *27*, 377–399.

Batiste, W. C., Olson, W. H., and Berlowitz, A. Codling moth: Influence of temperature and daylight intensity on periodicity of daily flight in the field. *Journal of Economic Entomology*, 1973, *66*, 883–892.

Behrens, M. Photomechanical changes in the ommatidia of the *Limulus* lateral eye during light and dark adaptation. *Journal of Comparative Physiology*, 1974, *89*, 45–57.

Beier, W., and Lindauer, M. Der Sonnenstand als Zeitgeber für die Biene. *Apidologie*, 1970, *1*, 5–28.

Bennett, M. F., and Reinschmidt, D. C. The diurnal cycle and locomotion in earthworms. *Zeitschrift für Vergleichende Physiologie*, 1965, *51*, 224–226.

Birukow, G. Innate types of chronometry in insect orientation. In *Biological Clocks—Cold Spring Harbor Symposia on Quantitative Biology*, 1960, *25*, 403–412.

Birukow, G. Aktivitäts- und Orientierungsrhythmik beim Kornkäfer (*Calandra granaria* L.). *Zeischrift für Tierpsychologie*, 1964, *21*, 279–301.

Blest, A. D. The rapid synthesis and destruction of photoreceptor membrane by a dinopid spider: The daily cycle. *Proceedings of the Royal Society of London*, 1978, *B. 200*, 463–483.

Brady, J. Spontaneous, circadian components of tsetse fly activity. *Journal of Insect Physiology*, 1972a, *18*, 471–484.

Brady, J. The visual responsiveness of the tsetse fly *Glossina morsitans* Westw. (Glossinidae) to moving objects: The effects of hunger, sex, host odour and stimulus characteristics. *Bulletin of Entomological Research*, 1972b, *62*, 257–279.

Brady, J. The physiology of insect circadian rhythms. *Advances in Insect Physiology*, 1974, *10*, 1–115.

Brady, J. Circadian changes in central excitability—The origin of behavioural rhythms in tsetse flies and other animals? *Journal of Entomology (A)*, 1975, *50*, 79–95.

Brady, J. *Biological Clocks* (Studies in Biology, No. 104). London: Edward Arnold, 1979.

Brady, J., and Crump, A. J. The control of circadian activity rhythms in tsetse flies: Environment or physiological clock? *Physiological Entomology*, 1978, *3*, 177–190.

Bregazzi, P. K., and Naylor, E. The locomotor activity rhythm of *Talitrus saltator* (Montagu) (Crustacea, Amphipoda). *Journal of Experimental Biology*, 1972, *57*, 375–391.

Brinkmann, K. Metabolic control of temperature compensation in the circadian rhythm of *Euglena gracilis*. In M. Menaker (Ed.), *Biochronometry*. Washington, D.C.: National Academy of Sciences, 1971, pp. 567–593.

Buck, J. B. Studies on the firefly. I. The effects of light and other agents on flashing in *Photinus pyralis*, with special reference to periodicity and diurnal rhythm. *Physiological Zoölogy*, 1937, *10*, 45–58.

Caldwell, R. L., and Rankin, M. A. Separation of migratory from feeding and reproductive behavior in *Oncopeltus fasciatus*. *Journal of Comparative Physiology*, 1974, *88*, 383–394.

Campan, R., Lacoste, G., and Morvan, R. Le rhythme journalier de l'orientation scototactique chez le grillon des bois *Nemobius sylvestris* (Bosc): Approche de la signification biologique. *Monitore Zoologico Italiano (N.S.)*, 1975, *9*, 119–136.

Cardé, R. T., Comeau, A., Baker, T. C., and Roelofs, W. L. Moth mating periodicity: Temperature regulates the circadian gate. *Experientia*, 1975, *31*, 46–48.

Charlwood, J. D., and Jones, M. D. R. Mating behaviour in the mosquito, *Anopheles gambiae* s.l. I. Close range and contact behaviour. *Physiological Entomology*, 1979, *4*, 111–120.

Cloudsley-Thompson, J. L. Entrainment of the "circadian clock" in *Buthotus minax* (Scorpiones: Buthidae). *Journal of Interdisciplinary Cycle Research*, 1973, *4*, 119–123.

Doube, B. M. Regulation of the circadian rhythm of detachment of engorged larvae and nymphs of the argasid kangaroo tick, *Ornithodoros gurneyi*. *Journal of Medical Entomology*, 1975, *12*, 15–22.

Dreisig, H. Environmental control of the daily onset of luminescent activity in glowworms and fireflies. *Oecologia*, 1975, *18*, 85–99.

Dreisig, H. The circadian rhythm of bioluminescence in the glowworm, *Lampyris noctiluca* L. (Coleoptera, Lampyridae). *Behavioral Ecology and Sociobiology,* 1978, *3,* 1–18.

Dumortier, B. Photoreception in the circadian rhythm of stridulatory activity in *Ephippiger* (Ins., Orthoptera). *Journal of Comparative Physiology,* 1972, *77,* 80–112.

Dürrwächter, G. Untersuchungen über Phototaxis und Geotaxis einiger *Drosophila*-Mutanten nach Aufzucht in verschiedenen Lichtbedingungen. *Zeitschrift für Tierpsychologie,* 1957, *14,* 1–28.

Edwards, D. K. Activity rhythms of lepidopterous defoliators. II. *Halisidota argentata* Pack. (Arctiidae), and *Nepytia phantasmaria* Stkr. (Geometridae). *Canadian Journal of Zoology,* 1964, *42,* 939–958.

Enright, J. T. When the beachhopper looks at the moon: The moon-compass hypothesis. In S. R. Galler, K. Schmidt-Koenig, G. J. Jacobs, and R. E. Belleville (Eds.), *Animal Orientation and Navigation.* Washington, D.C.: National Aeronautics and Space Administration, 1972, pp. 523–555.

Enright, J. T. Plasticity in an isopod's clockworks: Shaking shapes form and affects phase and frequency. *Journal of Comparative Physiology,* 1976, *107,* 13–37.

Enright, J. T., and Hamner, W. M. Vertical diurnal migration and endogenous rhythmicity. *Science,* 1967, *157,* 937–941.

Fatzinger, C. W. Circadian rhythmicity of sex pheromone release by *Dioryctria abietella* (Lepidoptera: Pyralidae (Phycitinae)) and the effect of a diel light cycle on its precopulatory behavior. *Annals of the Entomological Society of America,* 1973, *66,* 1147–1154.

Feldman, J. F., and Bruce, V. G. Circadian rhythm changes in autotrophic *Euglena* induced by organic carbon sources. *Journal of Protozoology,* 1972, *19,* 370–373.

Fleissner, G. Entrainment of the scorpion's circadian rhythm via the median eyes. *Journal of Comparative Physiology,* 1977, *118,* 93–99.

Fowler, D. J., and Goodnight, C. J. Physiological populations of the arachnid, *Leiobunum longipes* (Opiliones: Phalangiidae). *Systematic Zoology,* 1974, *23,* 219–225.

Gilhodes, J.-C. Étude du rythme d'activité locomotrice de *Callipus foetidissimus* Bröl (Diplopode) en libre cours. *Revue du Comportement Animal,* 1974, *8,* 63–70.

Gillett, J. D., Corbet, P. S., and Haddow, A. J. Observations on the oviposition-cycle of *Aedes (Stegomyia) aegypti* (Linnaeus). VI. *Annals of Tropical Medicine and Parasitology,* 1961, *55,* 427–431.

Gillies, M. T. The duration of the gonotrophic cycle in *Anopheles gambiae* and *Anopheles funestus,* with a note on the efficiency of hand catching. *East African Medical Journal,* 1953, *30,* 129–135.

Gould, J. L. Honey bee recruitment: The dance-language controversy. *Science,* 1975, *189,* 685–693.

Haddow, A. J., and Ssenkubuge, Y. Laboratory observations on the oviposition-cycle in the mosquito *Anopheles (Cellia) gambiae* Giles. *Annals of Tropical Medicine and Parasitology,* 1962, *56,* 352–355.

Hall, M. J. Circadian rhythm of proboscis extension responsiveness in the blowfly: Central control of threshold changes. *Physiological Entomology,* 1980, *5,* 223–233.

Hammack, L., and Burkholder, W. E. Circadian rhythm of sex pheromone-releasing behaviour in females of the dermestid beetle, *Trogoderma glabrum:* Regulation by photoperiod. *Journal of Insect Physiology,* 1976, *22,* 385–388.

Hauenschild, C., Fischer, A., and Hofmann, D. K. Untersuchungen am pazifischen Palolowurm *Eunice viridis* (Polychaeta) in Samoa. *Helgoländer Wissenschaftliche Meeresuntersuchungen,* 1968, *18,* 254–295.

Hawking, F., Gammage, K., and Worms, M. J. The periodicity of microfilariae. X. The relation between the circadian temperature cycle of monkeys and the microfilarial cycle. *Transactions of the Royal Society of Tropical Medicine and Hygiene,* 1965, *59,* 675–680.

Hunter, D. M. Eclosion and oviposition rhythms in *Simulium ornatipes* (Diptera: Simuliidae). *Journal of the Australian Entomological Society,* 1977, *16,* 215–220.

Jahn, T. L., and Wulff, V. J. Electrical aspects of a diurnal rhythm in the eye of *Dytiscus fasciventris. Physiological Zoölogy,* 1943, *16,* 101–109.

Jones, M. D. R., and Gubbins, S. J. Changes in the circadian flight activity of the mosquito *Anopheles gambiae* in relation to insemination, feeding and oviposition. *Physiological Entomology,* 1978, *3,* 213–220.

Jones, M. D. R., and Reiter, P. Entrainment of the pupation and adult activity rhythms during development in the mosquito *Anopheles gambiae. Nature* (London), 1975, *254,* 242–244.

Karakashian, M. W. The circadian rhythm of sexual reactivity in *Paramecium aurelia,* Syngen 3. In J. Aschoff (Ed.), *Circadian Clocks.* Amsterdam: North-Holland, 1965, pp. 301–304.

Keeble, F. *Plant Animals.* Cambridge: Cambridge University Press, 1910.

Klapow, L. A. Fortnightly molting and reproductive cycles in the sand-beach isopod, *Excirolana chiltoni. Biological Bulletin,* 1972, *143,* 568–591.

Koltermann, R. Periodicity in the activity and learning performance of the honeybee. In L. Barton Browne (Ed.), *Experimental Analysis of Insect Behaviour.* Berlin: Springer-Verlag, 1974, pp. 218–227.

Lickey, M. E., Block, G. D., Hudson, D. J., and Smith, J. T. Circadian oscillators and photoreceptors in the gastropod, *Aplysia. Photochemistry and Photobiology,* 1976, *23,* 253–273.

Lipton, G. R., and Sutherland, D. J. Feeding rhythms in the American cockroach, *Periplaneta americana*. *Journal of Insect Physiology*, 1970, *16*, 1757–1767.

Loher, W., and Chandrashekaran, M. K. Circadian rhythmicity in the oviposition of the grasshopper *Chorthippus curtipennis*. *Journal of Insect Physiology*, 1970, *16*, 1677–1688.

Lohmann, M. Zur Bedeutung der lokomotorischen Aktivität in circadianen Systemen. *Zeitschrift für Vergleichende Physiologie*, 1967, *55*, 307–332.

Martin, L. La mémoire chez *Convoluta roscoffensis*. *Compte Rendu Hebdomadaire des Séances de l'Académie des Sciences*. Paris, 1907, *145*, 555–557.

McCluskey, E. S., and Carter, C. E. Loss of rhythmic activity in female ants caused by mating. *Comparative Biochemistry and Physiology*, 1969, *31*, 217–226.

Meyer-Rochow, V. B., and Horridge, G. A. The eye of *Anoplognathus* (Coleoptera, Scarabaeidae). *Proceedings of the Royal Society of London*, 1975, *B. 188*, 1–30.

Minis, D. H. Parallel peculiarities in the entrainment of a circadian rhythm and photoperiodic induction in the pink boll worm *(Pectinophora gossypiella)*. In J. Aschoff (Ed.), *Circadian Clocks*. Amsterdam: North-Holland, 1965, pp. 333–343.

Minis, D. H., and Pittendrigh, C. S. Circadian oscillation controlling hatching: Its ontogeny during embryogenesis of a moth. *Science*, 1968, *159*, 534–536.

Mori, S. Influence of environmental and physiological factors on the daily rhythmic activity of a sea-pen. In *Biological Clocks—Cold Spring Harbor Symposia on Quantitative Biology*, 1960, *25*, 333–344.

Morton, B. The tidal rhythm and rhythm of feeding and digestion in *Cardium edule*. *Journal of the Marine Biological Association of the United Kingdom*, 1970, *50*, 488–512.

Nayar, J. K. The pupation rhythm in *Aedes taeniorhynchus* (Diptera: Culicidae). II. Ontogenetic timing, rate of development, and endogenous diurnal rhythm of pupation. *Annals of the Entomological Society of America*. 1967, *60*, 946–971.

Nayar, J. K., Samarawickrema, W. A., and Sauerman, D. M., Jr. Photoperiodic control of egg hatching in the mosquito *Mansonia titillans*. *Annals of the Entomological Society of America*, 1973, *66*, 831–835.

Neumann, D. Adaptations of chironomids to intertidal environments. *Annual Review of Entomology*, 1976, *21*, 387–414.

Nielsen, E. T. Activity patterns of *Eugaster* (Orthoptera: Ensifera). *Entomologia Experimentalis et Applicata*, 1974, *17*, 325–347.

Ollason, J. C., and Slater, P. J. B. Changes in the behaviour of the male zebra finch during a 12-hr day. *Animal Behaviour*, 1973, *21*, 191–196.

Palmer, J. D. A persistent, light-preference rhythm in the fiddler crab, *Uca pugnax*, and its possible adaptive significance. *American Naturalist*, 1964, *98*, 431–434.

Palmer, J. D. Tidal rhythms: The clock control of the rhythmic physiology of marine organisms. *Biological Reviews*, 1973, *48*, 377–418.

Palmer, J. D., and Round, F. E. Persistent, vertical-migration rhythms in benthic microflora. VI. The tidal and diurnal nature of the rhythm in the diatom *Hantzschia virgata*. *Biological Bulletin*, 1967, *132*, 44–55.

Payne, T. L., Shorey, H. H., and Gaston, L. K. Sex pheromones of noctuid moths: Factors influencing antennal responsiveness in males of *Trichoplusia ni*. *Journal of Insect Physiology*, 1970, *16*, 1043–1055.

Phelps, R. J., and Jackson, P. J. Factors influencing the moment of larviposition and eclosion in *Glossina morsitans orientalis* Vanderplank (Diptera: Muscidae). *Journal of the Entomological Society of South Africa*, 1971, *34*, 145–157.

Pittendrigh, C. S. The circadian oscillation in *Drosophila pseudoobscura* pupae: A model for the photoperiodic clock. *Zeitschrift für Pflanzenphysiologie*, 1966, *54*, 275–307.

Pittendrigh, C. S., and Skopik, S. D. Circadian systems. V. The driving oscillation and the temporal sequence of development. *Proceedings of the National Academy of Sciences, USA*, 1970, *65*, 500–507.

Polcik, B., Nowosielski, J. W., and Naegele, J. A. Daily rhythm of oviposition in the two-spotted spider mite. *Journal of Economic Entomology*, 1965, *58*, 467–469.

Rankin, M. A., Caldwell, R. L., and Dingle, H. An analysis of a circadian rhythm of oviposition in *Oncopeltus fasciatus*. *Journal of Experimental Biology*, 1972, *56*, 353–359.

Rao, K. P. Tidal rhythmicity of rate of water propulsion in *Mytilus*, and its modifiability by transplantation. *Biological Bulletin*, 1954, *106*, 353–359.

Rensing, L. Tagesperiodik von Aktivität und Phototaxis bei *Corixa punctata* und *Anticorixa sahlbergi*. *Zeitschrift für Vergleichende Physiologie*, 1965, *50*, 250–253.

Riddiford, L. M. The role of hormones in the reproductive behavior of female wild silkmoths. In L. Barton Brown (Ed.), *Experimental Analysis of Insect Behaviour*. Berlin: Springer-Verlag, 1974, pp. 278–285.

Ringelberg, J., and Servaas, H. A circadian rhythm in *Daphnia magna*. *Oecologia*, 1971, *6*, 289–292.

Roberts, S. K. Circadian rhythms in cockroaches—effects of optic lobe lesions. *Journal of Comparative Physiology*, 1974, *88*, 21–30.

Saunders, D. S. *Insect Clocks*. Oxford: Pergamon Press, 1976.

Schnabel, G. Der Einfluss von Licht auf die circadiane Rhythmik von *Euglena gracilis* bei Autotrophie und Mixotrophie. *Planta*, 1968, *81*, 49–63.

Shorey, H. H., and Gaston, L. K. Sex pheromones of noctuid moths. V. Circadian rhythm of pheromone-responsiveness in males of *Autographa californica, Heliothis virescens, Spodoptera exigua*, and *Trichoplusia ni* (Lepidoptera: Noctuidae). *Annals of the Entomological Society of America*, 1965, *58*, 597–600.

Sokolove, P. G. Locomotory and stridulatory circadian rhythms in the cricket, *Teleogryllus commodus*. *Journal of Insect Physiology*, 1975, *21*, 537–558.

Sokolove, P. G., and Loher, W. Rôle of eyes, optic lobes, and pars intercerebralis in locomotory and stridulatory circadian rhythms of *Teleogryllus commodus*. *Journal of Insect Physiology*, 1975, *21*, 785–799.

Sokolove, P. G., Beiswanger, C. M., Prior, D. J., and Gelperin, A. A circadian rhythm in the locomotor behaviour of the giant garden slug *Limax maximus*. *Journal of Experimental Biology*, 1977, *66*, 47–64.

Spangler, H. G. Role of light in altering the circadian oscillations of the honey bee. *Annals of the Entomological Society of America*, 1973, *66*, 449–451.

Stier, T. J. B. Diurnal changes in activities and geotropism in *Thyone briareus*. *Biological Bulletin*, 1933, *64*, 326–332.

Sukumar, R. Learning behavior and changes in the levels of RNA during learning in grasshopper, *Poecilocera picta*. *Behavioral Biology*, 1975, *14*, 343–351.

Traynier, R. M. M. Sexual behaviour of the Mediterranean flour moth, *Anagasta kühniella:* Some influences of age, photoperiod, and light intensity. *Canadian Entomologist*, 1970, *102*, 534–540.

Treherne, J. E., Foster, W. A., Evans, P. D., and Ruscoe, C. N. E. Free-running activity rhythm in the natural environment. *Nature* (London) 1977, *269*, 796–797.

Truman, J. W. Hour-glass behavior of the circadian clock controlling eclosion of the silkmoth *Antheraea pernyi*. *Proceedings of the National Academy of Sciences, USA*, 1971, *68*, 595–599.

Truman, J. W. Temperature sensitive programming of the silkmoth flight clock: A mechanism for adapting to the seasons. *Science*, 1973, *182*, 727–729.

Truman, J. W. Development and hormonal release of adult behavior patterns in silkmoths. *Journal of Comparative Physiology*, 1976, *107*, 39–48.

Truman, J. W. Hormonal release of stereotyped motor programmes from the isolated nervous system of the cecropia silkmoth. *Journal of Experimental Biology*, 1978, *74*, 151–173.

Tsutsumi, C. Characteristics of the daily behavior and activity patterns of the adult housefly with special reference to time-keeping device. *Japanese Journal of Medical Science and Biology*, 1973, *26*, 119–141.

Tychsen, P. H. The effect of photoperiod on the circadian rhythm of mating responsiveness in the fruit fly, *Dacus tryoni*. *Physiological Entomology*, 1978, *3*, 65–69.

Tychsen, P. H., and Fletcher, B. S. Studies on the rhythm of mating in the Queensland fruit fly, *Dacus tryoni*. *Journal of Insect Physiology*, 1971, *17*, 2139–2156.

Vick, K. W., Drummond, P. C., and Coffelt, J. A. *Trogoderma inclusum* and *T. glabrum:* Effects of time of day on production of female pheromone, male responsiveness, and mating. *Annals of the Entomological Society of America*, 1973, *66*, 1001–1004.

Von Frisch, K. *The Dance Language and Orientation of Bees*. London: Staples, 1967.

Wigglesworth, V. B. *The Principles of Insect Physiology* (7th ed.). London: Chapman and Hall, 1972.

Wright, J. E., Kappus, K. D., and Venard, C. E. Swarming and mating behavior in laboratory colonies of *Aedes triseriatus* (Diptera: Culicidae). *Annals of the Entomological Society of America*, 1966, *59*, 1110–1112.

Zann, L. P. Relationships between intertidal zonation and circatidal rhythmicity in littoral gastropods. *Marine Biology*, 1973, *18*, 243–250.

Zimmerman, W. F., and Ives, D. Some photophysiological aspects of circadian rhythmicity in *Drosophila*. In M. Menaker (Ed.), *Biochronometry*. Washington, D.C.: National Academy of Sciences, 1971, pp. 381–391.

9

Neural and Endocrine Control of Circadian Rhythmicity in Invertebrates

TERRY L. PAGE

INTRODUCTION

The importance of the nervous and neuroendocrine systems in the control of daily rhythms in invertebrates did not escape the notice of early workers in the field. As early as 1911, Demoll suggested that color changes in arthropods were controlled by a periodic phenomenon in the nervous system. Kalmus, in 1938, concluded that the eyestalk neurosecretory system was the source of control of the crayfish activity rhythm, and Welsh (1941) proposed that "a regular variation in the activity of nervous inhibitory centers" was the major factor in the hormonal control of the rhythmic migration of retinal shielding pigments in the crayfish. In the past two decades, a large body of evidence has been obtained that firmly establishes the proposition, implicit in much of this early work, that it is the central nervous and neuroendocrine systems that are responsible for the generation and coordination of the circadian rhythmicity of many behavioral and physiological functions.

The primary focus of research on the neural basis of circadian rhythmicity has been to identify, or at least to localize, the various components of the timing system. Research in this area, particularly in the past 15 years, has been fruitful. In the invertebrates, circadian oscillators have been localized in restricted portions of the nervous system in representatives of the mollusks, crustaceans, and insects; in many cases, photoreceptive structures involved in entrainment have been localized to visual organs or to the central nervous system, and in a few cases, the pathways by which pacemakers impose rhythmicity on some process have been specified. The successful "dissection" of the circadian system in several organisms

TERRY L. PAGE   Department of Biology, Vanderbilt University, Nashville, Tennessee 37235.

has had two major consequences. First, we have gained a greater appreciation of the complexity of circadian organization—in many cases, efforts to find "the" circadian pacemaker have revealed the existence of several pacemakers within the individual. The results have helped clarify the concept, first made explicit in studies of the formal properties of circadian rhythmicity (e.g., Pittendrigh, 1960), that there are several oscillators, and that the organism's temporal organization depends not only on the properties of individual pacemakers but on their integrative relationships as well. The second important consequence of the emerging descriptions of the anatomical organization of circadian systems is that it has made experimentally tractable many questions about the functional organization. Some progress has already been made in this area. In both *Aplysia* and the cockroach, we are beginning to understand the coupling relationships between bilaterally paired oscillators in the circadian system (Jacklet, 1971; Lickey, Block, Hudson, and Smith, 1976; Hudson and Lickey, 1977; Page, Caldarola, and Pittendrigh, 1977; Page, 1978); Truman (Truman and Riddiford, 1970; Truman, 1972; Truman and Sokolove, 1972) has been able to detail some aspects of the mechanism by which the circadian pacemaker triggers eclosion in the silkmoth; and Eskin (1972, 1977a,b) has made progress in elucidating the pathway and mechanism of entrainment in the isolated *Aplysia* eye.

In general, however, basic functional processes of the circadian system have not yet been linked to specified cells in the nervous system. This remains as a fundamental problem, central to progress in understanding circadian organization in the metazoa on a cellular level. The invertebrates—particularly mollusks and arthropods, with their simpler nervous systems, large identifiable neurons, and wealth of background neurophysiological information—would appear to offer the most promise for the precise identification of those cells that constitute the various components and pathways in the circadian system. As a consequence, they may also hold the most promise for the investigation of the cellular mechanisms by which these components are physiologically linked into an organized regulatory system.

The purpose of this review is to summarize the current state of progress in our efforts to understand the neurophysiological basis of circadian organization in the invertebrates. The first section is devoted to circadian pacemakers and entails a discussion of their location, numbers, and interactions in several organisms. The effects of circadian pacemakers on sensorimotor integration—both by their direct influence on CNS pathways and by modulation of sensory input—are discussed in the second section. The final section is concerned with entrainment of circadian pacemakers—about the location and properties of photoreceptors involved in entrainment, and about the mechanism by which they exert their effects.

Circadian Pacemakers in the Nervous System

Pacemakers in Vitro

The relative ease with which small portions of invertebrate nervous systems can be kept alive for several days, or even weeks, *in vitro,* either in a physiological saline or in culture medium, has led to the identification of a few neuronal circadian pacemakers. The best and most thoroughly studied example of these is the circadian rhythm in the isolated eye of the marine gastropod *Aplysia,* now described for several species (Jacklet, 1971, 1974), but first discovered by Jacklet (1969a) in *Aplysia californica.* The eye, which is about 0.5–1.0 mm in diameter and contains several thousand cells is complex, both morphologically and in its synaptic organization (Jacklet, 1969b; Jacklet, Alvarez, and Bernstein, 1972; Luborsky-Moore and Jacklet, 1977). The retina contains several cell types, including possibly two classes of primary receptors, secondary cells, neurosecretory cells, and pigmented support cells. The optic nerve, which attaches the eye to the cerebral ganglion, is about a centimeter long and is composed of the axons of secondary cells from the retina as well as a number of small efferent fibers from the cerebral ganglion to the eye (Eskin, 1971). The activity of the eye occurs as compound action potentials (CAPs) in the optic nerve. These may either be spontaneously generated or evoked by light. When the eye is removed from the animal and placed in constant darkness in filtered seawater or in culture medium, the frequency (Jacklet, 1969a) and amplitude (Jacklet and Geronimo, 1971; Jacklet, 1974) of CAPs exhibit a circadian rhythm that persists for several days (Figure 1). The phase of the peak activity of the eye corresponds quite closely with the time of subjective dawn when the animal has been maintained on LD 12:12 prior to eye removal. The eye can also be entrained by light cycles presented *in vitro* (Eskin, 1971). Thus, the *Aplysia* eye contains both a circadian pacemaker and a photoreceptor for entrainment. This preparation has proved especially useful as a model system for a number of pharmacological studies investigating both the mechanism of entrainment, discussed in detail below, and the molecular basis of the circadian oscillation, which is largely beyond the scope of this review.

A similar, although apparently less robust, rhythm of spontaneous neural activity has recently been discovered in the optic nerve of the predatory marine gastropod *Navanax inermis* (Eskin and Harcombe, 1977). A potential advantage of the *Navanax* eye over that of *Aplysia* is that the receptor cells are substantially larger (30 μm vs. 10 μm) and about

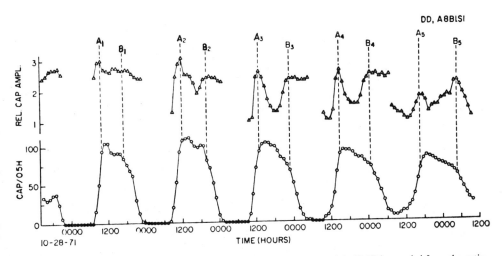

Fig. 1. The circadian rhythms in the spontaneous compound action potentials (CAPs) recorded from the optic nerve of an isolated *Aplysia* eye. The eye is maintained in constant darkness in culture medium. The lower record plots CAP frequency as a function of time. The upper record shows the rhythm of CAP amplitude that exhibits two peaks (A and B) during the subjective day. (From Jacklet, 1974. Reprinted with permission of Springer-Verlag, Heidelberg.)

$\frac{1}{10}$ as numerous. Therefore, interactions between cells may be more easily studied with intracellular recording techniques.

Circadian rhythms in frequency of action potentials have also been reported in multiunit recordings of activity in nerve roots of isolated ganglia. Strumwasser (1967) reported a circadian rhythm in continuous recordings of pericardial nerve activity of the *Aplysia* abdominal ganglion (also called the *parietovisceral ganglion*) maintained for several weeks in organ culture. He also found evidence for rhythmicity in single, unidentified units in the genital nerve of the abdominal ganglion (Strumwasser, 1974). Circadian rhythms in multiunit recordings from motor roots of the isolated abdominal nerve cords of crayfish have been recently described (Block, 1976).

These *in vitro* studies demonstrate that small, isolated portions of the nervous system can sustain circadian oscillations. However, there are still uncertainties about whether or not the circadian periodicities evident in these isolated tissues arise from a single cell or emerge from interactions among a few, several, or a large number of cells. This particular question has been examined in both the eye and the abdominal ganglion of *Aplysia* without resolution. Attempts at surgical reduction of the *Aplysia* eye to isolate the pacemaking cells have yielded conflicting results (Jacklet and Geronimo, 1971; Strumwasser, 1974); and extensive efforts to demonstrate that a single, identifiable neuron, cell R15, in the abdominal ganglion of *Aplysia* is a circadian pacemaker have not been conclusive (see reviews by Strumwasser, 1974; Lickey *et al.*, 1976).

LOCALIZATION VIA TRANSPLANTATION

Most of the research directed toward localizing neural circadian pacemakers has involved efforts to identify the oscillator that controls the timing of some particular, overtly expressed rhythm. These investigations as a rule have employed lesions as a technique, at least in early stages. Since the rhythmic expression of a behavior may involve pathways and processes quite distinct from the pacemaker, loss of rhythmicity as a consequence of some lesion is not necessarily a result exclusive to pacemaker destruction, and interpretations of experiments utilizing surgical or electrolytic lesions to the nervous system must be made cautiously.

One experimental technique that has been used to overcome these interpretive obstacles is that of tissue transplantation. In at least one instance in which the pacemaker exerts its effects hormonally, it has been possible by transplantation of putative pacemaker tissue to demonstrate the location of a circadian pacemaker. In a series of now classic experiments on silkmoths, Truman and Riddiford (1970; Truman, 1972) convincingly demonstrated that the circadian pacemaker that controls the time of eclosion is located in the brain. They worked with two species of silkmoth, *Hyalophora cecropia* and *Antheraea pernyi*. In both species, the emergence of the pharate adult from the pupal case is "gated" by a circadian oscillator; and when placed in constant darkness, populations will exhibit a daily peak of eclosion (Truman, 1971b). The time of day that each species emerges is different, however. When raised on 24-hr light cycles consisting of 17 hr of light followed by 7 hr of darkness, *H. cecropia* emerges during a gate approximately 8 hr in duration, which opens 1 hr after lights-on. *A. pernyi*, on the other hand, emerges in the last 5.5 hr before lights-off (Figure 2A). While removal of the brains of these animals did not prevent eclosion, "brainless" moths emerged at random times throughout the day (Figure 2B). If the brain was removed from the head but reimplanted in the abdomen, normal rhythmicity was restored: populations exhibited a freerunning eclosion rhythm in constant conditions (Truman, 1972) and emerged at the appropriate time of day in a light cycle (Figure 2C) (Truman and Riddiford, 1970; Truman, 1972). These results implicated the brain as the site of a clock that controlled the time of emergence via release of an eclosion hormone. The conclusive evidence, however, was provided by experiments in which brains were removed from the head of one species and transplanted into the abdomen of the other. Moths that had received these "switched-brain" transplants exhibited the normal stereotypic eclosion behavior for the host species; however, the phase of the eclosion rhythm in LD 17:7 was characteristic of the donor and not the host: *A. pernyi* that had received *H. cecropia* brains emerged just after dawn, while *H. cecropia* receiving *A. pernyi* brains emerged near dusk (Figure 2D).

The demonstration that the transplanted brains not only restored rhythmicity but *also determined the phase* of the rhythm in the host moths leaves virtually no doubt that the circadian pacemaker that controls the time of emergence is located in the brain. In an attempt to determine which part of the brain is responsible for timing the eclosion behavior, the brain was subdivided prior to transplantation (Truman, 1972, 1974a). The results suggested that the optic lobes are unnecessary since intact cerebral lobes adequately gated eclosion. When the cerebral lobes were subdivided, however, by cuts made laterally to the medial neurosecretory cell groups that are the site of production of the hormone that triggers eclosion behavior (Truman, 1973—see below), the isolated median piece did not gate the emergence. This suggested the possibility that the lateral portion of the cerebral lobes contains the pacemaker.

Similar transplantation experiments have been attempted in the cockroach with controversial results. The evidence for hormonal involvement in the control of the locomotor activity rhythm of the cockroach, *Periplaneta americana*, originated with a short report by Harker (1954). She found that when an arrhythmic roach was parabiotically linked (back

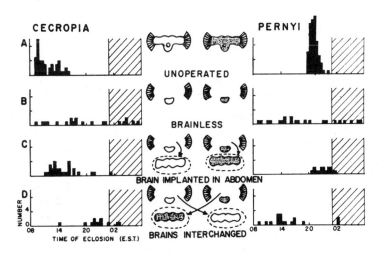

Fig. 2. The time of eclosion of *Hyalophora cecropia* and *Antheraea pernyi* moths in a 17-hr light: 7-hr dark regimen showing the effects of brain removal, transplantation of the brain to the abdomen, and interchange of brains between two species. After brain exchange, the host emerges at the eclosion time characteristic of the donor species. (From Truman, 1971a. Reprinted with permission of the Centre for Agricultural Publishing and Documentation, Wageningen, The Netherlands.)

to back) with a normally rhythmic but immobilized roach, rhythmicity was restored for about a week. The design and interpretation of this experiment has come under a great deal of criticism for several reasons, including (1) there were no control pairs with unconnected hemocoels and (2) the host animal was made arrhythmic by exposing it for several days to constant light, although it is now clear that cockroaches may remain rhythmic indefinitely in LL (Cymborowski and Brady, 1972). Nevertheless, the result led Harker to search for a hormonal clock. Harker had discovered that beheaded roaches no longer exhibited an activity rhythm, and she attempted to restore rhythmicity by implanting the subesophageal ganglion (SEG) of one donor animal into another, headless host. It was reported that the procedure did restore rhythmicity for at least a few days (Harker, 1956), and that the phase of the newly restored host rhythm was the same as that of the donor prior to transplantation (Harker, 1960).

Unfortunately, attempts to repeat these very important transplantation experiments have failed (Roberts, 1966; Brady, 1967), and a large body of other evidence (reviewed by Brady, 1971, 1974; also see next section) argues convincingly against a hormonal primary clock mechanism in the SEG. Furthermore, it has been shown that destruction of the neurosecretory cells *in situ* in the SEG by microcautery (Brady, 1967) or by surgical removal (Nishiitsutsuji-Uwo and Pittendrigh, 1968b) does not affect the rhythm in otherwise intact animals.

While these results are difficult to reconcile with Harker's hypothesis, it is interesting to note that the original parabiosis experiments have been successfully repeated recently. Cymborowski and Brady (1972), cognizant of several objections to the design of Harker's original experiments, have convincingly demonstrated in both *P. americana* and the cricket, *Acheta domesticus,* that rhythms could be driven in headless animals by a blood-borne factor released by a parabiotically coupled donor. They were, however, cautious in their interpretation and suggested several alternatives to Harker's conclusion that the rhythm is normally hormonally controlled.

LOCALIZATION VIA LESIONS

The apparent failure of Harker's hypothesis that the SEG contained the circadian pacemaker that controlled the activity rhythm in the cockroach led the search elsewhere in the CNS. In 1968, Nishiitsutsuji-Uwo and Pittendrigh (1968b) focused attention on the optic lobes of the brain. They reported that complete ablation of these structures, or section of the optic tracts, caused persistent arrhythmicity without significantly affecting the level of activity and suggested that they may contain the circadian pacemaker that controls the activity rhythm. Loher (1972) has made a similar observation in the cricket. He found that bilateral ablation of the optic lobes in *Teleogryllus commodus* completely disrupted the rhythm in stridulation (Figure 3), and it was later shown that lobe ablation also abolished both the circadian rhythms of spermatophore formation (Loher, 1974) and locomotion (Sokolove and Loher, 1975). These results, while suggestive, did not demonstrate that the optic lobes were the site of the pacemaker, only that they were necessary to sustain the rhythm. Subsequent experiments, however, have provided finer localization of the crucial cells and further evidence that these cells are involved in pacemaker function.

In both the cricket and the cockroach, unilateral optic-lobe ablation does not abolish rhythmicity (Nishiitsutsuji-Uwo and Pittendrigh, 1968b; Loher, 1972; Page *et al.,* 1977).

This fact was exploited by both Roberts and Sokolove to further localize the putative optic-lobe pacemaker in the cockroach. Roberts (1974), working with both *Leucophaea maderae* and *Periplaneta americana,* removed all of one optic lobe and with surgical lesions removed various amounts of the contralateral optic lobe. He found the most distal neuropil area, the lamina, to be dispensable for the maintenance of the freerunning rhythm. However, more proximal cuts that removed the medulla invariably caused arrhythmicity. Animals that had part of the medulla removed gave an intermediate result, with 1 animal being clearly rhythmic, 7 being clearly arrhythmic, and 17 being possibly rhythmic. Roberts also obtained similar results with electrolytic lesions and concluded that "normal freerunning rhythmicity depends on an intact medulla–lobula complex." Sokolove (1975a) published a similar study on *Leucophaea* in which he utilized small electrolytic rather than surgical lesions. His results were similar to Roberts's in that he found no evidence that the lamina was involved, but in contrast only 3 of 31 animals with lesions in the medulla were clearly aperiodic. On the other hand, lesions in the ventral half of the lobe in the region of the second optic chiasm and lobula were frequently effective in abolishing the rhythm. Sokolove hypothesized that it was the somata of cells in this area that were crucial and suggested that Roberts's surgical lesions through the medulla were likely to have damaged these cells.

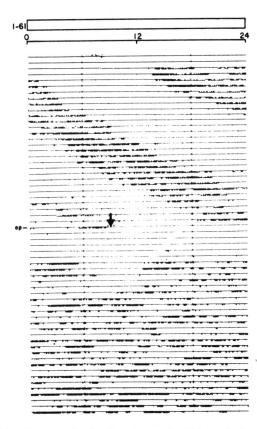

Fig. 3. Effects of optic lobe ablation on the circadian rhythm of stridulation in the cricket, *Teleogryllus commodus.* The event record begins with the intact animal freerunning in constant light. On Day 30 (arrow), bilateral destruction of the optic lobes abolishes rhythmicity. (From Loher, 1972. Reprinted with permission of Springer-Verlag, Heidelberg.)

More recently, Page (1978) has obtained results essentially identical to those of Sokolove, and has also concluded that the cells in the ventral half of the lobe near the lobula are critical to maintenance of rhythmicity, and that the medulla is not involved.

The finer localization of the portion of the optic lobe involved in sustaining rhythmicity did not alleviate the uncertainty that these cells may be necessary only for the expression of the rhythm and do not necessarily constitute the pacemaker that times it. Two recent studies (described in more detail in the next section), however, have provided evidence that strongly supports the notion that the optic lobes are involved in pacemaker activity. It has been shown that although either the right or the left lobe alone is sufficient to maintain rhythmicity, ablation of either one of the lobes has the consistent effect of lengthening the period of the freerunning rhythm, while control operations such as optic nerve section have no effect on period (Page et al., 1977). Furthermore, utilizing electrolytic lesions, it was found that the same region of the optic lobe (ventral and near the lobula) that is necessary to sustain rhythmicity also contains the cells crucial to maintaining the normal freerunning period (Page, 1978). The fact that both the maintenance and the normal period of the rhythm depends on these cells suggests that this region of the optic lobes contains at least part of the pacemaking system that controls the activity rhythm in the cockroach.

Although the evidence for involvement of the optic lobes in pacemaker function is reasonably convincing, lesions to other regions of the brain can also evoke arrhythmicity, and their involvement in the circadian timing process remains uncertain. Of particular interest is the pars intercerebralis. Lesions to the pars of cockroaches often results in arrhythmicity in locomotor activity (Roberts, 1966; Nishiitsutsuji-Uwo, Petropulos, and Pittendrigh, 1967), and in crickets, destruction of the pars frequently abolishes rhythmicity in spermatophore production (Loher, 1974), stridulation (Loher, 1974; Sokolove and Loher, 1975), and locomotor activity (Cymborowski, 1973; Sokolove and Loher; 1975). Whether or not these results reflect a participatory role for the pars in generating the circadian oscillation or whether this region merely couples the oscillator to the overt rhythms (generally the most favored hypothesis) is not certain (Loher, 1974; Sokolove and Loher, 1975). The possible role of the pars in driving overt rhythms is discussed more fully in the next section.

Several lesion studies have been undertaken in an effort to localize pacemakers that control circadian and tidal rhythmicity in decapod Crustacea. The results of early studies implicated the eyestalks in the control of locomotor activity. These structures contain a substantial portion of the protocerebrum (the optic lobes) as well as the X-organ-sinus gland complex, a major neurosecretory organ.

Much of the work has been done on crayfish, and Hans Kalmus (1938) first drew attention to the eyestalks of decapods when he reported that ablation of these structures in the crayfish, Potamobius and Cambarus, resulted in an apparent loss of circadian activity rhythm. Similar results were obtained in subsequent ablation experiments on Cambarus by both Schalleck (1942) and Roberts (1944). These studies demonstrated that eyestalk removal disrupts the normal control of locomotor activity and, in most cases, totally obscures periodicity. There is, however, reason to be cautious in the interpretation of these results—particularly with respect to the location of the pacemaker. First, in a recent study on the activity rhythm of the crayfish, Procambarus clarkii, it was found that a large proportion of animals exhibited rhythmicity following eyestalk ablation (Page and Larimer, 1975a). Clearly, the eyestalks are not the only pacemaker locus. Second, there are complicating factors that make the aperiodicity frequently seen following eyestalk removal difficult to interpret. The optic lobes and eyestalk neurosecretory system have been implicated in a large number of physiological and behavioral processes, and their removal is certain to have major effects exclusive of any role they may play in circadian organization. Furthermore, eyestalk removal in crayfish results in a pronounced increase in activity levels, which tends to obscure rhythmicity (Schalleck, 1942; Roberts, 1944; Page and Larimer, 1975a). Page and Larimer found, for example, that *P. clarkii* were almost continuously active following eyestalk ablation; rhythmicity was expressed as a modulation in the amount of activity, apparent only in a quantitative analysis.

Although eyestalk ablation does not consistently abolish locomotor rhythmicity in the crayfish, neural isolation of thoracic motor centers from the supraesophageal ganglion by section of the circumesophageal connectives (CEC) invariably results in aperiodic behavior (Page and Larimer, 1975a; Gordon, Larimer, and Page, 1977). This observation suggests that the pacemaker controlling the rhythm is located in the brain and drives the rhythm via neuronal pathways in the CEC. The data, however, are more complex than is indicated by this simple hypothesis. Although eyestalk structures are not required for rhythmicity, they do have a significant effect on the circadian organization of locomotor activity exclusive of their effect on activity levels. First, the frequent loss of rhythmicity following eyestalk ablation, observed in all studies, should not be completely disregarded. Second, in crayfish, the eyestalks have a major influence on the phase relationship between peak activity of the entrained rhythm and the ambient light cycles. In intact animals, peak activity occurs within 1–2 hr of the light-to-dark transition (in LD 12:12). In contrast, in the eyestalk-ablated animals, the peak generally occurs 6–10 hr later, and the phase angle appears to be much less stable within the individual and much more variable between individuals (Page and Larimer, 1975a).

Further data on the role of the eyestalks in the organization of the circadian system in crayfish has come from studies on the rhythm of migration of the retinal shielding pigments. In the crayfish, there are two sets of mobile retinal pigments, the proximal and the distal shielding pigments, which rhythmically migrate to shield or expose the ommatidia from light scattered within the eye (Welsh, 1941; Bennitt, 1932). The position of the pigments appears to be accurately reflected in the amplitude of the electroretinogram (ERG) (Aréchiga and Fuentes, 1970). It has been reported that the rhythm of retinal pigment migration is abolished when the supraesophageal ganglion is removed (Aréchiga, Fuentes, and Barrera, 1973), when the eyestalk is neurally isolated from the ganglion by cutting the optic tract (Page and Larimer, 1975b), or when the eyestalk is removed from the animal, although in the latter case, an ERG rhythm does persist (Sanchez and Fuentes-Pardo, 1977). Rhythmic migration is unaffected, however, when the CEC are cut, isolating the supraesophageal ganglion–optic lobe complex from the remainder of the CNS (Page and Larimer, 1975b). As in the case of locomotor activity, the simplest interpretation of the results is that the driving oscillator resides in the supraesophageal ganglion. Recently, however, it has been reported that in "brainless" *P. bouveri* maintained in dim light a rhythm of retinal pigment migration can be detected, although it is greatly reduced in amplitude (Barrera-Mera, 1976).

Thus, in the case of both locomotor activity and retinal pigment migration, an intact supraesophageal ganglion–optic lobe complex is necessary to maintain *normal* rhythmicity. On the other hand, both the brain and the optic lobe are apparently independently able to sustain rhythmicity. Before discussing the implications of these findings, it will be useful to summarize work on other decapods.

In a study on the tidal activity rhythm of the crab, *Carcinus,* Naylor and Williams (1968) found that ablation of the eyestalks invariably abolished rhythmicity. This aperiodicity was accompanied by an initial period of hyperactivity (about 12 hr) followed by a reduction in activity to below normal levels. They also made the interesting discovery that in intact individuals that were aperiodic following damping of the tidal rhythm in constant conditions, rhythmicity could be reinitiated by chilling the animal (10–12 hr at 4°C). Furthermore, while induction of rhythmicity could be accomplished by local chilling of the eyestalks alone, chilling had no effect on animals made aperiodic by eyestalk ablation. This observation yields to several alternative explanations, and Naylor and Williams (1968) were cautious in their interpretation.

Work on several other crabs has reiterated the effects of eyestalk ablation on rhythmicity. For example, Bliss (1962) was unable to detect the normal circadian activity rhythm in most *Gecarcinus* following this operation. Interestingly, however, in one individual, rhythmicity persisted, but with a greatly reduced freerunning period (Bliss, 1962).

Most of the results obtained from decapods can be accommodated by a simple scheme in which the oscillator is assumed to reside in the supraesophageal ganglion, and eyestalk structures function as a major output pathway coupling the pacemaker to the overt rhythms. There are three observations, however, that do not readily yield to this model. First is the reduction in freerunning period in *Gecarcinus* following eyestalk removal (Bliss, 1962); second is the major effect of eyestalk ablation on entrainment in *P. clarkii,* particularly with respect to the phase angle in steady state (Page and Larimer, 1975a); and finally is the persistence of the rhythm of retinal pigment migration in "brainless" crayfish (Barrera-Mera, 1976) and of ERG amplitude in isolated eyestalks (Sanchez and Fuentes-Pardo, 1977). The first two observations are perhaps most easily dealt with by postulating that an oscillatory component of the circadian system resides in the eyestalks; the last observation demands it.

The concept of two oscillators in decapods is not new. It was alluded to by both Bliss (1962) and Naylor and Williams (1968) and was presented in a formal model by Page and Larimer (1975a). Nevertheless, we still have only a vague impression of the organization of the circadian system in decapods, and few observations are currently available that clarify the functional roles of the two oscillators—one residing in the supraesophageal ganglion, the other in the eyestalks—in the control of rhythmicity.

The circadian rhythm in frequency of compound action potentials observed in the isolated eyes of *Aplysia* (see above) represents, perhaps, the clearest demonstration that a restricted portion of the nervous system can function as a self-sustained circadian pacemaker. The fact that *Aplysia* also exhibit a circadian rhythm of locomotor activity (Kupferman, 1968; Strumwasser, 1967) prompts the question of what role, if any, the ocular oscillator plays in the behavioral rhythm. The answer is not yet clear.

Aplysia californica are predominantly diurnal. When they are placed in a light cycle (LD 12:12), the majority of the activity occurs during the periods of lights-on, although there is often some activity just prior to the dark–light transition. In short photoperiods (LD 8:16), the positive phase angle between activity onset and dawn can be as much as 4 hr (Lickey *et al.,* 1976; Lickey, Wozniak, Block, Hudson, and Augter, 1977). Lickey and his co-workers (1976, 1977) found that subsequent to surgical removal of the eyes, the predawn activity is lost and the onset of the major peak of activity becomes tightly synchronized to lights-on. The essentially diurnal pattern of activity is retained, however, and persists, apparently indefinitely.

Some eyeless *Aplysia* also retain the ability to express a freerunning rhythm in constant conditions, although the clarity of the rhythms appears to be at least qualitatively impaired (Block and Lickey, 1973; Lickey *et al.*, 1976, 1977). Lickey *et al.* (1977) have subjectively scored a large number of activity records of both eyeless and intact *Aplysia* freerunning in constant conditions. They classified 9 of 20 records from intact animals as "good" freeruns, 8 were "average," and 3 were considered "poor." In contrast, only 2 of 33 eyeless animals were "good" freerunners, 11 were "average," and 20 were "poor." The results demonstrated that a circadian pacemaker competent to drive an activity rhythm in constant conditions exists somewhere outside the eyes, but the data also implicated eyes in the control of rhythmic activity. The exact function of the eye in this context is not certain. There are many alternative hypotheses that could accommodate the data—some of which do not involve the eye as a pacemaker—though it seems likely that the eyes do contribute significantly in the capacity of a circadian clock (Lickey *et al.*, 1977).

Multiple Pacemakers

The results described in the previous section illustrate one point rather decisively—that the circadian systems of invertebrates are comprised of more than one oscillator. The evidence for bilaterally paired oscillators is incontrovertible in *Aplysia* and *Navanax*, where it has been possible to isolate the two eyes from a single animal and show that each, independently, can sustain a circadian rhythm. In the cockroach, the data are also reasonably strong for a bilaterally paired system; each optic lobe, independently, is capable of sustaining rhythmicity. Finally, there is evidence from the beetle, *Blaps gigas*, for bilateral distribution of pacemakers that control the ERG rhythms in the two eyes (Koehler and Fleissner, 1978).

The data reviewed in the last section also point to the fact that multiple and, in contrast to the bilateral case, "nonredundant" (both functionally and anatomically) circadian pacemakers are an ubiquitous feature of invertebrate circadian systems. In *Aplysia*, besides the ocular oscillators, it appears that there is at least one other pacemaker located in the abdominal ganglion. In crayfish, the isolated abdominal ganglia and eyestalks account for two separate oscillators, and another apparently resides in the supraesophageal ganglion. Finally, in cockroaches and crickets, there is evidence that there may be a circadian pacemaker outside the optic lobes. Rence and Loher (1975) reported that the stridulatory behavior of crickets in which the optic lobes had been removed was rhythmic in a 24-hr temperature cycle of 10°C amplitude. In the temperature cycle, these lobeless crickets, which were aperiodic in constant conditions, restricted their stridulatory activity to the first several hours after the transition from high temperature (W) to low temperature (C). Two suggestive, though not compelling, observations suggested that the periodicity reflected the entrainment of an oscillatory system. First, a few transient cycles in the stridulatory rhythm were observed upon initiation of the temperature cycle (W:C 12:12) or following a single 12-hr low-temperature pulse. Second, lobeless animals were not rhythmic when subjected to a temperature cycle with a period outside the circadian range (W:C 15:15). Lobeless cockroaches will also exhibit a rhythm of locomotor activity when placed in a temperature cycle of 6°C amplitude (Page, unpublished). Furthermore, the phase-angle difference between the onset of activity and the W to C transition varies as a function of the period of the temperature cycle. These results on lobeless crickets and cockroaches are difficult to explain as simple reflexive behavior to a change in ambient temperature, and they are at least consistent with the hypothesis that the temperature cycle is acting through a strongly damped oscillator.

Thus, with the exception of the silkmoth, in every invertebrate where a careful search for "the" biological clock has been made, evidence for the existence of multiple (and "non-redundant") pacemakers has been found. This fact prompts a number of questions about the organization of circadian systems in these organisms in particular and in multicellular forms in general (Block and Page, 1978). Perhaps one of the most important questions is whether the "residual" rhythmicity often observed following removal of a putative driving oscillator reflects the presence of a pacemaker that is a major part of the timing system, or whether it simply represents the ability of many cells or tissues to exhibit circadian behavior under appropriate conditions. If these "residual" pacemakers do play a functional role in the circadian system, are they secondary slave oscillators controlled hierarchically by a primary driving oscillator—similar to the formal description of the *Drosophila* system (e.g., Pittendrigh, 1960)—or alternatively, are they components of a pacemaking system composed of a distributed network of mutually coupled oscillators?

There are three cases in which the bilateral distribution of circadian pacemakers in bilaterally symmetric animals has made possible investigations of the coupling relationships between pacemakers in a multioscillator system. Two questions with regard to the bilaterally distributed pacemakers have been examined in some detail. First, are the two pacemakers, left and right, functionally equivalent? and second, are they in some way coupled to form a compound pacemaker that formally behaves as though it were a single oscillator?

In *Aplysia,* it appears in simultaneous recordings from two eyes of the same animal that the two rhythms of CAP activity are virtually identical in phase, period, and waveform (for example, see Figure 1 in Jacklet, 1974). In the cockroach, it has not been possible to measure the frequencies of both the left and the right pacemakers in the same individuals. Nevertheless, systematic measurements of the freerunning periods of the activity rhythms of a number of individuals with only one optic lobe intact have shown that, at least as measured by their *average* frequency, left and right pacemakers are not significantly different: both have periods of about 23.95 hr at 24.5°C (Page *et al.*, 1977). Although firm conclusions are premature, the data from these studies suggest that at least to a first approximation, these anatomically redundant pacemakers are also functionally redundant.

A priori, it would seem reasonable to expect bilaterally paired oscillators to be mutually coupled; thus, any frequency instability or differences in freerunning period would be shared between the two pacemakers. In both *Aplysia* and the cockroach, there is evidence to suggest that the pacemakers are coupled. In the beetle, *Blaps gigas,* however, recent evidence suggests independent left and right pacemakers.

Hudson and Lickey (1977) examined the phase relationships between eyes of individual *Aplysia* that had been freerunning in DD or very dim LL. The phase difference for pairs of eyes removed 0–7 days after the initiation of constant conditions ranged between

0 and 1 hr—the eyes remained in phase. The phase angle between the majority of pairs of eyes dissected after 8 days, however, was 10–12 hr, while only a few pairs remained nearly synchronous. In no instance were pairs of eyes observed to have a phase angle within the range of 4–7.5 hr. The results suggest there are two stable phase relationships between the two ocular pacemakers in an animal, either in phase or in antiphase. This, in turn, implies that the eyes are coupled. However, it has been shown that one eye can be easily driven out of phase with the other eye *in vivo* by monocularly applied light cycles, a fact that suggests the coupling between the two eyes must be relatively weak (Jacklet, 1971; Lickey *et al.*, 1976).

Evidence in cockroaches also suggests that the bilaterally paired pacemakers are mutually coupled. The hypothesis that the optic lobes function as the circadian pacemaker controlling the activity rhythm was first prompted by the observation that ablation of the optic lobes or section of the optic tracts invariably causes persistent arrhythmicity (Nishiit-sutsuji-Uwo and Pittendrigh, 1968b). In a more recent study, Page *et al.* (1977) found that while either the left or the right lobe is sufficient to sustain rhythmicity, destruction of either one of the lobes consistently lengthened the freerunning period ($\overline{\Delta \tau} = 0.23$ hr) (Figure 4). On the basis of these results, it was proposed that the optic lobe pacemakers are mutually coupled and accelerate each other to form a compound pacemaker whose freerunning period is shorter than either constitutent oscillator. It was also suggested that mutual coupling could account for the fact, illustrated in Figure 4, that either of the compound eyes, which are the sole photoreceptors for entrainment (see below), can readily entrain both pacemakers (Page *et al.*, 1977).

The validity of the hypothesis of mutual coupling rested heavily on the assumption that the same optic lobe cells that were involved in sustaining rhythmicity were also responsible for maintaining the normal period and for mediating entrainment of the contralateral pacemaker. This was shown in a subsequent study utilizing small electrolytic lesions. The sufficiency of one compound eye to entrain the pacemaker of the contralateral lobe and the normal freerunning period depended on the integrity of cells in the ventral portion of the

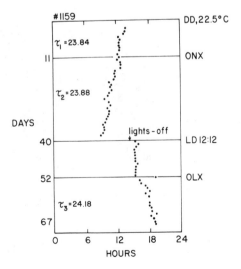

Fig. 4. Record of the activity rhythm of the cockroach, *Leucophaea maderae,* that illustrates the sufficiency of either compound eye (here the left eye) to mediate entrainment of the contralateral pacemaker and shows the effects of optic lobe ablation on the freerunning period. Onsets of daily activity peaks are shown by filled circles. The record begins with the animal freerunning in constant darkness (DD). Section of the right optic nerve (ONX) has no significant effect on the period. On Day 40, the animal was placed in an LD cycle that imposed a large phase delay on the rhythm. On Day 52, the left optic lobe was removed (OLX). The roach began to freerun in the light cycle, driven by the right-optic-lobe pacemaker, with an initial phase determined by the light cycle—the left eye was sufficient to entrain the right pacemaker. The freerunning period after removal of one lobe was significantly longer than the period in the earlier DD freerun. (From Page *et al.,* 1977.)

lobe near the lobula (Page, 1978), the same region identified as being crucial to the maintenance of rhythmicity (Sokolove, 1975a; Page, 1978). These results strongly support the
notion that cells in this region of the optic lobe function as bilaterally paired pacemaker
elements in a mutually coupled system.

Results from a recent study on the beetle, *Blaps gigas*, suggest that the ERG rhythms
in the two eyes of a single individual are controlled by independent pacemakers. The
rhythms from the eyes, monitored in constant darkness, have been found to freerun with
different periods (Koehler and Fleissner, 1978). Furthermore, the phase and period of the
rhythm in one of the eyes can be controlled in local illumination of the eye (either LD or
LL) without any consistent effect on the rhythm in the contralateral eye (Figure 5). The
results suggest that the rhythm in each eye is controlled by its own pacemaker, and that
the two pacemakers are either independent or only very weakly coupled.

The desynchronization of pacemakers in *Aplysia* and *Blaps* suggests that these organisms must rely on daily cues from the environment to maintain the appropriate phase relationship (Hudson and Lickey, 1977; Koehler and Fleissner, 1978). In the cockroach, however, there is no evidence that the optic lobe pacemakers either spontaneously desynchronize
or that they can be driven out of phase with unilateral illumination (Page *et al.*, 1977). In
this case, maintenance of synchrony appears to be accomplished by mutual entrainment
between the optic lobe pacemakers.

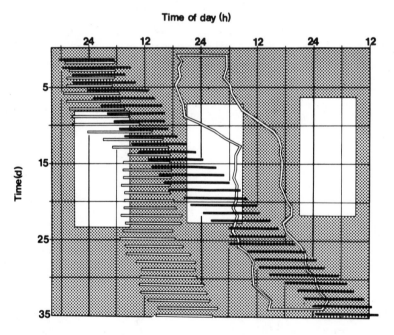

Fig. 5. The independence of the circadian ERG amplitude rhythms in the beetle *Blaps gigas*. The horizontal
bars mark the time during which the ERG of the left eye (open bars) and right eye (closed bars) were in the
night phase (high amplitude). Desynchronization begins almost immediately in DD (Days 1–5). On Days 9–
23, the left eye was exposed and entrained by an LD cycle. The right eye, which remained in DD throughout
the experiment, was unaffected. The envelope of night phases of the left eye is repeated once. (From Koehler
and Fleissner, 1978. Reprinted with permission of Macmillan Journals Ltd., London.)

Circadian Modulation of CNS and Neurosecretory Activity

In the previous section, the problem of pacemaker localization was considered. The results from work on several organisms suggest that restricted portions of the nervous system can function as circadian pacemakers; and in a number of cases, the site of the pacemaker(s) that appeared to exert primary control over the timing of certain overt rhythms was reasonably well localized. In this section, another question central to understanding circadian organization is examined. How do these circadian oscillators impose periodicity on various physiological and behavioral processes? With few exceptions, this question appears to have been asked only within the context of identifying the location of the oscillator, without addressing the more general and equally intriguing question of how the circadian system is able to impose rhythmicity on a large number of diverse processes and behaviors simultaneously. This problem will be difficult to approach experimentally until we have identified the pathways by which the circadian system exerts its effects. What purely neural pathways are involved? Is the neuroendocrine system utilized? At what level in the sensorimotor organization does the pacemaker begin to exert control?

Rhythmicity within cells of the neurosecretory and endocrine systems has been examined in a number of organisms (Brady, 1974). Rhythms of nuclear size, histological appearance, RNA synthesis, spectrophotometric absorbance, and ultrastructural changes have been described. In many instances, these results have prompted various hypotheses concerning the hormonal control of circadian rhythmicity. However, the relationship between these rhythms and the overt behavior and physiology of the organisms is obscure. As Brady (1974) has taken pains to point out, any two processes that exhibit a daily rhythm are inevitably temporally correlated but are not necessarily causally related. Furthermore, in all but one study, no convincing evidence is offered that the rhythms persist in constant conditions. In the one exception, Aréchiga and Mena (1975; Aréchiga, 1974) have examined the amount of distal retinal pigment light adapting hormone (DPLH) in the crayfish optic lobe. Utilizing gel electrophoresis, they isolated the hormone from the optic lobes of animals that had been maintained in constant darkness for 72 hr and sacrificed at various times throughout the subsequent 24-hr period. The density of the DPLH band in the gel covaried with the rhythm of retinal pigment migration, and as expected, the lowest concentration in the lobe occurred during the subjective day, when the hormone is postulated to be released into the circulatory system and to cause the pigments to move to a light-adapted position.

Although the study of rhythmicity in neurosecretory cells has revealed little about their role in circadian organization, in the invertebrates there are several cases in which there is almost certainly a neuroendocrine link in the pathway by which the circadian oscillator normally imposes rhythmicity on some processes. There is, however, only one case in which this link is well documented: the control of eclosion behavior in the silkmoth. The importance of the silkmoth brain in gating eclosion, as well as the hormonal nature of the trigger, was demonstrated in the transplantation experiments described in the previous section (Truman and Riddiford, 1970; Truman, 1972). The eclosion hormone is probably produced in the medial neurosecretory cells of the pars intercerebralis and released via neurohemal organs, the corpora cardiaca (Truman, 1973). During the larval and pupal stages, extracts of the brains and corpora cardiaca exhibit almost no hormonal activity, but as adult development takes place, the activity levels in the brain and corpora cardiaca gradually increase (Truman, 1973). The onset of the eclosion gate is accompanied by a rapid decrease in the brain and corpora cardiaca levels of hormone and an appearance of activity in the blood.

The release of the eclosion hormone triggers a stereotyped sequence of behavior, primarily involving abdominal movements, which ultimately results in emergence of the adult (Truman, 1971c). There is evidence to suggest that the motor score is preprogrammed in the abdominal nerve cord. The isolated abdomen injected with crude hormone extract performs the preeclosion behavior (Truman, 1971c), and the motor neuron activity responsible can be recorded with suction electrodes on the motor roots of a completely deafferented nerve cord (Truman and Sokolove, 1972). It appears, then, that the circadian pacemaker triggers the release of the eclosion hormone at the appropriate time of day. This hormone, in turn, initiates a motor program, present in the neural circuitry of the abdomen, that subsequently results in the emergence of the adult.

Neuroendocrine control of locomotor activity rhythms has also been postulated for a wide range of invertebrates, including various decapod Crustacea (Kalmus, 1938; Roberts, 1944; Bliss, 1962; Naylor and Williams, 1968); cockroaches (Harker, 1954, 1960; Nishiitsutsuji-Uwo and Pittendrigh, 1968b); crickets (Cymborowski, 1973); and scorpions (Rao and Gropalakrishnareddy, 1967). However, in none of these instances is the evidence particularly compelling, and in cockroaches and crayfish specifically, the data suggest that the coupling pathway is neuronal, not hormonal.

Harker (1954) was the first to suggest that the cockroach activity rhythm was hormonally controlled. Her specific hypothesis involving neurosecretory cells of the subesophageal ganglion was not substantiated by later work (see above). However, in the mid- to late 1960s, an alternative hypothesis implicating a hormonal pathway that involved the neurosecretory cells of the pars intercerebralis was developed.

Roberts (1966) first focused attention on the pars with a report that surgical lesions in the area "generally evoke arrhythmicity." Shortly afterward, in a systematic study on the effects of surgical ablation of the pars, it was found that lesions often resulted in arrhythmicity (Nishiitsutsuji-Uwo et al., 1967). Furthermore, there was a correlation between the presence or absence of neurosecretory cells in the pars region of lesioned animals and the postoperative regeneration of rhythmicity. In a subsequent study, Nishiitsutsuji-Uwo and Pittendrigh (1968b) reported that bilateral section of the circumesophageal connectives (CEC) isolating the brain from the rest of the central nervous system did not affect the activity rhythm.

On the basis of these results, it was suggested that a hormonal pathway, involving neurosecretory cells in pars, coupled the thoracic locomotor circuits to a circadian pacemaker, presumably located in the optic lobes (Nishiitsutsjui-Uwo and Pittendrigh, 1968b). More recent data, however, suggest that this hypothesis is unlikely. Roberts, Skopik, and Driskill (1971) have found that complete severance of the CEC invariably led to arrhythmicity in *Leucophaea*. They also reported that following the surgical procedure outlined in the Nishiitsutsuji-Uwo and Pittendrigh paper led them to cut nerves to the mouth parts instead of to the CEC. That CEC section does cause arrhythmicity has been verified (Brady, 1967; Page, unpublished observation; and see Pittendrigh's comment in Roberts *et al.,* 1971). Thus, it seems likely that the link between the pacemaker (optic lobes) and thoracic motor centers does involve a neuronal pathway in the CEC. This does not necessarily rule out the involvement of a neurosecretory step; on the other hand, the correlation between the presence or absence of stainable neurosecretory cells and the presence or absence of rhythmicity in animals with lesions of the pars reported by Nishiitsutsuji-Uwo *et al.* (1967) might have simply reflected the completeness of ablation of both neurosecretory and nonneurosecretory cells in that region; and one might also expect such a correlation even if the nonneurosecretory cells were mediating rhythmicity (Sokolove and Loher, 1975).

The involvement of the pars intercerebralis in the control of circadian rhythmicity in the cricket has been the subject of numerous investigations. As discussed above, lesions in the pars frequently abolish the circadian rhythms of stridulation, locomotion, and spermatophore production. In the case of locomotor activity, this result has led to the proposal that the rhythm is humorally controlled (Cymborowski, 1973). However, the arguments for a humoral control mechanism involving the pars intercerebralis are based mainly on the effects of lesions and on the observed rhythms (in LD) of intracellular processes of the neurosecretory cells and are not really compelling (see discussion in Sokolove and Loher, 1975). Sokolove and Loher (1975), on the other hand, have proposed an intermediary role for the pars in the control of rhythmicity that emphasizes the presence of nonneurosecretory neurons in this region. They suggested that different cells in the pars, driven by a circadian pacemaker located elsewhere in the brain, subserve different periodicities, some of which may be hormonally driven (e.g., spermatophore production) while others are driven by purely neuronal (electrical) signals (e.g., locomotion and stridulation). This hypothesis is attractive since it seems to accommodate the major experimental observations on both crickets and cockroaches. At this point, the evidence to support this specific hypothesis is limited; however, in some individuals, differential effects of pars lesions on locomotion and stridulation have been observed (Sokolove and Loher, 1975). Some lesions were found to abolish stridulation without disturbing the locomotor rhythm ($n = 1$), abolish locomotion but leave the stridulatory rhythm intact ($n = 2$), or cause arrhythmicity in locomotor activity with no effect on stridulation ($n = 1$). Although the numbers of observations are small, the data do support the suggestion that different cells in the pars control different behaviors.

Neuroendocrine control of rhythmic locomotor activity in decapod Crustacea has also been proposed. The hypothesis is that a hormone that inhibits activity is periodically released by the eyestalk neurosecretory system. The evidence primarily consists of two observations: (1) eyestalk ablation disrupts the normal periodicity of locomotor activity and usually results in hyperactivity (see p. 152); and (2) injections of eyestalk extracts inhibit activity (Roberts, 1944; Naylor and Williams, 1968). Furthermore, it has been suggested that in *Carcinus,* which exhibits a tidal activity rhythm, extracts made from animals at the time of high tide are less inhibiting than those made at low tide (Naylor, Smith, and Williams, 1973). More recent evidence strongly supports the notion of an activity-inhibiting hormone in the eyestalks of crayfish, but the results suggest that the inhibition is not periodic and that the rhythm of activity is driven via axons in the circumesophageal connectives (CEC). Page and Larimer (1975a) found that section of the CEC of crayfish consistently abolished the activity rhythm. Furthermore, subsequent removal of the eyestalks (which no longer had any neuronal connections with the thoracic nervous system) still resulted in marked hyperactivity. The data demonstrated that there is a blood-borne factor originating in the eyestalks that can directly inhibit the thoracic motor system, but there was no evidence that this inhibition is rhythmic. While it could be argued that the severance of the CEC caused a loss of rhythmicity in hormone release, this seems unlikely since this operation has no effect on the retinal pigment migration rhythm, which is also believed to be controlled via eyestalk hormones (Page and Larimer, 1975b).

It has been suggested that the locomotor activity rhythm in the scorpion may be hormonally controlled. Rao and Gropalakrishnareddy (1967) found that extracts of either the brain or the blood of scorpions strongly affected the spontaneous activity of the isolated ventral nerve cord. Furthermore, the effect could be either to increase activity or to decrease activity, depending on the phase of the donor's locomotor activity cycle (in LD) at which the sample was taken. The results are interesting, but further work is required to demonstrate this finding in the normal mechanism of control of rhythmic activity.

The clearest and most convincing demonstration of an identified neural link between pacemaker and overt rhythm comes from some recent work on the horseshoe crab, *Limulus polyphemus*. Barlow, Balanowski, and Brachman (1977) found that the lateral eyes of *Limulus* exhibit a circadian rhythm in the amplitude of the electroretinogram (ERG) evoked by a standard light pulse. They also observed a circadian rhythm in the efferent activity of the optic nerve, with the efferents being most active during the subjective night, when the ERG was maximal. When the optic nerve was cut, the ERG rhythm was abolished, and the amplitude remained at low, daytime levels. Furthermore, stimulating the optic nerve distal to the cut (presumably simulating the efferent activity) was effective in increasing the ERG amplitude to high night-time levels; and finally, activity recorded in the nerve proximal to the cut was shown to remain rhythmic. Evidently rhythmic efferent activity was modulating and imposing rhythmicity on the ERG response. This excellent piece of work is thus perhaps the only case in which a neural pathway has been shown to be not only necessary to sustain rhythmicity but also to exhibit rhythmic activity itself *in situ*.

CIRCADIAN MODULATION OF SENSORY INPUT

It is clear that the circadian system exerts a considerable degree of control over the effector pathways of the nervous system. There is also some evidence to suggest that there is a circadian modulation of the excitability of the sensory system, particularly with respect to visual input.

Probably the earliest demonstration of a circadian rhythm in a sensory response to a standard stimulus was the demonstration in 1940 of a rhythm in the amplitude of the electroretinogram of carabid beetles (Jahn and Crescitelli, 1940). Since then, ERG amplitude rhythms have been described in several invertebrates (see Figures 5, 7) including the crayfish (Aréchiga and Wiersma, 1969); the crab *Carcinus* (Aréchiga, Huberman, and Naylor, 1974); the scorpion *Androtonus australis* (Fleissner, 1974); and *Limulus polyphemus* (Barlow *et al.*, 1977). Frequently these rhythms in sensitivity reflect daily changes in the position of the retinal shielding pigments, which modulate the amount of light that reaches the photoreceptors (e.g., Aréchiga and Fuentes, 1970; Barlow *et al.*, 1977). However, there is evidence that a change in sensitivity of the primary photoreceptors (retinula cells) may, in some cases, contribute to the rhythm (Sanchez and Fuentes-Pardo, 1977; Barlow *et al.*, 1977) or be its primary basis (Jahn and Wulff, 1943).

In both the crayfish, *Procambarus clarkii,* (Aréchiga and Wiersma, 1969), and the crab, *Carcinus* (Aréchiga *et al.,* 1974), there is also a rhythm in the responsiveness of a class of visual interneurons, the sustaining fibers, that react tonically to changes in the level of illumination. The activity of sustaining fibers, recorded with chronically implanted microelectrodes, exhibits a variation in response to a standard light pulse that closely parallels the rhythm in ERG amplitude. Furthermore, in crayfish, the spontaneous activity of these cells in constant darkness exhibits a circadian rhythm, being higher during the subjective night than during the subjective day. The origin of this rhythm may lie with another class of neurons in the optic tract, the activity fibers. These are efferent mechanoreceptive interneurons that exhibit a rhythmic variation in activity that presumably reflects the animal's locomotor activity rhythm, and that have a facilatory influence on the sustaining fibers' response to light (Aréchiga and Wiersma, 1969).

There has been little effort to determine whether or not sensory systems responsive to stimuli other than light exhibit circadian rhythms of sensitivity. There is some evidence for rhythms in the sensitivity of primary mechanoreceptors and mechanoreceptive interneurons in decapod Crustacea (Aréchiga, 1974; Aréchiga *et al.,* 1974).

PHOTORECEPTION AND ENTRAINMENT

PHOTORECEPTOR LOCALIZATION

The fact that circadian rhythms can be entrained by an environmental light cycle demonstrates that the pacemaker must have access to a photoreceptor. Although some information is available on the general location of photoreceptors involved in entrainment, there are a number of important questions that concern both the properties of the photoreceptors and the transductional and translational events that lead to entrainment that remain. Future progress in this area will depend heavily on the precise identification of the photoreceptors and pathways involved. Attempts have been made in several organisms to identify those photoreceptors involved in entrainment. Some animals seem to rely solely on "organized" photoreceptive structures (e.g., compound eyes); in other cases, it appears that only extraretinal photoreception is utilized; and in some organisms, there are multiple photoreceptors adequate for entrainment.

Generally, efforts to localize these photoreceptors have involved attempts to disrupt known photoreceptive pathways either by placing an opaque covering over the photoreceptive structure or by surgical ablation of the receptor pathways. Results obtained with the former technique are especially fraught with interpretive difficulties. Only in cases in which opaquing a particular photoreceptor abolishes entrainment (but leaves an intact freerunning rhythm) is the result convincing. When opaquing has no effect, it is virtually impossible to rule out the possibility that the covering is imperfect or that light is not reaching the photoreceptor indirectly via other pathways (see also discussion in Brady, 1974; Truman, 1976).

Although "organized" photoreceptors are frequently bypassed in entrainment in invertebrates, there are at least two cases, the cockroach and the cricket, in which the compound eyes appear to be the exclusive photoreceptors for entrainment. Roberts (1965) provided the original evidence. He showed that when the eyes of intact roaches that were entrained to an LD cycle were painted over with black lacquer, the animals began to free-run, even though the single pair of ocelli remained intact and exposed to the LD cycle (Figure 6). On the other hand, surgical ablation of the ocelli had no effect on entrainment. Roberts's conclusion that the eyes were the necessary photoreceptive pathway for entrainment was subsequently verified by Nishiitsutsuji-Uwo and Pittendrigh (1968a), who were able to repeat Roberts's observations on the effect of painting the compound eyes and furthermore showed that the surgical ablation of the eyes by section of the optic nerve also abolishes entrainment by light. They confirmed that the ocelli were not involved. Finally, Driskill (1974) has shown that even at very high light intensities of 22,700 lux, optic nerve section effectively abolishes entrainment.

Similar results have been obtained with the cricket, *Teleogryllus commodus*. Severance of the optic nerves abolishes entrainment of the stridulatory rhythm, but destruction of the ocelli has no effect (Loher, 1972). There is also limited evidence that entrainment of the activity rhythm involves the compound eyes (Sokolove and Loher, 1975).

There is one other case in which it has been shown that retinal photoreceptors are involved in entrainment. In the scorpion, it appears that the median eyes are sufficient for entrainment of the rhythm in ERG amplitude of the median eyes. Fleissner (1977a) demonstrated that following surgical ablation of the lateral eyes, light cycles applied locally to one of the median eyes could successfully entrain the ERG rhythm in the contralateral median eye. When the illuminated eye was covered, the rhythm began to freerun even though the prosoma was illuminated. Fleissner (1977b) has also reported that the median eye rhythm can be entrained via localized, dim illumination of the lateral eyes.

There are several cases where extraretinal photoreceptors appear to be the primary pathway for entrainment, including the silkmoth, *Drosophila*, the grasshopper *Chorthippus curtipennis*, and the crayfish.

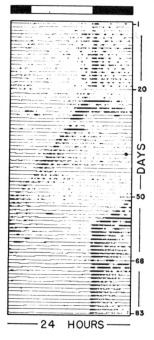

Fig. 6. Record of the locomotor activity of the roach, *Leucophaea maderae*, illustrating the necessity of the compound eyes for entrainment. The animal is maintained on a light–dark cycle indicated by the bar at the top of the record. On Day 20, the compound eyes were painted with black lacquer and the animal began to freerun. On Day 50, the paint was peeled off and the roach became entrained. Surgical ablation of the ocelli on Day 68 had no effect on entrainment. (From Roberts, 1965. Copyright 1965, by the American Association for the Advancement of Science. Reprinted with permission.)

In the silkmoth, there is good evidence that a photoreceptor in the brain is utilized in entrainment of the eclosion rhythm. Truman and Riddiford (1970; Truman, 1972) have shown that the neurally isolated brain can sustain an entrainable rhythm of eclosion in *A. pernyi* and *H. cecropia* (see p. 149). Furthermore, if the isolated brain is transplanted to the abdomen, the rhythm will entrain to light cycles presented only to the posterior end of the pupae. When brains of *H. cecropia* are removed and replaced in the head region, the rhythm is entrained by light cycles presented to the anterior end (Truman and Riddiford, 1970; Truman, 1972). The optic lobes are not required for entrainment, and thus, the photoreceptor is probably located in the main cerebral lobes (Truman, 1972). There is also further evidence that the flight rhythm of silkmoths is extraretinally entrained (Truman, 1974b).

Entrainment in *Drosophila* pupae and adults appears to involve extraretinal photoreception. The eclosion rhythm of the eyeless (and ocelli-less) mutant of *D. melanogaster, sine oculis,* entrains normally to light cycles (Engelmann and Honegger, 1966), and the activity rhythm of adult *sine oculis* can be entrained by light (Konopka, personal communication). Also, the phase of the *Drosophila* eclosion rhythm can be set by light as early as the first larval instar—well before the development of the compound eyes (Zimmerman and Ives, 1971).

There is some evidence for the involvement of extraretinal photoreception in entrainment of the oviposition rhythm of the grasshopper, *Chorthippus curtipennis*. Loher and Chandrashekeran (1970) found that surgical ablation of either the ocelli or the compound eyes did not abolish entrainment. In attempting to show that both eyes and ocelli were not required, the entire head capsule of the grasshopper (except mouth parts) was painted with an opaque material. The animals entrained normally, but the conclusion that the photoreception is extracephalic was unwarranted since a relatively high light intensity (1500–2000 lux) was used and the complete absence of light conduction to the compound eyes, ocelli, or brain photoreceptors was not adequately demonstrated.

The involvement of extraretinal photoreception in entrainment in crayfish has also been shown. Removal of the compound eyes, or the compound eyes and the most distal optic neuropil (the lamina ganglionaris), has no effect on entrainment of the circadian rhythm of locomotor activity (Page and Larimer, 1972). The caudal photoreceptor, a well-known light-sensitive neuron in the sixth abdominal ganglion, was also found to be unnecessary for entrainment (Page and Larimer, 1972). Subsequent studies on the activity and ERG amplitude rhythm have suggested that the extraretinal–extracaudal photoreceptor is located in the supraesophageal ganglion. Page and Larimer (1975a) found that eyestalkless animals could be entrained by light and concluded that the photoreceptor was at least not confined to the optic lobes. Furthermore, they found that the ERG rhythm could be entrained via an extraretinal pathway (Figure 7). When one light cycle was presented locally to one eye using fiber optics, and another, 180° out of phase with the first, was presented to the supraesophageal ganglion, the ERG rhythm was invariably entrained by the light cycle presented to the brain (Page and Larimer, 1976). Although the possibility of light's scattering to the optic lobes was not completely excluded, the results provided further support for a brain-centered extraretinal photoreceptor.

In many cases where entrainment occurs via extraretinal photoreception, retinal photoreceptors can modify the behavior "reflexively" (masking) without actually being involved in entrainment. For example, Truman (1972) has shown that the time of eclosion in silkmoths is reflexively modified by retinal input; and bursts of activity that are synchronous with the onset of light but do not persist in DD are apparently driven by retinal elements in silkmoth flight (Truman, 1974b) and crayfish locomotor activity (Page and Larimer, 1972). In other instances, however, both retinal and extraretinal pathways may be involved in entrainment.

The circadian oscillator in the *Aplysia* eye can be entrained to white light cycles when the eye is isolated in culture medium (Eskin, 1971). Thus, the photoreceptors of the eye are sufficient for entrainment. On the other hand, entrainment by cycles of red light (>600 nm) may involve extraocular photoreceptive pathways. When animals with one optic nerve

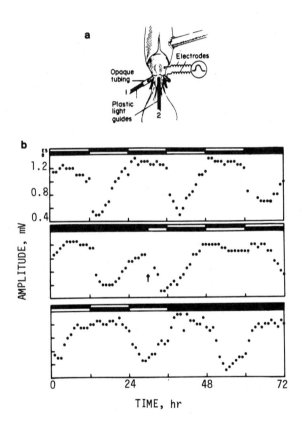

Fig. 7. Record of the ERG amplitude rhythm of the crayfish, *Procambarus clarkii,* illustrating extraretinal entrainment. (a) The animal was held by a plastic rod glued to the branchostegite. Two light guides were used to provide different light cycles to the right eye (1) and to the brain (2). The ERG response to a light pulse presented once an hour was monitored in the left eye. (b) The animal was entrained, prior to recording to an LD cycle that was in phase with the LD cycle initially presented to the right eye (illustrated in the top bar, ES). The record began 3 days subsequent to the beginning of the light regime provided by the light guides. During this time, the rhythm had entrained the light cycle directed to the brain (B) (lower bar); maximum ERG amplitude occurred during the time of lights-off of the brain LD cycle. When placed in DD, the rhythm freeran for 1 cycle with appropriate phase. When the positions of the probes were reversed (arrow), the ERG rhythm reentrained to the new LD cycle presented to the brain. The LD cycle presented to the eye was ineffective. (From Page and Larimer, 1976. Reprinted with permission.)

Fig. 8. Phase shifts in the *Aplysia* eye rhythm produced by 4-hr pulses of high potassium concentration (106.7 mM) in seawater. In (A) two panels show delay (*upper*) and advance (*lower*) phase shifts in the eye rhythm. The solid curves (FSW: filtered seawater) are from control eyes, and the broken curves are from eyes exposed to hi-K pulses. The eyes were maintained in constant darkness throughout the experiment. (B) The phase-response curve for hi-K pulses, showing the magnitude and sign of the phase shift as a function of the phase of the pulse. The horizontal bars are mean responses (number of experiments in parentheses) and span the time of exposure to hi-K. Vertical bars indicate the range of the phase shifts. The white bar indicates the time of projected lights-on. (From Eskin, 1972. Reprinted with permission of Springer-Verlag, Heidelberg.)

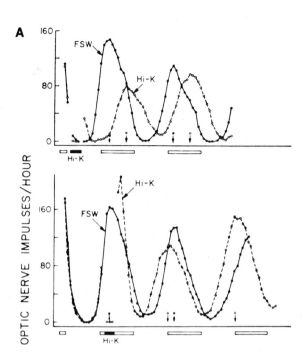

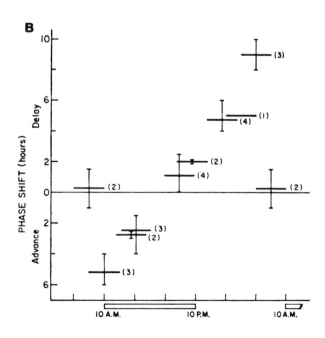

cut are placed on red light cycles, only the uncut eye will entrain; the isolated eye, which is entrainable by white light, appears to freerun (Block, Hudson, and Lickey, 1974). Although there are other explanations, the simplest interpretation of the data is that a red-sensitive, extraocular photoreceptor is sufficient for entrainment.

Dumortier (1972) has suggested (on the basis of experiments involving lesions and local illumination) that both retinal and extraretinal pathways are sufficient for entrainment in the tettigonid, *Ephippiger*. Unfortunately, he seems to have ignored the possibility of a reflexive, noncircadian component in the activity rhythm and did not assay the phase of the freerunning rhythm in DD following his various experimental manipulations (also see Brady's 1974 discussion of Dumortier's results); and conclusions about the roles of the various photoreceptors must be accepted only tentatively.

NEURAL MECHANISMS IN ENTRAINMENT

Some progress in understanding the nature of the transduction of the light signal and its subsequent translation into a phase shift has been made in one system, the *Aplysia* eye. Eskin (1972, 1977a,b) has begun to provide details on the physiological and anatomical pathway for entrainment of the isolated *Aplysia* eye by employing ion substitution and neuropharmacological techniques. The general procedure has been to assay the effects of various agents on the phase-shift response of the eye rhythm to a light pulse. It was found that treatments that blocked membrane depolarization (for example, solutions with very low sodium concentrations) also blocked the phase shift by light (Eskin, 1977b). Further-more, agents that cause depolarization of membranes (i.e., high $[K^+]$, strophanthidin) themselves cause phase shifts (both delays and advances) in the absence of light (Eskin, 1972, 1977a) (Figure 8). On the other hand, treatments that should have prevented transmission at chemical synapses (low $[Ca^{2+}]$, high $[Mg^{2+}]$) or that should have blocked action potentials (tetrodotoxin) did not affect the light-evoked phase shift. Eskin (1977b) has suggested that these results are consistent with one of two possible pathways for the translation of light into a phase shift: (1) the pacemaker might be located in the photoreceptor cells, and the entrainment process involves a nonregenerative photoreceptor potential; or (2) the pacemaker could be in the secondary cells and receive input from the photoreceptors via electrotonic synapses. Either explanation is consistent with the known structural and electrophysiological properties of the eye. For example, the photoreceptors in the *Aplysia* eye apparently do not generate action potentials (Jacklet, 1969b), and gap junctions do exist between receptors and second-order cells (Luborsky-Moore and Jacklet, 1977).

Recently, Corrent, McAdoo, and Erskin (1978) have also made the interesting discovery that the eye can be phase-shifted by a neurotransmitter, serotonin (5-hydroxytrypt-amine). The phase-response curve includes both advances and delays. The data suggest that although chemical transmission at synapses may not be necessary for entrainment, there may be serotonergic synapses that are sufficient. This could reflect an alternate pathway for ocular entrainment, or it may be the pathway for extraocular entrainment, either from extraocular photoreceptors (see p. 166) or from the contralateral ocular pacemaker (see p. 157). The eye is known to contain large amounts of serotonin, but the cells of origin have not been identified (Corrent *et al.*, 1978).

Aréchiga, H. Circadian rhythm of sensory input in the crayfish. In F. O. Schmitt and F. G. Worden (Eds.), *The Neurosciences: Third Study Program*. Cambridge, Mass.: MIT Press, 1974, pp. 517–523.

Aréchiga, H., and Fuentes, B. Correlative changes between retinal shielding pigments position and electro-retinogram in crayfish. *The Physiologist*, 1970, *13*, 137.

Aréchiga, H., and Mena, F. Circadian variations of hormonal content in the nervous system of the crayfish. *Comparative Biochemistry and Physiology*, 1975, *52A*, 581–584.

Aréchiga, H., and Wiersma, C. A. G. Circadian rhythm of responsiveness in crayfish visual units. *Journal of Neurobiology*, 1969, *1*, 71–85.

Aréchiga, H., Funetes, B., and Barrera, B. Circadian rhythm of responsiveness in the visual system of the crayfish. In J. Salánki (Ed.), *Neurobiology of Invertebrates*. Budapest: Akadémiai Kiadó, 1973, pp. 403–427.

Aréchiga, H., Huberman, A., and Naylor, E. Hormonal modulation of circadian neural activity in *Carcinus maenus* (L). *Proceedings of the Royal Society of London B.*, 1974, *187*, 299–313.

Barlow, R. B., Jr., Balanowski, S. J., Jr., and Brachman, M. L. Efferent optic nerve fibers mediate circadian rhythm in the *Limulus* eye. *Science*, 1977, *197*, 86–89.

Barrera-Mera, B. The effect of cerebroid ganglion lesions on ERG circadian rhythm in the crayfish. *Physiology and Behavior*, 1976, *17*, 59–64.

Bennitt, R. Diurnal rhythm in the proximal cells of the crayfish retina. *Physiological Zoology*, 1932, *5*, 65–69.

Bliss, D. E. Neuroendocrine control of locomotor activity in the land crab *Gecarcinus lateralis*. *Memoirs of the Society of Endocrinology*, 1962, *12*, 391.

Block, G. D. Evidence for an entrainable circadian oscillator in the abdominal ganglia of crayfish. *Neuroscience Abstracts*, 1976, *2*, 315.

Block, G. D., and Lickey, M. E. Extraocular photoreceptors and oscillators can control the circadian rhythm of behavioral activity in Aplysia. *Journal of Comparative Physiology*, 1973, *84*, 367–374.

Block, G. D., and Page, T. L. Circadian pacemakers in the nervous system, *Annual Review of Neuroscience*, 1978, *1*, 19–34.

Block, G. D., Hudson, D. J., and Lickey, M. E. Extraocular photoreceptors can entrain the circadian oscillator in the eye of *Aplysia*. *Journal of Comparative Physiology*, 1974, *89*, 237–250.

Brady, J. Control of circadian rhythm of activity in the cockroach. II. The role of the subesophageal ganglion and ventral nerve cord. *Journal of Experimental Biology*, 1967, *47*, 165–178.

Brady, J. The search for the insect clock. In M. Menaker (Ed.), *Biochronometry*. Washington, D.C.: National Academy of Sciences, 1971, pp. 517–524.

Brady, J. The physiology of insect circadian rhythms. *Advances in Insect Physiology*, 1974, 10, 1–115.

Corrent, G., McAdoo, D. J., and Eskin, A. Serotonin phase shifts the circadian rhythm from the *Aplysia* eye. *Science*, 1978, *202*, 977–979.

Cymborowski, B. Control of the circadian rhythm of locomotor activity in the house cricket. *Journal of Insect Physiology*, 1973, *19*, 1423–1440.

Cymborowski, B., and Brady, J. Insect circadian rhythms transmitted by parabiosis—A re-examination. *Nature* (London), 1972, *236*, 221–222.

Demoll, R. M. Über die Wanderung des Iris pigments in Facettenauge. *Zoologische Jahrbücher Abteilung für Allegemeine Zoologie und Physiologie der Tiere*, 1911, *30*, 159–180.

Driskill, R. J. The circadian locomotor rhythm of the cockroach: An examination of the photoreceptive system operative in entrainment. Master's thesis, University of Delaware, 1974.

Dumortier, B. Photoreception in the circadian rhythm of stridulatory activity in *Ephippiger* (Ins., Orthoptera): Likely existence of two photoreceptive systems. *Journal of Comparative Physiology*, 1972, *77*, 80–112.

Engelmann, W., and Honegger, H. W. Tagesperiodische Schlüpfrhythmik einer augenlosen Drosophila mel-anogaster-mutante. *Zeitschrift für Naturforschung*, 1966, *B: 22*, 1–2.

Eskin, A. Properties of the *Aplysia* visual system: *In vitro* entrainment of the circadian rhythm and centrifugal regulation of the eye. *Zeitschrift für Vergleichende Physiologie*, 1971, *74*, 353–371.

Eskin, A. Phase shifting a circadian rhythm in the eye of *Aplysia* by high potassium pulses. *Journal of Comparative Physiology*, 1972, *80*, 353–376.

Eskin, A. Entraining a circadian rhythm from the isolated eye of *Aplysia:* The involvement of changes in membrane potential. *Neuroscience Abstracts*, 1977a, *3*, 176.

Eskin, A. Neurophysiological mechanisms involved in photo-entrainment of the circadian rhythm from the *Aplysia* eye. *Journal of Neurobiology*, 1977b, *8*, 273–299.

Eskin, A., and Harcombe, E. Eye of *Navanax:* Optic activity, circadian rhythm and morphology. *Comparative Biochemistry and Physiology,* 1977, *57A,* 443–449.

Fleissner, G. Circadiane Adaptation und Schirmpigment—verlagerung in den Sehzellen der Medianaugen von *Androctonus australis* L. (Buthidae, Scorpiones). *Journal of Comparative Physiology,* 1974, *91,* 399–416.

Fleissner, G. Entrainment of the scorpion's circadian rhythm via the median eyes. *Journal of Comparative Physiology,* 1977a, *118,* 93–99.

Fleissner, G. Scorpion lateral eyes: Extremely sensitive receptors of zeitgeber stimuli. *Journal of Comparative Physiology,* 1977b, *118,* 101–108.

Gordon, W. H., Larimer, J. L., and Page, T. L. Circumesophageal interneurons required for reflexive and circadian locomotor behaviors in crayfish. *Journal of Comparative Physiology,* 1977, *116,* 227–238.

Harker, J. E. Diurnal rhythms in *Periplaneta americana* L. *Nature* (London) 1954, *173,* 689–690.

Harker, J. E. Factors controlling the diurnal rhythm of activity in *Periplaneta americana. Journal of Experimental Biology,* 1956, *33,* 224–234.

Harker, J. E. Internal factors controlling the subesophageal ganglion neurosecretory cycle in *Periplaneta americana. Journal of Experimental Biology,* 1960, *37,* 164–170.

Hudson, D., and Lickey, M. Weak negative coupling between the circadian pacemakers of the eyes of *Aplysia. Neuroscience Abstracts,* 1977, *3,* 179.

Jacklet, J. W. Circadian rhythm of optic nerve impulses recorded in darkness from isolated eye of *Aplysia. Science,* 1969a, *164,* 562–563.

Jacklet, J. W. Electrophysiological organization of the eye of *Aplysia. Journal of General Physiology,* 1969b, *53,* 21–42.

Jacklet, J. W. A circadian rhythm in the optic nerve impulses from an isolated eye in darkness. In M. Menaker (Ed.), *Biochronometry.* Washington, D.C.: National Academy of Sciences, 1971, pp. 351–362.

Jacklet, J. W. The effects of constant light and light pulses on the circadian rhythm in the eye of *Aplysia. Journal of Comparative Physiology,* 1974, *90,* 33–45.

Jacklet, J. W., and Geronimo, J. Circadian rhythm: Population of interacting neurons. *Science,* 1971, *174,* 299–302.

Jacklet, J. W., Alvarez, R., and Bernstein, B. Ultrastructure of the eye of *Aplysia. Journal of Ultrastructural Research,* 1972, *38,* 246–261.

Jahn, T. L., and Crescitelli, J. Diurnal changes in the electrical responses of the compound eye. *Biological Bulletin,* 1940, *78,* 45–52.

Jahn, T. L., and Wulff, V. J. Electrical aspects of a diurnal rhythm in the eye of *Dytiscus fasciventris. Physiological Zoology,* 1943, *16,* 101–109.

Kalmus, H. Das Aktogram des Flusskrebs und seine Beeinflussung durch Organextrakte. *Zeitschrift für Vergleichende Physiologie,* 1938, *25,* 689–802.

Koehler, W. K., and Fleissner, G. Internal desynchronization of bilaterally organized circadian oscillators in the visual system of insects. *Nature* (London), 1978, *274,* 708–710.

Kupfermann, I. A circadian locomotor rhythm in *Aplysia californica. Physiology and Behavior,* 1968, *3,* 179–182.

Lickey, M. E., Block, G. D., Hudson, D. J., and Smith, J. T. Circadian oscillators and photoreceptors in the gastropod, *Aplysia. Photochemistry and Photobiology,* 1976, *23,* 253–273.

Lickey, M., Wozniak, J., Block, G., Hudson, D., and Augter, G. The consequences of eye removal for the circadian rhythm of behavioral activity in *Aplysia. Journal of Comparative Physiology,* 1977, *118,* 121–143.

Loher, W. Circadian control of stridulation in the cricket, *Teleogryllus commodus* Walker. *Journal of Comparative Physiology,* 1972, *79,* 173–190.

Loher, W. Circadian control of spermatophore formation in the cricket *Teleogryllus commodus* Walker. *Journal of Insect Physiology,* 1974, *20,* 1155–1172.

Loher, W., and Chandrashekaran, M. K. Circadian rhythmicity in the oviposition of the grasshopper *Chorthippus curtipennis. Journal of Insect Physiology,* 1970, *16,* 1677–1688.

Luborsky-Moore, J. L., and Jacklet, J. W. Ultrastructure of the secondary cells in the *Aplysia* eye. *Journal of Ultrastructural Research,* 1977, *60,* 235–245.

Naylor, E., and Williams, B. G. Effects of eyestalk removal of rhythmic locomotor activity in *Carcinus. Journal of Experimental Biology,* 1968, *49,* 107–116.

Naylor, E., Smith, G., and Williams, B. The role of the eyestalk in the tidal activity rhythm of the shore crab, *Carcinus maenas* (L.). In J. Salanki (Ed.), *Neurobiology of Invertebrates.* Budapest: Publishing House of the Hungarian Academy of Sciences, 1973, pp. 423–429.

Nishiitsutsuji-Uwo, J., and Pittendrigh, C. S. Central nervous system control of circadian rhythmicity in the cockroach. II. The pathway of light signals that entrain the rhythms. *Zeitschrift für vergleichende Physiologie*, 1968a, *58*, 1–13.

Nishiitsutsuji-Uwo, J., and Pittendrigh, C. S. Central nervous system control of circadian rhythmicity in the cockroach. III. The optic lobes, locus of the driving oscillation? *Zeitschrift für vergleichende Physiologie*, 1968b, *58*, 14–46.

Nishiitsutsuji-Uwo, J., Petropulos, S. F., and Pittendrigh, C. S. Central nervous system control of circadian rhythmicity in the cockroach. I. Role of the pars intercerebralis. *Biological Bulletin Woods Hole*, 1967, *133*, 679–696.

Page, T. L. Interactions between bilaterally paired components of the cockroach circadian system. *Journal of Comparative Physiology*, 1978, *124*, 225–236.

Page, T. L., and Larimer, J. L. Entrainment of the circadian locomotor activity rhythm in crayfish. *Journal of Comparative Physiology*, 1972, *78*, 107–120.

Page, T. L., and Larimer, J. L. Neural control of circadian rhythmicity in the crayfish. I. The locomotor activity rhythm. *Journal of Comparative Physiology*, 1975a, *97*, 59–80.

Page, T. L., and Larimer, J. L. Neural control of circadian rhythmicity in the crayfish. II. The ERG amplitude rhythm. *Journal of Comparative Physiology*, 1975b, *97*, 81–96.

Page, T. L., and Larimer, J. L. Extraretinal photoreception in entrainment of crustacean rhythms. *Photochemistry and Photobiology*, 1976, *23*, 245–251.

Page T. L., Caldarola, P. C., and Pittendrigh, C. S. Mutual entrainment of bilaterally distributed circadian pacemakers. *Proceedings of the National Academy of Sciences, USA*, 1977, *74*, 1277–1281.

Pittendrigh, C. S. Circadian rhythms and the circadian organization of living systems. *Cold Spring Harbor Symposium on Quantitative Biology*, 1960, *25*, 159–182.

Rao, K. P., and Gropalakrishnareddy, T. Blood borne factors in circadian rhythms of activity. *Nature* (London), 1967, *213*, 1047–1048.

Rence, B., and Loher, W. Arrhythmically singing crickets: Thermoperiodic reentrainment after bilobectomy. *Science*, 1975, *190*, 385–387.

Roberts, S. K. Photoreception and entrainment of cockroach activity rhythms. *Science*, 1965, *148*, 958–959.

Roberts, S. K. Circadian activity rhythms in cockroaches. III. The role of endocrine and neural factors. *Journal of Cellular and Comparative Physiology*, 1966, *67*, 473–486.

Roberts, S. K. Circadian rhythms in cockroaches: Effects of optic lobe lesions. *Journal of Comparative Physiology*, 1974, *88*, 21–30.

Roberts, S. K., Skopik, S. D., and Driskill, R. J. Circadian rhythms in cockroaches: does brain hormone mediate the locomotor cycle? In M. Menaker (Ed.), *Biochronometry*. Washington, D.C.: National Academy of Sciences, 1971, pp. 505–515.

Roberts, T. W. Light, eyestalk chemical and certain other factors as regulators of the community activity for the crayfish, *Cambarus virilis* Hagen. *Ecological Monographs*, 1944, *14*, 361–385.

Sanchez, J. A., and Fuentes-Pardo, B. Circadian rhythm in the amplitude of the electroretinogram in the isolated eyestalk of the crayfish. *Comparative Biochemistry and Physiology*, 1977, *56A*, 601–605.

Schalleck, W. Some mechanisms controlling locomotor activity in the crayfish. *Journal of Experimental Zoology*, 1942, *91*, 155–166.

Sokolove, P. G. Localization of the cockroach optic lobe circadian pacemaker with microlesions. *Brain Research*, 1975a, *87*, 13–21.

Sokolove, P. G. Locomotory and stridulatory circadian rhythms in the cricket, *Teleogryllus commodus*. *Journal of Insect Physiology*, 1975b, *21*, 537–538.

Sokolove, P. G., and Loher, W. Role of eyes, optic lobes, and pars intercerebralis in locomotory and stridulatory circadian rhythms of *Teleogryllus commodus*. *Journal of Insect Physiology*, 1975, *21*, 785–799.

Strumwasser, F. Neurophysiological aspects of rhythms. In G. C. Quarton, T. Melnechuk, R. O. Schmitt (Eds.), *The Neurosciences, A Study Program*. New York: Rockefeller University Press, 1967, pp. 516–528.

Strumwasser, F. Neuronal principles organizing periodic behaviors. In F. O. Schmitt and F. G. Worden (Eds.), *The Neurosciences: Third Study Program*. Cambridge, Mass.: MIT Press, 1974, pp. 459–478.

Truman, J. W. Circadian rhythms and physiology with special reference to neuroendocrine processes in insects. In *Proceedings of the International Symposium on Circadian Rhythmicity*. Wageningen, Netherlands: Pudoc Press, 1971a, pp. 111–135.

Truman, J. W. Hour glass behavior of the circadian clock controlling eclosion of the silkmoth, *Antherea pernyi*. *Proceedings of the National Academy of Sciences, USA*, 1971b, *68*, 595–599.

Truman, J. W. Physiology of insect ecdysis. I. The eclosion behavior of silkmoths and its hormonal control. *Journal of Experimental Biology*, 1971c, *54*, 805–814.

Truman, J. W. Physiology of insect rhythms. II. The silk moth brain as the location of the biological clock controlling eclosion. *Journal of Comparative Physiology*, 1972, *81*, 99–114.

Truman, J. W. Physiology of insect ecdysis. II. The assay and occurrence of the eclosion hormone in the chinese oak silkmoth, *Antheraea pernyi. Biological Bulletin*, 1973, *114*, 200–211.

Truman, J. W. Circadian release of a prepatterned neural program in silkmoths. In F. O. Schmitt and F. G. Worden (Eds.), *The Neurosciences: Third Study Program*. Cambridge, Mass.: MIT Press, 1974a, pp. 525–529.

Truman, J. W. Physiology of insect rhythms. IV. Role of the brain in the regulation of the flight rhythm of the giant silkmoths. *Journal of Comparative Physiology*, 1974b, *95*, 281–296.

Truman, J. W. Extraretinal photoreception in insects. *Photochemistry and Photobiology*, 1976, *23*, 215–225.

Truman, J. W., and Riddiford, L. M. Neuroendocrine control of ecdysis in silkmoths. *Science*, 1970, *167*, 1624–1626.

Truman, J. W., and Sokolove, P. J. Silkmoth eclosion: Hormonal triggering of a centrally programmed pattern of behavior. *Science*, 1972, *175*, 1491–1493.

Welsh, J. H. The sinus glands and twenty-four hour cycles of retinal pigment migration in the crayfish. *Journal of Experimental Zoology*, 1941, *86*, 35–49.

Zimmerman, W. F., and Ives, D. Some photophysiological aspects of circadian rhythmicity in *Drosophila*. In M. Menaker (Ed.), *Biochronometry*. Washington, D.C.: National Academy of Science, 1971.

10

Genetics and Development of Circadian Rhythms in Invertebrates

Ronald J. Konopka

Developmental Ontogeny of the Pacemaker and Overt Rhythms

The scope of this review includes the developmental ontogeny and genetics of the driving oscillator and overt rhythms in invertebrates. The discussion is generally confined to metazoan organisms, except in cases where comparison with data from lower organisms is useful. The terms *pacemaker* and *oscillator* are usually used in the singular, although the actual physiological pacemaker may be made up of components—a population of coupled oscillators—or, at least, represented bilaterally in the two hemispheres of the brain. Only true circadian rhythms—those that persist in constant conditions—are covered; diel rhythms, which are expressed in LD but not in constant conditions, are not discussed.

A major question that arises in considering the developmental ontogeny of circadian rhythms is: Can any information be transmitted through the egg from a parent? Or, in other words, is there any coding or memory for phase or period information that persists from one generation to the next? Heritable mutations that alter the freerunning period of circadian rhythms exist and are discussed below. Specification of period length can therefore be encoded in the form of DNA and reexpressed in the next generation. Otherwise, there is very little information that bears on this question. A most intriguing report concerns the Queensland fruitfly, *Dacus,* in which Bateman (1955) claimed that the phase of the pupal ecdysis rhythm could be transmitted from mother to offspring. This report is as yet

Ronald J. Konopka   Division of Biology, 216-76, California Institute of Technology, Pasadena, California 91125.

unconfirmed. Such transmission of phase would imply either a continuing oscillation in the egg, which was set in the mother, or the coding of phase information in the absence of an ongoing oscillation, which could later be reencoded into the proper phase. A similar coding of phase information may operate in the honeybee, where it has been reported that a learned feeding time, a particular point in the circadian activity cycle, could be temporarily transplanted into a host bee by using frozen donor brain tissue (Martin, Martin, and Lindauer, 1978). In a noncircadian system, an interval timer controlling the ability of the aphid *Megoura* to respond to short photoperiods has been shown by Lees (1960) to persist through several generations. Thus, independent of the number of generations, a non-temperature-compensated timing mechanism determines when the switch from production of parthenogenetic offspring to production of male and female offspring will occur. Maternal induction of diapause in the next generation is well known (for review see Saunders, 1976).

Another major question concerns the relationship between the appearance of an overt rhythm and the development of the oscillator controlling it. In *Drosophila,* for example, the eclosion of the adult from the pupal case is a gated developmental event controlled by a circadian oscillator. Light to dark steps administered during the larval stage, as well as light pulses and temperature steps administered during the pupal stage, are capable of determining the ultimate phase of the eclosion rhythm (Pittendrigh, 1954; Brett, 1955; Zimmerman, 1969; Zimmerman and Ives, 1971). Phase information may in principle be stored in larval and pupal stages in the absence of an oscillation and expressed later in development, or an ongoing oscillation may be present in these stages whose expression as an overt rhythm is delayed until the pharate adult stage. That the latter situation is indeed the case has been elegantly shown by measuring the phase-response curve for light pulses administered at regular intervals during the pupal stage (Pittendrigh, 1966). A similar response curve is obtained on each of five days during the pupal stage, indicating that there is indeed an ongoing oscillation at this time. It is of interest that oxygen consumption of individual *Drosophila* larvae apparently is not rhythmic in constant conditions, while that of individual adult flies is rhythmic (Kayser and Heusner, 1967). This finding implies that although an ongoing oscillation most likely exists in larvae, it does not drive oxygen consumption in larvae, though oxygen consumption does become rhythmic at a later developmental stage. Since no phase-response curves have been determined for the adult oxygen-consumption rhythm, it is not possible to determine whether a similar or identical oscillator to that controlling the eclosion rhythm governs the oxygen consumption rhythm. Perhaps the driving oscillator is uncoupled from its output at early developmental stages and is later coupled by the developmentally regulated synthesis of one of more coupling factors—the same factor for rhythms of similar phase and a different factor for rhythms with a different phase. Other mechanisms are possible.

Circadian oscillators are capable of gating specific developmental events. In *Drosophila pseudoobscura,* for example, the time of pupariation, appearance of yellow eye pigment, and appearance of ocellar bristle pigment are not controlled by a circadian oscillator, even though an ongoing oscillation is present (Pittendrigh and Skopik, 1970), as determined by phase-response-curve measurements in a separate experiment (Pittendrigh, 1966). The time of eclosion, however, is under circadian control. A similar situation holds for *D. melanogaster* (Handler and Postlethwait, 1977). This observation can be explained by the coupling mechanism described above—a factor necessary for coupling the driving oscillator to a developmental event is not synthesized until late in the pupal stage. The case is very different, however, with *D. victoria*. Here, pupariation is indeed rhythmic, as is eclosion, but developmental events occurring between pupariation and eclosion, including head eversion and appearance of yellow eye pigment and ocellar bristle pigment, are not (Rensing and Hardeland, 1967; Pittendrigh and Skopik, 1970). Thus, separate oscillators, perhaps with similar properties, or one oscillator with two distinct coupling mechanisms may be operating in *D. victoria*.

Since the duration of the embryonic period in *Drosophila* is relatively short (about 24 hr at 25° for *D. melanogaster*), no systematic attempt has been made to localize the time of appearance of the oscillator controlling the eclosion or activity rhythms during development. A single light pulse or step administered to embryos does not synchronize the eclosion rhythm of the population (Brett, 1955). However, embryos that have seen a white-light-to-dark transition and have been raised in constant red light ($\lambda > 600$ nm) hatch into adults that individually exhibit freerunning locomotor activity rhythms, which are not, however, synchronized within the population (Konopka, unpublished experiments).

In *Pectinophora*, the duration of the embryonic stage is long enough (10–13 days at 20°) that the ontogeny of the oscillator controlling the hatching rhythm can be studied. Minis and Pittendrigh (1968) showed that light steps and pulses as well as temperature steps are not capable of synchronizing the hatching rhythm of a population of eggs until the sixth day of embryonic development. The environmental information is therefore able to be encoded at this time and expressed several days later when the eggs hatch. Most probably, the sixth day of development represents the day on which the oscillator controlling the egg hatch rhythms becomes active.

An important aspect of the control of circadian rhythms in holometabolous insects is the relationship between oscillators controlling rhythms at different stages of development. Data from four organisms are relevant to this problem. In studying the physiological control of ecdysis and adult flight-activity rhythms in silkmoths, Truman (1974) obtained evidence that the output of the clock controlling the ecdysis rhythm is hormonal, while the output controlling the flight activity rhythm may be electrical, since an intact pathway from the brain to the thoracic ganglia is necessary for expression of rhythmicity. Separate oscillators may be involved in the control of the two rhythms, or else one pacemaker may be coupled to separate output systems.

Three rhythms have been studied in the moth *Pectinophora:* egg hatch, ecdysis, and oviposition (Pittendrigh and Minis, 1971). In comparing the systems that control each rhythm, care must be taken to distinguish properties of overt rhythms from those of the pacemaker that controls them. The same pacemaker may be coupled differently (by means of slave oscillators or nonoscillatory coupling mechanisms) to different rhythms, resulting in distinct phase relationships and waveforms. In *Pectinophora*, oviposition normally occurs during the dark portion of an LD 14:10 cycle, while egg hatch and eclosion occur during the light portion, the egg hatch peak occurring about 3 hr earlier than the eclosion peak. Each rhythm thus has a unique phase relationship to the LD cycle. The response to genetic selection for early and late phases over several generations differs for these three rhythms. The selection was exerted on the eclosion rhythm, and the phase difference between early and late strains is most marked for this rhythm.

The egg hatch rhythm also shows a pronounced phase difference, while the phase of the oviposition rhythm is identical for early, late and wild-type strains. The effect of the selection can be interpreted either as a genetic alteration of pacemaker properties or as an alteration in an output system, perhaps in the mechanism by which the pacemaker is coupled to its output. Since the phase-response curves of the early and late strains were not measured, one cannot distinguish between these possibilities. Likewise, the phase differences among the three rhythms may be due to coupling and output systems rather than pacemaker differences. One observation that suggests that the pacemaker controlling the egg hatch rhythm is different from that controlling the other two rhythms is that the free-running period of the egg hatch rhythm is close to 24 hr, while that of the other two rhythms is about 22.5 hr. However, this period difference may be due to the same oscillator's running at different periods in the embryo and in later developmental stages, as a result of postembryonic maturation of input sensory cells or additional clock cells.

A dietary effect may also be involved, since the egg is a closed system, the embryo feeding off a very specialized yolk, while the larva is fed on laboratory medium. Thus, there may be differences in the protein or lipid composition of embryonic and larval membranes, accounting for the period difference. Dietary effects on photoperiodically induced diapause are well known in *Pectinophora* (Adkisson, 1961; Bull and Adkisson, 1960, 1962; Adkisson, Bell, and Wellso, 1963). Alternatively, the oscillators controlling the egg hatch and the eclosion and oviposition rhythms may be anatomically separate. Phase-response curves have been determined for the three rhythms, and all have a similar waveform and amplitude (Pittendrigh and Minis, 1971). Thus, the basic properties of the oscillators, if they are separate, are very similar.

In *Drosophila melanogaster,* mutants have been isolated that affect the periodicity of eclosion and adult locomotor activity rhythms; their properties are described in detail below, but here it is important to note that all three mutations affect both rhythms in a similar manner (Konopka and Benzer, 1971). Another mutation recently isolated at a separate locus lengthens the period of both rhythms by 1.5 hr (Smith and Konopka, unpublished). In addition, both rhythms can be entrained in the larval and pupal stages, and the phase-response curves of the wild-type pacemaker for each rhythm are similar in shape and amplitude (Konopka, unpublished experiments). These results, like those from *Pectinophora,* suggest that the oscillators controlling the two rhythms are similar, if not identical.

In the mosquito, *Aedes,* the adult flight activity rhythm is not carried over from rhythms in earlier developmental stages (Nayar and Sauerman, 1971). If larvae are exposed to an LD 12:12 cycle, the population will exhibit a pupal ecdysis rhythm, but individual adult females will not show a flight rhythm unless they are exposed to a light stimulus, of at least 6 hr duration, 24–36 hr after ecdysis. This is in contrast to the situation in *Drosophila melanogaster* and *Pectinophora* and suggests that separate oscillators govern the pupal ecdysis and flight activity rhythms in *Aedes.*

In *Drosophila pseudoobscura,* the freerunning periods of the pupal ecdysis and adult locomotor activity rhythms appear to be significantly different (Engelmann and Mack, 1978). Here, dietary influences seem unlikely, since larvae and adults feed on the same medium, consuming the yeast and sugars present in the medium. It is more likely that some alteration in the pacemaker system has taken place during development, perhaps a maturation of additional cells as suggested above. The two rhythms may be controlled by separate oscillators, although, as in *D. melanogaster,* arrhythmic mutants isolated in *D. pseudoobscura* affect both rhythms similarly (see below), implying that at least one component is common to the two oscillators. Precise anatomical localization of the oscillators controlling the two rhythms is required to resolve this issue.

Two approaches have been used to study genetic effects on circadian rhythms: multigene analysis, including determination of phenotypic differences among strains of a particular species, as well as selection of strains exhibiting a particular phenotype, and single-gene analysis, whereby the effects of mutations at single genetic loci on rhythmic parameters are studied. The former approach is limited by the difficulty in sorting out effects of single genes. In selection experiments, for example, the combined effects of several genes may be necessary to produce a particular effect on a rhythm, but the contribution of each selected gene may be difficult to determine. Consequently, little information can be obtained concerning the effects of individual genes on rhythms using this approach. However, correlations among the various effects of selected genes on rhythmic parameters, such as phase and period, can be analyzed, yielding information about the general organization of the circadian system. The latter approach, in contrast, involves the isolation, usually after chemical mutagenesis, of mutations at single genetic loci that have an effect on some aspect of a rhythm. In this way, the control exerted by a particular gene on the rhythm can be studied. In addition, since wild-type and mutant strains differ by a single gene, it is theoretically possible to isolate the mutant gene product and thereby identify a molecule that, when altered in structure or amount by a mutation, produces a definite, reproducible effect on a circadian rhythm. Examples of both approaches are discussed below.

MULTIGENE ANALYSIS

Neumann (1967) has analyzed strain differences in the time of eclosion of natural populations of the midge *Clunio,* a dipteran that inhabits the intertidal zone. Strains obtained from various regions of the European coast differ in their emergence times, since they are adapted to the local timing of the tides. When two strains differing in their daily emergence times were crossed, the emergence of the F_1 occurred at a time intermediate between the emergence times of the parental strains. A backcross of the F_1 generation with one parental strain likewise yielded an intermediate emergence time. Thus, the timing of emergence in *Clunio* is controlled by the activity of the products of one or more genetic loci. In the heterozygote, the emergence time is apparently a function of the average activity of the products of the loci, rather than a function of the noninteractive summation of the separate effects of each locus, which would have given a bimodal rhythm with peaks at both parental emergence times.

Rensing, Brunken, and Hardeland (1968) studied strain differences in the daily pattern of oxygen consumption of adult *Drosophila melanogaster.* By using strains with various ratios of the number of X chromosomes to the number of autosomes, they concluded that the X chromosome was important in the timing of the evening maximum of oxygen consumption in an LD 12:12 cycle.

In both *Drosophila* and *Pectinophora,* selection experiments have been carried out resulting in strains with early and late eclosion times. In *D. melanogaster* (Clayton and Paietta, 1972), selection of a laboratory wild-type strain resulted in wider variation between the early and late strains than did selection of a wild-caught strain, possibly indicating a relaxation of selection pressures as a result of laboratory breeding for many generations. In

D. pseudoobscura, selection over 50 generations resulted in two stable strains with relatively early and late eclosion times (Pittendrigh, 1967); the phase difference between the two strains was about 4 hr. When the phase-response curve of each strain was measured, however, there was no detectable difference between the strains. The selection therefore must have operated on some aspect of a driven system, which may itself be oscillatory, rather than the light-sensitive driving oscillator. Selection of early- and late-emerging strains in the moth *Pectinophora* yielded two strains whose emergence peaks differed in phase by 5 hr (Pittendrigh and Minis, 1971). Phase-response curves for these strains were not measured; however, since three rhythms were available for study, a comparison could be made of the effects of selection on the phase of the three rhythms. It was found that the egg hatch rhythm and eclosion rhythm exhibited a similar response to selection, the phases of early and late strains differing by 5 hr in an LD 14:10 cycle. In the case of the oviposition rhythm, however, there was no difference in phase between the two strains. The selection experiments revealed that some aspect of the pacemaker system controlling the oviposition rhythm is different from that controlling the egg hatch and pupal ecdysis rhythm.

SINGLE-GENE ANALYSIS

In two species of *Drosophila,* single-gene mutations affecting the eclosion and locomotor rhythms have been isolated. In *D. pseudoobscura,* five X-chromosome mutations have been isolated that produce arrhythmia in constant conditions (Pittendrigh, 1974). The eclosion rhythms of these mutants show varying degrees of forced rhythmicity in an LD cycle. These five mutations fall into two complementation groups. Double heterozygotes of mutations within each group are arrhythmic in constant conditions, while double heterozygotes of mutations in separate groups exhibit rhythms in constant conditions, but the freerunning period is longer than that of the wild-type strain, and the phase of the rhythm is about 5 hr later than that of wild-type both in an LD cycle and in constant conditions after entrainment. Thus, the complementation between these two groups of arrhythmic mutants is incomplete. These results suggest that at least two distinct gene products are required for expression of normal rhythmicity. They also indicate that both phase and period are under genetic control, and that gene products involved in maintenance of rhythmicity are also involved in determination of the phase of the rhythm. The observation that both eclosion and activity rhythms are arrhythmic in these mutants indicates that there is at least one component common to the oscillators controlling each rhythm, though the freerunning period of the activity rhythm is significantly shorter in wild-type flies than that of the eclosion rhythm (Engelmann and Mack, 1978).

In *D. melanogaster,* four X-chromosome mutations affecting the period of the eclosion and adult activity rhythms have been isolated (Konopka and Benzer, 1971; Konopka, 1972; Smith and Konopka, unpublished); three of these are allelic and located in region 3B1-2, while the fourth is located in region 10 and lengthens the period of both rhythms by 1.5 hr. The three mutations in 3B1-2 are at the *per* locus; this locus can be mutated to shorten the period of the rhythms to 19 hr (*per^s*), lengthen the period to 29 hr (*per^l*), and abolish rhythmicity completely (*per^0*). The freerunning periods of the eclosion and activity rhythms are not significantly different in *D. melanogaster* as they are in *D. pseudoobscura.*

The *per^l* and *per^0* alleles are almost completely recessive to the wild-type gene, while the *per^s* allele shows incomplete dominance; the periods of *per^s*/+ and *per^s*/*per^l* heterozygotes are intermediate between those of the respective homozygotes. The per^0 allele, in general, behaves genetically like a deficiency for the 3B1-2 region, suggesting that the per^0 allele lacks a functional gene product.

Although the periods of the eclosion and activity rhythms are drastically altered by the per^s and per^l alleles, the periods are still relatively temperature-compensated in the region of $18°-25°$. However, the dependence of period length on temperature is of opposite sign for the two alleles; the period of per^l increases with increasing temperature, while that of per^s decreases with increasing temperature (Konopka and Pittendrigh, unpublished experiments). In other words, the period lengths of both alleles approach that of wild-type at low temperatures; these mutations therefore have something of a temperature-sensitive character.

The region of the X chromosome to which the per alleles map has been intensively studied by Judd and his co-workers (Judd, Shen, and Kaufman, 1972). In this region, there is an approximately one-to-one correspondence between the number of lethal complementation groups and the number of cytologically visible chromosome bands. Genetic analysis suggests that each lethal complementation group maps to a particular chromosome band. The per locus, however, is not allelic to any of the lethal mutations in this region; it is therefore a "nonessential" locus that apparently does not mutate to lethality (Young and Judd, 1978). This finding raises the possibility that the per locus may be a regulatory gene rather than a structural gene.

A phase-response curve has been determined for the per^s allele (Konopka, 1972; Winfree and Gordon, 1977); remarkably, the per^s mutation, in addition to shortening the period length, increases the amplitude of the phase-response curve; the per^s response curve is a Winfree Type 0, whereas that of wild-type is a Type 1 (Winfree, 1973). This mutant, like wild-type *D. pseudoobscura,* can be given a critical stimulus of light at a particular phase that results in near arrhythmicity. The per^s pacemaker differs from that of *D. pseudoobscura,* however, in that its period is shorter, its delaying transients are more sluggish, and there is no dark adaptation in the interval between presentations of the first and second critical stimuli that induce near arrhythmicity (Winfree and Gordon, 1977).

The eclosion rhythm of the per^0 mutant can be entrained to a temperature cycle but not to a light cycle. However, the bistability phenomenon observed in temperature entrainment of the wild-type pacemaker, whereby the entrained rhythm in a temperature cycle can assume either of two phases about 3 hr apart, is absent in the mutant (Konopka, 1972). In addition, when the temperature cycle is removed, the eclosion pattern of the per^0 mutant rapidly becomes arrhythmic. Thus, the per^0 mutation has effectively abolished the self-sustaining character of the pacemaker.

Since the per locus is located on the X chromosome, the per^s mutation can be used as a marker in mapping the focus of this clock gene with respect to cuticular structures in mosaic flies that are composed of part male and part female tissue. Mosaic mapping yields a focus close to head cuticle, consistent with a brain location for the clock cells (Konopka, 1972). The ability of the brain to control the adult activity rhythm has been shown by experiments in which a donor per^s brain produced a short-period activity rhythm after transplantation into the abdomen of a genetically arrhythmic (per^0) host (Handler and Konopka, 1979). The brain can therefore produce a humoral factor, possibly made and secreted by neurosecretory cells, which controls the period of the activity cycle. It is interesting that arrhythmic mutations in both *D. melanogaster* and *D. pseudoobscura* increase the percentage of abnormally located cells belonging to a posterior neurosecretory cell cluster in the fly brain (Konopka and Wells, 1980). This cell group may be involved in the circadian system of the fly, possibly as the source of the humoral substance controlling the activity rhythm. The study of mosaic flies whose nerve cells are marked histochemically should help elucidate the role of this neurosecretory cell group in the control of circadian rhythmicity.

A genetic locus with certain properties similar to that of the *per* locus has been described in *Neurospora* (Feldman and Hoyle, 1973, 1976). This locus can also be mutated to short and long period lengths. Heterokaryons containing short-period and long-period nuclei have an intermediate period, as does the per^s/per^l heterozygote in *Drosophila*. Thus, there may exist loci with similar functions in both *Drosophila* and *Neurospora;* it is possible that the circadian pacemakers in these organisms are constructed similarly on the molecular level.

Thus far, genetic investigations of circadian pacemakers have provided new insights into the organization of the circadian system in several organisms; however, no concrete mechanism has yet been established. The biochemical identification of the products of mutant genes that affect the basic properties of circadian pacemakers will be the next step in the use of genetic techniques to elucidate a molecular mechanism for a circadian pacemaker.

REFERENCES

Adkisson, P. L. Effect of larval diet on the seasonal occurrence of diapause in the pink bollworm. *Journal of Economic Entomology,* 1961, *54,* 1107–1112.

Adkisson, P. L., Bell, R. A., and Wellso, S. G. Environmental factors controlling the induction of diapause in the pink bollworm, *Pectinophora gossypiella* (Saunders). *Journal of Insect Physiology,* 1963, *9,* 299–310.

Bateman, M. A. The effect of light and temperature on the rhythm of pupal ecdysis in the Queensland fruit-fly *Dacus (Strumeta) tryoni* (Frogg). *Australian Journal of Zoology,* 1955, *3,* 22–33.

Brett, W. J. Persistent diurnal rhythmicity in *Drosophila* emergence. *Annals of the Entomological Society of America,* 1955, *48,* 119–131.

Bull, D. L., and Adkisson, P. L. Certain factors influencing diapause in the pink bollworm, *Pectinophora gossypiella. Journal of Economic Entomology,* 1960, *53,* 793–798.

Bull, D. L., and Adkisson, P. L. Fat contents of the larval diet as a factor influencing diapause and growth rate of the pink bollworm. *Annals of the Entomological Society of America,* 1962, *55,* 499–502.

Clayton, D. L., and Paietta, J. V. Selection for circadian eclosion time in *Drosophila melanogaster. Science,* 1972, *178,* 994–995.

Engelmann, W., and Mack, J. Different oscillators control the circadian rhythm of eclosion and activity in *Drosophila. Journal of Comparative Physiology,* 1978, *127,* 229–237.

Feldman, J. F., and Hoyle, M. N. Isolation of circadian clock mutants of *Neurospora crassa. Genetics,* 1973, *75,* 605–613.

Feldman, J. F., and Hoyle, M. N. Complementation analysis of linked circadian clock mutants of *Neurospora crassa. Genetics,* 1976, *82,* 9–17.

Handler, A. M., and Konopka, R. J. Transplantation of a circadian pacemaker in *Drosophila. Nature,* 1979, *279,* 236–238.

Handler, A. M., and Postlethwait, J. H. Endocrine control of vitellogenesis in *Drosophila melanogaster:* Effects of the brain and corpus allatum. *Journal of Experimental Zoology,* 1977, *202,* 389–402.

Judd, B. H., Shen, M. W., and Kaufman, T. C. The anatomy and function of a segment of the X chromosome of *Drosophila melanogaster. Genetics,* 1972, *71,* 139–156.

Kayser, C., and Heusner, A. A. Le rhythme nycthéméral de la dépense d'énergie: Étude de physiologie comparée. *Journal de Physiologie,* 1967, *59*(1 Supplement), 3–116.

Konopka, R. J. Circadian clock mutants of Drosophila melanogaster. Ph.D. thesis, California Institute of Technology, Pasadena, 1972.

Konopka, R. J., and Benzer, S. Clock mutants of *Drosophila melanogaster. Proceedings of the National Academy of Sciences, USA,* 1971, *68,* 2112–2116.

Konopka, R. J., and Wells, S. *Drosophila* clock mutations affect the morphology of a brain neurosecretory cell group. *Journal of Neurobiology,* 1980, *11,* 411–415.

Lees, A. D. The role of photoperiod and temperature in the determination of parthenogenetic and sexual forms in the aphid *Megoura viciae* Buckton. II. The operation of the "interval timer" in young clones. *Journal of Insect Physiology,* 1960, *4,* 154–175.

Martin, U., Martin, H., and Lindauer, M. Transplantation of a time-signal in honeybees. *Journal of Comparative Physiology,* 1978, *124,* 193–201.

Minis, D. H., and Pittendrigh, C. S. Circadian oscillation controlling hatching: Its ontogeny during embryogenesis of a moth. *Science,* 1968, *159,* 534–536.

Nayar, J. K., and Sauerman, D. M. The effect of light regimes on the circadian rhythm of flight activity in the mosquito *Aedes taeniorhynchus. Journal of Experimental Biology,* 1971, *54,* 745–756.

Neumann, D. Genetic adaptation in emergence time of *Clunio* populations to different tidal conditions. *Helgoländer Wissenschaftliche Meeresuntersuchungen,* 1967, *15,* 163–171.

Pittendrigh, S. C. On temperature independence in the clock system controlling emergence time in *Drosophila. Proceedings of the National Academy of Sciences, USA,* 1954, *40,* 1018–1029.

Pittendrigh, C. S. The circadian oscillation in *Drosophila pseudoobscura* pupae: A model for the photoperiodic clock. *Zeitschrift für Pflanzenphysiologie,* 1966, *54,* 275–307.

Pittendrigh, C. S. Circadian systems. I. The driving oscillation and its assay in *Drosophila pseudoobscura. Proceedings of the National Academy of Sciences, USA,* 1967, *58,* 1762–1767.

Pittendrigh, C. S. Circadian oscillations in cells and the circadian organization of multicellular systems. In F. O. Schmitt and F. G. Worden (Eds.), *The Neurosciences Third Study Program.* Boston: MIT Press, 1974.

Pittendrigh, C. S., and Minis, D. H. The photoperiodic time measurement in *Pectinophora gossypiella* and its relation to the circadian system in that species. In M. Menaker (Ed.), *Biochronometry.* Washington, D.C.: National Academy of Sciences, 1971.

Pittendrigh, C. S., and Skopik, S. D. Circadian systems. V. The driving oscillation and the temporal sequence of development. *Proceedings of the National Academy of Sciences, USA,* 1970, *65,* 500–507.

Rensing, L., and Hardeland, R. Zur Wirkung der circadianen Rhythmik auf die Entwicklung von *Drosophila. Journal of Insect Physiology,* 1967, *13,* 1547–1568.

Rensing, L., Brunken, W., and Hardeland, R. On the genetics of a circadian rhythm in *Drosophila. Experientia,* 1968, *15,* 509–510.

Saunders, D. S. *Insect Clocks.* New York: Pergamon Press, 1976.

Truman, J. W. Physiology of insect rhythms. IV. Role of the brain in the regulation of the flight rhythm of the giant silkmoths. *Journal of Comparative Physiology,* 1974, *95,* 281–296.

Winfree, A. T. The investigation of oscillatory processes by perturbation experiments. In B. Chance, E. K. Pye, A. K. Ghosh, and B. Hess (Eds.), *Biological and Biochemical Oscillators.* New York: Academic Press, 1973.

Winfree, A. T., and Gordon, H. The photosensitivity of a mutant circadian clock. *Journal of Comparative Physiology,* 1977, *122,* 87–109.

Young, M. W., and Judd, B. H. Nonessential sequences, genes, and the polytene chromosome bands of *Drosophila melanogaster. Genetics,* 1978, *88,* 723–742.

Zimmerman, W. F. On the absence of circadian rhythmicity in *Drosophila pseudoobscura* pupae. *The Biological Bulletin,* 1969, *136,* 494–500.

Zimmerman, W. F., and Ives, D. Some photophysiological aspects of circadian rhythmicity in *Drosophila.* In M. Menaker (Ed.), *Biochronometry.* Washington, D.C.: National Academy of Sciences, 1971.

11

Vertebrate Behavioral Rhythms

Benjamin Rusak

Introduction

Interest in rhythms of animal behavior derives from the recognition that the biological value of a behavior depends as much on when it occurs as on the particular form it takes (see Enright, 1970, and Chapter 15). It follows that a meaningful ethogram of any species should describe both species-typical motor patterns and species-typical timing of behavior. This chapter surveys the variety of behavioral rhythms that have been studied and the range of species in which they have been described.

There are several problems with most of the available descriptions of behavioral rhythmicity. One is analogous to a classical problem in descriptive ethology: that of determining appropriate units of analysis. Ethologists have recognized that significant features of behavior, such as the degree of apparent stereotypy, are to a large extent determined by the temporal and spatial resolution of the recording procedure (Barlow, 1968). Reports of behavioral rhythms have generally ignored this issue and have included data that are grouped in a great variety of ways across hours, days, and individuals. The temporal resolution of such behavioral recording can determine whether particular rhythms are detected and what their apparent characteristics are. A simple example is that recording only the degree of "nocturnality" of a behavior may lead to the erroneous conclusion that a rhythm has been lost when only its phase relation to the light cycle has changed.

In other situations the appropriateness of particular units of analysis is more ambiguous. In a field study of monkey troops (Nilgiri langurs, *Presbytis johnii*), Horwich (1976) recorded hourly means of feeding and calling averaged over several days; the data obtained showed clear dawn and dusk peaks, especially of feeding. However, a finer-grained analysis of individual troops during a single day revealed previously undetected ultradian behavioral

Benjamin Rusak   Department of Psychology, Dalhousie University, Halifax, Nova Scotia, B3H 4J1 Canada. Preparation of the manuscript was aided by support from the NSERC of Canada.

cycles. Horwich concluded that the presence of significantly different individual (or troop) patterns and day-to-day variations can be obscured by grouping data across individuals and over days in search of the population mean. But the most detailed analysis is not always the best, since excessive attention to detail and individual differences can obscure biologically significant population trends and prevent the formulation of meaningful generalizations.

In order to choose among these possible descriptive strategies, it is useful first to identify some of the sources of behavioral variability among individuals and across time. If individual variability is generated as the sum of independent, stochastic determinants, then the average pattern in the population will also be the modal (i.e., most common) pattern. But if individual variability reflects the presence of naturally separate subpopulations, then the "species-typical pattern" may have little biological meaning. To take an extreme example, a bimodal activity pattern in a population might result from one subpopulation's preying on dawn-active species and another's utilizing dusk-active prey. The population average (dawn-and-dusk activity) may not reflect the actual activity pattern of any single animal on any day. Such individual specialization is familiar to naturalists and has received some analytic attention (e.g., McFarland, 1977), but most studies of behavioral rhythmicity have not dealt explicitly with sources of variability within populations.

A second issue in the description of behavioral rhythms is the appropriate definition of behavioral categories. The most frequently reported rhythm in both field and laboratory studies is that of *activity*. This term is used to refer to a diverse array of behaviors recorded by equally diverse methods. In the laboratory, behavioral criteria for defining the active phase generally include the occurrence of locomotion or other gross body movements, while physiological criteria may include metabolic rate, body temperature, and electroencephalographic activity. In field studies, the active phase may be defined by locomotion, absence from a roost or retreat, presence in a feeding area, or evidence of recent feeding.

These measures are presumed to be highly correlated on the assumption that each overt rhythm reflects a common, underlying cycle, which may be loosely defined as one of general arousal or of engagement with the environment. This supposition is reinforced by the finding that several behavioral rhythms recorded simultaneously in one animal have very similar parameters (Richter, 1967; Aschoff and von Saint Paul, 1973; Morin, 1978). In addition, the behavioral changes shown by rats subjected to supposedly nonspecific, arousal-producing manipulations (food/water deprivation or amphetamine injections) are very similar to those shown by rats as they enter their most active daily phase (Prescott, 1970).

However, some animals show clear dissociations among simultaneously recorded behaviors; for example, hamsters *(Mesocricetus auratus)* and opossums *(Didelphis marsupialis)* regularly eat during both the "active" and "rest" phases of their daily cycles, as defined by locomotion and other measures (Zucker and Stephan, 1973; Bombardieri and Johnson, 1969). In addition, the correspondence of several measures recorded under one set of conditions does not imply that these parameters will respond similarly to either internal or environmental changes. A variety of conditions may produce dissociations of rhythms that are normally synchronized (see Chapters 12 and 17), and the apparent "activity-type" may change dramatically with developmental stage or season (see below).

These considerations dictate caution in assuming that all measures of behavioral rhythmicity are roughly equivalent assays of a unitary underlying mechanism, and that a single activity type characterizes a species or even an individual. The descriptions of species-characteristic behavioral rhythms reviewed in this chapter do not adequately address these issues. Ideally, the descriptive categories, temporal units, and demographic units appropriate for describing behavioral rhythms would be derived from an understanding of the sources of behavioral variability in vertebrate populations; in practice, such information is generally unavailable. As a step toward identifying these sources of variability, this chapter emphasizes the role of environmental factors (other than the primary zeitgeber) in the production and modification of vertebrate behavioral rhythms.

Mammals

This section reviews in detail two topics about which there is substantial information available for mammals, namely, the influence of social and other environmental factors on activity rhythms, and the role of the circadian system in learning and memory. Other aspects of mammalian behavioral rhythms are reviewed elsewhere in this volume. Table I provides a partial list of the many mammalian species whose activity rhythms have been reported, as well as a sampling of other behavioral rhythms.

Activity

INTRODUCTION. Activity rhythms recorded in the laboratory have been our main (in many cases, exclusive) source of information about endogenous aspects of biological rhythms, including such species-characteristic features as period length, entrainment range, and light responsiveness. Information about these aspects is extensively reviewed in Chapters 6 and 7. The controlled conditions that permit observation of these aspects of rhythmicity necessarily preclude observation of the influence of many environmental factors that are major determinants of activity patterns in the field (Kavanau, 1969; Ashby, 1972). These factors include physical aspects of the environment that are predictable across generations (seasonal, lunar, and tidal cycles); physical aspects that are relatively unpredictable (terrain, weather); biological features such as quality and availability of food; and the presence of other organisms that may act as competitors, cooperators, predators, mates, or prey.

These exogenous factors have not been the object of the same sustained experimental attack as has been directed at the endogenous features of rhythmicity. In many cases, information about the role of exogenous factors can only be gleaned from reports aimed primarily at other subjects. But the contribution of the endogenous features of rhythmicity to fitness can be understood only in an environmental context: it is the degree to which these features meet, or are adaptively modified by, the exigencies of the field environment that determines the biological value of rhythmicity to the animal. It is therefore important to examine the degree to which environmental factors influence the expression of behavioral rhythmicity in mammals.

Environmental Influences

Social Stimuli. The efficacy of social stimuli in synchronizing mammalian activity rhythms has been the subject of anecdotal reports more often than of experimental studies. Sufficient evidence exists to warrant the conclusion that stimulation provided by conspecif-

TABLE I. BEHAVIORAL RHYTHMS: MAMMALS[a]

Behavior	Species	Type of study	Reference
Activity			
Norway rat	*Rattus norvegicus*	R	Richter (1922)
Deer mouse	*Peromyscus maniculatus*	R	Johnson (1926)
California vole	*Microtus californicus*	F	Pearson (1959)
Harvest mouse	*Reithrodontomys megalotis*	F	Pearson (1959)
Wood mouse	*Apodemus sylvaticus*	R	Miller (1954)
Flying squirrel	*Glaucomys volans*	R	DeCoursey (1960)
House mouse	*Mus musculus* (12 strains)	R	Ebihara and Tsuji (1976)
Birch mouse	*Sicista betulina*	R	Johansen and Krog (1959)
Richardson's ground squirrel	*Citellus richardsoni*	F	Quanstrom (1971)
Gray squirrel	*Sciurus carolinensis*	F	Thompson (1977)
Kangaroo rats	*Dipodomys merriami*	F	Kenagy (1973)
	D. microps	F	Kenagy (1973)
Beaver	*Castor canadensis*	F	Bovet and Oertli (1974)
Muskrat	*Ondatra zibethicus*	F	Stewart and Bider (1977)
Antelope ground squirrels	*Ammospermophilus leucurus*	R	DeCoursey (1973)
	A. harrisi	R	DeCoursey (1973)
Brewer's mole	*Parascalops breweri*	F	Hamilton (1939)
Lesser short-tailed shrew	*Cryptotis parva*	R	Allison, Gerber, Breedlove, and Dryden (1977)
Tree shrew	*Tupaia belangeri*	R	Hoffmann (1971)
Two-toed sloth	*Choloepus hoffmanni*	R	Howarth and Toole (1973)
Little brown bat	*Myotis lucifugus*	R	Griffin and Welsh (1937)
Greater European horseshoe bat	*Rhinolophus ferrum-equinum*	R	DeCoursey and DeCoursey (1964)
Jamaican fruit bat	*Artibeus jamaicensis*	F	Morrison (1978)
African false vampire bat	*Cardioderma cor*	F	Vaughan (1976)
Opossum	*Didelphis marsupialis*	R	Bombardieri and Johnson (1969)
Red kangaroo	*Macropus rufus*	F	Caughley (1964)
Gray kangaroo	*M. canguru*	F	Caughley (1964)
European badger	*Meles meles*	F	Canivenc, Croizet, Blanquet, and Bonnin-Laffargue (1960)
Sea otter	*Enhydra lutris*	F	Shimek and Monk (1977)
Dog	*Canis domesticus*	F	Scott and Causey (1973)
Least weasel	*Mustela rixosa*	R	Kavanau (1969)
African elephant	*Loxodonta africana*	F	Wyatt and Eltringham (1974)
Dorcas gazelle	*Gazella dorcas*	R	Ghobrial and Cloudsley-Thompson (1976)
African chevrotain	*Hyemoschus aquaticus*	F/R	Dubost (1975)
Boar	*Sus scrofa*	F	Gundlach (1968)
Merino sheep	*Ovis*	R	Squires (1971)
Bottle-nose dolphin	*Tursiops aduncus*	F/R	Saayman, Tayler, and Bower (1973)
Sperm whale	*Physeter catodon*	F	Matsushita (1955)
Slow loris	*Nycticebus coucang*	R	Tenaza, Ross, Tantichroenyos, and Berkson (1969)
Thick-tailed bushbaby	*Galago crassicaudatus*	R	Randolph (1971)
Squirrel monkey	*Saimiri sciureus*	R	Richter (1968)
Night monkey	*Aotus trivirgatus*	R	Erkert (1976)
Red colobus monkey	*Colobus badius tephrosceles*	F	Clutton-Brock (1974)
Japanese macaque	*Macaca fuscata*	F	Yotsumoto (1976)
Human	*Homo sapiens*	R	Aschoff, Fatranska, and Giedke (1971)

TABLE I. *(continued)*

Behavior		Species	Type of study	Reference
Aggression				
	House mouse	*Mus musculus*	R	Sofia and Salama (1970)
	House mouse	*Mus musculus*	R	Ziesenis (1974)
	House mouse	*Mus musculus*	R	Hyde and Sawyer (1977)
	Golden hamster	*Mesocricetus auratus*	R	Lerwill and Makings (1971)
	Golden hamster	*Mesocricetus auratus*	R	Landau (1975)
	Rat	*Rattus norvegicus*	R	Lonowski, Levitt, and Dickinson (1975)
Coprophagy				
	Cottontail rabbit	*Sylvilagus floridanus*	R	Heisinger (1965)
	Rat	*Rattus norvegicus*	R	Lutton and Chevalier (1973)
	Rabbit	*Oryctolagus cuniculus*	R	Jilge (1976)
Eating or drinking				
	Rat	*Rattus norvegicus*	R	Richter (1922)
	Guinea pig	*Cavia porcellus*	R	Horton, West, and Turley (1975)
	Chinchilla	*Chinchilla laniger*	R	Burdick and Luz (1973)
	Red colobus	*Colobus badius tephrosceles*	F	Clutton-Brock (1974)
	Dog	*Canis domesticus*	R	Ardisson, Dolisi, Camous, and Gastaud (1975)
	Sheep	*Ovis*	R	Squires (1971)
	Elephant	*Loxodonta africana*	F	Wyatt and Eltringham (1974)
Food selection				
	Gibbons	*Hylobates lar*	F	Raemaekers (1978)
		H. syndactylus	F	Raemaekers (1978)
Gnawing				
	Golden hamster	*Mesocricetus auratus*	R	Morin (1978)
Intracranial self-stimulation				
	Rat	*Rattus norvegicus*	R	Terman and Terman (1970)
	Rat	*Rattus norvegicus*	R	Dark, Chiodo, and Asdourian (1977)
Maternal behavior				
	Rat	*Rattus norvegicus*	R	Ader and Grota (1970)
Nest building				
	House mouse	*Mus musculus*	R	Roper (1975)
Sexual behavior				
	Male rat	*Rattus norvegicus*	R	Beach and Levinson (1949)
	Male rat	*Rattus norvegicus*	R	Larsson (1958)
	Male rat	*Rattus norvegicus*	R	Dewsbury (1968)
Tonic immobility				
	Rat	*Rattus norvegicus*	R	Hennig and Dunlap (1977)
Vocalization				
	Harp seal	*Pagophilus groenlandicus*	F	Terhune and Ronald (1976)
	Nilgiri langur	*Presbytis johnii*	F	Horwich (1976)

[a]This table lists behaviors that have been reported to show daily rhythms and the species in which these rhythms have been described. It is intended not to be exhaustive but to give some idea of the range of behavioral rhythms and species that have been studied. The first column lists the behavior involved; the second gives the common name of the species studied; the third gives the Latin name; the fourth indicates whether the study was of free-living (F) or restricted (R) animals (the latter category comprises both laboratory studies and field studies involving caged animals); the final column gives the reference. No attempt has been made to differentiate among the various measures used to yield "activity" patterns.

ics or by heterospecific predators or competitors can influence behavioral rhythmicity in many mammalian species.

Social synchronization among conspecifics was suggested by Johnson (1926), who reported that mice of the genus *Peromyscus* that were housed together tended to adopt similar activity rhythms. Kavanau (1963) also reported that the distinctive activity patterns of two singly caged female *Peromyscus* converged when they were housed together. Another report claimed that blinded *Mus musculus* were synchronized to LD cycles only if sighted mice were housed in the same room; this finding indicated an olfactory or auditory mechanism for synchronization among mice (Halberg, Visscher, and Bittner, 1954).

Male chevrotains (*Hyemoschus aquaticus,* a small antelope) penned outdoors without access to females had a bimodal activity pattern, while the females showed three activity peaks each night. When the sexes were separated by only a wire fence, the males adopted the female activity pattern, apparently by tracking the females' arousals (Dubost, 1975). Sexually isolated groups of red wolf–coyote hybrids (*Canis* sp.) showed distinctive activity patterns that converged on a single pattern when the full pack was reunited (Roper and Ryon, 1977). The activity patterns of beaver colonies *(Castor canadensis)* were recorded with microphones inserted into the lodges throughout the winter when ice and snow cover produced extended periods of effective DD. Several records showed clear evidence of stable, freerunning rhythms that could have been generated only if all members of the colony (2–5 individuals) were roughly synchronized (Bovet and Oertli, 1974; Potvin and Bovet, 1975). It is possible that all members of these family groups had similar natural periods, but the persistence of these rhythms intact over many weeks demands some form of social synchronization.

There is weak evidence for social synchronization among macaque monkeys in the laboratory (Fuselier, 1973; Rohles and Osbaldiston, 1969). In the latter study, monkeys *(Macaca mulatta)* were apparently synchronized when permitted only to see and hear each other, but there was inadequate evidence of freeruns in isolation to permit assessment of the effects of the social condition. Another study of this species reported ultradian cycles of social interaction in pairs of monkeys introduced to each other for the first time; in most cases, the period of the interaction cycle corresponded to that of the dominant monkey's cycle of exploratory behavior (Maxim, Bowden, and Sackett, 1976).

Sexual cyclicity of female mammals, which is controlled in part by a circadian mechanism (Alleva, Waleski, and Alleva, 1971; see Rusak and Zucker, 1979), is well known to be sensitive to social influences. The odor of male mice can synchronize estrous cycles of females, presumably by initiating ovulation simultaneously (Bronson, 1971), and groups of female humans and rats show a degree of social synchronization of their respective menstrual and estrous cycles. In the case of rats, the synchronizing cue appears also to be olfactory and may operate by affecting the timing of ovulation; in each species, synchrony is normally induced in individuals living in close contact with each other (McClintock, 1971, 1978).

It has been suggested that the rhythmicity of a mammalian mother may influence the rhythmicity of her offspring (Ader and Grota, 1970); some evidence exists to support this suggestion (Deguchi, 1975; Levin and Stern, 1975). However, it is also clear that this social influence is not critical to the development of rhythmicity, since rats (Folk, 1966) and monkeys (Miller, Caul, and Mirsky, 1971) not exposed to maternal rhythmicity still develop adult rhythms that are normal insofar as they have been studied.

Rather than promoting mutual synchrony, social contact may instead promote avoidance and thereby synchronize behavior through exclusion. In a rat colony studied under seminatural conditions, dominant rats appeared to exclude subordinate animals from a feeding site at one time of day, presumably on the basis of aggressive interactions (Calhoun, 1962). Similar effects of social interaction have been reported in laboratory studies of house mice (*Mus musculus;* Crowcroft and Rowe, 1963) and field mice (*Apodemus sylvaticus;* Bovet, 1972). Large kangaroo rats *(Dipodomys microps)* aggressively excluded smaller *D. merriami* from a favored feeding site early in the night; the latter returned to feed later in the night when *microps* were less active above ground (Kenagy, 1973).

There are many anecdotal reports of animals undergoing dramatic changes in activity pattern as a result of contact with other species, notably with humans (Kavanau, 1969). The activity of the wild boar *(Sus scrofa)* is diurnal in a protected environment but is altered by human predation (Gundlach, 1968); rats that feed nocturnally in the laboratory may in some situations feed almost exclusively by day in the absence of human interference (Taylor, 1975).

The long-term influence of human interference may be mediated by selection pressure exerted on a population with a heterogeneous activity type, but individual plasticity may also play a role. Rawson (1960) has reported phase delays of activity in *Peromyscus* handled by humans during the night; a mechanism that could mediate this effect or the influence of conspecifics has not been described. It may be that individuals of highly social species are sensitive to the disturbance produced by the activity of group members, much as humans are sensitive to the disturbance produced by an alarm clock or other social cues (Aschoff, Fatranska, and Giedke, 1971). If social synchronization does not represent a simple masking effect, it implies susceptibility of a central timekeeper either to social events as zeitgebers or to feedback from activity that is stimulated by social contact. Either possibility suggests a significant and largely unexplored sensitivity in the circadian system.

Lunar Cycles. Activity patterns of a number of animals, particularly those affected by the tides, are modulated by lunar cycles (see Chapter 19), but terrestrial mammals are not generally regarded as being influenced by the moon. However, some retrospective studies have described the use of lunar cycles as timing cues for mammalian reproduction (Menaker and Menaker, 1959; Sinclair, 1977), and many field and laboratory studies provide evidence for the modulation of activity patterns by moonlight in nocturnal mammals.

Many small mammals reduce activity levels on brightly moonlit nights; these include voles (*Microtus californicus;* Pearson, 1960) and bats (*Artibeus liturtatus, Rousettus aegyptiacus, Phyllostomus hastatus;* Erkert, 1974). Artificial illumination of the roost exit delayed the evening departure of myotid bats (*Myotis myotis* and *M. nattereri*), which usually leave when twilight intensities have reached a characteristic level (DeCoursey and DeCoursey, 1964; Laufens, cited in Voûte, Sluiter, and Grimm, 1974). By contrast, the night monkey *(Aotus trivirgatus)* was most active at the highest moonlight intensities, and around new moon, activity was restricted to bursts around dawn and dusk (Erkert, 1974). This species was also most active when the D phase of an artificial cycle was illuminated with about 0.1 lux (= full moonlight) and was less active at lower or higher light intensities (Erkert, 1976).

Two species of kangaroo rat (*Dipodomys spectabilis* and *D. nitratoides*) were found to be least active in the field at full moon and most active at new moon. When tested in running wheels under artificial solar and lunar cycles, these species showed exactly the opposite response, becoming most active when the artifical "moon" shone at night (Lockard and Owings, 1974). Such findings cast doubt on the significance of earlier results obtained using artificial light cycles to study the responses of *Peromyscus californicus* and *P. eremicus* to moonlight. The activity of *californicus* was reported to be inhibited by illumination at night, while that of *eremicus* was stimulated by such illumination (Owings and Lockard, 1971).

During the lunar half-cycle around new moon, Jamaican fruit bats *(Artibeus jamaicensis)* departed from their day roost after sunset and remained at a "feeding roost" throughout the night. From this site, they made frequent flights into nearby trees to feed. During the lunar half-cycle around full moon, they departed at a similar time (before the moon was high) but returned to their day roost after only a few feeding flights; they did not return to feed again until shortly before dawn. The bats followed this pattern of returning to their day roost for most of the night even when the near-full moon was obscured by heavy overcast. This finding was offered as one indication that bats time their activity in part using an endogenous lunar clock (Morrison, 1978).

Other evidence for endogenous lunar timing of activity is less compelling. The fact that bats (or rodents) are active near dawn and dusk at light intensities that they avoid when produced by the moon may suggest a lunar influence that is independent of moonlight, but other interpretations are possible (Morrison, 1978). The intensity of light may be less important than its source; diffuse twilight illumination may not increase the visibility of small mammals, but less intense, highly directional moonlight can cast stark shadows, which would act to a predator's advantage (Lockard and Owings, 1974; Morrison, 1978). Despite some claims of nonlight lunar influences on the activity of mammals (Brown and Park, 1967; see Mills, Lockard, and Owings, 1975, for references), most of the reported evidence suggests only responsiveness to moonlight (Klinowska, 1972; Mills *et al.,* 1975; Erkert, 1976). This represents a significant ecological factor, but the persistence of overt lunar activity cycles in mammals isolated from moonlight remains to be convincingly demonstrated.

Seasonal Cycles. The dramatic environmental changes associated with seasonal cycles often entail dramatic behavioral changes such as those involved in hibernation and migration (see Chapters 20 and 21). But seasonal cycles of food availability, photoperiod, temperature, and ground cover may produce more subtle changes in the activity patterns of many animals. The activity patterns of these species cannot be described as being of a single type, at least in the natural environment. Seasonal variability itself varies with latitude and other local conditions; the range of adaptability of most animals to these influences remains unexplored.

Seasonal changes in activity have been described in various temperate-zone species, including several species of vole (Eibl-Eibesfeldt, cited in Vaughan, 1972; Erkinaro, 1961; Grodziński, 1963; Stebbins, 1972), deer mice (*Peromyscus maniculatus;* Stebbins, 1971), woodchucks (*Marmota monax;* Bronson, 1962), ground squirrels (*Spermophilus richardsoni;* Quanstrom, 1971), gray squirrels (*Sciurus carolinensis;* Thompson, 1977), and macaques (Yotsumoto, 1976). These changes are sometimes quite extreme and may include switching from strongly nocturnal to diurnal patterns with the seasons (e.g., Grodziński, 1963). The complexities involved in trying to describe a species-typical activity pattern are exemplified by a study of the vole *Clethrionymus gapperi* (Stebbins, 1972). Voles studied near Edmonton, Alberta (near 53°N) were diurnally active, with a peak near dawn throughout the study period (November–June). The same species studied further north (near 61°N) showed a single nocturnal peak in winter, a bimodal nocturnal pattern in spring, and a polycyclic pattern in June, with activity extending into the long daylight phase (see also pp. 200 and 204).

In equatorial regions, photoperiod is relatively stable, but there are large seasonal changes in rainfall and temperature that influence activity patterns. The reported changes are not extreme and may be attributable to variations in food availability and to the disruptive effects of very heavy rainfall. Species for whom significant seasonal changes have been reported include the red colobus monkey (*Colobus badius tephrosceles;* Clutton-Brock, 1974), Dorcas gazelle (*Gazella dorcas;* Ghobrial and Cloudsley-Thompson, 1976), and the African false vampire bat (*Cardioderma cor;* Vaughan, 1976).

Other Environmental Conditions. Ambient weather conditions, particularly temperature and precipitation, affect behavioral expression in mammals (e.g., Bernstein, 1972). Rainfall delayed the evening roost-departure of myotid bats (DeCoursey and DeCoursey, 1964) and the midday feeding of red colobus monkeys (Clutton-Brock, 1974). By contrast, rainfall increased the activity of *Microtus californicus* (Pearson, 1960) and caused muskrats *(Ondatra zibethicus)* to become active earlier in the day and to increase the amount of nocturnal activity (Stewart and Bider, 1977). When exposed to the weather in rooftop enclosures, bushbabies *(Galago senegalensis)* and a night monkey *(Aotus trivirgatus)* decreased their running-wheel activity in the rain, but precipitation encouraged longer active phases in slow lorises (*Nycticebus coucang;* Kavanau and Peters, 1976).

Laboratory housing conditions may modify activity patterns; the availability of a secure retreat or other cover is of particular significance to feral animals (see below, p. 204). Food intake of a South American rodent *(Oxymycterus rutilans)* became less strictly nocturnal when a darkened nest box was added to its cage (Vilchez and Echave Llanos, 1971). Similarly, the addition of a darkened burrow and nest box modified the activity, drinking, and feeding patterns of albino rats housed under an illumination cycle (Rusak and Block, unpublished observations, 1973).

Some more subtle environmental stimuli have been reported to modulate activity patterns in the laboratory. Artificial electric fields (Wever, 1971) and cycles of atmospheric pressure (Hayden and Lindberg, 1969) modified various circadian parameters and even produced entrainment in humans and mice, respectively, but the influence of variations in these parameters on activity in the natural environment has not been documented.

Food and Water Restriction. Obtaining sufficient food and water appears to be a primary goal of much animal activity in the field. It is not surprising, therefore, to find that the pattern of availability of food and water is a significant determinant of the pattern of activity in the laboratory. The continuous availability of excess food in "normal" laboratory conditions is a departure from usual field conditions that undoubtedly influences an animal's behavior. Similarly, experimental restriction of food availability to a limited amount and/or time affects not only motivation for food but also a variety of rhythmic behavioral and physiological parameters.

It is well established that the quantity of food consumed by rats is not a simple function of the length of prior deprivation. Rather, the effectiveness of deprivation in promoting feeding depends on the time of day at which it occurs (e.g., Lawrence and Mason, 1955; Bare and Cicala, 1960; Bellinger and Mendel, 1975). Similarly, the effectiveness of food intake in reducing subsequent feeding depends on its phasing (Quartermain, Kissileff, Shapiro, and Miller, 1971; Panksepp, 1973). Apparently, during both sustained food deprivation (Bellinger and Mendel, 1975) and continuous food infusion (Quartermain *et al.*, 1971), the substrate underlying the feeding rhythm remains relatively normally entrained to the illumination cycle.

When food deprivation is repeated on a daily basis and food is available only during brief periods outside the normal feeding time, several, but not all, behavioral and physiological rhythms are reported to be phase-shifted relative to the illumination cycle (e.g., Philippens, von Mayersbach, and Scheving, 1977: Krieger and Hauser, 1978). Interpretation of these phase shifts depends on a careful reexamination of the evidence.

There is substantial evidence to support the following conclusions: (1) rats become active on a daily basis in anticipation of the time of limited daily food availability, regardless of its relation to the illumination cycle; (2) rats can anticipate 24-hr restriction schedules but not 19- or 29-hr schedules (Bolles and Stokes, 1965); (3) they can anticipate more than one restriction phase per day (Bolles and Moot, 1973); and (4) normal nocturnal entrainment (in LD) or a freerun (in LL) of activity may coexist with anticipatory activity accompanying the restricted feeding or drinking phase (Bolles and Duncan, 1969; Bolles and Moot, 1973; Panksepp and Krost, 1975; Moore and Ziegler, 1978; Boulos, Rosenwasser, and Terman, 1980).

These results fall short of establishing that cycles of food availability entrain circadian rhythms as do cycles of illumination. A rigorous demonstration of such an entrainment function would require (1) establishment of a stable freerun in the dependent parameter with food freely available; (2) demonstration of stable phase and period control by the cycle of restricted food availability; and (3) evidence that the phase of food availability predicts the phase of a subsequent freerun better than does the phase of the extrapolated prior freerun (cf. Menaker and Eskin, 1966; Boulos *et al.*, 1980). Recent claims that feeding restriction acts as a zeitgeber to entrain activity, drinking, or other rhythms in rats (Edmonds and Adler, 1977a,b; Krieger and Hauser, 1978; Krieger, Hauser, and Krey, 1977) and squirrel monkeys (Sulzman, Fuller, and Moore-Ede, 1977a,b) have not been supported by such evidence.

One study of rats has demonstrated that while food restriction causes drinking to occur mainly during and after the time of food availability, the phase of the subsequent freerun of drinking is not predicted by the phase of food restriction (Boulos *et al.*, 1980). The same study, however, indicated that there are unambiguous circadian constraints on anticipatory (nonreinforced) lever pressing, as there are on anticipatory activity (Bolles and Stokes, 1965). These and earlier data support two conclusions: that a circadian oscillator is involved in the production of anticipatory behavior in response to food restriction, and that this oscillator is not the dominant, light-entrained system that dictates the phase of the intact freerunning rhythm. A necessary corollary to these conclusions is that a single behavioral function is multiply controlled by an ensemble of oscillators that may be dissociated under some conditions (cf. Rusak, 1977; see Chapters 12 and 17).

This mechanism may permit rats to "mark" significant phases in a daily cycle using a circadian mechanism without resynchronizing the entire circadian system to those phases (see p. 194 and Chapter 15). In the field, this ability may permit rats to take advantage of short-lived resources that are available at unusual times of day without disrupting solar-day entrainment that is essential for other functions, such as photoperiodism. The efficacy of food restriction in shifting rhythms in most mammals is not known; since other mammals do not respond to food restriction as rats do (e.g., Silverman and Zucker, 1976), the validity of these conclusions for them remains to be established.

LEARNING AND MEMORY

DAILY VARIATIONS. The performance of laboratory animals on a learning task varies with the phase of an LD cycle at which they are tested; such variations have been reported for conditioned suppression (Stroebel, 1967; Evans and Patton, 1970); avoidance learning (Davies, Navaratnam, and Redfern, 1973; Ghiselli and Patton, 1976; Gordon and Scheving, 1968); maze learning (Hostetter, 1966; Stavnes, 1972); and taste-aversion learning (Rusak and Zucker, 1974; Ternes, 1976). Daily rhythms might influence learning and performance in several ways; (1) variations in arousal, motivation (e.g., hunger), or sensory thresholds during acquisition and/or testing could modify the salience of discriminative cues as well as the value of rewards or punishments; (2) the ability to consolidate and store acquired information might vary with time of training; and (3) the ability to retain and recall stored information might vary with time of testing.

In the majority of studies, no attempt has been made to discriminate among the many factors that might contribute to rhythmic differences in performance. In one study, performance efficiency, but not acquisition, was affected by time of day of testing (Ghiselli and Patton, 1976); in another, initial performance was equivalent among groups, but resistance to extinction varied dramatically with time of training (Ternes, 1976). Electroconvulsive shock (ECS) given to mice immediately after training disrupted memory equally well at two times of day, but ECS given 3 min after training disrupted memory only in mice tested during the D phase and not in those tested in L (Stephens, McGaugh, and Alpern, 1967). It is possible that memory consolidation proceeds at different rates at different times of day. Indirect evidence suggests that both sensory and central processing rhythms could play significant roles in producing learning and memory rhythms. Daily variations have been described in sensitivity to environmental stimuli (Grabfield and Martin, 1913; Martin, Bigelow, and Wilbur, 1914; Henkin, 1970; Wada and Asakura, 1970; Rusak and Zucker, 1974; Zihl, Poppel, and von Cramon, 1977) and in the function of neural systems, some of which may be involved in memory (e.g., Schmitt, 1973; Barnes, McNaughton, Goddard, Douglas, and Adamec, 1977).

The type of performance rhythm obtained depends on the type of learning task used. Rats trained to inhibit activity in a passive avoidance task performed better when tested during L rather than D (Sandman, Kastin, and Schally, 1971); rats trained in an active avoidance task performed better late in L than early in L (Pagano and Lovely, 1972). Predictably, conclusions about the influence of drugs on learning and performance also depend on the time of drug administration relative to endogenous hormonal, neurochemical, and performance cycles. Administration of melanocyte-stimulating hormone (MSH) improved performance (i.e., increased step-through latencies) on a passive avoidance task during D but was completely ineffective during L (Sandman et al., 1971). By contrast, adrenocorticotrophic hormone (ACTH), which is structurally similar to MSH, improved performance on an active avoidance task early in L but failed to affect performance late in

L when peak levels of endogenous ACTH normally occur (Pagano and Lovely, 1972). Assessing drug affects on learning at only a single phase could easily lead to erroneous conclusions.

CIRCADIAN TIME MEMORY. The anticipatory activity of rats on a restricted feeding schedule bears at least a strong formal similarity to the well-studied *Zeitgedächtnis* of honeybees (see above p. 191 and Chapter 15). This phenomenon is not a direct response to lengthening deprivation and subsequent satiation, as indicated by several kinds of evidence. Only circadian intervals can be anticipated (Bolles and Stokes, 1965), more than one daily phase can be anticipated (Bolles and Moot, 1973), and both activity levels (Bolles and Moot, 1973) and corticosterone levels (Coover, Sutton, and Haybach, 1977) fall after the scheduled mealtime even if feeding is omitted on one day. The mechanism involved in learning to anticipate particular daily phases is unknown, but it may involve the restriction-induced shift of a circadian oscillator (see above pp. 191–193).

Learning and performance are modulated by a circadian mechanism that is completely independent of time-of-day effects. Rats trained in active or passive avoidance tasks at various times of day performed well at circadian intervals after training, and moderately well 12 hr after training and at its circadian multiples; however, at 6, 18, and 30 hr after training, performance was very poor (Holloway and Wansley, 1973a,b). Similar temporal effects have been reported for performance on tasks involving conditioned suppression (Stroebel, 1967; Hunsicker and Mellgren, 1977). The function of circadian modulation of learning that is independent of time of day is unknown; perhaps such a mechanism permits temporally selective avoidance of, or attraction to, environments whose valence changes with time, but unpredictably with respect to the illumination cycle. For example, rats may learn to avoid a feeding site when local predators or competitors are likely to be present, but not at other times (cf. Calhoun, 1962). Independence of this mechanism from time of day would permit such learned place attraction and avoidance in situations where the critical phases cannot be predicted in the absence of specific learning (see Rusak and Zucker, 1975).

BIRDS

INTRODUCTION

Activity rhythms have been described for a large number of avian species in the field; these descriptions are often based on the times of singing (Palmgren, 1949; Leopold and Eynon, 1961) or of feeding (Morton, 1967). Laboratory studies have also concentrated on rhythms of activity and their regulation by light (see Gwinner, 1975, for a review). Few other avian rhythms have been studied, although a number have been reported incidentally; Table II lists some of these rhythms and the species in which they were observed.

Most avian species are diurnal, but many of these same species are also nocturnal migrants (Palmgren, 1949), and some groups are characteristically dusk- or night-active (Strigiformes and Caprimulgiformes). Although the results of both laboratory and field studies indicate the dominance of light in the control of avian circadian rhythms, other environmental factors also play a significant role. There has been little attempt to under-

TABLE II. BEHAVIORAL RHYTHMS: BIRDS[a]

Behavior		Species	Type of study	Reference
Activity				
	House sparrow	*Passer domesticus*	R	Menaker and Eskin (1966)
	Greenfinch	*Chloris chloris*	R	Aschoff and Wever (1965)
	Bullfinch	*Pyrrhula pyrrhula*	R	Aschoff and Wever (1965)
	Chicken	*Gallus domesticus*	R	Aschoff and von Saint Paul (1973)
Copulation/courtship				
	Ring dove	*Streptopelia risoria*	R	Martinez-Vargas and Erickson (1973)
	Great-tailed grackle	*Quiscalus mexicanus*	F	Kok (1971)
	Great spotted woodpecker	*Dendrocopos major*	—	Pynnönen, cited in Palmgren (1949)
	Laughing gull	*Larus atricilla*	F	Burger(1976)
Drumming				
	Ruffed grouse	*Bonasa umbellus*	F	Archibald (1976)
Egg laying				
	Willow warbler	*Phyloscopus trochilus*	—	Kuuisisto, cited in Palmgren (1949)
Feeding				
	White-crowned sparrow	*Zonotrichia leucophrys*	F/R	Morton (1967)
	Mourning dove	*Zenaidura macroura*	F	Schmid (1965)
Food storage				
	Yellow-billed magpie	*Pica nuttalli*	F	Verbeek (1972)
Incubation				
	Pigeons	—	—	Lorenz, cited in Palmgren (1949)
	Ring dove	*Streptopelia risoria*	R	Gerlach, Heinrich, and Lehrman (1975)
Nest building				
	Yellow-billed magpie	*Pica nuttalli*	F	Verbeek (1972)
	Laughing gull	*Larus atricilla*	F	Burger (1976)
	Willow warbler	*Phyloscopus trochilus*	—	Kuuisisto, cited in Palmgren (1949)
	Ring dove	*Streptopelia risoria*	R	Martinez-Vargas and Erickson (1973)
Nest departure				
	Brunnich's guillemot	*Uria lomvia*	F	Cullen (1954)
Parental feeding				
	Meadow pipit	*Anthus pratensis*	F	Hillman and Young (1977)
	White-backed woodpecker	*Dendrocopos leucotos*	—	Franz, cited in Palmgren (1949)
Predation				
	Kestrel	*Falco sparverius*	R	Mueller (1973)
	Barn owl	*Tyto alba*	F	Bunn (1972)
Preening				
	Kittiwake	*Rissa tridactyla*	F	Cullen (1954)
	Ring dove	*Streptopelia risoria*	R	Martinez-Vargas and Erickson (1973)
Singing				
	20 species	—	F	Leopold and Eynon (1961)
Territorial defense				
	Great-tailed grackle	*Quiscalus mexicanus*	F	Kok (1971)
	Yellow-billed magpie	*Pica nuttalli*	F	Verbeek (1972)
	Laughing gull	*Larus atricilla*	F	Burger (1976)
Tonic immobility				
	Chicken	*Gallus domesticus*	R	Rovee, Kaufman, and Collier (1977)

[a]This table is intended to provide an overview of the variety of behavioral rhythms that have been reported among birds; it does not attempt to review the immense literature available on activity patterns in the field and laboratory. For reviews on these topics, see Gwinner (1975), Palmgren (1949), and Leopold and Eynon (1961). For further information see Table I.

stand how birds (or other vertebrates) combine photic and nonphotic control mechanisms, but the evidence reviewed below indicates that birds are capable of some remarkable feats of behavioral rhythm integration.

ACTIVITY

Among diurnal species, a typical daily pattern includes a peak of activity following dawn and one preceding dusk (Aschoff, 1966; Gwinner, 1975; Leopold and Eynon, 1961; Palmgren, 1949). A similar bimodal pattern characterizes many other behaviors, including feeding (Morton, 1967; Zeigler, Green, and Lehrer, 1971); singing and calling (Palmgren, 1949; Leopold and Eynon, 1961; Kok, 1971); courtship and copulation (Pynnönen, cited in Palmgren, 1949; Burger, 1976); and territorial defense (Burger, 1976). The dawn peak of activity is usually larger and may include behaviors, such as nest building, that are rare at other times of day (Palmgren, 1949; Verbeek, 1972; Burger, 1976). Some species may, however, ingest the largest volume of food late in the day (see Savory, 1976, for references).

The timing of these daily peaks of activity in the field is closely related to the changing times of dawn and dusk (Leopold and Eynon, 1961; Aschoff, Gwinner, Kureck, and Muller, 1970; see Gwinner, 1975, for additional references). Ambient light intensity at other times is also a significant factor: robins *(Turdus migratorius)* sing earlier when bright moonlight precedes dawn (Leopold and Eynon, 1961); several species are reported to take advantage of artificial illumination to feed before dawn and after dusk (see Bakken and Bakken, 1977, for references); territorial drumming of grouse *(Bonasa umbellus)*, which is normally diurnal, is strongly stimulated by bright moonlight (Archibald, 1976); and petrels *(Pterodroma* sp.) extend their feeding time and reduce breeding on moonlit nights (Imber, 1975).

Effects of illumination on behavior are modulated by other factors: singing at dawn may be extended and feeding delayed after a warm night that helps conserve metabolic energy (Kok, 1971); wind or rain may inhibit singing (Leopold and Eynon, 1961); and sparrows *(Zonotrichia leucophrys)* stop feeding early in the afternoon during the phase of premigratory fattening, even if they are first experimentally food-deprived (Morton, 1967). The metabolic demands of preparation for and recovery from a night without feeding may appear to account for the normal dawn and dusk feeding peaks, but other factors are also involved. Morton (1967) recorded such feeding patterns in the field but failed to find them in sparrows when they were housed as outdoor captives. These same birds simultaneously generated typical, bimodal patterns of perch hopping, with a large peak occurring after dawn. The lack of the typical feeding pattern in these captive birds exposed to their natural photoperiod suggests that food quality, social interactions, and the opportunity to move among microniches may all play a role in generating the normal field pattern (Morton, 1967).

Laboratory studies have shown that conspecific sound can act as an entraining agent for several species (Gwinner, 1966; Menaker and Eskin, 1966; Cain and Wilson, 1974; Savory, 1976). Social synchronization of behavioral rhythms probably plays a significant role in the field as well. Several studies of doves, especially ring doves *(Streptopelia risoria)*, showed that the male and female alternate egg incubation with a diurnal rhythm (Lorenz, cited in Palmgren, 1949; Gerlach, Heinrich, and Lehrman, 1975). A similar phenomenon has been reported in the ostrich (*Struthio* sp.; McLaughlin and Liversidge, 1958) and is probably a common feature in birds that share incubation duties.

Herring gulls *(Larus argentatus)* also show a rhythm of nest relief that permits each partner to feed (McFarland, 1977, and personal communication, 1978). The situation in the colony studied by McFarland was complicated by the fact that various colony members specialized in feeding on different, rhythmically available resources. These included refuse at a dump site (diurnally available, except weekends), worms (nocturnally available, but dependent on weather), and mussels and starfish (available on a complex lunar–tidal cycle). Each gull would have had to adjust its incubation time to permit both itself and its partner to take advantage of the temporally limited resources that each specialized in exploiting, without leaving the nest unattended. (Gulls are notoriously cannibalistic.) The successful development of a breeding partnership would require considerable learning about the rhythmicity of each bird by its partner. Successful incubation by these gulls indicates remarkable behavioral synchronization to a complex pattern of stimuli associated with solar, lunar–tidal, and social rhythms.

Such complexity is not unique to this species. Laughing gulls *(Larus atricilla)* show solar-day rhythms in many behaviors but follow tidal rhythms in their foraging (Burger, 1976). Guillemots *(Uria aalge)* feed with a tidal rhythm at one season but not when food availability becomes maximal at another season (Slater, 1976). Kittiwakes *(Rissa tridactyla)* also switch from a tidal feeding rhythm to a diurnal pattern as prey availability increases seasonally (O'Connor, 1974). In the latter case, the kittiwakes follow a rhythm of effluent release from a sewer that is synchronized to high tide; their feeding is delayed relative to the peak tidal flow because of competition from larger, more aggressive birds (especially herring gulls). The kittiwakes abandon this resource as the density of herring gulls feeding on the effluent increases and fish become increasingly available nearby (O'Connor, 1974). Another example of interspecific synchronization is the limited daily period during which glaucous gulls *(Larus hyperboreus)* patrol an open beach in order to hunt fledgling guillemots *(Uria lomvia)* as the latter drop from their nesting ledges on their way to the sea (Cullen, 1954). Presumably, flight synchrony among the guillemots serves to "flood" their predators (see Chapter 15).

Social interactions very likely play a significant role in determining the time of roosting or migration while birds live in flocks. Rooks *(Corvus frugilegus)* from a wide region gather at a variety of assembly sites before dusk and converge in groups on secondary assembly areas, then to a final assembly site from which they enter a compact roosting area. While light intensity is important in cuing assembly, other factors must play a role, since rooks using an assembly area remote from the final roost begin to assemble earlier than those using more proximate sites. Light intensity, social cues, and learned habits all appear to modulate a circadian mechanism that signals departure for assembly areas (Swingland, 1976).

These observations on birds reinforce the conclusion that overt behavioral cycles in the field can be understood only as the consequence of the meshing of endogenous mechanisms and environmental pressures. The rhythms of shorebirds are particularly striking examples of how these complex behavioral integrations are related to temporal constraints in the environment.

BENJAMIN RUSAK

There are few reports of behavioral cycles in reptiles except for those of general loco-motor activity (See Table III). Exceptions include rhythms of movement between shore and water in crocodilians (Cott, 1961; Lang, 1976), burrowing and emergence in a snake (*Chionactis occipilalis;* Norris and Kavanau, 1966), and mouth gaping (a thermoregulatory behavior) in the crocodile (*Crocodilus niloticus;* Cott, 1961).

The existence of endogenous circadian rhythmicity in reptiles has long been recognized (Barden, 1942; Marx and Kayser, 1949), but most discussions have emphasized the over-riding importance of behavioral thermoregulation in dictating the activity patterns of these poikilotherms. This emphasis is particularly apparent in discussion of seasonal changes in activity pattern of snakes. For example, the viper *Aspis cerastes* is sluggish and inactive in a burrow during the winter and becomes diurnally active in spring and fall and nocturnally active in summer (Saint Girons, 1959). Similar seasonal changes are reported for garter snakes *(Thamnophis radix)* and water snakes (*Natrix sipedon;* Heckrotte, 1962). A simple interpretation of these findings is that snakes seek optimal temperature ranges and avoid activity when the temperature becomes too high or too low.

The role of a circadian mechanism in achieving optimal seasonal patterns of activity was emphasized by the findings of Heckrotte (1962, 1975) on garter snakes and water snakes. When maintained in LD cycles at various constant temperature levels, the snakes were diurnally active at low constant temperatures but became nocturnal at high constant temperatures. The modifications in activity pattern were remarkably similar to those reported to occur seasonally under fluctuating daily temperature cycles, although, in the study, the shift from diurnal to nocturnal activity was completely ineffective in changing the snakes' exposure to heat. The changes occurred and persisted as if increased mean temperatures dictated a shift in activity pattern quite independently of the consequence of the shift. The details of these activity patterns suggest the existence of oscillators that are shifted by changes in ambient temperature relative to each other as well as relative to the illumination cycle. A parallel effect was observed in response to changes in constant humid-ity levels; female garter snakes became more nocturnally active as humidity was lowered even though the environment was equally moist in L and D (Heckrotte, 1962).

In this case, adaptive regulation of behavior in relation to temperature was accom-plished not by direct responses to ambient temperature but by temperature-induced changes in the entrainment pattern of a circadian rhythm. However, reptiles also respond directly to temperature changes and can be entrained by temperature cycles (Hoffmann, 1968). Gopher tortoises *(Gopherus polyphemus)* become active earlier at higher than at lower temperatures (Gourley, 1972). Crocodiles and alligators *(Alligator mississippiensis)* usu-ally spend the entire day on shore, but they return to the water at midday if heat is extreme; large individuals, which have the greatest difficulty dissipating heat, are most likely to return to the water (Cott, 1961; Lang, 1976).

Too few data are available to permit any meaningful generalizations about reptiles, but the results summarized here suggest caution in assuming that adaptive synchronization of behavior to an environmental variable necessarily implies direct responsiveness to fluc-tuations in that variable (cf. Pittendrigh, 1958). Other environmental variables may also influence behavior by affecting circadian rhythmicity rather than by functioning as cuing stimuli; for example, permitting tortoises in LL access to partial cover reduced both the

TABLE III. BEHAVIORAL RHYTHMS: REPTILES[a]

Behavior		Species	Type of study	Reference
Activity				
	Six-lined racerunner	*Cnemidophorus sexlineatus*	R	Barden (1942)
	Caucasian rock lizard	*Lacerta sicula*	R	Hoffmann (1968)
	Sand lizard	*L. agilis*	R	Marx and Kayser (1949)
	Wall lizard	*L. muralis*	R	Marx and Kayser (1949)
	Texan spiny lizard	*Sceloporus olivaceus*	R	Underwood (1973)
	Desert spiny lizard	*S. magister*	R	Underwood (1973)
	Clark's spiny lizard	*S. clarkii*	R	Underwood (1973)
	Carolina anole	*Anolis carolinensis*	R	Underwood (1973)
	Ground gecko	*Coleonyx variegatus*	R	Underwood (1973)
	Warty gecko	*Hemidactylus turcicus*	R	Underwood (1973)
	Desert night lizard	*Xantusia vigilis*	R	Underwood (1973)
	Gopher tortoise	*Gopherus polyphemus*	R	Gourley (1972)
	Plains garter snake	*Thamnophis radix*	R	Heckrotte (1962, 1975)
	Western shovel-nosed snake	*Chionactis occipitalis*	R	Norris and Kavanau (1966)
	Horned viper	*Aspis cerastes*	R	Saint Girons (1959)
	Snub-nosed viper	*Vipera latastei*	R	Saint Girons (1954)
Shore–water movements				
	Nile crocodile	*Crocodilus niloticus*	F	Cott (1961)
	American alligator	*Alligator mississippiensis*	R	Lang (1976)

[a]See footnote in Table I.

TABLE IV. BEHAVIORAL RHYTHMS: AMPHIBIANS[a]

Behavior		Species	Type of study	Reference
Activity				
	American toad	*Bufo americanus*	R	Higginbotham (1939)
	Fowler's toad	*B. fowleri*	R	Higginbotham (1939)
	Axolotl	*Ambystoma tigrinum* (larvae)	R	Kalmus (1940)
	Colorado River toad	*Bufo alvarius*	F	Arnold (1943)
	Spadefoot toad	*Scaphiopus couchii*	F	Arnold (1943)
	Red-backed salamander	*Plethodon cinereus*	R	Ralph (1957)
	Spotted newt	*Triturus viridiscens*	R	Bennett and Staley (1960)
	Leopard toad	*Bufo regularis*	R	Cloudsley-Thompson (1967)
	Slimy salamander	*Plethodon glutinosus*	R	Adler (1969)
	Green frog	*Rana clamitans*	R	Adler (1971)
	Smooth newt	*Triturus vulgaris*	R	Himstedt (1971)
	Alpine newt	*T. alpestris*	R	Himstedt (1971)
	Crested newt	*T. cristatus*	R	Himstedt (1971)
	Fire salamander	*Salamandra salamandra*	R	Himstedt (1971)
	Leopard frog	*Rana pipiens*	R	Robertson (1978)
Immobility response				
	Marine toad	*Bufo marinus*	R	Ternes (1977)
Migration				
	Woodhouse's toad	*Bufo woodhousii fowleri*	F	Stille (1952)
	Frogs	*Rana* sp.	F	Stille (1952)
	American toad	*Bufo americanus*	F	Fitzgerald and Bider (1974a,b)
Water imbibition				
	Woodhouse's toad	*Bufo woodhousii fowleri*	F	Stille (1952)

[a]See footnote in Table I.

intra- and the interindividual variability of their freerunning rhythms (Gourley, 1972; see also pp. 191 and 204). Reptiles seem to be a particularly appropriate group in which to study the interactions of environmental stimuli that have a direct cuing function for behavior with those that act indirectly to influence behavior through a circadian mechanism.

AMPHIBIANS

Amphibian behavioral rhythms have not been extensively studied; a recent review (Adler, 1976) listed only about 13 species whose activity pattern had been described (see Table IV). Early reports on toads (*Bufo* sp.; Higginbotham, 1939) and salamanders (*Ambystoma tigrinum* larvae; Kalmus, 1940) described the "persistence" of 24-hr rhythms rather than freeruns in constant illumination. Several more recent studies have also described persistence of solar-day or 24-hr rhythms in LL or DD (Ralph, 1957; Bennett and Staley, 1960; Cloudsley-Thompson, 1967). These reports should be regarded with great caution since amphibians may share with other poikilotherms (see p. 198) the capacity to entrain to very-small-amplitude temperature cycles that may not have been detected or controlled (cf. Hoffmann, 1968). When temperature is effectively controlled, activity rhythms freerun in DD with a circadian period for at least a few cycles (Adler, 1969, 1971).

A number of environmental factors that influence activity have been described in both the field and the laboratory. These include temperature (Fitzgerald and Bider, 1974b); rainfall (Arnold, 1943; Fitzgerald and Bider, 1974b); barometric pressure (Robertson, 1978); and moonlight (Fitzgerald and Bider, 1974b; Robertson, 1978). There are also claims based on scant evidence that lunar cycles exert an influence on animals isolated from moonlight (Ralph, 1957; Bennett and Staley, 1960).

The best-documented evidence for rhythm lability in amphibians deals with developmental and seasonal changes in behavior. Aquatic larval newts *(Triturus vulgaris, T. cristatus)* were diurnally active, while adults that were aquatic during the breeding season were primarily nocturnal; during their nonbreeding, terrestrial stage, adults remained nocturnal but were phase-shifted relative to their aquatic stage activity (Dolmen, 1976). Himstedt (1971) described activity patterns in aquatic larval and adult salamanders and in terrestrial adults (three species of *Triturus* and *Salamandra salamandra*). Terrestrial adults were narrowly crepuscular; the patterns of aquatic adults and larvae varied from the strict nocturnality and bimodal pattern of larval *S. salamandra* to the weak rhythmicity and high levels of L activity of *T. vulgaris*. Juvenile toads were also reported to be less strictly nocturnal than adults (Fitzgerald and Bider, 1974a).

Some of the differences in activity pattern shown by amphibians at different life stages may be accounted for by the variety of ecological conditions they experience. Differences between adults and young in the same environment may serve to partially isolate the young from competition with adults for food and from the adults' cannibalism (Fitzgerald and Bider, 1974a). The dramatic changes in activity pattern shown by some developing amphibians may provide a useful model for studying rhythm development in general, and for investigating the physiological mechanisms that produce diverse forms of entrainment at different life stages (see Adler, 1976).

INTRODUCTION

Although behavioral rhythms in fish have been studied in the laboratory for many years (Spencer, 1939; Harden Jones, 1956), "field" studies are the only source of information about most species. Three techniques are commonly used in field studies: daily movements of populations are inferred from changes in the composition of catches made at several depths and/or at several times of day (e.g., Carlander and Cleary, 1949; Turuk, 1973); feeding patterns are inferred from changes in stomach content of fish caught at different times of day (e.g., Harmelin-Vivien and Bouchon, 1976); and fish movements and feeding are observed directly by divers (e.g., Collette and Talbot, 1972).

General reviews of fish rhythmicity are available (Woodhead, 1965; Schwassmann, 1971), and several studies have investigated rhythmicity in a wide range of species at densely populated coral reefs (Collette and Talbot, 1972; Harmelin-Vivien and Bouchon, 1976; Ogden and Buckman, 1973). Nevertheless the amount of available information is very limited compared with the immense diversity of structural and behavioral adaptations among fish; the majority of published reports have dealt with a few commercially important species, game fish, and coral reef dwellers.

There is substantial evidence that an endogenous circadian mechanism underlies rhythmicity in many species (Spencer, 1939; Lissmann and Schwassmann, 1965; Nelson and Johnson, 1970; see also Schwassmann, 1971; Beitinger, 1975, for references), but such a mechanism is not universal. In careful studies of two nocturnal sharks, Nelson and Johnson (1970) found clear evidence of endogenous circadian rhythmicity in swell sharks *(Cephaloscyllium ventriosum)* and equally good evidence for strictly exogenous control of rhythmicity in horn sharks *(Heterodontus francisci)*. If any generalization can be made, it is that under natural conditions virtually all species studied show daily rhythms of swimming, migration, or feeding at some life stages. A few other rhythms have been described, and these are listed in Table V.

ACTIVITY

DAILY MIGRATION AND FEEDING. The availability of commercially important fish species at particular ocean depths varies predictably with the time of day. Marine scientists have generally concluded that this finding reflects species-characteristic patterns of vertical movement ("migration") through the water column (e.g., Woodhead, 1965). In lakes (Carlander and Cleary, 1949; Baumann and Kitchell, 1974), in pools (Barlow, 1958), and at coral reefs (Collette and Talbot, 1972), relatively minor changes in vertical distribution may be accompanied by substantial lateral displacements, such as from the shallows near shore (littoral zone) to open water near the lake center (limnetic zone). An understanding of these daily rhythms and their causation is a major concern of those involved in fisheries management.

One view is that these migrations are roughly analogous to the daily movements of terrestrial vertebrates, such as birds and bats, between exposed feeding areas and secure roost sites (Woodhead, 1965). Although migration undoubtedly has many additional functions, the activity patterns of many fish fit this model well. Perch *(Perca flavescens)* are reported to form large schools high in the water column during daytime feeding and to disperse to the sea bottom during their nocturnal rest phase (Hasler and Villemonte, 1953). Parrotfish *(Scarus croicensis)* feed on a shallow reef shelf by day and swim several hundred meters into deep water at sunset; there they retreat to a rock crevice and spend the night hidden behind a mucous cocoon they form around the opening (Ogden and Buckman, 1973). An extensive report on dozens of coral reef species has described alternate movements into and out of limited feeding niches by diurnal and nocturnal species (Collete and Talbot, 1972).

In some freshwater species, daily migration may be a means of tracking cyclically available prey. Bluegill *(Lepomis macrochirus)* feed in the littoral zone on night-active insect nymphs and larvae but return to the limnetic zone to feed on zooplankton by day when their insect prey are inactive (Baumann and Kitchell, 1974). Bulldog fish *(Gnathonemus macrolepidotus)*, which apparently are exclusive bottom feeders, take chaoborid lar-

TABLE V. BEHAVIORAL RHYTHMS: FISH[a]

Behavior		Species	Type of study	Reference
Activity				
	Sunfish	*Eupomotis gibbosus*	R	Spencer (1939)
	Goldfish	*Carassius auratus*	R	Spencer (1939)
	Minnow	*Phoxinus phoxinus*	R	Harden Jones (1956)
	Swell shark	*Cephaloscyllium ventriosm*	R/F	Nelson and Johnson (1970)
	35+ coral reef species	—	F	Collette and Talbot (1972)
Agonistic behavior				
	Snakeskin gourami	*Trichogaster pectoralis*	R	Robison and Miller (1972)
Color change				
	Common killifish	*Fundulus heteroclitus*	R	Kavaliers and Abbott (1977)
	Golden pencil fish	*Nannostomus beckfordi anomalus*	R	Reed (1968)
Electric discharge				
	Sandfish	*Gymnorhamphichthys hypostomus*	R	Lissmann and Schwassmann (1965)
Food preference				
	Scorpion fish	*Dentrochirus brachypterus*	F	Harmelin-Vivien and Bouchon (1976)
Lateral migration				
	Striped parrotfish	*Scarus croicensis*	F	Ogden and Buckman (1973)
	Bluegill	*Lepomis macrochirus*	F	Baumann and Kitchell (1974)
	Desert pupfish	*Cyprinodon macularius*	F	Barlow (1958)
	Common sucker	*Catostomus commersoni*	F	Carlander and Cleary (1949)
Spawning				
	Pupfish	*Cyprinodon rubrofluviatilis*	F	Echelle (1973)
	Annual killifish	*Nothobranchius guentheri*	R	Haas (1976)
	Sardine	*Sardina pilchardus*	F	Gamulin and Hure (1956)
Temperature preference				
	Common (white) sucker	*Catostomus commersoni*	R	Reynolds and Casterlin (1978)
Territorial defense				
	Snakeskin gourami	*Trichogaster pectoralis*	R	Robison and Miller (1972)
	Pupfish	*Cyprinodon rubrofluviatilis*	F	Echelle (1973)
Vertical migration				
	Perch	*Perca flavescens*	F	Hasler and Villemonte (1953)
	Cod	*Gadus morhua*	F	Turuk (1973)
	Various species	—	F/R	Woodhead (1965)
	Norway pout	*Trisopterus esmarki*	F	Bailey (1975)

[a]See footnote in Table I.

vae from the central lake floor by day; in the evening, these larvae migrate upward and the fish simultaneously migrate laterally to the littoral zone to feed on chironomid larvae that remain available on the bottom at night (Kruger, 1973). Different species in the same environment can migrate simultaneously in opposite directions (Carlander and Cleary, 1949).

Cod *(Gadus morhua)* may adopt different migratory patterns depending on their primary prey. Those feeding heavily on bottom-dwelling sand lances *(Ammodytes dubius)* feed near the bottom at night and move up into the pelagic zone by day; those feeding primarily on free-swimming capelin *(Mallotus villosus)* follow the latter's migration into the pelagic zone at night and feed on sand lances near the bottom by day (Turuk, 1973). Unfortunately, the available data do not discriminate between the possibility that cod modify their patterns in response to local conditions and the possibility that different cod populations show diverse migratory patterns independently of food availability (see p. 184).

Daily migration patterns serve additional functions, such as facilitating thermoregulation and increasing the physiological efficiency of food utilization (Brett, 1971; Echelle, 1973). Desert pupfish *(Cyprinodon macularius)* show seasonally variable migratory movements that appear to be adaptively related to water temperature (Barlow, 1958). For some fish, vertical movements may be a means of gaining access to horizontal currents, which are used for dispersal or for following tidal cycles (Woodhead, 1965). Both the pattern and the function of daily migration may vary with age, feeding strategy, and season (Woodhead, 1965; Baumann and Kitchell, 1974).

Some species restrict most feeding to limited daily periods (Brett, 1971; Elston and Bachen, 1976; Haas, 1976; Moriarty, Darlington, Dunn, Moriarty, and Tevlin, 1973), while others feed both day and night (Harmelin-Vivien and Bouchon, 1976; Wallace, 1976). Many species appear to be relatively unspecialized and to feed on any available prey of appropriate size; daily cycles of availability may then dictate apparent cycles of food preference (Elston and Bachen, 1976; Wallace, 1976). One species *(Menidia audens)* appears to feed whenever L intensity is sufficient for prey detection (Elston and Bachen, 1976). However, opportunism alone cannot explain some feeding rhythms; among sympatric reef-dwelling scorpion fish (Scorpaenidae), one species eats mostly shrimp by day and brachyuran crustaceans at night, while another species shows the opposite pattern. Differences in hunting pattern that depend on size, crypticity, and resting habits may be important factors; sea basses (Serranidae) strike from ambush during the day but swim actively to hunt prey at night (Harmelin-Vivien and Bouchon, 1976). Mechanisms controlling the diverse and flexible feeding strategies of fish are generally poorly understood, but cycles of light intensity, predator migration, and prey availability seem to play important roles.

ENVIRONMENTAL INFLUENCES. While feeding and activity are closely connected, it is not clear to what extent the availability of food influences the activity pattern of fish. Swift (1964) reported that brown trout *(Salmo trutta)* that were fed every 2 hr both day and night showed normal diurnal activity patterns. He concluded that feeding in trout was controlled by the time of activity rather than the converse; Andreasson (1969) reached a similar conclusion for sculpins *(Cottus* sp.). Peaks of activity anticipating feeding time have been recorded in several species (Davis, 1964; Davis and Bardach, 1965; Myrberg and Gruber, 1974), but the simultaneous presence of LD cycles confounded interpretation of these findings. When the LD cycle and food restriction were unconfounded, activity remained synchronized to the LD cycle (Davis, 1964). In a later study, feeding time apparently synchronized the activity of killifish *(Fundulus heteroclitus)* in LL, but in LD, activity occurred both in anticipation of feeding and in normal phase relation to the LD cycle (Davis and Bardach, 1965). These findings are not conclusive, but they are similar to those obtained in food restriction studies of mammalian activity rhythms (see p. 192).

Both light intensity and temperature may influence activity without exerting classic zeitgeber effects (Brett, 1971; Echelle, 1973). Storm-caused increases in water turbidity delayed the morning departure of nocturnal fish and the arrival of diurnal fish at a reef (Collette and Talbot, 1972). Turbid water also influenced the cohesion of schooling fish (Harden Jones, 1956; Ogden and Buckman, 1973). Bright moonlight stimulated feeding (Elston and Bachen, 1976) and activity (Stickney, 1972) in diurnally active species, while artificial light at night inhibited activity of a nocturnal shark (Nelson and Johnson, 1970) and of a gymnotid fish (Lissmann and Schwassmann, 1965).

The influence of light on behavior may depend on the availability of shelter (cf. mammals, p. 191). Both flounders and minnows *(Phoxinus phoxinus)* kept in aquaria under LD cycles were active throughout the cycle, but particularly during the L phase. When sand was added to the aquaria, the flounders dug in by day and became exclusively nocturnal; similarly, the addition of hollow bricks for cover almost completely eliminated activity in L by the minnows (Harden Jones, 1956; Woodhead, 1965). Artificial light inhibited electric discharges and swimming in a gymnotid sandfish *(Gymnorhamphichthys hypostomus)* at night only if sand were available for digging into; otherwise, vigorous swimming continued despite the illumination (Lissmann and Schwassmann, 1965).

Tidal cycles entrain the activity of some fish that live in the intertidal zone (Gibson, 1976); for the blenny *(Blennius pholis)*, the most effective signal for inducing tidal rhythmicity is apparently a cycle of hydrostatic pressure (Gibson, 1971). Longer-period behavioral cycles may also occur, particularly in relation to breeding; seasonal changes have been reported in activity level and rhythmicity (Harden Jones, 1956), feeding substrate (Wallace, 1976), and feeding pattern (Arntz, 1973).

The activity patterns of two species of sculpin were nocturnal throughout the year in southern Sweden. However, populations of one of these species *(Cottus poecilopus)* from northern Sweden were nocturnal only in summer and became diurnally active in winter; they continued to show this seasonal reversal when transported to southern Sweden. Their conspecifics native to the south, which did not change activity pattern seasonally, did respond to dimming of either a natural or an artificial L-phase by becoming diurnally active, a pattern not found in a closely related species *(C. gobio;* Andreasson, 1969). The similarity of rhythm shifts shown by northern *poecilopus* to those shown by far-northern vole populations (Stebbins, 1972; see p. 190) suggests that dramatic seasonal changes in behavioral rhythms may occur in many populations exposed to extreme photoperiods.

CONCLUSION

An obvious conclusion that emerges from this survey is that rhythmicity is a common feature of behavioral systems in a great variety of vertebrate species. The investigation of most of these rhythms has not progressed beyond description, and little is known of either the mechanisms that produce them or their functional significance. If one can extrapolate from the few well-studied rhythms, most vertebrate rhythms are endogenously generated and their expression is dominated by illumination cycles (see Chapters 6 and 7).

However, these rhythms are also sensitive to a number of other environmental factors. In some cases, environmental stimuli may affect behavior by modifying or overriding behavioral tendencies that are the product of an ongoing biological rhythm. So, an animal may be induced to eat at an unusual daily phase when attractive food becomes available, without disruption of the circadian organization of feeding. An alternative is that responsiveness to such stimuli is not simply a behavioral adjustment that is independent of underlying biological oscillators but may reflect an adaptive feature of the oscillators themselves.

Such a mechanism is suggested by the behavior of rats exposed to temporally limited feeding (see p. 191) or place-avoidance learning (see p. 194) and of fish on restricted feeding schedules (see p. 204). In each case, an oscillatory process may be synchronized by the manipulated stimuli while light entrainment of other oscillators remains unaffected. The apparent reorganization of daily rhythms in garter snakes at different constant temperature levels (see p. 198) and the synchronization of gulls to a complex of tidal, solar, and social cues (see p. 197) also suggest that biological oscillators are sensitive to a variety of external stimuli.

If these speculations are correct, then the remarkable regularity of biological rhythms studied under uniform laboratory conditions may mask an important adaptive feature of the vertebrate multioscillator system. Outside the laboratory, the responsiveness of portions of this oscillatory complex to environmental events may contribute significantly to the adaptive behavioral flexibility that characterizes many vertebrates.

Acknowledgments

I am grateful to Gail Eskes for her many helpful comments and criticisms, to Lise Marois-Chabot for bibliographic assistance, and to Nancy Feener, Carol McAulay, and Nancy Beattie for typing the manuscript.

REFERENCES

Ader, R., and Grota, L. J. Rhythmicity in the maternal behaviour of *Rattus norvegicus*. *Animal Behavior*, 1970, *18*, 144–150.

Adler, K. Extraoptic phase shifting of circadian locomotor rhythm in salamanders. *Science*, 1969, *164*, 1290–1292.

Adler, K. Pineal end organ: Role in extraoptic entrainment of circadian locomotor rhythms in frogs. In M. Menaker (Ed.), *Biochronometry*. Washington, D.C.: U.S. National Academy of Sciences, 1971, pp. 342–350.

Adler, K. Extraocular photoreception in amphibians. *Photochemistry and Photobiology*, 1976, *23*, 275–298.

Alleva, J. J., Waleski, M. V., and Alleva, F. R. A biological clock controlling the estrous cycle of the hamster. *Endocrinology*, 1971, *88*, 1368–1379.

Allison, T., Gerber, S. D., Breedlove, S. M., and Dryden, G. L. A behavioral and polygraphic study of sleep in the shrews *Suncus murinus*, *Blarina brevicauda*, and *Cryptotis parva*. *Behavioral Biology*, 1977, *20*, 354–366.

Andreasson, S. Locomotory activity patterns of *Cottus poecilopus* Heckel and *C. gobio* L. (Pisces). *Oikos*, 1969, *20*, 78–94.

Archibald, H. L. Spring drumming patterns of ruffed grouse. *Auk*, 1976, *93*, 808–829.

Ardisson, J.-L., Dolisi, C., Camous, J.-P., and Gastaud, M. Rhythmes spontanés des prises alimentaire et hydrique chez le chien: Étude préliminaire. *Physiology and Behavior*, 1975, *14*, 47–52.

Arnold, L. W. Notes on two species of desert toads. *Copeia*, 1943, *2*, 128.

Arntz, W. E. Periodicity of diel food intake of cod *Gadus morhua* in the Kiel Bay. *Oikos*, 1973, Supplement *15*, 138–145.

Aschoff, J. Circadian activity pattern with two peaks. *Ecology*, 1966, *47*, 657–662.

Aschoff, J., and von Saint Paul, U. Brain temperature as related to gross motor activity in the unanesthetized chicken. *Physiology and Behavior*, 1973, *10*, 529–533.

Aschoff, J., and Wever, R. Circadian rhythms of finches in light–dark cycles with interposed twilights. *Comparative Biochemistry and Physiology*, 1965, *16*, 507–514.

Aschoff, J., Gwinner, E., Kureck, A., and Muller, K. Diel rhythms of chaffinches *Fringilla coelebs* L., tree shrews *Tupaia glis* L. and hamsters *Mesocricetus auratus* L. as a function of season at the Arctic circle. *Oikos*, 1970, Supplement *13*, 91–100.

Aschoff, J., Fatranska, M., and Giedke, H. Human circadian rhythms in continuous darkness: Entrainment by social cues. *Science*, 1971, *171*, 213–215.

Ashby, K. R. Patterns of daily activity in mammals. *Mammal Review*, 1972, *1*, 171–185.

Bailey, R. S. Observations on diel behaviour patterns of North Sea gadoids in the pelagic phase. *Journal of the Marine Biological Association of the United Kingdom*, 1975, *55*, 133–142.

Bakken, L. E., and Bakken, G. S. American redstart feeding by artificial light. *Auk*, 1977, *94*, 373–374.

Barden, A. Activity of the lizard, *Cnemidophorus sexlineatus*. *Ecology*, 1942, *23*, 336–344.

Bare, J. K., and Cicala, G. Deprivation and time of testing as determinants of food intake. *Journal of Comparative and Physiological Psychology*, 1960, *53*, 151–154.

Barlow, G. W. Daily movements of desert pupfish, *Cyprinodon macularius*, in shore pools of the Salton Sea, California. *Ecology*, 1958, *39*, 580–587.

Barlow, G. W. Ethological units of behavior. In D. Ingle (Ed.), *Central Nervous System and Fish Behaviour*. Chicago: University of Chicago Press, 1968, 217–232.

Barnes, C. A., McNaughton, B. L., Goddard, G. V., Douglas, R. M., and Adamec, R. Circadian rhythm of synaptic excitability in rat and monkey central nervous system. *Science*, 1977, *197*, 91–92.

Baumann, P. C., and Kitchell, J. F. Diel patterns of distribution and feeding of bluegill *(Lepomis macrochirus)* in Lake Wingra, Wisconsin. *Transactions of the American Fisheries Society*, 1974, *103*, 255–260.

Beach, F. A., and Levinson, G. Diurnal variations in the mating behavior of male rats. *Proceedings of the Society for Experimental Biology and Medicine*, 1949, *72*, 78–80.

Beitinger, T. L. Diel activity rhythms and thermoregulatory behavior of bluegill in response to unnatural photoperiods. *Biological Bulletin*, 1975, *149*, 96–108.

Bellinger, L. L., and Mendel, V. E. Effect of deprivation and time of refeeding on food intake. *Physiology and Behavior*, 1975, *14*, 43–46.

Bennett, M. F., Staley, J. Cycles of motor activity in the newt, *Triturus viridiscens*. *Anatomical Record*, 1960, *137*, 339.

Bernstein, I. S. Daily activity cycles and weather influences on a pigtail monkey group. *Folia Primatologica*, 1972, *18*, 390–415.

Bolles, R. C., and Duncan, P. M. Daily course of activity and subcutaneous body temperature in hungry and thirsty rats. *Physiology and Behavior*, 1969, *4*, 87–89.

Bolles, R. C., and Moot, S. A. The rat's anticipation of two meals a day. *Journal of Comparative and Physiological Psychology*, 1973, *83*, 510–514.

Bolles, R. C., and Stokes, L. W. Rat's anticipation of diurnal and a-diurnal feeding. *Journal of Comparative and Physiological Psychology*, 1965, *60*, 290–294.

Bombardieri, R. A., and Johnson, J. I., Jr. Daily activity schedule of captive opossums. *Psychonomic Science*, 1969, *17*, 135–136.

Boulos, Z., Rosenwasser, A., and Terman, M. Feeding schedules and the circadian organization of behavior in the rat. *Behavioral Brain Research*, 1980, *1*, 39–65.

Bovet, J. On the social behavior in a stable group of long-tailed field mice *(Apodemus sylvaticus)*. II. Its relations with distribution of daily activity. *Behaviour*, 1972, *41*, 55–67.

Bovet, J., and Oertli, E. Free-running circadian activity rhythms in free-living beaver *(Castor canadensis)*. *Journal of Comparative Physiology*, 1974, *92*, 1–10.

Brett, J. R. Energetic responses of salmon to temperature: A study of some thermal relations in the physiology and freshwater ecology of sockeye salmon *(Onchorhynchus nerka)*. *American Zoologist*, 1971, *11*, 99–113.

Bronson, F. H. Daily and seasonal activity patterns in woodchucks. *Journal of Mammalogy*, 1962, *43*, 425–427.

Bronson, F. H. Rodent pheromones. *Biology of Reproduction*, 1971, *4*, 344–357.

Brown, F. A., Jr., and Park, Y. H. Synodic monthly modulation of the diurnal rhythm of hamsters. *Proceedings of the Society for Experimental Biology and Medicine,* 1967, *125,* 712–715.

Bunn, D. S. Regular daylight hunting by barn owls. *British Birds,* 1972, *65,* 26–30.

Burdick, C. K., and Luz, G. A. Consummatory drinking of the chinchilla. *Bulletin of the Psychonomic Society,* 1973, *2,* 266–268.

Burger, J. Daily and seasonal activity patterns in breeding laughing gulls. *Auk,* 1976, *93,* 308–323.

Cain, R. J., and Wilson, W. O. The influence of specific environmental parameters on the circadian rhythms of chickens. *Poultry Science,* 1974, *53,* 1438–1447.

Calhoun, J. B. *The Ecology and Sociology of the Norway Rat.* Bethesda, Md.: U.S. Public Health Service, 1962.

Canivenc, R., Croizet, J., Blanquet, P., and Bonnin-Laffargue, M. Mesure de l'activité journalière du blaireau européen *Meles meles* L. *Comptes rendus de l'Académie des Sciences,* 1960, *250,* 1915–1917.

Carlander, K. D., and Cleary, R. E. The daily patterns of some freshwater fishes. *American Midland Naturalist,* 1949, *41,* 447–452.

Caughley, G. Social organization and daily activity of the red kangaroo and the grey kangaroo. *Journal of Mammalogy,* 1964, *45,* 429–436.

Cloudsley-Thompson, J. L. Diurnal rhythm, temperature and water relations of the African toad, *Bufo regularis. Journal of Zoology,* London, 1967, *152,* 43–54.

Clutton-Brock, T. H. Activity patterns of red colobus *(Colobus badius tephrosceles). Folia Primatalogica,* 1974, *21,* 161–187.

Collette, B. B., and Talbot, F. H. Activity patterns of coral reef fishes with emphasis on nocturnal–diurnal changeover. *Bulletin of the Natural History Museum of Los Angeles County,* 1972, *14,* 98–124.

Coover, G. D., Sutton, B. R., and Heybach, J. P. Conditioning decreases in plasma corticosterone level in rats by pairing stimuli with daily feedings. *Journal of Comparative and Physiological Psychology,* 1977, *91,* 716–726.

Cott, H. B. Scientific results of an inquiry into the ecology and economic status of the Nile crocodile *(Crocodilus niloticus)* in Uganda and Northern Rhodesia. *Transactions of the Zoological Society of London,* 1961, *29,* 211–356.

Crowcroft, P., and Rowe, F. P. Social organization and territorial behaviour in the wild house mouse *(Mus musculus* L.). *Proceedings of the Zoological Society of London,* 1963, *140,* 517–531.

Cullen, J. M. The diurnal rhythm of birds in the Arctic summer. *Ibis,* 1954, *96,* 31–46.

Dark, J. G., Chiodo, L. A., and Asdourian, D. Long-term analysis of hypothalamic self-stimulation in the rat: Is a circadian rhythm present? *Physiological Psychology,* 1977, *5,* 76–80.

Davies, J. A., Navaratnam, V., and Redfern, P. H. A 24-hour rhythm in passive avoidance behaviour in rats. *Psychopharmacologia* (Berl.), 1973, *32,* 211–214.

Davis, R. E. Daily "predawn" peak of locomotion in fish. *Animal Behaviour,* 1964, *12,* 272–283.

Davis, R. E., and Bardach, J. E. Time-coordinated prefeeding activity in fish. *Animal Behaviour,* 1965, *13,* 154–162.

DeCoursey, G., and DeCoursey, P. J. Adaptive aspects of activity rhythms in bats. *Biological Bulletin,* 1964, *126,* 14–27.

DeCoursey, P. J. Phase control of activity in a rodent. *Cold Spring Harbor Symposia on Quantitative Biology,* 1960, *25,* 49–54.

DeCoursey, P. J. Free-running rhythms and patterns of circadian entrainment in three species of diurnal rodent. *Journal of Interdisciplinary Cycle Research,* 1973, *4,* 67–77.

Deguchi, T. Ontogeny of a biological clock for serotonin: Acetyl coenzyme A *N*-acetyltransferase in pineal gland of rat. *Proceedings of the National Academy of Sciences, USA,* 1975, *72,* 2814–2818.

Dewsbury, D.A. Copulatory behavior of rats—Variations within the dark phase of the diurnal cycle. *Communications in Behavioral Biology,* Part A, 1968, *1,* 373–377.

Dolmen, D. Diel rhythm of *Triturus vulgaris. Norwegian Journal of Zoology,* 1976, *24,* 234.

Dubost, G. Le comportement du Chevrotain africain, *Hyemoschus aquaticus* Ogilby (Artiodactyla, Ruminantia). *Zeitschrift für Tierpsychologie,* 1975, *37,* 403–448.

Ebihara, S., and Tsuji, K. Strain differences in the mouse's wheel-running behavior. *Japanese Psychological Research,* 1976, *18,* 20–29.

Echelle, A. A. Behavior of the pupfish, *Cyprinodon rubrofluviatilis. Copeia,* 1973, *1,* 68–76.

Edmonds, S. C., and Adler, N. T. Food and light as entrainers of circadian running activity in the rat. *Physiology and Behavior,* 1977a, *18,* 915–919.

Edmonds, S. C., and Adler, N. T. The multiplicity of biological oscillators in the control of circadian running activity in the rat. *Physiology and Behavior,* 1977b, *18,* 921–930.

Elston, R., and Bachen, B. Diel feeding cycle and some effects of light on feeding intensity of the Mississippi silverside, *Menidia audens,* in Clear Lake, California. *Transactions of the American Fisheries Society,* 1976, *105,* 84–88.

Enright, J. Ecological aspects of endogenous rhythmicity. *Annual Review of Ecology and Systematics,* 1970, *1,* 221–238.

Erkert, H. G. Der Einfluss des Mondlichtes auf die Aktivitätsperiodik nachtaktiver Saugetiere. *Oecologia* (Berl.), 1974, *14,* 269–287.

Erkert, H. G. Beleuchtungsabhangiges Aktivitätsoptimum bei Nachtaffen *(Aotus trivirgatus). Folia primatologica,* 1976, *25,* 186–192.

Erkinaro, E. The seasonal change of the activity of *Microtus agrestis. Oikos,* 1961, *12,* 157–163.

Evans, H. L., and Patton, R. A. Scopolamine effects on conditioned suppression: Influence of diurnal cycle and transitions between normal and drugged states. *Psychopharmacologia* (Berl.), 1970, *17,* 1–13.

Fitzgerald, G. J., and Bider, J. R. Evidence of a relationship between age and activity in the toad *Bufo americanus. Canadian Field Naturalist,* 1974a, *88,* 499–501.

Fitzgerald, G. J., and Bider, J. R. Influence of moon phase and weather factors on locomotor activity in *Bufo americanus. Oikos,* 1974b, *25,* 338–340.

Folk, G. E., Jr. *Introduction to Environmental Physiology.* Philadelphia: Lea & Febiger, 1966.

Fuselier, P. H. Status as a variable in determination of social entrainment. *Dissertation Abstracts,* 1973, *34,* 2966B–2967B.

Gamulin, T., and Hure, J. Spawning of the sardine at a definite time of day. *Nature,* 1956, *177,* 193–194.

Gerlach, J. L., Heinrich, W., and Lehrman, D. S. Quantitative observations of the diurnal rhythm of courting, incubation, and brooding behavior in the ring dove *(Streptopelia risoria). Verhandlungen der Deutschen zoologischen Gesellschaft,* 1975, *1974,* 351–357.

Ghiselli, W. B., and Patton, R. A. Diurnal variation in performance of free-operant avoidance behavior of rats. *Psychological Reports,* 1976, *38,* 83–90.

Ghobrial, L. I., and Cloudsley-Thompson, J. L. Daily cycle of activity of the dorcas gazelle in the Sudan. *Journal of Interdisciplinary Cycle Research,* 1976, *7,* 47–50.

Gibson, R. N. Factors affecting the rhythmic activity of *Blennius pholis* L. (Teleostei). *Animal Behaviour,* 1971, *19,* 336–343.

Gibson, R. N. Comparative studies on the rhythms of juvenile flatfish. In P. J. DeCoursey (Ed.), *Biological Rhythms in the Marine Environment.* Columbia: University of South Carolina Press, 1976, pp. 199–213.

Gordon, P., and Scheving, L. E. Covariant 24-hour rhythms for acquisition and retention of avoidance learning and brain protein synthesis in rats. *Federation Proceedings,* 1968, *27,* 223.

Gourley, E. V. Circadian activity rhythm of the gopher tortoise *(Gopherus polyphemus). Animal Behaviour,* 1972, *20,* 13–20.

Grabfield, G. P., and Martin, E. G. Variations in the sensory threshold for faradic stimulation in normal human subjects. I. The diurnal rhythm. *American Journal of Physiology,* 1913, *31,* 300–308.

Griffin, D. R., and Welsh, J. H. Activity rhythms in bats under constant external conditions. *Journal of Mammalogy,* 1937, *18,* 337–342.

Grodziński, W. Seasonal changes in the circadian activity of small rodents. *Ekologia Polska,* 1963, *B9,* 3–17.

Gundlach, H. Brutfürsorge, Brutplege, Verhaltenontogenese and Tagesperiodik beim Wildschwein *(Sus scrofa* L.). *Zeitschrift für Tierpsychologie,* 1968, *25,* 955–995.

Gwinner, E. Entrainment of a circadian rhythm in birds by species-specific song cycles (Aves, Fringillidae: *Carduelis spinus, Serinus serinus). Experientia,* 1966, *22,* 765.

Gwinner, E. Circadian and circannual rhythms in birds. In D. S. Farner, J. R. King, and K. C. Parkes (Eds.), *Avian Biology.* Vol. 5. New York: Academic Press, 1975, pp. 221–285.

Haas, R. Behavioral biology of the annual killifish, *Nothobranchius guentheri. Copeia,* 1976, *1,* 80–91.

Halberg, F., Visscher, M. B., and Bittner, J. J. Relation of visual factors to eosinophil rhythm in mice. *American Journal of Physiology,* 1954, *179,* 229–235.

Hamilton, W. J., Jr. Activity of Brewer's mole *(Parascalops breweri). Journal of Mammalogy,* 1939, *20,* 307–310.

Harden Jones, F. R. The behaviour of minnows in relation to light intensity. *Journal of Experimental Biology,* 1956, *33,* 271–281.

Harmelin-Vivien, M. L., and Bouchon, C. Feeding behavior of some carnivorous fishes (Serranidae and Scorpaenidae) from Tuléar (Madagascar). *Marine Biology,* 1976, *37,* 329–340.

Hasler, A. D., and Villemonte, J. R. Observations on the daily movements of fishes. *Science,* 1953, *118,* 321–322.

Hayden, P., and Lindberg, R. G. Circadian rhythm in mammalian body temperature entrained by cyclic pressure changes. *Science,* 1969, *165,* 1288–1289.

Heckrotte, C. The effect of the environmental factors in the locomotory activity of the plains garter snake *(Thamnophis radix radix). Animal Behavior,* 1962, *10,* 193–207.

Heckrotte, C. Temperature and light effects on the circadian rhythm and locomotory activity of the plains garter snake *(Thamnophis radix hayendi)*. *Journal of Interdisciplinary Cycle Research*, 1975, *6*, 279–290.

Heisinger, J. F. Analysis of the reingestion rhythm in confined cottontails. *Ecology*, 1965, *46*, 197–201.

Henkin, R. I. The effect of cortcosteroids and ACTH on sensory systems. In D. DeWied and J. A. W. M. Weijnen (Eds.), *Pituitary, Adrenal and the Brain*. Amsterdam: Elsevier, 1970, pp. 270–294.

Hennig, C. W., and Dunlap, W. P. Circadian rhythms of tonic immobility in the rat: Evidence of an endogenous mechanism. *Animal Learning and Behavior*, 1977, *5*, 253–258.

Higginbotham, A. C. Studies of amphibian activity. I. Preliminary report on the rhythmic activity of *Bufo americanus americanus* Holbrook and *Bufo fowleri* Hinckley. *Ecology*, 1939, *20*, 58–70.

Hillman, A. K. K., and Young, C. M. A. Observations of the breeding behaviour of the meadow pipit *Anthus pratensis* under continual daylight. *Ibis*, 1977, *119*, 206–207.

Himstedt, W. Die Tagesperiodik von Salamandriden. *Oecologia*, 1971, *8*, 194–208.

Hoffmann, K. Synchronisation der circadianen Aktivitätsperiodik von Eidechsen durch Temperaturcyclen verschiedener Amplitude. *Zeitschrift für vergleichende Physiologie*, 1968, *58*, 225–228.

Hoffmann, K. Splitting of the circadian rhythm as a function of light intensity. In M. Menaker (Ed.), *Biochronometry*. Washington, D.C.: U.S. National Academy of Sciences, 1971, pp. 134–148.

Holloway, F. A., and Wansley, R. A. Multiphasic retention deficits at periodic intervals after passive avoidance learning. *Science*, 1973a, *180*, 208–210.

Holloway, F. A., and Wansley, R. A. Multiple retention deficits at periodic intervals after active and passive avoidance learning. *Behavioral Biology*, 1973b, *9*, 1–14.

Horton, B. J., West, C. E., and Turley, S. D. Diurnal variation in the feeding pattern of guinea pigs. *Nutrition and Metabolism*, 1975, *18*, 294–301.

Horwich, R. H. The whooping display in Nilgiri langurs: An example of daily fluctuations superimposed on a general trend. *Primates*, 1976, *17*, 419–431.

Hostetter, R. C. Time of day effects on learning and open field activity. *Psychonomic Science*, 1966, *5*, 257–258.

Howarth, S. T., and Toole, J. F. Some observations on the circadian rhythm of *Choloepus hoffmanni*, the two toed sloth. *Laboratory Animal Science*, 1973, *23*, 377–379.

Hunsicker, J. P., and Mellgren, R. L. Multiple deficits in the retention of an appetitively motivated behavior across a 24-hr period in rats. *Animal Learning and Behavior*, 1977, *5*, 14–16.

Hyde, J. S., and Sawyer, T. F. Estrous cycle fluctuations in aggressiveness of house mice. *Hormones and Behavior*, 1977, *9*, 290–295.

Imber, M. J. Behaviour of petrels in relation to the moon and artificial lights. *Notornis*, 1975, *22*, 302–306.

Jilge, B. The entrainment of the circadian soft faeces excretion in the rabbit. *Journal of Interdisciplinary Cycle Research*, 1976, *7*, 229–235.

Johansen, K., and Krog, J. Diurnal body temperature variations and hibernation in the birchmouse, *Sicista betulina*. *American Journal of Physiology*, 1959, *196*, 1200–1204.

Johnson, M. S. Activity and distribution of certain wild mice in relation to biotic communities. *Journal of Mammalogy*, 1926, *7*, 245–275.

Kalmus, H. Diurnal rhythms in the axolotl larva and in Drosophila. *Nature*, 1940, *145*, 72–73.

Kavaliers, M., and Abbott, F. S. Rhythmic colour change of the killifish, *Fundulus heteroclitus*. *Canadian Journal of Zoology*, 1977, *55*, 553–561.

Kavanau, J. L. The study of social interaction between small animals. *Animal Behaviour*, 1963, *11*, 263–273.

Kavanau, J. L. Influences of light on activity of small mammals. *Ecology*, 1969, *50*, 548–557.

Kavanau, J. L., and Peters, C. R. Activity of nocturnal primates: Influences of twilight zeitgebers and weather. *Science*, 1976, *191*, 83–86.

Kenagy, G. J. Daily and seasonal patterns of activity and energetics in a heteromyid rodent community. *Ecology*, 1973, *54*, 1201–1219.

Klinowska, M. A comparison of lunar and solar activity rhythms of the golden hamster (*Mesocricetus auratus* Waterhouse). *Journal of Interdisciplinary Cycle Research*, 1972, *3*, 145–150.

Kok, O. B. Vocal behavior of the great-tailed grackle *(Quiscalus mexicanus prosopidicola)*. *Condor*, 1971, *73*, 328–363.

Krieger, D. T., and Hauser, H. Comparison of synchronization of circadian corticosteroid rhythms by photoperiod and food. *Proceedings of the National Academy of Sciences USA*, 1978, *75*, 1577–1581.

Krieger, D. T., Hauser, H., and Krey, L. C. Suprachiasmatic nuclear lesions do not abolish food-shifted circadian adrenal and temperature rhythmicity. *Science*, 1977, *197*, 393–399.

Kruger, E. J. Autumn feeding cycle of the bull-dog fish, *Gnathonemus macrolepidotus* (Pisces, Mormyridae). *Zoologica Africana*, 1973, *8*, 25–34.

Landau, I. T. Light-dark rhythms in aggressive behavior of the male golden hamster. *Physiology and Behavior*, 1975, *14*, 767–774.

Lang, J. W. Amphibious behavior of *Alligator mississippiensis:* Roles of a circadian rhythm and light. *Science,* 1976, 191, 575–577.

Larsson, K. Age differences in the diurnal periodicity of male sexual behavior. *Gerontologia,* 1958, 2, 64–72.

Lawrence, D. H., and Mason, W. A. Food intake in the rat as a function of deprivation intervals and feeding rhythms. *Journal of Comparative and Physiological Psychology,* 1955, 48, 267–271.

Leopold, A., and Eynon, A. E. Avian daybreak and evening song in relation to time and light intensity. *Condor,* 1961, 63, 269–293.

Lerwill, C. J., and Makings, P. The agonistic behavior of the golden hamster *Mesocricetus auratus* (Waterhouse). *Animal Behaviour,* 1971, 19, 714–421.

Levin, R., and Stern, J. M. Maternal influences on ontogeny of suckling and feeding rhythms in the rat. *Journal of Comparative and Physiological Psychology,* 1975, 80, 711–721.

Lissmann, H. W., and Schwassmann, H. O. Activity rhythm of an electric fish, *Gymnorhamphichthys hypostomus,* Ellis. *Zeitschrift für vergleichende Physiologie,* 1965, 51, 153–171.

Lockard, R. B., and Owings, D. H. Moon-related surface activity of bannertail *(Dipodomys spectabilis)* and Fresno *(D. nitratoides)* kangaroo rats. *Animal Behaviour,* 1974, 22, 262–273.

Lonowski, D. J., Levitt, R. A., and Dickinson, W. A. Carbachol-elicited mouse killing by rats: Circadian rhythm and dose response. *Bulletin of the Psychonomic Society,* 1965, 6, 601–604.

Lutton, C., and Chevalier, F. Copraphagie chez le rat blanc: Aspects quantitatifs et relation chronologique avec les prises alimentaires. *Journal de Physiologie* (Paris), 1973, 66, 219–228.

Martin, E. G., Bigelow, G. H., and Wilbur, G. B. Variations in the sensory threshold for faradic stimulation in normal human subjects. II. The nocturnal variation. *American Journal of Physiology,* 1914, 33, 415–422.

Martinez-Vargas, M. C., and Erickson, C. J. Some social and hormonal determinants of nest-building behaviour in the ring dove *(Streptopelia risoria).* *Behaviour,* 1973, 45, 12–37.

Marx, C., and Kayser, C. Le rhythme nycthéméral de l'activité chez le lézard *(Lacerta agilis, Lacerta muralis).* *Comptes rendus de la Société de Biologie,* 1949, 143, 1375–1377.

Matsushita, T. Daily rhythmic activity of the sperm whale in the Antarctic Ocean. *Bulletin of the Japanese Society for Scientific Fisheries,* 1955, 20, 770–773.

Maxim, P. E., Bowden, D. M., and Sackett, G. P. Ultradian rhythms of solitary and social behavior in rhesus monkeys. *Physiology and Behavior,* 1976, 17, 337–344.

McClintock, M. K. Menstrual synchrony and suppression. *Nature,* 1971, 229, 244–245.

McClintock, M. K. Estrous synchrony and its mediation by airborne chemical communication *(Rattus norvegicus).* *Hormones and Behavior,* 1978, 10, 264–276.

McFarland, D. J. Decision making in animals. *Nature,* 1977, 269, 15–21.

McLaughlin, G. R., and Liverside, R. *Roberts Birds of South Africa.* Cape Town: Cape Times Ltd., 1958.

Menaker, M., and Eskin, A. Entrainment of circadian rhythms by sound in *Passer domesticus. Science,* 1966, 154, 1579–1581.

Menaker, W., and Menaker, A. Lunar periodicity in human reproduction: A likely unit in biological time. *American Journal of Obstetrics and Gynecology,* 1959, 77, 905–914.

Miller, R. E., Caul, W. E., and Mirsky, I. A. Patterns of eating and drinking in socially isolated rhesus monkeys. *Physiology and Behavior,* 1971, 7, 127–134.

Miller, R. S. Activity rhythms in the wood mouse, *Apodemus sylvaticus,* and the bank vole, *Clethrionomys glareolus. Proceedings of the Zoological Society of London,* 1954, 125, 505–519.

Mills, K. E., Lockard, R. B., and Owings, D. H. Search for lunar periodicity in the bannertail kangaroo rat *(Dipodomys spectabilis). Journal of Interdisciplinary Cycle Research,* 1975, 6, 323–333.

Moore, R. Y., and Ziegler, B. Secondary synchronizing stimuli, the suprachiasmatic nucleus (SCN) and the entrainment of circadian rhythms in the rat. *Society for Neuroscience Abstracts,* 1978, 4, 349.

Moriarty, D. J. W., Darlington, J. P. E., Dunn, I. G., Moriarty, C. M., and Tevlin, M. P. Feeding and grazing in Lake George, Uganda. *Proceedings of the Royal Society of London* B, 1973, 184, 299–319.

Morin, L. P. Rhythmicity of hamster gnawing: Ease of measurement and similarity to running activity. *Physiology and Behavior,* 1978, 21, 317–320.

Morrison, D. W. Lunar phobia in a neotropical fruit bat, *Artibeus jamaicensis (Chiroptera: Phyllostomatidae). Animal Behaviour,* 1978, 26, 852–855.

Morton, M. L. Diurnal feeding patterns in white-crowned sparrows, *Zonotrichia leucophrys gambelii. Condor,* 1967, 69, 491–512.

Mueller, H. C. The relationship of hunger to predatory behaviour in hawks *(Falco sparverius* and *Buteo platypterus). Animal Behaviour,* 1973, 21, 513–520.

Myrberg, A. A., Jr., and Gruber, S. H. The behavior of the bonnethead shark, *Sphyrna tiburo. Copeia,* 1974, 2, 358–374.

Nelson, D. R., and Johnson, R. H. Diel activity rhythms in the nocturnal bottom-dwelling sharks, *Heterodontus francisci* and *Cephaloscyllium ventriosum*. *Copeia*, 1970, *4*, 732–739.

Norris, K. S., and Kavanau, J. L. The burrowing of the Western shovel-nosed snake, *Chionactis occipilalis* Hallowell, and the undersand environment. *Copeia*, 1966, *4*, 650–664.

O'Connor, R. J. Feeding behaviour of the kittiwake. *Bird Study*, 1974, *21*, 185–192.

Ogden, J. C., and Buckman, N. S. Movements, foraging groups and diurnal migrations of the striped parrotfish *Scarus croicensis* Bloch (Scaridae). *Ecology*, 1973, *54*, 589–596.

Owings, D. H., and Lockard, R. B. Different nocturnal activity patterns of *Peromycus californicus* and *Peromyscus eremicus* in lunar lighting. *Psychonomic Science*, 1971, *22*, 63–64.

Pagano, R. R., and Lovely, R. H. Diurnal cycle and ACTH facilitation of shuttlebox avoidance. *Physiology and Behavior*, 1972, *8*, 721–723.

Palmgren, P. On the diurnal rhythm of activity and rest in birds. *Ibis*, 1949, *91*, 561–576.

Panksepp, J. Reanalysis of feeding patterns in the rat. *Journal of Comparative and Physiological Psychology*, 1973, *82*, 78–94.

Panksepp, L., and Krost, K. Modification of diurnal feeding patterns by palatability. *Physiology and Behavior*, 1975, *15*, 673–677.

Pearson, O. P. A traffic survey of *Microtus-Reithrodontomys* runways. *Journal of Mammalogy*, 1959, *40*, 169–180.

Pearson, O. P. Habits of harvest mice revealed by automatic photographic recorders. *Journal of Mammalogy*, 1960, *41*, 58–74.

Philippens, K. M. H., von Mayersbach, H., and Scheving, L. E. Effects of scheduling of meal-feeding at different phases of the circadian system in rats. *Journal of Nutrition*, 1977, *107*, 176–193.

Pittendrigh, C. S. Adaptation, natural selection, and behavior. In A. Roe and G. G. Simpson (Eds.), *Behavior and Evolution*. New Haven, Conn.: Yale University Press, 1958, pp. 390–416.

Potvin, C. L., and Bovet, J. Annual cycle of patterns of activity rhythms in beaver colonies *(Castor canadensis)*. *Journal of Comparative Physiology*, 1975, *98*, 243–256.

Prescott, R. G. W. Some behavioral effects of variables which influence the "general level of activity." *Animal Behaviour*, 1970, *18*, 791–796.

Quanstrom, W. R. Behaviour of Richardson's ground squirrel *Spermophilus richardsonii richardsonii*. *Animal Behaviour*, 1971, *19*, 646–652.

Quartermain, D., Kissileff, H., Shapiro, R., and Miller, N. E. Suppression of food intake with intragastric loading: Relation to natural feeding. *Science*, 1971, *173*, 941–943.

Raemaekers, J. Changes through the day in the food choice of wild gibbons. *Folia Primatologica*, 1978, *30*, 194–205.

Ralph, C. L. A diurnal activity rhythm in *Plethodon cinereus* and its modification by an influence having a lunar frequency. *Biological Bulletin*, 1957, *113*, 188–197.

Randolph, M. Role of light and circadian rhythms in the nocturnal behavior of *Galago crassicaudatus*. *Journal of Comparative and Physiological Psychology*, 1971, *74*, 115–123.

Rawson, K. S. Effects of tissue temperature on mammalian activity rhythms. *Cold Spring Harbor Symposia on Quantitative Biology*, 1960, *25*, 105–113.

Reed, B. L. The control of circadian pigment changes in the pencil fish: A proposed role for melatonin. *Life Sciences*, 1968, *7*, 961–973.

Reynolds, W. W., and Casterlin, M. E. Behavioral thermoregulation and diel activity in white sucker *(Catostomus commersoni)*. *Comparative Biochemistry and Physiology*, 1978, *59A*, 261–262.

Richter, C. P. A behavioristic study of the activity of the rat. *Comparative Psychology Monographs*, 1922, *1*.

Richter, C. P. Sleep and activity: Their relation to the 24-hour clock. *Proceedings of the Association for Research on Nervous and Mental Diseases*, 1967, *45*, 8–27.

Richter, C. P. Inherent twenty-four hour and lunar clocks of a primate—the squirrel monkey. *Communications in Behavioral Biology*, 1968, *1*, 305–332.

Robertson, D. R. The light–dark cycle and a nonlinear analysis of lunar perturbations and barometric pressure associated with the annual locomotor activity of the frog, *Rana pipiens*. *Biological Bulletin*, 1978, *154*, 302–321.

Robinson, H. W., and Miller, R. J. Diel activity patterns of the male snakeskin gourami, *Trichogaster pectoralis* (Regan) (Pisces, Belontiidae). *Proceedings of the Oklahoma Academy of Sciences*, 1972, *52*, 27–33.

Rohles, F. H., Jr., and Osbaldiston, G. Social entrainment of biorhythms in rhesus monkeys. In F. H. Rohles (Ed.), *Circadian Rhythms in Nonhuman Primates*. Basel/New York: Karger, 1969, pp. 39–51.

Roper, T. Diurnal rhythm in the nest-building behaviour of female mice. *Behaviour*, 1975, *52*, 95–103.

Roper T. J., and Ryon, C. J. Mutual synchronization of diurnal activity rhythms in groups of red-wolf/coyote hybrids. *Journal of Zoology*, 1977, *182*, 177–185.

Rovee, C. K., Kaufman, L. W., and Collier, G. H. Components of predation defense behavior in chickens: Evidence for endogenous rhythmicity. *Physiology and Behavior,* 1977, *19,* 663–671.

Rusak, B. The role of the suprachiasmatic nuclei in the generation of circadian rhythms in the golden hamster, *Mesocricetus auratus. Journal of Comparative Physiology,* 1977, *188,* 145–164.

Rusak, B., and Zucker, I. Fluid intake of rats in constant light and during feeding restricted to the light or dark portion of the illumination cycle. *Physiology and Behavior,* 1974, *13,* 91–100.

Rusak, B., and Zucker, I. Biological rhythms and animal behavior. *Annual Review of Psychology,* 1975, *26,* 137–171.

Rusak, B., and Zucker, I. Neural regulation of circadian rhythms. *Physiological Reviews,* 1979, *59,* 449–526.

Saayman, G. S., Tayler, C. K., and Bower, D. Diurnal activity cycles in captive free-ranging Indian Ocean bottlenose dolphins (*Tursiops aduncus* Ehrenburg). *Behaviour,* 1973, *44,* 212–233.

Saint Girons, H. Le cycle d'activité et ses facteurs chez *Vipera latastei* Bosca. *Vie et Milieu,* 1954, *5,* 513–528.

Saint Girons, H. Les facteurs du rhythme nychthéméral d'activité chez *Aspis cerastes* (L.). *Vie et Milieu,* 1959, *10,* 353–366.

Sandman, C. A., Kastin, A. J., and Schally, A. V. Behavioral inhibition as modified by melanocyte-stimulating hormone (MSH) and light dark conditions. *Physiology and Behavior,* 1971, *6,* 45–48.

Savory, C. J. Effects of different lighting regimes on diurnal feeding patterns of the domestic fowl. *British Poultry Science,* 1976, *17,* 341–350.

Schmid, W. D. Energy intake of the mourning dove *Zenaidura macroura marginella. Science,* 1965, *150,* 1171–1172.

Schmitt, M. Circadian rhythmicity in responses of cells in the lateral hypothalamus. *American Journal of Physiology,* 1973, *225,* 1096–1101.

Schwassmann, H. O. Biological rhythms. In W. S. Hoar and D. J. Randall (Eds.), *Fish Physiology,* Vol. 6: *Environmental Relations and Behavior.* New York: Academic Press, 1971, pp. 371–428.

Scott, M. D., and Causey, K. Ecology of feral dogs in Alabama. *Journal of Wildlife Management,* 1973, *37,* 253–265.

Shimek, S. J., and Monk, A. Daily activity of sea otter off the Monterey Peninsula, California. *Journal of Wildlife Management,* 1977, *41,* 277–283.

Silverman, H. J., and Zucker, I. Absence of post-fast food compensation in the golden hamster (*Mesocricetus auratus*). *Physiology and Behavior,* 1976, *17,* 271–285.

Sinclair, A. R. E. Lunar cycle and timing of mating season in Serengeti wildebeest. *Nature,* 1977, *267,* 832–833.

Slater, P. J. B. Tidal rhythm in a seabird. *Nature,* 1976, *264,* 636–638.

Sofia, R. D., and Salama, A. I. Circadian rhythm for experimentally-induced aggressive behavior in mice. *Life Sciences,* 1970, *9,* 331–338.

Spencer, W. P. Diurnal activity rhythms in fresh-water fishes. *Ohio Journal of Science,* 1939, *39,* 119–132.

Squires, V. R. Temporal patterns of activity in a small flock of Merino sheep as determined by an automatic recording technique. *Animal Behaviour,* 1971, *19,* 657–660.

Stavnes, K. L. State-dependent learning: Its relation to brain amines and natural states. *Dissertation Abstracts,* 1972, *32,* 4265B.

Stebbins, L. L. Seasonal variations in circadian rhythms of deer mice in northwestern Canada. *Arctic,* 1971, *24,* 124–131.

Stebbins, L. L. Seasonal and latitudinal variations in circadian rhythms of red-backed vole. *Arctic,* 1972, *25,* 216–224.

Stephens, G., McGaugh, J. L., and Alpern, H. P. Periodicity and memory in mice. *Psychonomic Science,* 1967, *8,* 201–202.

Stewart, R. W., and Bider, J. R. Summer activity of muskrats in relation to weather. *Journal of Wildlife Management,* 1977, *41,* 487–499.

Stickney, A. P. The locomotor activity of juvenile herring (*Clupea harengus harengus*) in response to changes in illumination. *Ecology,* 1972, *53,* 438–445.

Stille, W. T. The nocturnal amphibian fauna of the southern Lake Michigan beach. *Ecology,* 1952, *33,* 149–162.

Stroebel, C. F. Behavioral aspects of circadian rhythms. In J. Zubin and H. F. Hunt (Eds.), *Comparative Psychopathology: Animal and Human.* New York: Grune & Stratton, 1967, pp. 158–172.

Sulzman, F. M., Fuller, C. A, and Moore-Ede, M. C. Environmental synchronizers of squirrel monkey circadian rhythms. *Journal of Applied Physiology,* 1977a, *43,* 795–800.

Sulzman, F. M., Fuller, C. A., and Moore-Ede, M. C. Feeding time synchronizes primate circadian rhythms. *Physiology and Behavior,* 1977b, *18,* 775–779.

Swift, D. R. Activity cycles in the brown trout (*Salmo trutta* L.). II. Fish artifically fed. *Journal of the Fisheries Research Board of Canada,* 1964, *21,* 133–138.

Swingland, I. R. The influence of light intensity on the roosting time of the rook *(Corvus frugilegus)*. *Animal Behaviour,* 1976, *24,* 154–158.

Taylor, K. D. An automatic device for recording small mammal traffic on runways. *Journal of Zoology,* 1975, *176,* 274–277.

Tenaza, R., Ross, B. A., Tanticharoenyos, P., and Berkson, G. Individual behaviour and activity rhythms of captive slow lorises. *Animal Behaviour,* 1969, *17,* 664–669.

Terhune, J. M., and Ronald, K. Examining harp seal behavioural patterns via their underwater vocalizations. *Applied Animal Ethology,* 1976, *2,* 261–264.

Terman, M., and Terman, J. S. Circadian rhythm of brain self-stimulation behavior. *Science,* 1970, *168,* 1242–1244.

Ternes, J. W. Resistance to extinction of a learned taste aversion varies with time of conditioning. *Animal Learning and Behavior,* 1976, *4,* 317–321.

Ternes, J. W. Circadian susceptibility to animal hypnosis. *Psychological Record,* 1977, *27,* 15–19.

Thompson, D. C. Diurnal and seasonal activity of the grey squirrel *(Sciurus carolinensis)*. *Canadian Journal of Zoology,* 1977, *55,* 1185–1189.

Turuk, T. N. Diurnal periodicity in feeding and the vertical movements of the Atlantic cod (*Gadus morhua* L.). *Journal of Ichthyology,* 1973, *13,* 275–288.

Underwood, H. Retinal and extraretinal photoreceptors mediate entrainment of the circadian locomotor rhythm in lizards. *Journal of Comparative Physiology,* 1973, *83,* 187–222.

Vaughan, T. A. *Mammalogy.* Philadelphia: Saunders, 1972.

Vaughan, T. A. Nocturnal behavior of the African false vampire bat *(Cardioderma cor)*. *Journal of Mammalogy,* 1976, *57,* 227–248.

Verbeek, N. A. M. Daily and annual time budget of the yellow-billed magpie. *Auk,* 1972, *89,* 567–582.

Vilchez, C. A., and Echave Llanos, J. M. Circadian rhythm in the feeding activity of *Oxymycterus rutilans:* Role played by light and food availability. *Journal of Interdisciplinary Cycle Research,* 1971, *2,* 73–77.

Voûte, A. M., Sluiter, J. W., and Grimm, M. P. The influence of the natural light–dark cycle on the activity rhythm of pond bats (*Myotis dasycneme* Boie, 1825) during summer. *Oecologia* (Berl.), 1974, *17,* 221–243.

Wada, J. A., and Asakura, T. Circadian alteration of audiogenic seizure susceptibility in rats. *Experimental Neurology,* 1970, *29,* 211–214.

Wallace, D. C. Feeding behavior and developmental, seasonal and diel changes in the food of the silverjaw minnow, *Ericymba buccata* Cope. *American Midland Naturalist,* 1976, *95,* 361–376.

Wever, R. Influence of electric fields on some parameters of circadian rhythms in man. In M. Menaker (Ed.), *Biochronometry.* Washington, D.C.: U.S. National Academy of Science, 1971, pp. 117–132.

Woodhead, P. M. J. Effects of light upon behaviour and distribution of demersal fishes of the North Atlantic. *International Commission for the Northwest Atlantic Fisheries Special Publication,* 1965, *6,* 267–287.

Wyatt, J. R., and Eltringham, S. K. The daily activity of the elephant in the Rwenzori National Park, Uganda. *East African Wildlife Journal,* 1974, *12,* 273–289.

Yotsumoto, N. The daily activity rhythm in a troop of wild Japanese monkey. *Primates,* 1976, *17,* 183–204.

Zeigler, H. P., Green, H. L., and Lehrer, R. Patterns of feeding behavior in the pigeon. *Journal of Comparative and Physiological Psychology,* 1971, *76,* 468–477.

Ziesensis, J. S. Diel variation in the aggressive behavior of the mouse, *Mus musculus. Dissertation Abstracts,* 1974, *35,* 1132B.

Zihl, J., Poppel, E., and von Cramon, D. Diurnal variation of visual field size in patients with postretinal lesions. *Experimental Brain Research,* 1977, *27,* 245–249.

Zucker, I., and Stephan, F. K. Light–dark rhythms in hamster eating, drinking, and locomotor behaviors. *Physiology and Behavior,* 1973, *11,* 239–250.

12

Internal Temporal Order

MARTIN C. MOORE-EDE AND FRANK M. SULZMAN

The temporal organization of physiological events within an animal may often be as important as their spatial organization. Mutually interdependent events must not only occur at precise spatial locations but must also occur with appropriate timing. Similarly, incompatible processes, which may require different physicochemical conditions for their completion, can be separated just as effectively in time as in space.

This chapter first examines the normal temporal order of biochemical, physiological, and behavioral events over the course of the circadian day, looking at animals both entrained to 24-hr environmental time cues and freerunning in constant conditions. Second, the anatomy and physiology of the system that maintains this internal temporal order is discussed. Finally, we consider the advantages of maintaining a cyclic environment and the consequences of disturbing internal synchrony.

INTERNAL TEMPORAL ORDER IN STEADY-STATE-ENTRAINED CONDITIONS

When animals are maintained in an environment with a strong zeitgeber, such as a 24-hr light–dark cycle, each circadian rhythm in the organism assumes a stable relationship with that zeitgeber. An obvious consequence is that the various circadian rhythms within the organism assume stable phase relationships with each other. In this section, we discuss the structure of the entrained system.

MARTIN C. MOORE-EDE AND FRANK M. SULZMAN   Department of Physiology, Harvard Medical School, Boston, Massachusetts 02115. This work was supported by NASA Grants NAS9-14249 and NSG-9054; NSF Grant PCM76-19943; and NIH Grants GN-22085, NS-13921, and MH 28460. Dr. Moore-Ede is the recipient of NIH Career Development Award NS-00247.

MARTIN C. MOORE-
EDE AND FRANK M.
SULZMAN

Some idea of the problem of description of the internal temporal order of the circadian system can be gained by examining Figure 1, where a number of different rhythmic patterns in physiological functions are displayed. It is apparent that not only do they reach their peaks and troughs at different phases of the circadian day, but also the waveforms are dramatically different. Some are sinusoidal; others approach square wave patterns; and still others resemble more a single short-lived pulse once every 24 hr.

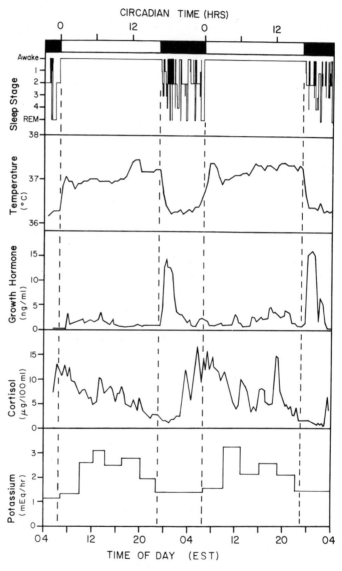

Fig. 1. Entrained circadian patterns of sleep, colonic temperature, plasma growth-hormone concentration, plasma cortisol concentration, and urinary potassium excretion of a human subject. Two consecutive days are shown with lights on from 0630 to 2300 both days. The vertical dashed lines indicate the times of change in illumination. Colonic temperature is plotted at 30-min intervals, and plasma samples were taken at approximately 20-min intervals. (Replotted data from Czeisler, 1978.)

The complexities of the waveforms are due to many types of components. The genetically determined structure of the organism and the tissues that generate the rhythm obviously contribute a major component. Thus, the rhythm of plasma cortisol concentration is a combined function of the inherent rhythmicity of the adrenal cortex, the rhythmicity in the volume of the body fluid in which it is distributed (Cranston and Brown, 1963), and the rhythms in hepatic degradation (Marotta, Hiles, Lanuza, and Boonayathap, 1975) and renal excretion (Kobberling and Muhlen, 1974). In addition, environmental influences contribute both entraining (e.g., LD cycles; Krieger and Hauser, 1977) and masking (e.g., stress; Czeisler, Moore-Ede, Regestein, Kisch, and Fang, 1976) effects on the plasma cortisol rhythm. Superimposed on a waveform may be other frequency oscillations that are beyond the scope of this review. Particularly prominent, for example, are the episodic bursts of cortisol secretion at approximately 90-min intervals (Weitzman, Fukushima, Nogeire, Roffwarg, Gallagher, and Hellman, 1971).

To analyze the organization of the circadian system, we must reduce these complex waveforms to some common descriptor. The one that is most useful is phase, defining the positioning of various marker points of a rhythm with respect to an externally defined time scale. In animals entrained to zeitgebers with 24-hr periods, such as shown in Figure 1, the time scale used is that of the environmental light–dark cycle.

What characteristic point on each cycle should then be used as a marker of phase? It should be a well-defined and accurate characterization of the positioning of a whole complex waveform with respect to the external time scale. With growth hormone, the maximum may be useful, but with complex patterns such as plasma cortisol concentration, or more square wave patterns such as body temperature, the actual timing of the maximum may vary quite widely within the total pattern of the waveform. Activity onset has been frequently used in studies of mammals since this is often a well-defined point (Pittendrigh and Daan, 1976). However, in an effort to find a common feature of the waveform, the practice of fitting by least-squares to the data a sine wave with the period of the waveform has been widely used (Rummel, Lee, and Halberg, 1974; Batschelet, 1974). The maximum (acrophase) of this sine wave is then used as the descriptor of phase for each of the rhythms. This approach, too, has problems, since while the urinary potassium rhythm may reasonably be described by a sine wave, the rhythm of growth hormone secretion clearly is not.

PHASE MAPS OF THE CIRCADIAN SYSTEM

Phase maps produced by plotting the acrophase of each rhythmic variable provide a ready way of documenting the internal temporal order of an organism. An example of an extensive phase map that has been produced for the mouse by Szabó, Kovats, and Halberg (1978) is shown in Figure 2. This phase map shows that the rhythms in a wide variety of physiological and pharmacological variables reach their acrophases at various times throughout the 24-hr day. Thus, while all these rhythms are synchronized to the 24-hr cycle and to each other, they demonstrate a dispersion of phase throughout the 24 hr. As an indicator of biological variability, each acrophase is plotted with its standard error around the mean. However, in light of the previous discussion, it should be realized that the variability is partly composed of a true variance in circadian phase and partly due to exogenous effects on the waveform that influence the timing of the acrophase from cycle to cycle.

MARTIN C. MOORE-
EDE AND FRANK M.
SULZMAN

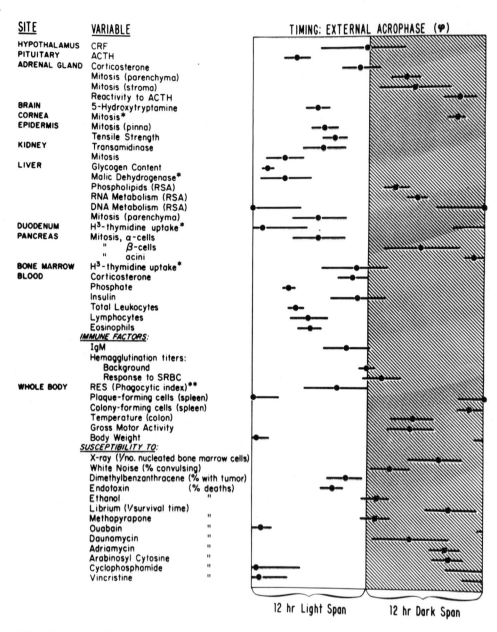

Fig. 2. Phase map of the circadian system of the mouse. The acrophase ± SEM for the various rhythms of animals maintained in LD 12:12 cycles are plotted. Original data from Chronobiology Laboratories, University of Minnesota, Minneapolis; *Department of Anatomy, University of Arkansas Medical Sciences, Little Rock; and **University Medical School of Szeged, Hungary. (Figure 3 in Szabó et al., 1978. Reprinted with permission of Casa Editrice "Il Ponte," Milan.)

Different species and different individuals within a species are coupled with their own typical phases to the natural 24-hr environmental cycle. Most obvious is the division of animals into diurnal, nocturnal, or crepuscular. Yet, when one examines the internal phase relationships between rhythms in nocturnal and diurnal animals (Figure 3), one observes striking similarities. The maximum of plasma corticosteroids coincides with the beginning of activity in both species even though the animals are approximately 180° out of phase. In other words, the internal temporal order is comparable although the phasing with respect to the outside world is quite different.

The inherited differences in internal temporal order are much more subtle. Figure 3 shows the internal phase relationships of the nocturnal rat and the diurnal squirrel monkey. An example of differences in internal phase relationships is that body temperature phase-lags urinary potassium excretion in the rat but phase-leads it in the squirrel monkey. Just as phase relationships to the zeitgeber are inherited (see Chapter 7), presumably internal phase relationships between rhythms are to some extent an inherited feature of the organism's physiology.

It is worth distinguishing between two genetically inherited features of rhythms that contribute toward the specific phase of a rhythm being observed. The first feature is the coupling of the rhythm to entraining cycles, which thus directly influences phase. Mutations in this aspect of the temporal system need not affect the period (τ) of the timekeeping mechanism. This has been demonstrated by the isolation of phase mutants in lower organisms where τ is unchanged (see Chapter 10). A second genetically determined characteristic is the endogenous period of the rhythm as demonstrated by period mutants.

The difference between the period of the driven oscillator and the period of the entraining oscillation ($\tau - T$) in any given system, whether the entraining oscillation is an environmental zeitgeber or another oscillator within the animal, is a determinant of phase, since a driven rhythm with a naturally shorter freerunning period tends to be phase-advanced and one with a naturally longer freerunning period, phase-delayed with respect to the phase of the driving oscillation. As a consequence, not only are external phase-angle relationships dependent on $\tau - T$, but also the internal phase-angle relationships in a

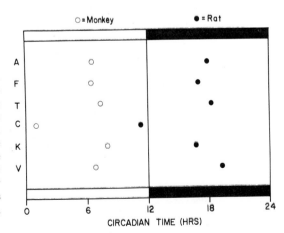

Fig. 3. Comparison of acrophases for several rhythms of squirrel monkeys (O) and rats (●) maintained on LD 12:12 cycles. The dark portion of the cycle is represented by the box from hours 12 to 24. The rhythms compared are activity (A), feeding (F), body temperature (T), urinary potassium excretion (K), urine volume (V), and plasma cortisol (in monkeys) and corticosterone (in rats) (C). (The data for rats are from Halberg, 1969; for monkeys from Sulzman et al., 1978a, and Hiles et al., unpublished observations.)

coupled multi-oscillator system are dependent on the respective $\tau - T$ at each point of entrainment within the system.

PLASTICITY OF PHASE

Circadian systems demonstrate significant plasticity of phase. There are a number of causes, the most trivial of which are the passive responses of rhythms to masking effects from factors in both the external and the internal environments of the animal. Thus, the apparent phase of the body temperature rhythm is influenced by when a human subject might have a hot shower and to a smaller extent by the timing of feeding. Similarly, a stress applied on the organism may produce a large outpouring of cortisol at times other than the normal circadian maxima (Czeisler, Moore-Ede et al., 1976). Such exogenous influences may be circadian phase-dependent, which makes their separation from underlying endogenous rhythms somewhat complicated. For example, the magnitude of the increase in plasma corticosterone in response to the masking effect of handling stress is dependent on circadian phase (Mayersbach, Philippens, and Schering, 1977). Because of these influences on the waveform of the observed rhythm, the measured phase will vary from cycle to cycle.

Variations in each of the factors that influence endogenous circadian phase also contribute to plasticity of phase. Thus, fluctuations in the frequency of the endogenous oscillator generating the rhythm will alter the function $\tau - T$, so that the phase of a measured rhythm with respect to entraining cycles will vary. Such changes in endogenous circadian period may be brought about by changes in the hormonal concentration in the internal milieu, for example (Morin, Fitzgerald, and Zucker, 1977). Similarly, changes in coupling strength will cause phase plasticity. The two factors that contribute to coupling strength are discussed below.

COUPLING STRENGTH

NATURE OF THE ZEITGEBER. While the light–dark cycle is the predominant zeitgeber in most vertebrate species, other zeitgebers have been shown to play some role. For example, sound, social cues, and feeding cycles (see Chapter 6) have been shown to be capable of synchronizing circadian rhythms in various vertebrate species. Sulzman, Fuller, and Moore-Ede (1978a) have compared the phase maps of squirrel monkeys entrained by either food availability cycles (EF = eating–fasting) or light–dark (LD) cycles (Figure 4). It can

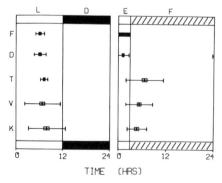

Fig. 4. Timing of the acrophase for each rhythm with its standard error (boxes) and standard deviation (lines). *(Left)* Shows the acrophase for monkeys entrained to an LD 12:12 cycle. *(Right)* Acrophase for monkeys entrained to an EF 3:21 cycle. Data for the rhythms of feeding (F), drinking (D), temperature (T), urine volume (V), and urinary potassium excretion (K) are shown. Feeding during the EF 3:21 cycle is represented by a dark box in the top of the right panel since no precise acrophase could be calculated. (Figure 2 in Sulzman et al., 1978a. Reprinted with permission of the American Physiological Society.)

be seen that although in each case all rhythms are synchronized to the 24-hr zeitgeber period, the internal phase relationships between the rhythms are different. Thus, in animals entrained to LD cycles, the body temperature rhythm on average phase leads the rhythm of urinary potassium excretion by 0.6 hr but phase-lags it by 1.9 hr when the animals are entrained to the EF cycle.

The different internal temporal order in the same animals synchronized to either light–dark cycles or eat–fast cycles is a consequence of the illumination and feeding zeitgebers apparently being coupled at different loci to the circadian timing system. This differential coupling is discussed in more detail below.

CONTRAST IN THE ZEITGEBER CYCLE. Coupling strength is also a function of the ratio in intensity of the contrasting portions of the zeitgeber signal. Thus, animals are less strongly entrained by light–dark cycles where the illumination is at a relatively low intensity during the lights-on portion of the cycle. This may be assayed, for example, by comparing the rate of phase shift of the animal's rhythms after a shift in the entraining zeitgeber (Aschoff *et al.*, 1975). Changes in coupling strength as the strength of the zeitgeber signal is varied cause alterations in the phase relationships between the entrained rhythms and the zeitgeber (Aschoff, 1960, 1965b). The phase plasticity of rhythms is in part caused by such changes in the coupling strength both to external environmental zeitgeber cycles and to internal neural and endocrine zeitgeber cycles within the circadian system (see below).

TEMPORAL ORDER IN THE ABSENCE OF ENVIRONMENTAL TIME CUES

INTERNAL SYNCHRONY BETWEEN RHYTHMS

The maintenance of stable phase relationships between the various rhythmic variables within an organism does not depend on the presence of an environmental zeitgeber. Animals freerunning in an environment without effective time cues nevertheless tend to demonstrate internal synchrony between the various rhythms. In rats, for example, the freerunning rhythms of plasma corticosterone, pineal *N*-acetyltransferase activity, and serotonin remain synchronized with the rest–activity cycle in blinded rats over at least 60 days of observation (Gibbs and Van Brunt, 1975; Pohl and Gibbs, 1978). Similarly, in the squirrel monkey, internal synchronization between the freerunning rhythms of feeding, temperature, and urinary potassium excretion is usually seen in animals maintained in constant illumination (LL) (Sulzman, Fuller, and Moore-Ede, 1979). Studies in man, such as that shown in Figure 5, indicate that such rhythms as sleep–wake, body temperature, and plasma cortisol concentration usually all maintain freerunning rhythms with the same periodicity and stable phase relationships with each other (Czeisler, Weitzman, Moore-Ede, and Fusco, 1976; Czeisler, 1978).

Such internal synchrony between circadian rhythms freerunning in constant conditions has been observed over considerable periods of time. For example, human subjects have been maintained in isolation for a month or more with each rhythm maintaining stable phase relationships throughout the period of study in most of the individuals examined (Aschoff, 1965a; Czeisler, Weitzman *et al.*, 1976; Czeisler, 1978). Such studies provide evidence that there is a reasonably strong internal coupling mechanism between the various circadian rhythms within the animal, and that internal entrainment is not dependent on the presence of strong environmental time cues.

INTERNAL PHASE-ANGLE SHIFTS

The organization of the circadian system is not identical in freerunning and entrained states. Wever (1973) has pointed out that there are internal phase-angle shifts between circadian rhythms when human subjects are freerunning in time-cueless environments. This is apparent in Figure 5, where the acrophase of plasma cortisol is phase-delayed 4.4 hr from midsleep in the entrained situation, but it is phase-delayed by only 2.3 hr when freerunning. Similarly, the acrophase of body temperature is phase-delayed by 11.1 hr from the time of midsleep in the entrained state and by 6.8 hr in the freerunning conditions.

ALTERATIONS IN CIRCADIAN WAVEFORM

Phase shifts in computed acrophases provide only a single-dimensional analysis of the circadian response to the change in the environmental state. An analysis of waveform changes reveals much more complex responses. Figure 6 shows the waveforms of the feeding, temperature, and urinary potassium rhythms in monkeys entrained to LD 12:12 or freerunning in LL. Each educed pattern represents the mean and standard error of the mean of 30–40 cycles from eight animals. There is a reduction in amplitude evident in each rhythm in LL and some significant changes in waveform. For example, the feeding rhythm that in LD has two discrete maxima is much more sinusoidal in LL. Each rhythm in LL shows relatively more time above the mean than below it as compared with the LD entrained state (Sulzman et al., 1979).

What phenomena underlie these changes in waveform? A major component appears to be the passive response of physiological systems to ambient light intensity. A 2-hr pulse of light during the dark portion of an LD 12:12 cycle will elevate body temperature, for example (Fuller, Sulzman, and Moore-Ede, 1978), to the level associated with subjective night in LL of the same intensity. In addition, the response is graded, depending on the intensity of ambient light (Sulzman et al., 1979). Other changes in endogenous circadian oscillations (as entraining signals are removed and as their period reverts to a freerun) may also contribute to changes in waveform, but these are less well understood (Wever, 1973).

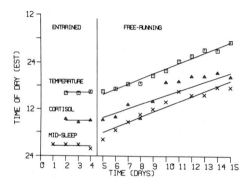

Fig. 5. Comparison of the daily timing of the acrophase of the rhythms of body temperature (□), plasma cortisol (△), and the time of midsleep (X) of a human subject in entrained and freerunning conditions. The time of occurrence (in EST) of the point is plotted against elapsed experimental time in days. (Replotted data from Czeisler, 1978.)

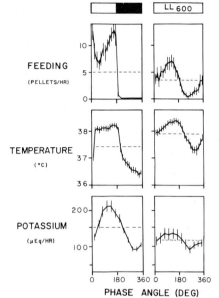

Fig. 6. Comparison of the educed waveforms of the feeding, colonic temperature, and urinary potassium excretion rhythms of squirrel monkeys either entrained to an LD 12:12 cycle or freerunning in constant light. The light intensity of both the light portion of the LD cycle and constant light was 600 lux. Plotted are the mean values ($\pm$ SEM) at each time point. Each educed pattern represents 30–40 cycles from eight monkeys. The horizontal dashed lines represent the daily mean values. (Redrawn from Figure 6 in Sulzman *et al.,* 1979.)

Increased Plasticity of Phase

Although the internal coupling between circadian rhythmic variables in an organism is usually sufficient to maintain internal synchronization, there is evidence of increased plasticity of phase in animals when they are no longer entrained by environmental zeitgebers. An example can be seen in Figure 5, where there is more variability in internal phase-angle relationships from cycle to cycle in the freerunning than in the entrained state. Studies in squirrel monkeys by Fuller, Sulzman, and Moore-Ede (1979) have shown that this phase plasticity can be considerable. For example, the circadian rhythms of core body temperature and skin temperature may show up to ±6 hr variability in internal phase relationship. In contrast, in the entrained state, the variability in internal phase relationship is never more than 0.5 hr.

On occasion, the internal coupling is sufficiently weak so that different variables may uncouple and oscillate quite independently of one another. This condition, called *internal desynchronization,* is discussed in greater detail in the next section because of its particular significance in the organization of the circadian system.

Anatomical and Physiological Basis of Internal Temporal Order

The compendiums (Conroy and Mills, 1970) and the comprehensive phase maps (Halberg, 1969; Ehret, Groh, and Meinert, 1978) have demonstrated how widespread is circadian rhythmicity throughout the physiological functions of an animal. Because of this ubiquity, it is now interesting to find a physiological variable that does not show circadian rhythms, suggesting that there may be some particular advantage to strict internal constancy. The mechanisms that maintain such internal constancy in the face of an intrinsically rhythmic system may require particularly elaborate physiological strategies.

In this section, we turn to the anatomical and physiological basis of circadian time-keeping. Previous formal models (Pittendrigh and Bruce, 1957, 1959; Pittendrigh, 1974) have treated the entire circadian system somewhat as an engineer's black box. The inputs were environmental zeitgebers and the outputs were rhythms in whatever behavioral or physiological variable it was most convenient to measure. We now move to the next step: the examination of the contents of that black box.

Abstract Models of Internal Organization

Some time ago, we published three alternative models of the circadian timing system (Moore-Ede, Schmelzer, Kass, and Herd, 1976; Moore-Ede and Sulzman, 1977). Each of the models can account for the phenomenon of internal synchronization between rhythms and for the known formal properties of the interaction between zeitgebers and physiological rhythms. The models are presented in Figure 7. We recognized that minor variants of these models, or combinations of their features, are entirely possible, but the models we chose emphasized the contrasts between certain possible organizations of the circadian system.

Model I, which has been assumed in many investigations of the circadian timing system (e.g., Mills, 1966), consists of a network of cellular systems (A, B, C, etc.) that passively oscillate as a forced response to a single self-sustained driving pacemaker (P). Where these cellular units are noncontiguous in a multicellular animal, the model requires that oscillating levels of physical or chemical mediators be postulated (a, b, c, etc.), with the period of P, but not necessarily the same phase. These mediating systems, which would presumably be nervous (neurotransmitter release) or endocrine (hormonal concentration), would transmit the oscillations from P to the various passively responding cellular units. The

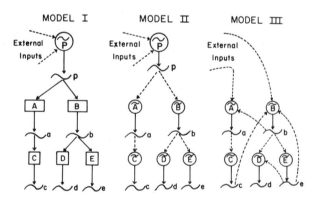

Fig. 7. Three alternative models of the mammalian circadian timing system. The symbol ⊖ represents an active cellular unit capable of maintaining a self-sustained oscillation with its own independent period; □ represents a cellular unit that responds passively to an oscillating driving force; ∼ indicates the oscillating concentration of a chemical mediator; — — → indicates the entrainment of a self-sustained oscillator by a phase-response mechanism; and ⟶ is the direction of flow of passive responses to an oscillating driving force. P = pacemaker. Model 1 is therefore a single oscillator system, whereas the other models are multioscillator systems arranged in a hierarchical (Model II) or nonhierarchical (Model III) manner. (Redrawn from Figure 2 in Moore-Ede *et al.*, 1976.)

entire circadian system would be entrained by environmental time cues via exteroceptive sensory inputs to the pacemaker.

Model II describes a network of cellular units that are each themselves self-sustained oscillators, able to maintain oscillations with an independent period in the absence of periodic inputs. One oscillator (P) acts as a pacemaker and is entrained by exteroceptive sensory inputs from environmental time cues. As in Model I, it is necessary to postulate oscillating nervous or endocrine mediators that maintain synchronization within the animal. However, the mediators in this model actively entrain the self-sustained cellular oscillators by a phase-control mechanism similar to the entrainment of the organism's circadian system by cycles of environmental illumination (Pittendrigh, 1960).

Model III also describes a multioscillator model, but in this case, no one oscillator consistently acts as a pacemaker. Instead, the various exteroceptive sensory inputs entrain different oscillators. Internal synchronization within the system is maintained by the feedback action of mediators (a, b, c, etc.) on the separate oscillating units (A, B, C, etc.). As in Model II, the mediators synchronize the oscillators by active entrainment.

SINGLE OR MULTIOSCILLATOR SYSTEM? There are several ways in which it is possible to differentiate between the single-oscillator system (Model I) and a multiple-oscillator system (Model II or III). This evidence strongly suggests that the circadian timekeeping is a product of a multioscillator system, particularly in man and nonhuman primates.

Internal Desynchronization. We have discussed above how circadian rhythms in physiological variables measured simultaneously within the same animal are normally internally synchronized, with each oscillating variable demonstrating identical periods and stable phase relationships. In higher animals, however, a state called *internal desynchronization* can occasionally be observed, where the separate monitored variables show oscillations with independent periods and, therefore, constantly changing phase relationships. Such independence between the oscillations in different physiological variables is incompatible with a single-oscillator model (Model I) and strongly suggests that Model II or III is more applicable.

The first reports of internal desynchronization were from human subjects isolated from time cues. Aschoff, Gerecke, and Wever (1967) reported that about 10% of their subjects demonstrated a circadian rhythm of rest–activity that would spontaneously freerun with a period distinctly different from that of the body temperature rhythm (see Chapter 17). Subsequent studies demonstrated that internal desynchronization could also be forced by entraining the subject to zeitgeber periods of longer than 26 hr (Wever, 1975). The body temperature rhythm would not entrain, while the rest–activity cycle would. More recently, studies by Czeisler, Weitzman, *et al.* (1976) and Czeisler (1978) have shown that spontaneous internal desynchronization in man can also occur between the rhythm of plasma cortisol and the sleep–wake cycle.

Internal desynchronization has also been reported in the squirrel monkey by Sulzman, Fuller, and Moore-Ede (1977c) (Figure 8.) When maintained in constant light (LL) of 600 lux, approximately 25% of monkeys show an internal desynchronization between the renal rhythms of potassium and water excretion, on the one hand, and the rhythms of body temperature and feeding activity, on the other. Forced internal desynchronization could also be induced in squirrel monkeys by light–dark cycles with periods of 26–30 hr, which usually entrain the circadian rhythms of body temperature and feeding, but not the rhythms of urinary potassium excretion (Sulzman, Fuller, and Moore-Ede, 1980).

Wever (1975) has argued that to demonstrate that two circadian rhythms are driven by independent oscillators requires that one rhythm complete at least one full cycle more than the other over the period of observation and thereby show an internal phase-angle shift of at least 360° with respect to the other. In this situation, it would be difficult to envisage both rhythms being driven by the same circadian oscillator. To date, internal desynchronization by this criterion has been demonstrated only in humans and the squirrel monkey. In large part, however, this is due to the dearth of animal preparations where multiple and diverse circadian rhythms can be monitored continuously in an individual animal for long enough to document internal desynchronization.

It is interesting to note that even when two rhythms are internally desynchronized, there is still some residual interaction. When the rhythms pass through a certain phase relationship, there can be a slowing down of the oscillation and then a subsequent speeding up as a nonpreferred phase relationship is again reached (see Figure 8). This interaction Czeisler (1978) termed "relative internal coordination" since it is strictly analogous to the relative external coordination seen between an environmental zeitgeber and the circadian system when the coupling strength is not sufficient to permit entrainment (von Holst, 1939).

Splitting. Not only do different physiological systems appear to be timed by separate circadian oscillators, but also within a system there may be multiple oscillators. There are a number of situations, particularly where external or internal time cues are confusing or

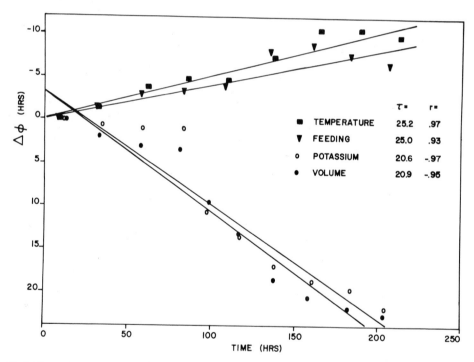

Fig. 8. Phase plots of the rhythms of feeding (▼), colonic temperature (■), and urinary potassium (○) and water (●) excretion of a squirrel monkey displaying internal desynchronization. Acrophase values obtained from the band-pass filter analysis of the raw data are normalized so that the beginning of constant light equals zero. The differences between the acrophase for the first cycle and the acrophase for each subsequent cycle are plotted against the experimental time in hours at which each acrophase occurred. (Redrawn from Figure 3 in Sulzman *et al.*, 1977c. Reprinted with permission of Pergamon, Press, Inc.)

insufficient, in which multiple components can be observed within a rhythmic function. Probably the best-documented example is called *splitting*. Two or more components become clearly visible in the waveform of a circadian rhythm, and these freerun with independent periods. Often they resynchronize at an alternate stable phase position 180° apart (see Chapter 5). This phenomenon was first reported in rest–activity patterns in rodents (Pittendrigh, 1960) and prosimians (Hoffmann, 1971). It has also been observed in body temperature rhythms in bats (Menaker, 1959) and squirrel monkeys (Fuller *et al.*, 1979). Often such splitting is induced by changes in the intensity of constant light, but a similar condition can be observed when lesions are placed in neural pathways that are important in the transduction of light information to the circadian system (Rusak, 1977b).

In Vitro Studies. If circadian rhythms are generated by multiple oscillators located in various body tissues, then it should be possible to isolate, *in vitro,* tissue containing one or more spontaneous circadian oscillators. A number of investigators have reported *in vitro* persisting circadian rhythmicity in such variables as adrenal corticosteroid production (Andrews, 1971), liver enzyme activity (Rensing, Goedeke, Wassman, and Broich, 1974) and pineal activity (Binkley, Riebman, and Reilly, 1977).

These studies are difficult to conduct because several days of *in vitro* culture are required and the culture medium demands of circadian systems are poorly understood. There have been some problems in repeating these experiments, but there is no doubt about the potential importance of this approach in probing the physiology of circadian oscillators.

Mechanisms of Oscillator Coupling. Since circadian rhythms are normally internally synchronized with each other as well as being externally synchronized with environmental zeitgebers, there must be mechanisms of temporal communication within the animal. The most obvious way to transmit period and phase information is through the rhythmic activity of neural and endocrine systems. Rhythms in hormone or neurotransmitter concentration in the milieu of a circadian oscillator could exert phase control by a mechanism analogous to the entrainment of circadian oscillators by light–dark cycles.

There is extensive evidence for the rhythmic activity of neural and endocrine systems. Circadian rhythms in neuronal firing rate (Schmitt, 1973; Koizumi and Nishino, 1976); the concentration of the neurotransmitters 5-hydroxy-tryptamine (Hery, Chouvet, Kan, Pujol, and Glowinski, 1977), norepinephrine (Manshardt and Wurtman, 1968; Reis, Weinbren, and Corvelli, 1968; Bobillier and Mouret, 1971), and dopamine (Bobillier and Mouret, 1971); and synaptic excitability (Barnes, McNaughton, Goddard, Douglas, and Adamec, 1977) have been reported. Furthermore, there is evidence for the transmission of circadian information by neural pathways from the hypothalamus to the pineal (Axelrod, 1974); liver (Black and Reis, 1971); and other hypothalamic and brain stem centers (Moore, 1978).

Similarly, there are prominent circadian rhythms in the plasma concentration of a variety of hormones, including growth hormone (Weitzman, 1976); prolactin (Sassin, Frantz, Weitzman, and Kapen, 1972); cortisol (Weitzman *et al.*, 1971); and testosterone (Lincoln, Rowe, and Racey, 1974). As we discussed earlier, the effective rhythm in plasma hormone concentration is a combined result of rhythms in secretion, body fluid compartment volume, degradation, and renal excretion.

Although circadian rhythms in neural and endocrine systems are well documented, the mechanism of transmission of phase and period information between circadian oscillators within an organism has received little attention. This is in obvious contrast to the attention paid the mechanism of entrainment by external zeitgebers (see Chapter 7). As we commence our analysis, it is first important to recognize the difference between internal synchrony in single oscillator and multioscillator systems. The transmission of temporal information to a passively responding tissue and the phase control of an active circadian oscillator are quite distinct. To illustrate this, let us examine as an example the element E, which produces the rhythm e, in each of the models in Figure 7.

If E were a passively responding tissue forced by the rhythm in b, as in Model I, then we would predict that (1) phase-shifting b will produce an equal and immediate phase shift in e; (2) e must cease to oscillate if b is maintained at a constant level; and (3) a change in the level of b must induce an equivalent change in e at any time in the 24-hr day.

In contrast, if E were a spontaneous circadian oscillator as in Models II or III, we would predict that (1) a phase shift in b will result in a phase shift in e, but only after a transient response; (2) if b is maintained at a constant level, e would continue to oscillate with a freerunning rhythm that is no longer synchronized to other circadian rhythms in the animal; and (3) an acute change in the level of b will not necessarily have an effect on e because the response will depend on the circadian phase at which the change occurs.

To distinguish between these models of coupling, Moore-Ede, Schmelzer, Kass, and Herd (1977) examined the control of the circadian rhythm of renal potassium excretion by the circadian rhythm of plasma cortisol concentration. Thus, b would represent the plasma cortisol rhythm, E the kidney (or rather the renal distal tubules), and e the urinary potassium rhythm. Using adrenalectomized squirrel monkeys with chronically implanted catheters so that plasma adrenal steroid rhythms could be artifically generated by infusions, they found (1) that phase shifts in the daily timing of the plasma cortisol rhythm would cause a comparable (though not equal) phase shift in urinary potassium excretion, but only after a transient response lasting several days (Figure 9); (2) the elimination of circadian

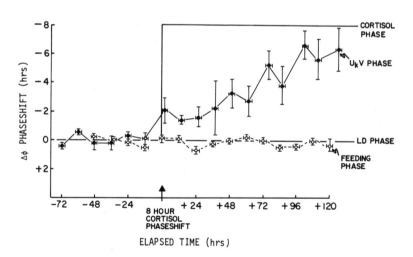

Fig. 9. Changes of phase (mean ± SEM) of circadian rhythms of urinary potassium excretion (U_kV, ●) and feeding (○) after an 8-hr phase delay of the timing of cortisol administration in adrenalectomized monkeys. Phase shift of each rhythm, as compared to mean phase over the control period prior to phase shift, is plotted against elapsed time, in hours. Urinary potassium rhythm resynchronized with a phase delay 80% that of the cortisol phase shift, but the feeding rhythm remained synchronized to light–dark cycle phase. (Figure 5 in Moore-Ede *et al.*, 1977. Reprinted with permission of the American Physiological Society.)

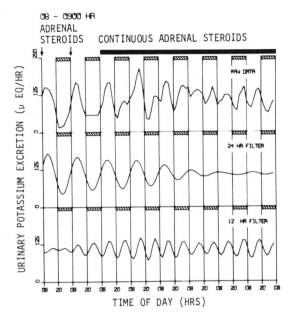

Fig. 10. Response to the continuous administration of adrenal steroids in a representative adrenalectomized monkey. For the first 2 days the daily dose of cortisol and aldosterone was administered between 0800 and 0900 hr. Then, for the remainder of the experiment, the same daily dose was evenly spread over each 24 hr. Top panel shows raw data, middle panel the output of a frequency filter centered at a 24-hr period, and lower panel the output of a filter centered at a 12-hr period. Circa 24-hr period damped out while circa 12-hr period gained strength during the continuous adrenal steroid administration. (Figure 3 in Moore-Ede *et al.*, 1977. Reprinted with permission of the American Physiological Society.)

rhythmicity in adrenal steroid administration in adrenalectomized animals results in the appearance of freerunning persistent oscillations in urinary potassium excretion (Figure 10); and (3) a pulse of cortisol administered in the evening hours to intact animals, approximately 12 hr phase-delayed from the endogenous peak of plasma cortisol concentration, did not induce an elevation in urinary potassium excretion equivalent to that induced by the endogenous cortisol peak. These results suggested that the action of cortisol as an internal synchronizer of the urinary potassium rhythm may involve a phase-control mechanism that is comparable to the well-documented action of light on circadian systems (see Chapter 7). The results also suggest that the circadian rhythm of urinary potassium excretion is the product of one or more autonomous renal oscillators that can persist and freerun in the absence of temporal information derived from the plasma cortisol rhythm.

It was significant that cortisol rather than the more potent mineralocorticoid aldosterone appeared to act as the hormonal mediator synchronizing the circadian rhythm of renal potassium excretion with the light–dark cycle. The urinary potassium rhythm was indistinguishable whether cortisol and aldosterone together, or cortisol alone, were administered in the adrenalectomized monkeys. Thus, cortisol would appear to be involved in the circadian synchronization of renal potassium (Moore-Ede *et al.*, 1977) and aldosterone in its moment-to-moment regulation (Moore-Ede, Meguid, Fitzpatrick, Boyden, and Ball, 1978). As the components of the circadian timing system and their internal zeitgebers are identified, it may turn out to be a general finding that circadian synchronization may be subserved by its own specialized set of hormones and neural pathways. We will return to discuss this point later.

ORGANIZATION OF THE MULTIPLE-OSCILLATOR SYSTEM. The discussion in the previous section makes clear that the circadian timing system in higher animals is composed of multiple potentially independent oscillators located in various body tissues, and that these oscillators are internally coupled with each other and externally coupled with the environment via circadian rhythms in neural and endocrine systems. We next turn our attention to the question of how these oscillators are organized. A number of the questions can be addressed by contrasting the structures of Models II and III in Figure 7.

Pacemakers in the Circadian Timing System. An analogy with the organization of the oscillating cells of the heart would lead us to expect a pacemaker that dictates period and phase to the constituent oscillators of the system. Such an organization is depicted in Model II. In contrast, in Model III, no one single oscillator consistently acts as a pacemaker to the circadian system. Rather, there are multiple interactions among the various circadian oscillators that mutually determine period and phase.

In the last few years, a candidate pacemaker for the circadian timing system has been identified: the suprachiasmatic nuclei of the hypothalamus (SCN). This work is discussed in detail in Chapter 13. Because lesions that destroy the SCN result in widespread disturbances of circadian rhythms, early workers suggested that the SCN might be acting as *the* circadian clock. This is very unlikely since there is extensive evidence indicating a multiple-oscillator system, and subsequently, more extended studies have shown that the observed rhythms may not be entirely lost but merely disorganized into multiple components (Rusak, 1977b) and that rhythms that were eliminated may reappear within several weeks (Lengvari and Liposits, 1977). Whether the SCN act as a true pacemaker or are merely involved as a way station coupling rhythmic functions with each other and with the light–dark cycle remains a subject for future investigation.

Differential Coupling to Environmental Zeitgebers. Another distinction between Models II and III is that Model II shows the pacemaker resolving all conflicting temporal information from the various zeitgebers in the environment, whereas Model III shows the zeitgebers impacting on separate oscillators within the organism so that no single oscillator receives all environmental phase and period information.

A series of studies in the squirrel monkey by Sulzman, Fuller, and Moore-Ede (1977a,b) has demonstrated that besides the light–dark cycle, cycles of food availability are a strong zeitgeber for this species. Rhythms with 3 hr of eating and 21 hr of fasting each day (EF 3:21) can synchronize all the documented circadian rhythms of the squirrel monkey when the animal is maintained in an environment with constant lighting (LL).

A comparison of the strength of coupling of each of these zeitgebers to the various rhythmic functions in the squirrel monkey made it apparent that there was differential coupling between each zeitgeber and the various rhythms. The coupling strength of each synchronized rhythm to the entraining zeitgeber can be assayed by a number of criteria, including (1) the rate of resynchronization of the rhythm after a shift of the zeitgeber phase; (2) the range of entrainment over which the rhythm will track the period of the zeitgeber; and (3) the stability of phase (and waveform) of the rhythm from cycle to cycle when entrained by the zeitgeber. Such studies indicated that the circadian rhythm of body temperature, for example, was more tightly synchronized to LD than EF cycles, whereas the reverse was true for the circadian rhythm of urinary potassium excretion (Sulzman *et al.*, 1978a).

To compare the strength of internal coupling between the circadian oscillators with the external coupling strength to the zeitgebers, conflicting period and phase information was given from the LD and EF zeitgebers. Each zeitgeber was applied (1) with different phases but the same period and (2) with different periods. In each of these situations, the body temperature rhythm remained entrained to the light–dark cycle, but the urinary potassium rhythm remained synchronized to the EF cycle (Sulzman *et al.,* 1978c). This finding demonstrated that there is no internal resolution of phase and period information by a single oscillator such as depicted in Model II. Rather, each zeitgeber impinged on a different site within the circadian timing system and thus was coupled with a different relative strength to the different constituent oscillators.

QUALITATIVE MODELS OF THE CIRCADIAN TIMING SYSTEM

The abstract models of Figure 7 served the purpose of focusing attention on different possible types of organization of the components within the circadian timing system. The next step is to turn to specific qualitative models of the circadian timing system where the different oscillators are localized and the neural and endocrine pathways that synchronize them are identified. This must be done before we can commence the quantitative description of the system with the precise behaviors of each oscillator measured and the strength of coupling determined.

The present state of understanding of the circadian system lags far behind the modeling detail that Guyton and his colleagues (1972) have published for the cardiovascular system. However, the modern study of the anatomy and physiology of the cardiovascular system started with Harvey (1628/1958), whereas the equivalent studies of the circadian timing system have started only in the last two decades!

BASIC PREMISES. In this section, we start a first, tentative approach to the qualitative modeling of the circadian timing system in higher animals. Using the same symbology as the models in Figure 7, we recognize several basic premises, the evidence for which has been discussed in the previous sections:

1. The circadian system is composed of multiple, potentially independent oscillators that when deprived of temporal information, from either the environment or the other oscillators in the body, can demonstrate independent, freerunning periods.

2. Besides these spontaneous oscillating elements, there are also passive elements such as those seen in Model I of Figure 7.

3. Many tissues demonstrate both active and passive components—the passive components, of course, being the subject of the vast majority of physiological studies. Both active and passive elements may contribute to the observed rhythmic outputs of that tissue.

4. We recognize that many tissues that contribute to a rhythm may be bilateral (e.g., adrenal glands, kidneys). It is possible for each member of a pair to behave independently and hence to complicate the waveform of the rhythm.

5. Two distinct time cues in the environment, light–dark cycles and cycles of food availability, are each capable of synchronizing the circadian system and, as discussed earlier, show differential coupling to the various elements within the system.

6. We recognize that there are many separate *subsystems* that comprise the circadian timing system. The criterion for a subsystem is that it is capable of oscillating independently *in vivo.* We consider rest–activity, body temperature, and the pituitary–adrenal axis as

subsystems because they can internally desynchronize from each other and show independent periodicities.

With this groundwork we can start to sketch an outline of the circadian timing system.
In Figure 11, we particularly focus on the pituitary–adrenal axis and the elements controlling renal potassium excretion because more information is available on these than on
the other subsystems. We will discuss the experimental evidence that underlines each of the
components shown in Figure 11 and the coupling links between them.

RECEPTION OF TEMPORAL INFORMATION FROM ZEITGEBERS

Light–Dark Cycles (LD). The entrainment of the circadian timing system by light–
dark cycles is reviewed in detail in Chapter 7. In mammals, this temporal information is
received primarily through the retina. Optical enucleation results in freerunning circadian
rhythms no longer entrainable to light–dark cycles (Richter, 1968). In other vertebrates,
however, there is evidence for additional extraretinal photoreceptors that can transduce
circadian LD information. Their physiology has been reviewed elsewhere (Menaker and
Underwood, 1976). The retina is shown as a passive element since there is no evidence of
independent oscillators in the retina of mammals, although there is such evidence for various invertebrate species (Menaker, Takahashi, and Eskin, 1978).

From the retina, circadian information is transmitted by the neural activity of the
retinohypothalamic tract (RHT) to the SCN (see Chapter 13). A much less important
pathway appears to be routed through the primary optic tract to the lateral geniculate
nucleus and from thence to the SCN (Rusak, 1977a).

The SCN, as discussed above, appear to contain important oscillators and maybe pacemakers of the circadian system that are normally synchronized to the light–dark cycle.
Temporal information from the SCN appears to pass to various circadian subsystems, some
of which are indicated in Figure 11.

Eat–Fast Cycles (EF). Another zeitgeber of major importance in primates is the timing of food availability (Sulzman *et al.*, 1977a,b). The evidence of food cycles entraining
rodents is more ambiguous (Boulos, Rosenwasser, and Terman, 1977; Edmonds and Adler,
1977). Subsequent work by Sulzman *et al.* (1978c) in primates and Krieger and Hauser
(1978) in rodents has shown that eat–fast cycles are coupled differently into the circadian
timing system than light–dark cycles and require that we postulate distinct pathways.

The ingestion of water with a circadian periodicity does not act as a zeitgeber (Sulzman *et al.*, 1977a), suggesting that it is some constituent of the diet that provides circadian
entrainment. The temporal information presumably passes through the passive elements
of the digestive system and then is absorbed into the extracellular compartment. We postulate that there is some component of the diet that synchronizes an oscillator separate from
the SCN (Figure 11). That the oscillator is separate is suggested by the work of Krieger
and Hauser (1977), who have shown that the synchronization of animals to eat–fast cycles
persists after bilateral destruction of the SCN.

The light–dark cycle also exerts some control over the timing of feeding. Thus, if food
is available *ad lib,* and the animal is placed in a light–dark cycle, two effects on feeding
can be distinguished. First, there is a direct passive response, so that feeding behaviors tend
to be confined to lights-on and cease when lights are off. This effect can be demonstrated
using high-frequency LD cycles beyond the circadian range of entrainment (Sulzman *et
al.*, unpublished observations). Second, there is an active circadian component that is

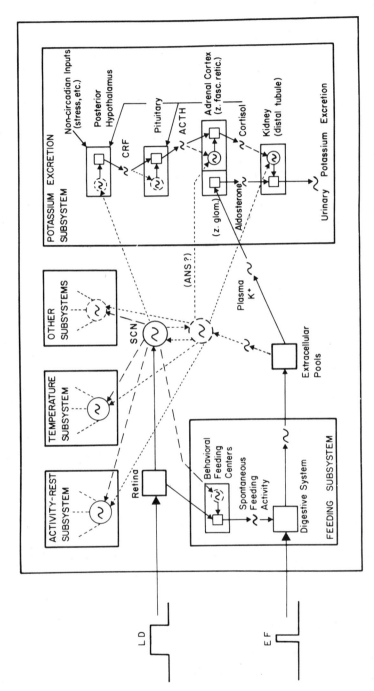

Fig. 11. Qualitative model of the circadian timekeeping system showing some subsystems and details of the urinary potassium excretion subsystem. Symbols are the same as in Figure 7 with the following additions: ——→ signifies passive control; — —→ indicates entrainment of a circadian oscillator; ·········→ represents hypothetical entrainment pathways; and ⊘ signifies a postulated self-sustained circadian oscillator.

entrainable by light–dark cycles within a limited range of entrainment (Sulzman *et al.*, 1980). This component is driven by one or more circadian oscillators, since it will freerun in the absence of temporal information from the retina (in LL or DD or optically enucleated animals). The circadian organization of feeding in situations where food is available *ad lib* is to a large extent under the control of the SCN, since after SCN lesions, there is a considerable breakdown of circadian organization in feeding rhythms (Fuller *et al.*, 1977).

Each of these passive and active components impinging on the behavioral feeding centers contributes to the rhythm of spontaneous feeding activity, which determines the input to the digestive system in *ad lib* food conditions. However, in situations where there is restricted availability of food (EF cycles), this restricted feeding dominates, so that temporal information is conveyed to the circadian system from EF cycles even when light–dark cycles with different temporal information are simultaneously applied (Sulzman *et al.*, 1978c).

ANALYSIS OF A CIRCADIAN SUBSYSTEM. The circadian timing system can be broken down into a number of subsystems that can measure time independently although they are normally synchronized with the other circadian timekeeping components. These subsystems can be identified because they desynchronize either spontaneously or when forced by manipulations of zeitgeber period (see above). Besides the body temperature and rest–activity subsystems that can be identified in this way, there is a subsystem that incorporates the pituitary–adrenal axis and the renal excretion of potassium. This we show in some detail in Figure 11. In man, the circadian rhythm of plasma cortisol can freerun independently of the sleep–wake rhythm (Czeisler, Weitzman *et al.*, 1976; Czeisler, 1978), and in squirrel monkeys the renal potassium rhythm can also desynchronize from the rhythm of rest-activity and body temperature (Sulzman *et al.*, 1977c).

Circadian rhythms in hypothalamic CRF activity (Hiroshige and Wada, 1974), plasma ACTH (Cheifetz, Gaffud, and Dingman, 1968), plasma cortisol (Weitzman, 1976), and renal potassium excretion (Moore-Ede and Herd, 1977) are well documented and present a plausible route for the flow of circadian information between the hypothalamus and the renal distal tubules, which control potassium excretion. Circadian information can flow centrifugally down this axis, since a persisting rhythm of plasma ACTH concentration is seen in the adrenalectomized rat (Cheifetz *et al.*, 1968) and the rhythm of CRF activity is still observed in hypophysectomized animals (Takebe, Sakahura, and Mashimo, 1972). In turn, the posterior hypothalamus is most likely the recipient of circadian information from the SCN, probably via the medial forebrain bundle.

We postulate that each tissue in this subsystem contains both passive elements and active circadian oscillators. The passive elements are the well-documented responders to noncircadian inputs, such as stress, which directly result in changes in CRF, ACTH, and cortisol secretion. The presence of endogenous circadian oscillators has been demonstrated in the adrenal cortex (Andrews, 1971) and the kidney (Moore-Ede *et al.*, 1978). However, studies to test for the presence of such oscillators have not yet been undertaken for the pituitary or posterior hypothalamus.

We presume that the mode of transmission of circadian information between the elements of the subsystem is by the phase control mechanism characteristic of circadian systems. We have discussed earlier how we have documented one example of such phase control, the synchronization of the circadian rhythm of renal potassium excretion by the rhythm of plasma cortisol concentration (Moore-Ede *et al.*, 1977). In contrast, present available evidence would suggest that plasma aldosterone concentration may influence the passive components controlling potassium excretion but does not play a major role in circadian synchronization (Moore-Ede *et al.*, 1977). Rhythms in plasma aldosterone concentration may be under the influence of rhythms in plasma potassium concentration, which influences the rate of aldosterone secretion (Moore-Ede *et al.*, 1978).

There is also evidence of a centripetal flow of information up the pituitary–adrenal axis that can modify circadian phase. Adrenalectomized (Hiroshige and Wada, 1974) or hypophysectomized (Takebe *et al.*, 1972) animals show a phase advance in CRF as compared with controls, and a phase advance in ACTH is seen in adrenalectomized rats (Cheifetz *et al.*, 1968). However, feedback from the rhythm of plasma cortisol does not influence the other circadian subsystems (Sulzman *et al.*, 1978b). In these studies, adrenalectomized monkeys were placed in an environment with no time cues (LL, EE) and were provided with a rhythmic cortisol infusion so that they maintained a circadian rhythm of plasma cortisol concentration with a 24-hr rhythm. It was found that while the rhythm of renal potassium excretion was synchronized by the plasma cortisol rhythm, the rest–activity and temperature cycles freeran. This finding suggests that there is only a unidirectional flow of information from the SCN to this subsystem.

The existence of an alternate pathway conveying circadian information to the adrenal cortex and to the kidney is indicated by the results of a number of studies. There are reports from Meier (1977) that the plasma corticosterone rhythm in fish and rodents will reset after phase shifts in environmental light–dark cycles, even after hypophysectomy. There is also a growing body of evidence from Dallman's group (Dallman, 1977; Dallman, Engeland, Rose, Wilkinson, Shinsako, and Siedenburg, 1978) that there is an alternate, probably neural, input to the adrenal cortex that can regulate cortisol secretion separately from plasma ACTH. Third, Krieger and Hauser (1978) have shown that EF cycles synchronize the plasma corticosterone rhythm in rats even when there is conflicting phase information from the light–dark cycle.

These findings lead us to postulate there may be an autonomic neural input from the putative central oscillator or oscillators that are synchronized by EF inputs. These oscillators then transmit temporal information to the adrenal cortex. There may be an additional direct input also to the kidney, which does not use the plasma cortisol rhythm as a mediator, since after a phase shift of the infused plasma cortisol rhythm in our studies of adrenalectomized animals (Moore-Ede *et al.*, 1977), the urinary potassium rhythm only phase-shifted by 80% of the expected value.

The structure of the circadian system outlined in Figure 11 is, of course, a first attempt to build a qualitative model of the circadian system. This effort may give rise to more questions than answers, but in doing so, we hope that it will serve a useful purpose.

Importance of Internal Temporal Order

In previous sections, we have described the elaborate counterpoint of rhythms in a host of physiological functions, and we have discussed the specialized physiological system that keeps internal temporal order. We turn now to discuss the teleonomical questions. What are the evolutionarily significant advantages of a periodic internal temporal structure, and what are the consequences of failures in this internal temporal order?

Advantages of a Periodic Internal System

The 24-hr period of the earth's rotation is correlated with major oscillations in many critical variables in the animal's environment, including ambient illumination and temperature, the availability of food, and the activity of predators. The periodicity of these challenges and opportunities demands a similar periodicity in the organization of the animal's behavior and physiology. Why animals should have evolved endogenous self-sustaining circadian oscillators rather than hourglass mechanisms that are initiated each day is less clear. One possible advantage may be that an internal temporal prediction capability provided by circadian oscillators enables organisms to anticipate the probability of a demand upon homeostatic systems however variable or confusing signals from the environment have been over the previous 24 hr. Thus, some effectors with long time delays (of the order of several hours) can be utilized in response to a daily environmental challenge because they are internally activated in advance of the challenge's occurring. When we examine the events that occur during the last portion of the daily sleep period, we see body temperature climbing and plasma corticosteroids rising in advance of the time when the animal awakes, and waking itself may be in advance of the time that lights-on occurs.

Besides the requirements of correlating circadian cycles with the periodicities in the environment, there are other apparent advantages to a periodic arrangement of the internal environment. For example, there appears to be a major advantage in separating mutually incompatible processes in time as well as in space. Physiologists are well accustomed to the specialization of different tissues and subcellular fractions that perform discrete physiological functions. However, it is also feasible to utilize the same cellular machinery at different times for the conduct of physiological functions that require different local ionic and pH conditions for their completion. There may also be a considerable significance in the rhythmic ingestion of food, with food intake being confined to a particular phase of the circadian day. The ensuing daily cycles of anabolism and catabolism may be essential for the proper handling and storage of body fuels. Thus, when patients are fed highly nutritious mixtures continuously throughout each 24 hr by vein (intravenous hyperalimentation), they show a number of undesirable sequelae, such as hepatic fat accumulation—a problem that has been reported to be less severe when intravenous feeding is given for only 12 hr in each day (Benotti, Bothe, Miller, Bistrian, and Blackburn, 1976).

Oatley and Goodwin (1971) have discussed other possible advantages of a periodic internal environment. For example, it may be an advantage for physiological control systems to have oscillating components that provide stability and enhance control of the whole system. Oscillating systems may be more capable of distinguishing positive from negative perturbations of a homeostatically controlled system. These considerations deserve much more detailed study.

Consequences of Failures in Strict Internal Temporal Order

Once highly periodic physiological systems were established, it became very important to maintain a strict internal synchrony. Mutually interdependent events require the constituent parties to be at the correct place at the correct time. Similarly, if there are multiple effectors in a homeostatic system, then their activity must be synchronized for an effective coordination of the homeostasis of the controlled variable. We discuss here two examples of coordinated systems with multiple rhythmic components and examine the consequences of failures in internal synchrony.

In man, there are major circadian variations in net potassium flux between intracellular and extracellular compartments so that potassium is moving out of the cells and into the extracellular fluid and plasma during the daytime hours, but is moving in the reverse direction at night (Moore-Ede, Brennan, and Ball, 1975). These fluxes are counterbalanced by a prominent circadian rhythm in renal potassium excretion that reaches its maximum in the middle of the day—the time at which the efflux from the intracellular compartment is maximal—and then falls to a minimum during the night. The most obvious assumption is that the two circadian rhythms are directly causally related. However, this is not the case; they are two independently generated circadian rhythms. The rate of renal potassium excretion is much more responsive to elevations in plasma potassium concentration in the middle of the day than it is at night, and therefore, the kidney is not responding passively to plasma potassium concentration (Moore-Ede *et al.*, 1978). Similarly, because there is a small circadian rhythm in plasma potassium concentration with a peak at the time of maximum potassium movement out of the extracellular fluid, the cellular fluxes cannot be secondary to any reduction in extracellular potassium concentration because of the renal fluxes.

Normally, the synchrony between these circadian rhythms of potassium flux means that changes in potassium concentration in the extracellular space are minimized. However, should the circadian rhythm in renal potassium excretion become desynchronized from the circadian rhythm in cellular potassium flux, then major changes in the extracellular potassium concentration could occur. Should the two circadian rhythms become out of phase by 180°, then the plasma potassium concentration at one phase of the cycle could fall to a level that is liable to induce severe cardiac effects.

Another example of a coordinated rhythmic system with multiple components is the thermoregulatory system. Circadian rhythms in heat gain (Aschoff and Pohl, 1970) and heat loss mechanisms (Aschoff, Biebach, Heise, and Schmidt, 1974) are well documented. Desynchronization of these elements could result in failures of the thermoregulatory system. Fuller *et al.* (1978b) have shown that when monkeys are entrained by either LD or EF cycles, an 8° reduction in ambient temperature produces no significant effect on body temperature. However, when animals are in conditions where there are no external time cues and where desynchronization of the circadian system occurs, this small reduction in environmental temperature results in a significant failure of thermoregulatory homeostasis so that body temperature falls as much as 2°C.

This is the first time the competency of a homeostatic system in an internally desynchronized animal has been examined. It indicates the importance of internal temporal order and the importance of examining other physiological systems for their dependence on strict internal synchrony.

Acknowledgments

We gratefully acknowledge the contributions made by Drs. Charles A. Fuller and Charles A. Czeisler in discussions of the subjects of this chapter and by Ms. Louise Kilham in preparing this manuscript.

MARTIN C. MOORE-
EDE AND FRANK M.
SULZMAN

Andrews, R. V. Circadian rhythms in adrenal gland cultures. *Gegenbaurs Morphologisches Jahrbuch*, Leipzig, 1971, *117*, 89–98.

Aschoff, J. Exogenous and endogenous components of circadian rhythms. *Cold Spring Harbor Symposia on Quantitative Biology*, 1960, *25*, 11–28.

Aschoff, J. Circadian rhythms in man. *Science*, 1965a, *148*, 1427–1432.

Aschoff, J. The phase-angle difference in circadian periodicity. In *Circadian Clocks*. Amsterdam: North Holland Publishing Co., 1965b, pp. 262–276.

Aschoff, J., and Pohl, H. Rhythmic variations in energy metabolism. *Federation Proceedings, Federation of American Societies for Experimental Biology*, 1970, *29*, 1541–1552.

Aschoff, J., Gerecke, V., and Wever, R. Desynchronization of human circadian rhythms. *The Japanese Journal of Physiology*, 1967, *17*, 450–457.

Aschoff, J., Biebach, H., Heise, A., and Schmidt, T. Day–night variation in heat balance. In J. C. Monteith and L. E. Mount (Eds.), *Heat Loss from Animals and Man*. London: Butterworths, 1974, pp. 147–172.

Aschoff, J., Hoffmann, K., Pohl, H., and Wever, R. Re-entrainment of circadian rhythms after phase-shifts of the zeitgeber. *Chronobiologia*, 1975, *2*, 23–78.

Axelrod, J. The pineal gland: A neurochemical transducer. *Science*, 1974, *184*, 1341–1348.

Barnes, C. A., McNaughton, B. L., Goddard, G. V., Douglas, R. M., and Adamec, R. Circadian rhythm of synaptic excitability in rat and monkey central nervous system. *Science*, 1977, *197*, 91–92.

Batschelet, E. Statistical Rhythm Evaluation. In F. Ferin, F. Halberg, R. M. Richart, and R. L. Van de Wiele (Eds.), *Biorhythms and Human Reproduction*. New York: Wiley, 1974, pp. 25–35.

Benotti, P. N., Bothe, A., Miller, J. D. B., Bistrian, B. R., and Blackburn, G. L. Cyclic hyperalimentation. *Comprehensive Therapy*, 1976, *2*, 27–36.

Binkley, S., Riebman, J. B., and Reilly, K. B. Timekeeping by the pineal gland. *Science*, 1977, *197*, 1181–1183.

Black, I. B., and Reis, D. J. Central neural regulation by adrenergic nerves of the daily rhythm in hepatic tyrosine transaminase activity. *Journal of Physiology*, 1971, *219*, 267–280.

Bobillier, P., and Mouret, J. R. The alterations of the diurnal variations of brain trytophane, biogenic amines and 5-hydroxyindole acetic acid in the rat under limited time feeding. *International Journal of Neuroscience*, 1971, *2*, 271–282.

Boulos, Z., Rosenwasser, A., and Terman, M. Limited daily access to food drives—but fails to entrain—circadian rhythms in rats. *Society for Neuroscience Abstracts 7th Annual Meeting*, 1977, *3*, 161.

Cheifetz, P., Gaffud, N., and Dingman, J. F. Effects of bilateral adrenalectomy and continuous light on the circadian rhythm of corticotrophin in female rats. *Endocrinology*, 1968, *82*, 1117–1124.

Conroy, R. T. W. L., and Mills, J. In *Human Circadian Rhythms*. London: J. & A. Churchill, 1970.

Cranston, W. I., and Brown, W. Diurnal variation in plasma volume in normal and hypertensive subjects. *Clinical Science*, 1963, *25*, 107–114.

Czeisler, C. A. Human circadian physiology: Internal organization of temperature, sleep-wake, and neuroendocrine rhythms monitored in an environment free of time cues. Ph.D. thesis, 1978, Stanford University.

Czeisler, C. A., Moore-Ede, M. C., Regestein, Q. R., Kisch, E. S., Fang, V. S., and Ehrlich, E. N. Episodic 24-hour cortisol secretory patterns in patients awaiting elective cardiac surgery. *The Journal of Clinical Endocrinology & Metabolism*, 1976, *42*, 273–283.

Czeisler, C. A., Weitzman, E. D., Moore-Ede, M. C., and Fusco, R. Phase angle and educed waveform relationships among the circadian rhythms of plasma cortisol, body temperature and sleep under free-running conditions in man. *Vth International Congress of Endocrinology*, 1976, Hamburg, Germany.

Dallman, M. F., Engeland, W. C., and McBride, M. H. The neural regulation of compensatory adrenal growth. *Annals of the New York Academy of Sciences*, 1977, *297*, 373–392.

Dallman, M. F., Engeland, W. C., Rose, J. C., Wilkinson, C. W., Shinsako, J., and Siedenburg, F. Nycthemeral rhythm in adrenal responsiveness to ACTH. *American Journal of Physiology*, 1978, *235*, 210–218.

Edmonds, S. C., and Adler, N. T. Food and light as entrainers of circadian running activity in the rat. *Physiology & Behavior*, 1977, *18*, 915–919.

Ehret, C. F., Groh, K. R., and Meinert, J. C. Circadian desynchronism and chronotypic ecophilia. In H. V. Samis and S. Capobianco (Eds.), *Aging and Biological Rhythms*. New York: Plenum Press, 1978, pp. 185–214.

Fuller, C. A., Sulzman, F. M., and Moore-Ede, M. C. The effect of suprachiasmatic nucleus lesions on circadian rhythms in the squirrel monkey *(Saimiri sciureus)*. *Society for Neuroscience*, 1977, *3*, 162.

Fuller, C. A., Sulzman, F. M., and Moore-Ede, M. C. Active and passive responses of circadian rhythms in body temperature to light-dark cycles. *Federation Proceedings, Federation of American Societies for Experimental Biology*, 1978, *37*, 832.

Fuller, C. A., Sulzman, F. M., and Moore-Ede, M. C. Thermoregulation is impaired in an environment without circadian time cues. *Science*, 1978b, *199*, 794–796.

Fuller, C. A., Sulzman, F. M., and Moore-Ede, M. C. Circadian control of thermoregulation in the squirrel monkey *(Saimiri sciureus)*. *American Journal of Physiology*, 1979, *236*(3), 153–161.

Gibbs, F. P., and Van Brunt, P. Correlation of plasma corticosterone ("B") levels with running activity in blinded rats. *Federation Proceedings, Federation of American Societies for Experimental Biology*, 1975, *34*, 301.

Guyton, A. C., Coleman, T. G., and Granger, H. J. Circulation: Overall regulation. *Annual Review of Physiology*, 1972, *34*, 13–46.

Halberg, F. Chronobiology. *Annual Review of Physiology*, 1969, *31*, 675–725.

Harvey, W. *Exercitatio Anatomica de Mortu Cordis et Sanguinis in Animalibus*, 1628, Frankfurt. From English translation by C. D. Leake (4th ed.). Springfield: Thomas, 1958, p. 42.

Hery, F., Chouvet, G., Kan, J. P., Pujol, J. F., and Glowinski, J. Daily variations of various parameters of serotonin metabolism in the rat brain. II. Circadian variations in serum and cerebral tryptophase levels: Lack of correlation with 5-HT turnover. *Brain Research*, 1977, *123*, 137–145.

Hiroshige, T., and Wada, S. Modulation of the circadian rhythm of CRF activity in the rat hypothalamus. In J. Aschoff, F. Ceresa, F. Halberg, and F. K. Schattauer (Eds.), *Chronobiological Aspects of Endocrinology*. Stuttgart: Verlag, 1974, pp. 51–63.

Hoffmann, K. Splitting of the circadian rhythm as a function of light intensity. In M. Menaker (Ed.), *Biochronometry*. Washington, D.C.: National Academy of Sciences, 1971, pp. 134–146.

Holst, E. von. Die relative Koordination als Phaenomen und als Methode zentralnervoeser Funktionsanalyse. *Ergebnisse der Physiologie, Biologischen Chemie und Experimentellen Pharmakologie*, 1939, *42*, 228–306.

Kobberling, J., and Muhlen, A. von zur. The circadian rhythm of free cortisol determined by urine sampling at two hour intervals in normal subjects and in patients with severe obesity or Cushing's syndrome. *The Journal of Clinical Endocrinology & Metabolism*, 1974, *38*, 313–319.

Koizumi, K., and Nishino, H. Circadian and other rhythmic activity of neurones in the ventromedial nuclei and lateral hypothalamic area. *Journal of Physiology*, 1976, *263*, 331–356.

Krieger, D. T., and Hauser, H. Suprachiasmatic nuclear lesions do not abolish food-shifted circadian adrenal and temperature rhythmicity. *Science*, 1977, *197*, 398–399.

Krieger, D. T., and Hauser, H. Comparison of synchronization of circadian corticosteroid rhythms by photoperiod and food. *Proceedings of the National Academy of Sciences of the United States of America*, 1978, *75*, 1577–1581.

Lengvari, I., and Liposits, Z. Return of diurnal plasma corticosterone rhythm long after frontal isolation of the medial basal hypothalamus in the rat. *Neuroendocrinology*, 1977, *23*, 279–284.

Lincoln, G. A., Rowe, P. H., and Racey, R. A. The circadian rhythm in plasma testosterone concentration in man. In J. Aschoff, F. Ceresa, and F. Halberg (Eds.), *Chronobiological Aspects of Endocrinology*. New York: Schattauer-Verlag, 1974, pp. 137–149.

Manshardt, J., and Wurtman, R. J. Daily rhythm in the noradrenaline content of rat hypothalamus. *Nature*, 1968, *217*, 574–575.

Marotta, S. F., Hiles, L. G., Lanuza, D. M., and Boonayathap, U. The relation of hepatic *in vitro* inactivation of corticosteroids to the circadian rhythm of plasma corticosterone. *Hormone and Metabolic Research*, 1975, *7*, 334–337.

Mayersbach, H. von, Philippens, K. M. H., and Schering, L. E. Light—A synchronizer of circadian rhythms. In *Proceedings XII International Conference of International Society for Chronobiology*. Milan: Il Ponte, 1977, pp. 503–510.

Meier, A. H. Daily variations in plasma corticosteroid concentrations in hypophysectomized fish and rats. In *Proceedings XII International Conference International Society for Chronobiology*. Milan: Il Ponte, 1977, pp. 235–238.

Menaker, M. Endogenous rhythms of body temperature in hibernating bats. *Nature*, 1959, *184*, 1251–1252.

Menaker, M., and Underwood, H. Extraretinal photoreception in birds. *Photochemistry and Photobiology*, 1976, *23*, 299–306.

Menaker, M., Takahashi, J. S., and Eskin, A. The physiology of circadian pacemakers. *Annual Review of Physiology*, 1978, *40*, 501–526.

Mills, J. N. Human circadian rhythms. *Physiological Reviews*, 1966, *46*, 128–171.

Moore, R. Y. Central neural control of circadian rhythms. In D. T. Krieger (Ed.), *Endocrine Rhythms*. New York: Raven Press, 1978.

Moore-Ede, M. C., and Herd, J. A. Renal electrolyte circadian rhythms: Independence from feeding and activity patterns. *American Journal of Physiology*, 1977, *232*, F128–F135.

Moore-Ede, M. C., and Sulzman, F. M. The physiological basis of circadian timekeeping in primates. *Physiologist*, 1977, *20*, 17–25.

Moore-Ede, M. C., Brennan, M. F., and Ball, M. R. Circadian variation of intercompartmental potassium fluxes in man. *Journal of Applied Physiology*, 1975, *38*, 163–170.

Moore-Ede, M. C., Schmelzer, W. S., Kass, D. A., and Herd, J. A. Internal organization of the circadian timing system in multicellular animals. *Federation Proceedings, Federation of American Societies for Experimental Biology*, 1976, *35*, 2333–2338.

Moore-Ede, M. C., Schmelzer, W. S., Kass, D. A., and Herd, J. A. Cortisol mediated synchronization of circadian rhythm in urinary potassium excretion. *American Journal of Physiology*, 1977, *233*, R230–R238.

Moore-Ede, M. C., Meguid, M. M., Fitzpatrick, G. F., Boyden, C. M., and Ball, M. R. Circadian variation in response to potassium infusion in man. *Clinical Pharmacology and Therapeutics*, 1978, *23*, 218–227.

Morin, L. P., Fitzgerald, K. M., and Zucker, I. Estradiol shortens the period of hamster circadian rhythms. *Science*, 1977, *196*, 305–307.

Oatley, K., and Goodwin, B. C. The explanation and investigation of biological rhythms. In W. P. Colquhoun (Ed.), *Biological Rhythms and Human Performance*. New York: Academic Press, 1971, pp. 1–38.

Pittendrigh, C. S. Circadian rhythms and the circadian organization of living systems. *Cold Spring Harbor Symposia on Quantitative Biology*, 1960, *25*, 159–184.

Pittendrigh, C. S. Circadian oscillations in cells and the circadian organization of multicellular systems. In F. O. Schmitt and F. G. Worden (Eds.), *The Neurosciences Third Study Program*. Cambridge, Mass.: MIT Press, 1974, pp. 437–458.

Pittendrigh, C. S., and Bruce, V. G. An oscillator model for biological clocks. In D. Rudnick (Ed.), *Rhythmic and Synthetic Processes in Growth*. Princeton, N.J.: Princeton University Press, 1957, pp. 75–109.

Pittendrigh, C. S., and Bruce, V. G. Daily rhythms as coupled oscillator systems and their relation to thermoperiodism and photoperiodism. In R. B. Withrow (Ed.), *Photoperiodism and Related Phenomena in Plants and Animals*. Washington, D.C.: American Association for the Advancement of Science, 1959, pp. 475–505.

Pittendrigh, C. S., and Daan, S. A functional analysis of circadian pacemakers in nocturnal rodents. I. The stability and lability of spontaneous frequency. *Journal of Comparative Physiology*, 1976, *106*, 223–252.

Pohl, C. R., and Gibbs, F. P. Circadian rhythms in blinded rats: Correlation between pineal and activity cycles. *American Journal of Physiology*, 1978, *234*(3), R110–R114.

Reis, D. J., Weinbren, M., and Corvelli, A. A circadian rhythm of norepinephrine regionally in cat brain: Its relationship to environmental lighting and to regional diurnal variations in brain serotonin. *Journal of Pharmacology and Experimental Therapeutics*, 1968, *164*, 135–145.

Rensing, L., Goedeke, K., Wassmann, G., and Broich, G. Presence and absence of daily rhythms of nuclear size and DNA synthesis of different normal and transformed cells in culture. *Journal of Interdisciplinary Cycle Research*, 1974, *5*, 267–276.

Richter, C. P. Inherent twenty-four hour and inner clocks of a primate—the squirrel monkey. *Communications in Behavioral Biology*, 1968, *1*, 305–332.

Rummel, J. A., Lee, J., and Halberg, F. Combined linear–nonlinear chronobiologic windows by least squares resolve neighbouring components in a physiologic rhythm spectrum. In F. Ferin, F. Halberg, R. M. Richart, and R. L. Van de Wiele (Eds.), *Biorhythms and Human Reproduction*. New York: Wiley, 1974, pp. 53–82.

Rusak, B. Involvement of the primary optic tracts in mediation of light effects on hamster circadian rhythms. *Journal of Comparative Physiology*, 1977a, *118*, 165–172.

Rusak, B. The role of the suprachiasmatic nuclei in the generation of circadian rhythms in the golden hamster, *Mesocricetus auratus*. *Journal of Comparative Physiology*, 1977b, *118*, 145–164.

Sassin, J. F., Frantz, A. G., Weitzman, E. D., and Kapen, S. Human prolactin: 24-hour pattern with increased release during sleep. *Science*, 1972, *177*, 1205–1207.

Schmitt, M. Circadian rhythmicity in responses of cells in the lateral hypothalamus. *American Journal of Physiology*, 1973, *225*, 1096–1101.

Sulzman, F. M., Fuller, C. A., and Moore-Ede, M. C. Environmental synchronizers of squirrel monkey circadian rhythms. *Journal of Applied Physiology*, 1977a, *43*(5), 795–800.

Sulzman, F. M., Fuller, C. A., and Moore-Ede, M. C. Feeding time synchronizes primate circadian rhythms. *Physiology & Behavior*, 1977b, *18*, 775–779.

Sulzman, F. M., Fuller, C. A., and Moore-Ede, M. C. Spontaneous internal desynchronization of circadian rhythms in the squirrel monkey. *Comparative Biochemistry and Physiology*, 1977c, *58A*, 63–67.

Sulzman, F. M., Fuller, C. A., and Moore-Ede, M. C. Comparison of synchronization of primate circadian rhythms by light and food. *American Journal of Physiology*, 1978a, *234*(3), R130–R135.

Sulzman, F. M., Fuller, C. A., and Moore-Ede, M. C. Extent of circadian synchronization by cortisol in the squirrel monkey. *Comparative Biochemistry and Physiology*, 1978b, *59A*, 279–283.

Sulzman, F. M., Fuller, C. A., Hiles, L. G., and Moore-Ede, M. C. Circadian rhythm dissociation in an environment with conflicting temporal information. *American Journal of Physiology*, 1978c, *235*(3), 175–180.

Sulzman, F. M., Fuller, C. A., and Moore-Ede, M. C. Tonic effects of light on the circadian system of the squirrel monkey. *Journal of Comparative Physiology*, 1979, *129*, 43–50.

Sulzman, F. M., Fuller, C. A., and Moore-Ede, M. C. Effects of phasic and tonic light inputs on the circadian organization of the squirrel monkey. *Photochemistry and Photobiology*, 1981, in press.

Szabó, I., Kovats, T. G., and Halberg, F. Circadian rhythm in murine reticuloendothelial function. *Chronobiologia*, 1978, *5*, 137–143.

Takebe, K., Sakakura, M., and Mashimo, K. Continuance of diurnal rhythmicity of CRF activity in hypophysectomized rats. *Endocrinology*, 1972, *90*, 1515–1520.

Weitzman, E. D. Circadian rhythms and episodic hormone secretion in man. *Annual Review of Medicine*, 1976, *27*, 225–243.

Weitzman, E. D., Fukushima, D. K., Nogeire, C., Roffwarg, H., Gallagher, T. F., and Hellman, L. Twenty-four hour pattern of the episodic secretion of cortisol in normal subjects. *The Journal of Clinical Endocrinology and Metabolism*, 1971, *33*, 14–22.

Wever, R. Internal phase angle differences in human circadian rhythms: Causes for changes and problems of determinations. *International Journal of Chronobiology*, 1973, *1*, 371–390.

Wever, R. The circadian multi-oscillator system of man. *International Journal of Chronobiology*, 1975, *3*, 19–55.

13

Neural and Endocrine Control of Circadian Rhythms in the Vertebrates

MICHAEL MENAKER AND SUE BINKLEY

INTRODUCTION

Although circadian oscillations may be generated at or below the cellular level, their behavioral expression in multicellular animals depends on neural and endocrine processes. This is true in the nontrivial sense that is implied by the fact that neural and endocrine structures have been identified that themselves oscillate, in a few cases independently of the rest of the organism. The nervous and endocrine systems are therefore not simply the output side of a circadian system, the interesting properties of which reside elsewhere, but rather *contain* the circadian system—its input sensors, its oscillators, and much of its output machinery. It would indeed be surprising if that were not the case. On the other hand, it is no longer necessary to accept that statement as a reasonable assumption. We have good evidence that it is true and can proceed to make it explicit by working out its details (Menaker, Takahashi, and Eskin, 1978). More importantly, we can begin to investigate the material basis of circadian organization and to search for general principles.

Rhythms of behavior are only one of the manifestations of the temporal organization imposed on multicellular organisms by their circadian systems and, because they are farthest removed from the central oscillators, are of interest to circadian physiologists or biochemists only if they offer unexcelled convenience of measurement. To the student of behavior, on the other hand, circadian rhythms offer a unique opportunity for analysis. They occur in the absence of environmental input, but such input, which can be accurately

MICHAEL MENAKER   Department of Biology, University of Oregon, Eugene, Oregon 97403.   SUE BINKLEY   Department of Biology, Temple University, Philadelphia, Pennsylvania 19122.

defined, does influence them. They are precise, stable, and unusually refractory to disruption by extraneous variables. Many circadian rhythms of behavior are easy to record automatically, and they often have clear meaning in the lives of the animals that perform them. For these reasons, it seems possible that we will have an understanding of the mechanisms that generate and control circadian behavior before such understanding is achieved for other behaviors of equal complexity and importance.

In this chapter we review what is presently known about (1) photoreceptive input to the circadian system of vertebrates; (2) neural and humoral oscillators; and (3) the hierarchy of control mechanisms that govern interactions among the various components. About the last of these, we still know very little, but encouragingly the questions have become considerably sharper in the past few years.

PERCEPTION OF ENTRAINING SIGNALS

Although social cues (Gwinner, 1966; Menaker and Eskin, 1966), temperature (Enright, 1966; Lindberg and Hayden, 1974), and magnetic fields (Bliss and Heppner, 1976) have been shown to entrain or at least to influence the circadian rhythms of various vertebrate species, light is the dominant environmental zeitgeber and also the only one about the perception of which we have much in the way of physiological information. The perceptual routes by which information contained in environmental light cycles reaches and entrains the circadian oscillators of vertebrates are multiple, complex, and distinct from those involved in the processing of visual information. The same is true of invertebrate circadian photoreceptors (see Chapter 9). The functional significance of such an arrangement is not at all clear but should be sought, as the phenomenon appears to be quite general. A clue may be contained in the now well-supported observation that the connection between circadian oscillators and their photoreceptors is more intimate than might be expected. Indeed, although perhaps there are counterexamples, a generalization is emerging from recent work to the effect that circadian oscillators are light-sensitive and that photoreceptors oscillate.

The brains of vertebrates contain photorecptors—in most cases, still unidentified—that directly mediate behavioral, physiological, and biochemical responses to light. In several species of amphibians (Adler, 1976), reptiles (Underwood and Menaker, 1976), and birds (Menaker and Underwood, 1976), it has been demonstrated that brain photoreceptors are functionally coupled to whatever mechanism exists for the generation of circadian rhythmicity. Brain photoreception has never been convincingly demonstrated in adult mammals despite repeated attempts to do so (Rusak and Zucker, 1975). It seems likely that photoreceptive input to circadian as well as other "nonvisual" processes is fundamentally different in mammals and the other classes of vertebrates. Interestingly, neonatal rats retain brain photoreception for the first two to to three weeks of life (Zweig, Snyder, and Axelrod, 1966).

Among birds, brain photoreceptive input to the circadian system has been most extensively studied in the house sparrow *(Passer domesticus)*. In this species, brain photoreceptors alone are sufficient for entrainment of the locomotor rhythm to light cycles of very low intensity (Figure 1) and for mediation of the effect of light intensity on the freerunning period of the locomotor rhythm in constant light (Menaker, 1968b). They are involved in, but are not sufficient for, the production of intense arrhythmic activity by bright constant light (McMillan, Elliott, and Menaker, 1975). Retinal photoreception is also involved in the control of these three circadian parameters. Although the pineal organ of some birds is clearly light-sensitive (see below), blinded, pinealectomized sparrows still entrain to environmental light cycles (Menaker, 1971). Photoperiodic time measurement, a circadian process with outputs to the hypothalamic–gonadal axis, is accomplished without retinal input in intact sparrows (Menaker, Roberts, and Elliott, 1970). Photoperiodic photoreception requires considerably higher intensities of light than does entrainment, and this, together

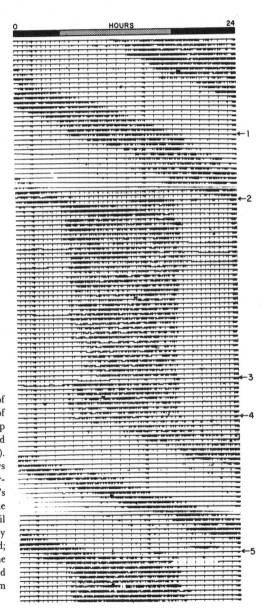

Fig. 1. Continuous record of the perching activity of a bilaterally enucleated sparrow in the presence of a light cycle (indicated diagrammatically at the top of the figure: black bars indicate darkness, stippled bar indicates green light of approximately 0.02 lux). Arrows at the right of the figure indicate the days on which various experimental treatments were performed: at 1, feathers were plucked from the bird's back; at 2, feathers were plucked from the head (the bird now becomes entrained to the light cycle until 7 or 8 days before 3); at 3, feathers, which had by now regenerated, were again plucked from the head; at 4, India ink was injected under the skin of the head; at 5, some of the head skin was removed and the ink deposit was scraped from the skull. (From Menaker, 1968a, p. 299.)

with light penetration measurements by Hartwig and van Veen (1979) and localization experiments of Yokoyama, Oksche, Darden, and Farner (1978) in white-crowned sparrows, suggests that photoperiodic photoreceptors may be hypothalamic and perhaps distinct from those involved in the control of locomotor rhythmicity. In sparrows, then, there is probably photoreceptive input to the circadian system from the eyes, the pineal organ, hypothalamic structures, and other as yet unidentified brain regions. Such complexity at the receptor level was unanticipated and remains puzzling but is confirmed by work on other birds and has also been found in the lizards.

Brain photoreceptors can effect entrainment of the circadian locomotor rhythm in several species of lizard (Underwood, 1973). Removal of the pineal organ and the parietal eye, both of which are well studied photoreceptors, does not prevent entrainment of blind lizards (Underwood and Menaker, 1976). Although blind lizards of all species tested entrained to light cycles, the freerunning period of the locomotor rhythm of blind but not of sighted *Lacerta sicula* was insensitive to changes in the level of constant illumination. *Sceloporus olivaceus,* when blinded in constant light, behaved as if the light intensity had been increased: they either shortened their freerunning periods or became arrhythmic. Photoperiodic control of the testis in *Anolis carolinensis* is largely unaffected by removal of the lateral eyes and the parietal organ (Underwood, 1975). Input to the circadian system from multiple photoreceptors is characteristic of some avian and reptilian species, and there is no reason to believe that it is not a general phenomenon in these two vertebrate classes. Although the direct evidence for similar input to the circadian systems of fish and amphibians is much less extensive, the widespread occurrence of extraretinal photoreceptors in these groups suggests that such receptors may function in the same general way with respect to the circadian system as in reptiles and birds.

The situation in the "lower" vertebrates is in marked contrast to that in mammals, where all known photic input to the circadian system is retinal. On the other hand, the retinal projections that carry information to the circadian system may be primarily nonvisual. Rats and hamsters with lesions of the primary optic and superior accessory optic tracts entrain to LD cycles. Lesions of the inferior accessory optic tracts likewise do not interfere with entrainment, although the original experiments are subject to some criticism (Moore and Klein, 1974; Moore and Eichler, 1976; Rusak and Zucker, 1979). In rodents, entrainment is severely affected although not always abolished by destruction of the retinohypothalamic tract, a direct projection from the retinae to the suprachiasmatic nuclei of the hypothalamus (Rusak and Zucker, 1979). Although the evidence is far from extensive, at the moment it appears reasonable to conclude that in mammals, the pathways for photic input to the circadian system are multiple, with a major route via the retinohypothalamic tract—a projection with no visual function—and perhaps secondary inputs from the primary and accessory optic tracts.

Granting the several assumptions that underlie the above discussion, we may tentatively conclude that photic inputs to vertebrate circadian systems are often distinct from the image-processing visual system whether they involve receptors in the retina, the pineal and related structures, the hypothalamus, or other brain regions. The specific details concerning which receptors are used in particular situations and how they interact with each other and with the visual system clearly vary from one group to another. As we increase our knowledge of this variability, we may begin to understand the selection pressures that produced it and how photic inputs relate to circadian mechanisms.

In order to account for the formal properties of vertebrate circadian systems, we must assume that environmental light cycles and other inputs act to entrain biological units that are themselves capable of self-sustained oscillation in the circadian range. Such units might exist at any level of organization, and it is a measure of our ignorance that we cannot yet make a well-founded guess as to whether they are fundamentally subcellular or, at the other extreme, dependent for their properties on interactions at the tissue level. We will call such structures *primary circadian pacemakers* in spite of the difficulties that are raised by such a definition. In using that definition, we assume that if a structure, or indeed a series of chemical reactions, can be shown to oscillate with circadian time constants in the absence of rhythmic input from either the environment or another part of the organism, then it has a pacemaking role in the overall circadian system. We further assume that such structures or reactions are relatively rare in multicellular organisms. When found, they are likely to be at or near the top of the circadian hierarchy. Neither of these assumptions is particularly well founded, and either one or both could easily be incorrect. However, defining primary pacemakers in such restrictive terms provides a framework for discussion of the available information and in particular underlines the difficulty of assigning a role in the circadian system to structures that have not been shown to be capable of self-sustained oscillation.

If we apply the above definition strictly, the only structure in multicellular animals that qualifies as a primary pacemaker is the eye of *Aplysia* (see Chapter 9). This structure oscillates robustly under constant conditions *in vitro* and so conforms to our limited definition. It is still not clear for what other structures or processes it acts as pacemaker or where it fits in the overall circadian organization of the animal. In the vertebrates, there are two strong candidates: the avian pineal organ and the mammalian suprachiasmatic nuclei (in the anterior hypothalamus). We know more about the roles played by each of these structures than about the eye of *Apalysia,* but neither has been unequivocally shown to be a self-sustained oscillator.

THE AVIAN PINEAL ORGAN

A great deal of circumstantial evidence supports the hypothesis that the pineal organ of the house sparrow is a primary pacemaker in that bird's circadian system. Pinealectomy abolishes the locomotor rhythm of *Passer domesticus* in constant conditions (Gaston and Menaker, 1968), but denervation of the pineal *in situ* leaves the rhythm unaffected. Rhythmicity can be restored to pinealectomized birds by implantation of a donor bird's pineal in the anterior chamber of the eye (Zimmerman and Menaker, 1975) (Figure 2), and the restored rhythm bears the phase of the donor (Zimmerman and Menaker, 1979) (Figure 3). Sparrows have a circadian rhythm of melatonin in the plasma, which in part is the result of pineal melatonin synthesis (Norris and Menaker, in preparation) and melatonin, administered at low levels, changes the freerunning period of the locomotor rhythms in constant darkness (Turek, McMillan, and Menaker, 1976). The simplest interpretation of these facts is that the pineal is a self-sustained oscillator that secretes melatonin rhythmically and that the melatonin rhythm in the blood (or possibly the cerebrospinal fluid) synchronizes that portion of the circadian system that is "downstream" from the pineal. We know that there are other, nonpineal, components in the sparrow circadian system because pinealectomized sparrows, while they will not freerun, do entrain to light cycles. Whether these components are really "downstream" from the pineal is unclear. In fact, lesions of the suprachiasmatic nuclei (SCN) also abolish freerunning rhythmicity in sparrows (Takahashi and Menaker, 1980) (Figure 4). Were it not for the evidence indicating a central role for the SCN in mammalian rhythms (see below), one would interpret the effects of SCN lesions in sparrows as resulting from the elimination of a downstream link, perhaps the target organ of pineal melatonin. This may yet prove to be the case, but the caution that one feels in advancing that interpretation attests to the importance of a comparative view. Alternative interpretations involving reciprocal interactions between the pineal and the SCN (Takahashi and Menaker, 1979) may be more complex, but they may also be correct.

Such complications underline the importance of the missing evidence. We do not yet have a direct demonstration of self-sustained oscillation by the isolated sparrow pineal. In fact, serious attempts to obtain such a demonstration have not been made because, for prac-

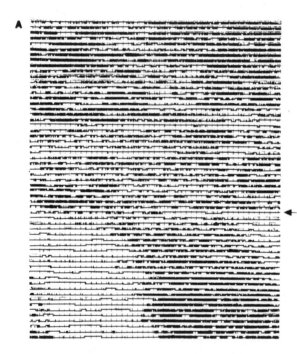

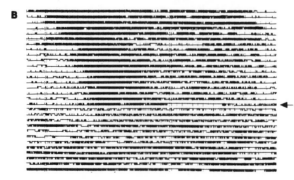

Fig. 2. (A.) Restoration of freerunning rhythmicity in an aperiodic pinealectomized sparrow following transplantation of a pineal. A pineal from a donor bird was transplanted on the day indicated by the arrow. Note the immediate appearance of rhythmicity in the activity of the host bird. The sparrow was in DD except for a brief exposure to light at the time of surgery. (B) Restoration of aperiodic locomotor activity following removal of a successful pineal transplant. On the day indicated by the arrow, the eye bearing the pineal transplant was removed. Except for a brief exposure to light at the time of surgery, the sparrow was in DD. (From Menaker and Zimmerman, 1976.)

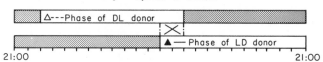

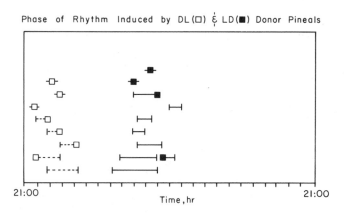

Fig. 3. Phases of activity onsets after pineal transplantations from donors on different entrainment schedules. All surgery was done during the 2-hr overlap of the light periods. The symbols indicate variability in the precision with which activity onset can be estimated. When activity onset was clearly defined, a square indicates the best estimate of its phase; a horizontal line indicates the limits of uncertainty. A horizontal line alone indicates an onset that is within that range but cannot be determined more precisely. (From Zimmerman and Menaker, 1979.)

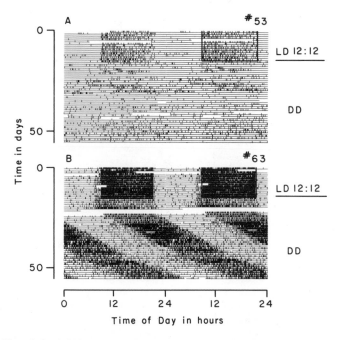

Fig. 4. Effects of hypothalamic lesions on circadian activity rhythms in sparrows. (A) Activity record of a sparrow bearing SCN lesions. The bird's activity is rhythmic in LD 12:12, but arrhythmic in constant darkness (DD). (B) Activity record of a sparrow with a lesion that missed the SCN. The bird is entrained in LD 12:12 and freeruns in constant darkness. Its behavior is similar to unoperated sparrows. (From Takahashi and Menaker, 1980.)

tical reasons, the biochemical and *in vitro* culture work on the avian pineal has focused on that of the chicken. Unfortunately, in this case, species differences may be significant since pinealectomy of chickens and of their relative, the Japanese quail, does not appear to abolish locomotor rhythmicity (Simpson and Follett, in press). Although the pineal organ of chickens has not yet been shown to play a role in that bird's circadian organization, it does display a very-large-amplitude circadian rhythm in the activity of the enzyme serotonin *N*-acetyltransferase (NAT), which is involved in the synthesis of melatonin (Binkley and Geller, 1975). Furthermore, that rhythm persists in pineal organs cultured *in vitro* in the presence of an environmental light cycle (Binkley, Hryshethyshyn, and Reilly 1978; Deguchi, 1979b; Kasal, Menaker, and Perez-Polo, 1978, 1979) and for at least two cycles in constant darkness (Kasal *et al.*, 1979) (Figure 5). In a recent study, Deguchi (1979a) has

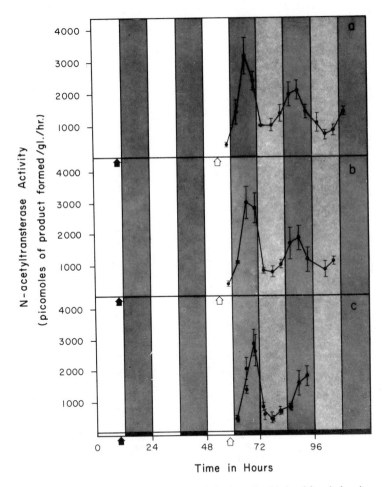

Fig. 5. *N*-acetyltransferase (NAT) activity in chick pineal glands on the third and fourth days in organ culture. Pineals were removed from the birds and placed in culture just prior to lights-off (solid arrow), and the light cycle was continued in culture during Days 1–3 (horizontal bar below graph and shaded and light areas above); the glands were refed with fresh media and regassed on Day 3 at the time indicated by the open arrow; at the onset of darkness on Day 3, the glands were placed in constant darkness (DD). Sampling at 4-hr intervals (four glands per point) revealed a circadian rhythm of NAT activity with peaks occuring during the projected night of Days 3 and 4 in culture (dark-shaded areas). Three replicate experiments are shown (a, b, and c). (From Kasal *et al.*, 1979.)

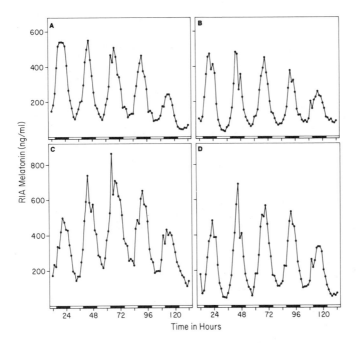

Fig. 6. Rhythms of melatonin release from four different individually isolated chicken pineals cultured in a flow-through superfusion system. The *in vitro* 12:12 (L = 350–500 lux cool white fluorescent: D = 0 lux) light cycle is indicated at the bottom of each panel. Samples of perfusate were collected for 90 min. Concentration of melatonin in the culture medium was determined by radioimmunoassay. Each point represents a single radioimmunoassay determination and is plotted at the onset of the collection interval. (From Takahashi *et al.,* 1980.)

shown that NAT continues to be rhythmic for 17 days in chicken pineal cell cultures held in a light cycle. Melatonin secretion from individual chicken pineals has been measured in a flow-through culture system. It is strongly rhythmic for at least five days in a light cycle (Figure 6). The rhythm persists in constant darkness but is heavily damped (Takahashi, Hamm, and Menaker, 1980). Clearly, the chicken pineal is rhythmic *in vitro*, at least in a light–dark cycle. It cannot yet be claimed that it is a self-sustained circadian oscillator as its rhythmicity may damp rapidly in constant conditions.

It is possible that in chickens some other structure is the dominant pacemaker in the circadian system. That suggestion is consistent with the reported lack of effect of pinealectomy on locomotor rhythmicity and with the apparent damping of pineal rhythmicity in culture. On the other hand, both of those results need confirmation before they are accepted. For this reason, reports of NAT rhythmicity in the chicken eye (Binkley, Riebman, and Reilly, 1979) that persists in constant darkness following pinealectomy and is accompanied by a rhythm of melatonin content (Hamm and Menaker, 1980) (Figure 7) are of particular interest.

Circadian organization in birds (and perhaps in lower vertebrates as well; Underwood, 1977) appears to revolve around the pineal organ. The reported species differences in the effect of its removal (Takahashi and Menaker, 1979) may reflect unresolved differences in experimental technique or real differences among species in the relative roles of the pineal, the SCN, and perhaps the retinae. Note that the retinae and the pineal are both photoreceptive organs and that the avian hypothalamus may also contain photoreceptors.

MICHAEL MENAKER
AND SUE BINKLEY

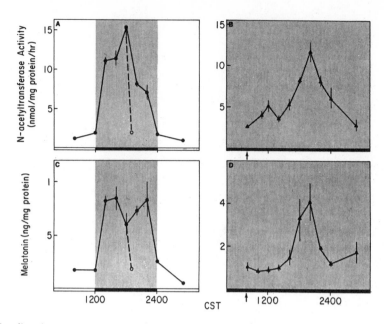

Fig. 7. Circadian changes in indoleamine metabolism in the retina-pigment epithelium complex of the chick. Shaded boxes represent darkness; closed circles, chicks killed every 2 hr; open circles, chicks pretreated with 1-hr light (1300–1400 lux) at mid-dark before sacrifice (A) NAT activity in LD 12:12; (B) NAT activity in DD; (C) Melatonin content in LD 12:12; (D) Melatonin content in DD. Arrow is placed 44 hr after animals were transferred to DD. NAT activity and melatonin were measured from the same eye in LD 12:12; in DD, NAT activity was measured from one eye, melatonin from the other eye of each chick. $N = 5$ chicks in all groups. The standard errors are indicated when they exceed the size of the symbol. (From Hamm and Menaker, 1980.)

If any of these structures is a primary pacemaker, it should be possible to demonstrate this with currently available techniques.

THE MAMMALIAN SUPRACHIASMATIC NUCLEI

An extensive literature demonstrates that lesions of the mammalian suprachiasmatic nuclei (SCN) cause the loss of normal circadian rhythms in a variety of functions in several mammalian species. Although mammals so treated are not completely arrhythmic—they often retain rhythms with short periods outside the circadian range and some still respond to LD cycles—freerunning circadian rhythms appear to be largely abolished by complete or almost complete SCN lesions.

The literature has recently been extensively reviewed by Rusak and Zucker (1979). As they pointed out, interpretation of lesion data is inherently difficult and particularly so when, as in this case, the lesioned structure is part of a complex and poorly understood system. Nonetheless, it is difficult to escape the conclusion that the mammalian SCN plays a central role in circadian organization. Three lines of evidence support this conclusion: (1) there is a separate fiber tract—the retinohypothalamic tract—connecting the SCN directly with the retina; (2) all circadian rhythms so far examined are disrupted to some extent by SCN lesions, ruling out the possibility of highly specific, limited effects of the lesions on only output parameters in a particular subsystem, such as wheel-running behavior; and (3) Kawamura and Inouye have shown that the circadian rhythms of multiunit electrical activity can be recorded from the SCN and from several other sites in the brains of intact rats, but only from the SCN itself when a hypothalamic island including this structure has been surgically produced (Inouye and Kawamura, 1979; Kawamura and Inouye, 1978). Of these three kinds of evidence, only the last suggests what specific role the SCN may play. Rhythmicity in an isolated island of neural tissue implies that the rhythm is generated from within the island. The strength of this interpretation depends only on the degree of certainty concerning isolation. If there were no remaining neural connections and if hormonal influences could be ruled out, then it would be safe to conclude that the island contained a primary pacemaker. The loss of rhythmicity in brain areas outside the island suggests that if a pacemaker exists in the SCN, it may drive or entrain other brain regions and, through them, physiological and behavioral rhythms. Clearly, it is of central importance to confirm and extend these experiments and to develop other analytical approaches that complement them.

DAMPED OSCILLATORS AND DRIVEN RHYTHMS

A central unanswered question about circadian organization in the vertebrates (and other multicellular organisms as well) is whether the total system is constructed of many primary pacemakers, each controlling a specific function or set of related functions, or rather is composed of many damped oscillators and/or directly driven rhythms maintained, entrained, or forced by a small number of centrally located primary pacemakers. As posed, the question is clearly a false dichotomy. A large number of possible specific answers exist that fall between the two stated poles. On the other hand, it is important to recognize the question and to realize that we have virtually no evidence that bears directly on it. The search to date has turned up only two putative primary pacemakers, but it has just begun. It will be very difficult to demonstrate that particular oscillators are *not* self-sustained *in vitro*. We are not entitled to assume, because machinery capable of generating circadian rhythms can be contained within a eucaryotic cell, that all, most, or even many cells of multicellular organisms contain or express such machinery. The great advantages in phase control that can be derived from interactions among oscillators (see Chapters 5 and 7) argue strongly for a multioscillator system, as does much of the physiology described here (see also Chapter 9). On the other hand, none of these considerations supports a particular view of the level of organization at which the multiplicity of oscillators occurs nor of whether most are damped or self-sustained.

Such questions are of particular importance to students of the neural and endocrine aspects of circadian systems. They are bound to arise again and again as attempts are made to understand how the many *rhythms* that are measured in neural and endocrine activity are controlled and integrated by underlying *oscillators*. At this stage of our knowledge, it seems as if there is no escape from the very difficult course of studying many particular cases in depth, eschewing easy *a priori* assumptions. Generalizations are bound to emerge from such work, however slowly.

REFERENCES

Adler, K. Extraocular photoreception in amphibians. *Photochemistry and Photobiology*, 1976, *23*, 275–298.

Binkley, S., and Geller, E. B. Pineal *N*-acetyltransferase in chickens: Rhythm persists in constant darkness. *Journal of Comparative Physiology*, 1975, *99*, 67.

Binkley, S., Riebman, J. B., and Reilly, K. G. The pineal gland: A biological clock in vitro. *Science*, 1978, *202*, 1198.

Binkley, S., Hryschethyshyn, M., and Reilly, K. *N*-acetyltransferase activity responds to environmental lighting in the eye as well as in the pineal gland. *Nature,* 1979, *281,* 479–481.

Bliss, V. L., and Heppner, F. H. Circadian activity rhythm influenced by near zero magnetic field. *Nature,* 1976, *261,* 411–412.

Deguchi, T. A circadian oscillator in cultured cells of chicken pineal gland. *Nature,* 1979a, *282,* 94–96.

Deguchi, T. Circadian rhythms of serotonin *N*-acetyltransferase activity in organ culture of chicken pineal gland. *Science,* 1979b, *203,* 1245.

Enright, J. T. Temperature and the free-running circadian rhythm of the house finch. *Comparative Biochemistry and Physiology,* 1966, *18,* 463–475.

Gaston, S., and Menaker, M. Pineal function: The biological clock in the sparrow? *Science,* 1968, *160,* 1125–1127.

Gwinner, E. Entrainment of a circadian rhythm in birds by species–species song cycles. *Experientia,* 1966, *22,* 765–768.

Hamm, H. E., and Menaker, M. Retinal rhythms in chicks: Circadian variation in melatonin and *N*-acetyltransferase activity. *Proceedings of the National Academy of Sciences, USA.* In press.

Hartwig, H. G., and van Veen, T. Spectral characteristics of visible radiation penetrating into the brain and stimulating extraretinal photoreceptors. *Journal of Comparative Physiology,* 1979, *130,* 277–282.

Inouye, S.-I. T., and Kawamura, H. Persistence of circadian rhythmicity in a mammalian hypothalamic "island" containing the suprachiasmatic nucleus. *Proceedings of the National Academy of Sciences, USA,* 1979, *76,* 5962–5966.

Kasal, C. A., Menaker, M., and Perez-Polo, J. R. Persistence of a circadian rhythm of *N*-acetyltransferase in the chick pineal in vitro. *Society of Neuroscience Abstracts,* 1978, *4,* 347.

Kasal, C., Menaker, M., and Perez-Polo, R. Circadian clock in culture: *N*-acetyltransferase activity of chick pineal glands oscillates in vitro. *Science,* 1979, *203,* 656–657.

Kawamura, H., and Inouye, S.-I. T. Circadian rhythm within the hypothalamic island containing the suprachiasmatic nucleus. *Naito International Symposium Abstracts,* 1978, 51.

Lindberg, R. G., and Hayden, P. Thermoperiodic entrainment of arousal from torpor in the little pocket mouse, *Perognathus longimembris. Chronobiologia,* 1974, *1,* 356–361.

McMillan, J. P., Elliott, J. A., and Menaker, M. On the role of the eyes and brain photoreceptors in the sparrow: Arrhythmicity in constant light. *Journal of Comparative Physiology,* 1975, *102,* 263–268.

Menaker, M. Light perception by extra-retinal receptors in the brain of the sparrow. *Proceedings of the 76th Annual Convention of the American Psychological Association,* 1968a.

Menaker, M. Extraretinal light perception in the sparrow. I. Entrainment of the biological clock. *Proceedings of the National Academy of Sciences, USA,* 1968b, *59,* 414–421.

Menaker, M. Synchronization with the photic environment via extraretinal receptors in the avian brain. In M. Menaker (Ed.), *Biochronometry.* Washington, D.C.: National Academy of Sciences, 1971, pp. 315–332.

Menaker, M., and Eskin, A. Entrainment of circadian rhythms by sound in *Passer domesticus. Science,* 1966, *154,* 1579–1581.

Menaker, M., and Underwood, H. Extratetinal photoreception in birds. *Photochemistry and Photobiology,* 1976, *23,* 299–306.

Menaker, M., and Zimmerman, N. Role of the pineal in the circadian DD system of birds. *American Zoologist,* 1976, *16.*

Menaker, M., Roberts, R., Elliott, J., and Underwood, H. Extraretinal light perception in the sparrow. III. The eyes do not participate in photoperiodic photoreception. *Proceedings of the National Academy of Sciences, USA,* 1970, *67,* 320–325.

Menaker, M., Takahashi, J. S., and Eskin, A. The physiology of circadian pacemakers. *Annual Reviews of Physiology,* 1978, *40,* 501–526.

Moore, R. Y., and Eichler, V. B. Central neural mechanisms in diurnal rhythm regulation and neuroendocrine responses to light *Psychoneuroendocrinology,* 1976, *1,* 265–279.

Moore, R. Y., and Klein, D. C. Visual pathways and the central neural control of a circadian rhythm in pineal serotonin *N*-acetyltransferase activity. *Brain Research,* 1974, *71,* 17–33.

Norris, C., and Menaker, M. Manuscript in preparation.

Rusak, B., and Zucker, I. Biological rhythms and animal behavior. *Annual Reviews in Psychology,* 1975, *26,* 137–171.

Rusak, B., and Zucker, I. Neural regulation of circadian rhythms. *Physiological Reviews,* 1979, *59,* 449–526.

Simpson, S. M., and Follett, B. K. The role of the pineal and the anterior hypothalamus in regulating the circadian rhythm of locomotor activity in Japanese quail. *Proceedings of the XVII International Ornithological Congress.* In press.

Takahashi, J. S., and Menaker, M. Physiology of avian circadian pacemakers. *Federation Proceedings,* 1979, *38,* 2583–2588.

Takahashi, J. S., and Menaker, M. Brain mechanisms in avian circadian systems. In M. Suda, O. Kayaishi, and H. Nakagawa (Eds.), *Biological Rhythms and Their Central Mechanism*. Amsterdam: Elsevier-North-Holland Biomedical Press, 1980, pp. 95–109.

Takahashi, J. S., Hamm, H., and Menaker, M. Circadian rhythms of melatonin release from individual superfused chicken pineal glands in vitro. *Proceedings of the National Academy of Sciences, USA*, 1980, *77*, 2319–2322.

Turek, F. W., McMillan, J. P., and Menaker, M. Melatonin: Effects on the circadian locomotor rhythm of sparrows. *Science*, 1976, *194*, 1441–1443.

Underwood, H. Retinal and extraretinal photoreceptors mediate entrainment of the circadian locomotor rhythm in lizards. *Journal of Comparative Physiology*, 1973, *83*, 187–222.

Underwood H. Extraretinal light receptors can mediate photoperiodic photoreception in the male lizard *Anolis carolinensis*. *Journal of Comparative Physiology*, 1975, *99*, 71–78.

Underwood, H. Circadian organization in lizards: the role of the pineal organ. *Science*, 1977, *195*, 587–589.

Underwood, H., and Menaker, M. Extraretinal photoreception in lizards. *Photochemistry and Photobiology*, 1976, *23*, 227–243.

Yokoyama, K., Oksche, A., Darden, T. R., and Farner, D. S. The sites of encephalic photoreception in photoperiodic induction of the growth of the testes in the white-crowned sparrow, *Zonotricia leucophrys gambeii*. *Cell and Tissue Research*, 1978, *189*, 441–467.

Zimmerman, N. H., and Menaker, M. Neural connections of sparrow pineal: Role in circadian control of activity. *Science*, 1975, *190*, 477–479.

Zimmerman, N. H., and Menaker, M. The pineal: A pacemaker withinthe circadian system of the house sparrow. *Proceedings of the National Academy of Sciences, USA*, 1979, *76*, 999–1003.

Zweig, M., Snyder, S. H., and Axelrod, J. Evidence for a non-retinal pathway of light to the pineal gland of new born rats. *Proceedings of the National Academy of Sciences, USA*, 1966, *56*, 515–520.

14

Ontogeny of Circadian Rhythms

FRED C. DAVIS

INTRODUCTION

Ontogeny is the life history of the individual organism, including its physical construction from a fertilized egg, the functional maturation of its behavioral, homeostatic and reproductive systems, and the decline of these systems with age. Because so many functions—behavioral, physiological, and biochemical—within an individual organism show circadian rhythmicity, the ontogeny of any particular function is likely to include the appearance of and changes in its rhythmic control. The ontogeny of circadian rhythms, as a set of biological questions, must, however, go beyond a simple cataloging of many rhythms and their ontogenic changes. Different circadian rhythms are not independent of one another. Whether controlled by a single circadian pacemaker or by many, overt rhythms are temporally organized with respect to each other and to the environment. The pacemakers, the pathways to overt rhythms, and the mechanisms of entrainment are all part of the "circadian system" that underlies not only internal temporal organization of multiple functions but also the remarkable ability of organisms to measure, precisely and adaptively, the passage of astronomical time.

The ontogeny of circadian rhythms, or more appropriately the ontogeny of the circadian system, should then include the means, both formal and physiological, by which the parts of the system emerge and become organized. It should include the mechanisms that guide this emergence as well as the causes and effects of a loss of organization with age. It is within this framework that the ontogeny of circadian rhythms is reviewed here, not only to discover certain generalities, but to exemplify this framework and the circadian system as a piece of complex and adaptive biological organization.

FRED C. DAVIS   Department of Anatomy and Brain Research Institute, University of California at Los Angeles, School of Medicine, Los Angeles, California 90024. The original experimental work reported here was supported by NIH grant HD–03803 to Michael Menaker.

Timing of developmental events—although measured in hours, weeks, and months—reflects the constancy of developmental processes and not control by a circadian timer. For example, the length of gestation in mice is approximately 21 days, not 21 circadian cycles but an absolute amount of time measured as 21 twenty-four hour periods. The duration of gestation, in hours, is the same whether female mice are entrained throughout gestation to a 21-hr or to a 24-hr day (Lanman and Seidman, 1977). Except for the first (fertilization; Everett, 1961) and final (birth; Smolensky, Halberg, and Sargent, 1972) events of prenatal life, which may occur at restricted times of day, the circadian system appears to have no input to developmental timing in vertebrates. The timing of developmental stages could, however, be influenced by daily variation in growth rate (Barr, 1973).

EMERGENCE OF ORGANIZATION

During development, different functions or states become organized in time. Descriptive accounts of how this occurs—gradually or abruptly, in the same way or differently in different rhythms, by changes in one or in all of rhythm form, phase, and amplitude—constitute the bulk of available information on the emergence of circadian rhythmicity. For the most part, these accounts provide few insights into the physiological changes underlying the development of the rhythms or into the development of the circadian mechanisms that control them. They do, however, delineate the basic phenomena of interest as well as expose questions and problems that merit attention in future studies.

MEASUREMENT OF DEVELOPING RHYTHMS

Overt circadian rhythmicity is primarily a postnatal phenomenon (see Tables I and II in Davis, 1980); for most rhythms studied, a lack of rhythmicity has been demonstrated at a postnatal age prior to that at which each rhythm is first detected. The absence of prenatal rhythms may be due, in part, to the lack of earnest attempts to discover them. The developing embryo and fetus are unquestionably subjected to a rhythmic intrauterine environment, not only from normal adult rhythms such as activity and temperature, but from placental hormones as well (Selinger and Levitz, 1969).

The initial detection and measurement of a developing rhythm in a particular function can be greatly influenced by the frequency with which the function is sampled. When only two time points 12 hr apart or day and night totals are compared, the age at which a rhythm appears may reflect a changing phase relationship relative to the sampling times or the development of entrainment mechanisms, rather than the development of the rhythm itself. For example, if the development of the sleep–wake rhythm in Figure 1 had been measured as a difference between day and night totals (environmental time), then a rhythm may not have been detected until much later than the age at which it can be seen freerunning, beginning at six weeks. Furthermore, a changing phase relationship between the rhythm and the environment would appear as changing amplitude. A prerequisite to the measurement of a population rhythm (e.g., blood samples from different individuals at different times) is the development of entrainment mechanisms and the synchronization of individuals in the population.

The earliest a circadian pacemaker can be detected, except under certain circumstances, is when the assayable function it drives has matured. An indirect method, however, for assaying the presence or absence of a circadian pacemaker has been used by Deguchi (1975). He has suggested that the prenatal entrainment of a pacemaker can be detected by the phase of an overt postnatal rhythm in constant conditions. Figure 2 is not related to Deguchi's findings but illustrates the approach used and its general utility. For 11 days after release into constant darkness (DD), the rats in Figure 2A appear to be arrhythmic. The same rats, if recorded for a longer time (Figure 2B), begin to show clear circadian rhythms, with the onset of their active periods occurring at the approximate time expected if they had been nocturnally entrained to the light–dark cycle or to their mother. Therefore, something in the rats was entrainable before 15 days of age even though it was not immediately observable in their overt activity.

In contrast, when an overt rhythm is initially measured in a rhythmic environment, one cannot be sure that it is under the control of and hence reflects a circadian pacemaker. The rhythmic environment may simply impose a rhythm on the overt function. This effect can in fact be seen in human sleep–wake rhythms, which are initially greatly influenced by daily feeding schedules (Hellbrügge, 1960).

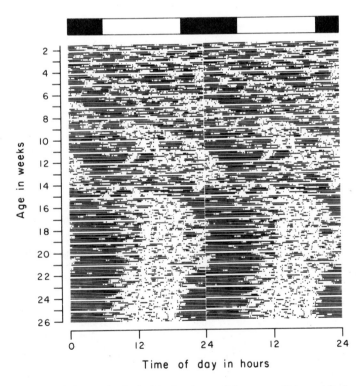

Fig. 1. The development of sleep–wake rhythmicity in a human infant on a self-demand feeding schedule and a light–dark cycle as indicated at the top of the figure. The black bars in the record indicate time asleep, and the dots represent feedings. The record is repeated and shifted up a day in the right half of the figure to aid visual appreciation of the freerunning rhythm. Weekly sets of data are separated by white gaps of no data. (From Kleitman and Englemann, 1953. Reprinted with permission of The American Physiological Society.)

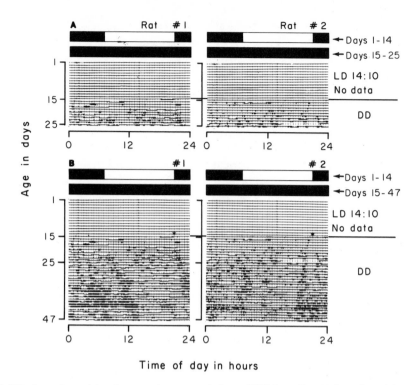

Fig. 2. Wheel-running activity of two rats in constant darkness (DD) from 15 to 25 days of age (A) and of the same two rats from 15 to 47 days of age (B). In both A and B, the first 14 days of age, during which the rats were with their mother on a light–dark cycle, are shown as "no data." The asterisk on Day 14 of B indicates the last seen transition from light to dark.

DEVELOPMENT OF OVERT RHYTHMICITY IN HUMANS

Two generalizations can be made about the development of daily rhythms in humans (see Table I in Davis, 1980). One is that different rhythms appear at different ages, and the other is that most of these rhythms pass through some period of maturation. For example, daily sleep–wake rhythmicity appears during the second postnatal month (Kleitman and Englemann, 1953), while that in plasma adrenal steroids may not appear until 2 years of age (Franks, 1967). Both of these rhythms may continue to mature at least into adolescence. Hence, it appears that in humans, temporal organization has an extended period of maturation. Any interpretation of the available information beyond this simple, but not trivial, generalization is tenuous and limited, in part by the constraints inherent in the problems of measurement as discussed above. Developmental changes in either the freerunning period of any single rhythm or in the phase relationships among rhythms (i.e., internal temporal order) have not been specifically studied in humans. There is, however, sufficient information on changes in the entrainment and in the amplitude of rhythms during development to warrant further discussion.

ENTRAINMENT. At least in the case of Figure 1, the development of a circadian rhythm precedes that of its mechanism of entrainment. Even though the 24-hr light–dark or social cycle appears to modulate the infant's freerunning sleep–wake rhythm as it scans the day and night (Weeks 6–15—although this may reflect a second freerunning rhythm), it does not stably entrain it until 22 weeks of age. Martin du Pan (1974) has shown, however, that an infant's sleep–wake rhythm rapidly entrains to a light–dark cycle when the infant is transferred to it from constant light at 11 weeks of age. Hellbrügge (1960) has reported changes in the entrained phase relationships to the environment of several rhythms (pulse rate, body temperature, wakefulness, and skin resistance) as a progressive delay with increasing age in their morning rise to daytime values.

AMPLITUDE. The maturation of a rhythm generally includes an increase in its amplitude. The change in amplitude may result from either a rise in peak values (e.g., urinary excretion; Hellbrügge, 1960), from a fall in trough values (e.g., heart rate and body temperature; Hellbrüge, 1960; Mullin, 1939), or from both simultaneously. The physiological basis of an amplitude change is not known (although see the following section), nor is the meaning of the differences among rhythms.

The development of a function such as sleep, measured as an all-or-none state and recorded as in Figure 1, occurs by a reorganization of episodic events that are initially observed throughout the day, either randomly or under the control of an ultradian mechanism. This reorganization, which is seen in the first weeks of the record in Figure 1 (but which may continue to a lesser extent for years), is descriptively the decrease of a state at one time of day and its simultaneous increase at another. The mechanism underlying this reorganization can be viewed in at least two different ways: as an actual coalescence of the events underlying episodes into one-half of the day, or as an increase in the amplitude or effectiveness of a circadian pacemaker that modulates the expression of the underlying events. The latter view is illustrated by Figure 3, in which the development of the locomotor activity rhythm of a rat comes about by an increasing daily modulation of an ultradian rhythm. Daily rhythms in human growth (Finkelstein, Roffwarg, Boyar, Kream, and Hellman, 1972) and luteinizing (Kapen, Boyar, Hellman, and Weitzman, 1975) hormones also appear by a time-of-day selective increase in ultradian episodes.

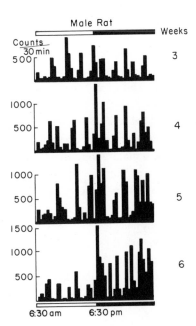

Fig. 3. Development of the daily locomotor activity rhythm in a male rat. (From Honma and Hiroshige, 1977. Reprinted with permission.)

That different rhythms appear at different ages or that their amplitudes increase in different ways does not mean that they are controlled by different circadian pacemakers. These differences may reflect when and how fast the overt functions are "plugged into" the same central pacemaker.

PHYSIOLOGY OF EMERGING RHYTHMICITY IN THE RAT

The development of circadian rhythms in vertebrates other than humans has been studied primarily in the rat and usually in the presence of a light–dark cycle (see Table II in Davis, 1980). As in humans, different rhythms in the rat appear at different ages and have some period of maturation. A review of these rhythms and the age at which they appear reveals a crude sequence in the maturation of daily rhythmicity as follows:

1. Rhythms associated with imposed feeding, such as weight gain
2. Rhythms in the pineal and sympathetic nervous system
3. Pituitary controlled endocrine rhythms
4. Rhythms in voluntary behaviors, such as drinking and locomotion, and in the cortical characteristics of sleep

This sequence does not necessarily reflect the inception of the functions themselves or the complete maturation of their rhythmicity. It may reflect a general maturational succession in adaptive and regulatory needs from autonomic and visceral to cortical and outwardly behavioral. If a single central circadian pacemaker (possibly the suprachiasmatic nucleus [SCN] of the hypothalamus) underlies many or all of these rhythms as evidence suggests (see Chapter 13), then the sequential appearance of different rhythms must reflect the sequential maturation of output pathways or control mechanisms somewhere distal to the pacemaker.

DEVELOPMENT OF PINEAL RHYTHMICITY. A great deal is known about the biochemistry and regulation of pineal rhythmicity in the adult rat (for a review, see Axelrod and Zatz, 1977). Briefly, control of rhythmicity in the activity of the pineal enzyme, serotonin N-acetyltransferase (NAT), is as follows. Rhythmicity originates in the central nervous system (possibly the SCN), reaching the pineal via sympathetic innervation from the superior cervical ganglia. Stimulation of β-adrenergic receptors in the pineal by norepinephrine activates an adenylate cyclase system leading to increased activity of NAT. Entrainment of the NAT rhythm is through the retina and a direct retinohypothalamic tract to the SCN.

The development of these components that underly the control of NAT activity roughly coincides with the appearance of rhythmicity, although the components may continue to mature long afterwards (see Table III in Davis, 1980). The left half of Figure 4 illustrates the development of the day–night difference in rat NAT activity, which, although significant on Day 4, shows a marked amplitude increase on Day 7 by a fall in daytime values. Yuwiler, Klein, Buda, and Weller (1977) have suggested that the important physiological event leading to the development of the rhythm on Day 7 is the functional maturation of pineal sympathetic innervation. In addition to supplying increased stimulation at night, these nerves provide uptake of basal levels of norepinephrine or an agonist (possibly in the blood from an unknown source) that, prior to neural maturation, chronically stimulates NAT activity.

If the manner in which the rat NAT rhythm develops reflects neural maturation, then the maturation of an NAT rhythm in chickens should be different. Although not understood, the role of sympathetic innervation to the chicken pineal is known to be different from that in rats (Binkley, 1976; Ralph, Binkley, MacBride, and Klein, 1975). As the right half of Figure 4 demonstrates, the manner in which the rhythm matures is indeed different; the amplitude increases primarily by a rise in nighttime values. It should be noted that if the appearance of a rhythm in an organ such as the pineal depended only on the synchronization of already rhythmic components (e.g., cells), then the appearance should occur by both an increase in high values and a decrease in low values.

Because the morphological maturation of the rat SCN is not complete until after the appearance of a rhythm in NAT activity (Lenn, Bruce, and Moore, 1977), it is likely that the completion of synaptogenesis in the SCN is not essential for it to have a role in the generation of circadian rhythms.

The preceding scheme for the development of pineal rhythmicity in the rat is oversimplified. Although Illnerova and Skopkova (1976) have shown that NAT rhythmicity in the neonate rat pineal depends on sympathetic innervation, as in the adult, there are reports that this is not the case for a rhythm in serotonin (Machado, Machado, and Wragg, 1969; Machado, Wragg, and Machado, 1969). Furthermore, recent evidence suggests that a serotonin rhythm may persist *in vitro* for at least one day in pineals from neonate, but not from adult, rats (Brammer, 1979). This possible developmental loss of autonomous rhythmicity to a dependency on a central pacemaker may prove to exemplify a general process in the ontogeny (as well as the phylogeny) of circadian organization, that is, progressive centralization of control mechanisms.

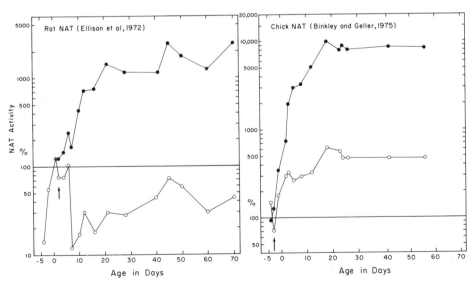

Fig. 4. Development of a day (○)–night(●) difference in enzyme activity of the pineal glands of rats (left) and chickens (right). *N*-acetyltransferase (NAT) activity is expressed as a percentage of the mean level of NAT activity on the day indicated by an arrow (↑). This day is the oldest age at which a significant day–night difference was not detected. (The data were replotted from the sources cited.)

DEVELOPMENT OF ADRENAL RHYTHMICITY. Figure 5 summarizes two studies on the development of morning and evening differences in plasma corticosterone levels in the rat. As in the development of the rat pineal NAT rhythm, the corticosterone rhythm becomes apparent following a drop in values to those at the time of adult low values (approximately lights-on). The peak values (at approximately lights-off) also contribute to the rhythm by continuing to rise. As shown by these and other studies (e. g. Takahashi, Hanada, Kobayashi, Hayafuji, Otani, and Takahashi, 1979), adrenal rhythmicity develops much later than that of the pineal gland.

Even though a good deal is known about the development of the hypothalamic–pituitary–adrenal axis, it is not possible to say what the final physiological event is that leads to the development of rhythmicity. The channels of information flow within the adrenal axis—at least with respect to a stress response—develop before rhythmicity (Hiroshige and Sato, 1970; Levin and Levine, 1975; Levine, 1970). Furthermore, if the same neural pacemaker underlies pineal and adrenal rhythmicity (e. g., the SCN; Moore and Eichler, 1972), then it is likely not to be the development of a pacemaker that is limiting. A possibility suggested by the development of a rhythm in corticotropin-releasing factor (Honma and Hiroshige, 1977) is that rhythmicity in the adrenal axis could depend on the maturation of circadian oscillators peripheral to a central pacemaker.

The precise course of the development of rhythmicity in the adrenal axis is complex and manipulable by both internal and external factors. Ramaley (1978) has described changes in the shape, amplitude, and phase relationship to the light–dark cycle of the plasma corticosterone rhythm in female rats. The rhythm continues to change from the time of its appearance around Day 18 (Ramaley, 1972) until puberty (Ramaley, 1978). Furthermore, the development of the adrenal rhythmicity can be accelerated by electric shock (Ader, 1969) or by thyroxine injections (Lengvari, Branch, and Taylor, 1977) given neonatally, and it can be suppressed or delayed by neonatal treatment with adrenal steroids or adrenocorticotropic hormone (Krieger, 1972; Lorenz, Branch, and Taylor, 1974; Miyabo and Hisada, 1975; Taylor and Lengvari, 1977).

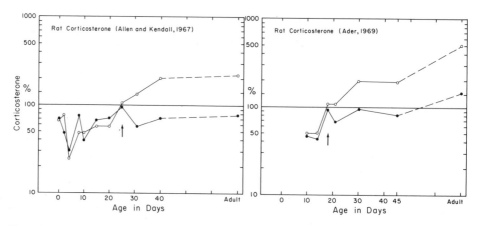

Fig. 5. Development of an evening (○) and morning (●) difference in plasma corticosterone levels in the rat. Corticosterone is expressed as a percentage of the mean value at the age indicated by the arrow (↑). This age is the oldest at which no significant rhythm was detected. (The data were replotted from the sources cited.)

Although the development of a corticotropin-releasing factor (CRF) rhythm parallels that of plasma corticosterone during the time that both rhythms are emerging (Hiroshige, Abe, Wada, and Kaneko, 1973), the CRF rhythm at puberty undergoes a phase change that the corticosterone rhythm does not (Honma and Hiroshige, 1977). This phase change, as well as an increase in the amplitude of the plasma corticosterone rhythm (Critchlow, Liebelt, Bar-Sela, Mountcastle, and Lipscomb, 1963; Ramaley, 1972), occurs specifically in female rats, resulting in a sex difference that persists into adulthood. A possible causal relationship between puberty and adrenal rhythmicity has been reviewed by Ramaley (1978).

DEVELOPING PHASE RELATIONSHIPS. Several rhythms, in addition to the CRF mentioned above, undergo dramatic phase changes during development. Two of these, liver tyrosine amino transferase (Honova, Miller, Ehrenkranz, and Woo, 1968; Ulrich and Yuwiler, 1971) and weight gain (Levin and Stern, 1975) show 180° phase reversals around the time of weaning, probably because of a change in feeding patterns. Rhythms in brain serotonin (Asano, 1971; Okada, 1971) and acetylcholinesterase (Mohan and Radha, 1974; Moudgil and Kanungo, 1973) show, if not reversals, at least significant changes in phase, but somewhat later and correlated with the development of locomotor activity. Neither the meaning nor the control of these phase changes is understood; there is no evidence that they affect other developmental events, nor is there evidence of any consequences of a disruption in these changes.

DEVELOPMENT OF THE CIRCADIAN SYSTEM

Once it is recognized that temporal organization—and hence, the circadian system—develops, the critical question inevitably arises: What determines the specific structure of the timing system that underlies the myriad overt rhythms of an individual? Or, more simply, why do events occur when they do? While questions such as why an animal is nocturnal rather than diurnal or why plasma corticosterone peaks when it does demand functional answers, they also demand developmental answers. They are analogous to asking anatomical questions, such as: Why does a lens form from ectoderm where it does? Can we assume that adult temporal organization is an emergent property of a genetically determined system, or does the environment play some role in shaping it? Surely, the answer to this question may include both of these alternatives. As with anatomical development, the system is likely to obtain its final form by a continuous interaction of its parts throughout its emergence.

A topic not discussed in the preceding sections is the development of a circadian pacemaker. Pacemaker properties such as freerunning period, lability, or mechanism of entrainment have not been studied during development, and it is not known to what extent the changing phase relationships that have been described reflect changes in underlying pacemakers. A complex neural pacemaker (complex in the sense of Pittendrigh and Daan, 1976b) that hypothetically functions as a population of interacting neurons must have some period, however brief, of development. One approach to understanding this development is to examine those factors that influence it. This approach is included in the following section, which examines environmental factors that may be important to the development of temporal organization.

FRED C. DAVIS

Circadian rhythms, although endogenous, are entrained by various rhythmic features of the environment; a response of the circadian system to the environment is an essential part of its mechanism. Even a long-lasting but temporary change in the circadian system (e.g., a change in the freerunning period) can be induced by a small change in the environment (e.g., a light pulse; Pittendrigh and Daan, 1976a). It is not known, however, to what extent the environment may have a guiding or permanent influence on the developing circadian system.

LIGHT–DARK CYCLES

Animals do not need to experience 24-hr light–dark cycles during development to show circadian rhythms as adults. This has been shown for rodents (Aschoff, 1955; Browman, 1952; Richter, 1971), chickens (Aschoff and Meyer-Lohmann, 1954), lizards (Hoffman, 1957), and humans (Martin du Pan, 1974; Miles, Raynal, and Wilson, 1977) by raising them in either constant light (LL) or constant dark (DD). Additional studies have shown that rats, having been raised in LL, will show rhythmicity, including normal phase and nocturnality, when placed in a light–dark cycle (Ramaley, 1975; Schild, 1974; Zucker, 1971). Hence, not only is the rhythmicity innate, but so is its general mechanism of entrainment. The demonstration that the infant in Figure 1 shows a freerunning rhythm in the

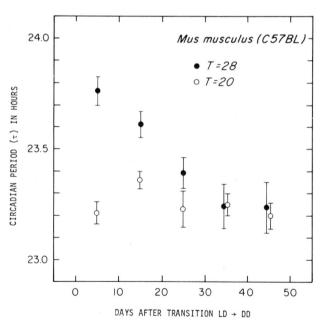

Fig. 6. Freerunning period (τ) measured at 10-day intervals following release (at 10 weeks of age) into constant darkness (DD) from light–dark cycles (LD) with periods (T) different from 24 hr. Open circles are means (n = 16) for mice raised from conception on $T = 20$ (L:D, 11.67:8.33), and closed circles are those for mice raised on $T = 28$ (L:D, 16.33: 11.67). Vertical lines indicate standard errors of the means. All animals as well as their mothers were known to have been entrained to the non-24-hr LD cycles. (From Davis and Menaker, in preparation).

presence of a light–dark cycle further indicates a developing rhythm's independence from the environment.

Depsite these findings, it has not been convincingly shown that light–dark cycles have no role in the development of circadian rhythms. Hoffman (1959) raised lizards on 18- and 36-hr days and found no effect on their freerunning periods as adults. An effect of such cycles may, however, depend on the animal's being entrained to them during some critical developmental period, and it is not known if the lizards in these experiments were ever entrained. Lanman and Seidman (1977) have mentioned that mice raised on a 21-hr day entrain more easily to it than those raised on a 24-hr day. Brown (1974) has suggested an effect on freerunning period of raising rats on a 27-hr day, but it is not clear if this effect is only temporary, as are the well-known "aftereffects" (Pittendrigh and Daan, 1976a) due to entrainment in adult rodents. Figure 6 shows that for at least one strain of mice, the effects of being raised on a 20- or 28-hr day on the freerunning period of the circadian pacemaker underlying locomotor activity are only temporary. Nonetheless, in view of the adaptive complexity of entrainment mechanisms postulated for rodents (Pittendrigh and Daan, 1976b), it is possible that the need for some degree of "fine tuning" of the circadian system by the environment may exist in some species.

In humans, the appearance of circadian rhythmicity appears to depend more on the level of maturity of the infant than on the time since birth and the period of exposure to environmental factors; premature infants develop rhythmicity later than do full-term infants (Hellbrügge, 1974).

The Mother as a Zeitgeber

In rats, maternal behavior is unquestionably rhythmic, although the strength (amplitude) of this rhythmicity appears to change during the development of the litter (Grota and Ader, 1970; Lee and Williams, 1977). This change in maternal rhythmicity raises the possibility that the mother adapts her rhythmicity to that of pups as it develops. Levin and Stern (1975) have shown, however, that a rat mother has a powerful influence on the daily rhythm of weight gain in her pups, not only when she is imposing a rhythm of food availability on them but also after weaning, when they are eating solid food. On the other hand, it is not known if the mother has actually entrained a circadian rhythm in feeding or is in some other way influencing the time of feeding. Deguchi (1975, 1977) has found that a mother rat does not entrain but may influence the rhythm in pineal NAT activity of her pups. Although a foster mother does not postnatally impose her phase on the pups' rhythm in constant darkness, she can influence its phase relationship to a light–dark cycle. The observed synchronization of pups when they are freerunning in constant lighting conditions (Deguchi, 1975; Takahashi et al., 1979) may be due to a maternal influence, prenatal light–dark cycles, the event of birth itself, or a combination of factors, including interactions among pups within a litter. Clearly, the questions of how strong a zeitgeber the mother is and to what extent mothers and pups adapt to each others' rhythmicity are still open.

Probably the most important feature of the newborn human infant's environment is the care and feeding it receives from a caretaker or its mother. Such attention can be either regimented, with clear effects on the infant's pattern of sleep and wakefulness (Hellbrügge, 1960; Martin du Pan, 1974), or given on infant demand. Sander, Stechler, Burns, and Julia (1970) have studied the effects of different caretaking methods on sleep–wake rhythmicity in newborn infants. They found that the less responsive attention and scheduled feedings of a nursery situation result in a more rapid appearance of a circadian rhythm than is seen in infants attended by a single caretaker. They also noted less overall regularity of sleep patterns in infants cared for by single caretakers than in those cared for by their natural mothers. The manner in which regular circadian or ultradian patterns emerge may be a function of the degree to which caretakers and infants adapt to each others' rhythms. Synchronization between a mother and an infant may begin before birth, but there is no conclusive evidence of this (Sterman, 1967).

The Internal Environment

The effects of corticosteroids and thyroxine on the development of circadian rhythms in rats have already been mentioned. There is only indirect evidence that other hormones, specifically gonadal steroids, may also in some way influence the development of rhythmicity. Sexual dimorphism of rhythms (in amplitude and phase) have been described (Critchlow *et al.*, 1963; Honma and Hiroshige, 1977; Ramaley, 1972; ter Harr, MacKinnon, and Bulmer, 1974), and the general role of gonadal steroids in sexual differentiation is well known (Gorski, 1971). Davis, Darrow, and Menaker (in preparation) have found evidence of sexual dimorphism (e. g., upper limit of entrainment) of the pacemaker underlying locomotor activity in hamsters, which persists in castrated adults, suggesting neonatal differentiation. Sexual dimorphisms of the suprachiasmatic nucleus (SCN) have been described in rats, but the degree to which they are dependent on gonadal steroids is not yet clear (Crowley, O'Donohue, and Jacobowitz, 1978; Gorski, Gordon, Shryne, and Southam, 1978; Nagamachi, 1977).

The general plasticity of the function presumably subserved by the SCN has been investigated by Mosko and Moore (1978), who have shown that the SCN and the role it plays in circadian organization are permanently abolished by neonatal lesions in the rat. That is, there is no recovery of function as is commonly observed in other brain areas (Stein, Rosen, and Butters 1974). Furthermore, in the absence of the SCN, a retinohypothalamic tract does not develop. It is as yet uncertain if deafferentation of the SCN early in development (e.g., blinding) has effects on the morphology of the SCN or, other than loss of entrainment, on circadian organization (Lenn *et al.*, 1977; Silver, 1977; Wenisch and Hartwig, 1973).

Aging

There is no doubt that temporal organization changes with age (Cahn, Folk, and Huston, 1968), the most common change being the same as that seen during development: a change in rhythm amplitude. With aging, amplitude decreases and a rhythm may even disappear, usually by a drop in peak values. This can be seen in rat and mouse body temperature (Yunis, Fernandez, Nelson, and Halberg, 1974), in mouse audiogenic convulsions (Halberg, Bittner, Gully, Albrecht, and Benny, 1955) and oxygen consumption (Sacher and Duffy, 1978), and, in humans, in potassium excretion (Lobban and Tredre, 1967), growth hormone (D'Agata, Vigneri, and Polosa, 1974; Finkelstein *et al.*, 1972) and testosterone and leutinizing hormones (Boyar, Rosenfeld, Kapen, Finkelstein, Roffwarg, Weitzman, and Hellman, 1974; Kapen *et al.*, 1975). In contrast, a rhythm in plasma cortisol may persist with undiminished amplitude (Serio, Piolanti, Romano, De Magistris, and Guisti, 1970). In a review of sleep patterns in aged humans, Webb (1978) has identified several age-related changes. These include an increase in daytime naps and in interruptions of nighttime sleep, and a phase relationship change in nighttime sleep, seen as an earlier, morning rise time.

More interesting than these changes in single rhythms, however, is the evidence in humans that the incidence of spontaneous internal desynchronization increases with age (Wever, 1975). Aschoff, Gerecke, and Wever (1967) have found that in humans in constant conditions, the sleep–wake rhythm and that in body temperature can freerun with different circadian periods. The age distribution of this internal desynchronization is skewed toward older age when compared to the distribution of the more common synchronized state (Wever, 1975). This finding suggests that the ability of the circadian system to maintain order may change with age, such a change possibly leading to changes in the phase relationships among rhythms and in a decreased ability of individuals to adjust to schedule changes (i. e., to phase shift). The idea that such changes occur with age in humans or other animals has been put forth a number of times in the literature (Halberg and Nelson, 1978; Samis, 1968), but without substantial supporting evidence. There is, however, evidence suggesting that rats phase-shift more slowly when they are older (Ehret, Groh, and Meinert, 1978; Quay, 1972). Furthermore, Mohan and Radha (1978) have evidence that the phase relationships among central nervous system rhythms in acetylcholine, acetylcholinesterase, and choline acetylase change throughout life in the rat, as do their relationships to the light–dark cycle. As pointed out by Wever (1975), changes in human temporal organization with age may in part be due to a lack of social contact or regimentation that normally serves as a zeitgeber.

Pittendrigh and Daan (1974) have shown that a circadian pacemaker can itself change with age. They observed a shortening of the freerunning period of the locomotor activity rhythm of mice and hamsters that occurred not only from maturity to old age, but in the hamster also from soon after puberty, throughout the mature life of the animal. This finding implies that aging with respect to the underlying pacemaker is a process that occurs throughout the ontogeny of the organism. The consequences of changing period in the overall temporal organization of the animal is not known, but may include internal disorder as well as a change in the animal's relationship to the environment.

Whether or not a change in temporal organization with age causes or reflects a loss of vigor is part of the larger question of the importance of temporal organization to the general well-being of the organism. For animals, this question has been most directly addressed in insects, where longevity as a function of temporal organization has been studied (Aschoff, Saint Paul, and Wever, 1971; Pittendrigh and Minis, 1972; Saint Paul and Aschoff, 1978; Wever, 1968). In these studies, temporal organization is presumably disrupted by maintaining flies on light cycles with periods different from 24 hr (in humans, such cycles have been shown to force internal desynchronization; Aschoff, Pöppel, and Wever, 1969; Wever, 1975) or in constant light, or by subjecting them to phase shifts of a 24-hr cycle every two weeks (i.e., simulating "jet lag"). In every case, flies in the disruptive conditions die sooner. Furthermore, although complicated by the detrimental light cycles, the results with non-24-hr cycles suggest that, as with the length of gestation in mice (see the first section of this chapter), age is not measured in circadian cycles but depends on the rate of some constant ontogenetic change.

PROSPECTUS

The circadian system that underlies an organism's temporal structure within a day changes throughout ontogeny. This change is well documented as an emergence of rhythmicity during development but is indicated only by the scarcity of work on aging and on changes that occur throughout the life of the organism. Progress in understanding the nature of temporal organization and its ontogeny will ultimately depend on a greater knowledge of the circadian system, particularly pacemaker mechanisms and the mechanisms of coupling among oscillators. The potential already exists, however, for fruitful ontogenetic work on select pieces of circadian organization. Examples include the mammalian pineal gland and suprachiasmatic nucleus, as well as a descriptive but thorough analysis of the relationships between two or more rhythms throughout an organism's life. Problems such as the nature of circadian organization in the aged and the characterization of factors that influence the course of events during development as well as during aging are among those in dire need of attention.

As the field of circadian rhythms evolves and expands, ontogenetic questions will become better defined in both their specific and their broad implications. From a medical standpoint, the discovery that temporal organization changes with age implies that the optimal timing of daily medical treatments also changes. Furthermore, the medical consequences of temporal disorder are of greater or lesser importance depending on an individual's age, possibly becoming critical in the very old. In a broader context, however, and more importantly, an understanding of circadian control mechanisms is demanded by the ubiquity of daily modulation in the control of function at all levels of organization. Such an understanding, including an appreciation of the role of temporal organization in the economy of living systems, will depend on a knowledge of both the phylogenetic and the ontogenetic origins of circadian rhythmicity.

Acknowledgments

This chapter is dedicated to Professor Colin Pittendrigh on the occasion of his 60th birthday, as an expression of my gratitude for the introduction he gave me to experimental science and to the field of circadian rhythms. I also want to thank Jane Kana for her contribution to the literature review.

REFERENCES

Ader, R. Early experiences accelerate maturation of the 24-hour adrenocortical rhythm. *Science,* 1969, *163,* 1225–1226.

Allen, C., and Kendall, J. W. Maturation of the circadian rhythm of plasma corticosterone in the rat. *Endocrinology,* 1967, *80,* 926–930.

Asano, Y. The maturation of the circadian rhythm of brain norepinephrine and serotonin of the rat. *Life Sciences,* 1971, *10,* 883–894.

Aschoff, J. Tagesperiodik von Mäusestämmen unter konstanten Umgebungsbedingungen. *Pflügers Archiv für die Gesamte Physiologie,* 1955, *262,* 51–59.

Aschoff, J., and Meyer-Lohmann, J. Angeborene 24-Stunden-Periodik beim Kücken. *Pflügers Archive*, 1954, *260*, 170–176.

Aschoff, J., Gerecke, U., and Wever, R. Desynchronization of human circadian rhythms. *Japanese Journal of Physiology*, 1967, *17*, 450–457.

Aschoff, J., Pöppel, E., and Wever, R. Circadiane Periodik des Menschen unter dem Einfluss von Licht-Dunkel-Wechseln unterschiedlicher Perioden. *Pflügers Archive*, 1969, *306*, 58–70.

Aschoff, J., Saint Paul, U. von, and Wever, R. Die Lebensdauer von Fliegen unter dem Einfluss von Zeitverschiebungen. *Naturwissenschaften*, 1971, *58*, 574.

Axelrod, J., and Zatz, M. The β-adrenergic receptor and the regulation of circadian rhythms in the pineal gland. In G. Litwack (Ed.), *Biochemical Actions of Hormones*. Vol. 4. New York: Academic Press, 1977.

Barr, M. Prenatal growth of Wistar rats: Circadian periodicity of fetal growth late in gestation. *Teratology*, 1973, *1*, 283–287.

Binkley, S. Comparative biochemistry of the pineal glands of birds and mammals. *American Zoologist*, 1976, *16*, 57–65.

Binkley, S., and Geller, E. B. Pineal enzymes in chickens: Development of daily rhythmicity. *General and Comparative Endocrinology*, 1975, *27*, 424–429.

Boyar, R. M., Rosenfeld, R. S., Kapen, S., Finkelstein, J. W., Roffwarg, H. P., Weitzman, E. D., and Hellman, L. Human puberty: Simultaneous augmented secretion of LH and testosterone during sleep. *Journal of Clinical Investigation*, 1974, *54*, 609–618.

Brammer, M. Daily serotonin changes persist in rat pineals in organ culture. *Life Sciences*, 1979, *24*, 967–972.

Browman, L. G. Artificial sixteen-day activity rhythms in the white rat. *American Journal of Physiology*, 1952, *168*, 694–697.

Brown, F. M. 27-hour effects on reproduction and circadian activity period in rats. In L. E. Scheving, F. Halberg, and J. E. Pauly (Eds.), *Chronobiology*. Tokyo: Igoku Shoin, 1974.

Cahn, A. A., Folk, G. E., and Huston, P. E. Age comparison of human day–night physiological differences. *Aerospace Medicine*, 1968, *39*, 608–610.

Critchlow, V., Liebelt, R. A., Bar-Sela, M., Mountcastle, W., and Lipscomb, H. S. Sex difference in resting pituitary–adrenal function in the rat. *American Journal of Physiology*, 1963, *205*, 807–815.

Crowley, W. R., O'Donohue, T. L., and Jacobowitz, D. M. Sex differences in catecholamine content in discrete brain nuclei of the rat; effects of neonatal castration or testosterone treatment. *Acta Endocrinologica*, 1978, *89*, 20–28.

D'Agata, R., Vigneri, R., and Polosa, P. Chronobiological study on growth hormone secretion in man: Its relation to sleep–wake cycles and to increasing age. In L. E. Scheving, F. Halberg, and J. E. Pauly (Eds.), *Chronobiology*. Tokyo: Iguku Shoin, 1974.

Davis, F. C. *Circadian rhythmicity in the wheel running activity of rodents: Factors affecting development of the pacemaker*. Ph.D. thesis, University of Texas, Austin, 1980.

Davis, F. C., and Menaker, M. Development of the mouse circadian pacemaker: Independence from environmental cycles. In preparation.

Davis, F. C., Darrow, J. M., and Menaker, M. Sexual dimorphism of the hamster circadian pacemaker. In preparation.

Deguchi, T. Ontogenesis of biological clock for serotonin: Acetyl coenzyme a *N*-acetyltransferase in pineal gland of rat. *Proceedings of the National Academy of Sciences USA*, 1975, *72*, 2814–2818.

Deguchi, T. Circadian rhythms of enzyme and running activity under ultradian lighting schedule. *American Journal of Physiology*, 1977, *232*, E375–E381.

Ehret, C. F., Groh, K. R., and Meinert, J. C. Circadian dyschronism and chronotypic ecophilia as factors in aging and longevity. In H. V. Samis, Jr., and S. Capobianco (Eds.), *Aging and Biological Rhythms*. New York and London: Plenum Press, 1978.

Ellison, N., Weller, J. L., and Klein, D. C. Development of a circadian rhythm in the activity of pineal serotonin N-acetyltransferase. *Journal of Neurochemistry*, 1972, *19*, 1335–1341.

Everett, J. W. The mammalian female reproductive cycle and its controlling mechanisms. In W. C. Young (Ed.), *Sex and Internal Secretions*. Baltimore: Williams & Wilkins, 1961.

Finkelstein, J. W., Roffwarg, H. P., Boyar, R. M., Kream, J., and Hellman, L. Age related changes in the 24-hour spontaneous secretion of growth hormone. *Journal of Clinical Endocrinology and Metabolism*, 1972, *35*, 665–670.

Franks, R. Diurnal variations of plasma 17-hydroxycorticosteroids in children. *Journal of Clinical Endocrinology and Metabolism*, 1967, *26*, 75–78.

Gorski, R. A. Gonadal hormones and the prenatal development of neuroendocrine function. In L. Martini and W. Ganong (Eds.), *Frontiers in Neuroendocrinology*. New York: Oxford University Press, 1971.

Gorski, R. A., Gordon, J. H., Shryne, J. E., and Southham, A. M. Evidence for a morphological sex difference within the medial preoptic area of the rat brain. *Brain Research*, 1978, *148*, 333–346.

Grota, L. J., and Ader, R. Rhythmicity of the maternal behavior in *Rattus norvegicus. Animal Behavior,* 1970, *18,* 144–150.

Halberg, F., and Nelson, W. Chronobiologic optimization of aging. In H. V. Samis, Jr., and S. Capobianco (Eds.), *Aging and Biological Rhythms.* New York and London: Plenum Press, 1978.

Halberg, F., Bittner, J. J., Gully, R. J., Albrecht, P. G., and Brackney, E. L. 24-hour periodicity and audiogenic convulsions in I mice of various ages. *Proceedings of the Society for Experimental Biology and Medicine,* 1955, *88,* 169–173.

Hellbrügge, T. The development of circadian rhythms in infants. *Cold Spring Harbor Symposia on Quantitative Biology,* 1960, *25,* 311–323.

Hellbrügge, T. The development of circadian and ultradian rhythms of premature and full-term infants. In L. E. Scheving, F. Halberg, and J. E. Pauly (Eds.), *Chronobiology.* Tokyo: Iguku Shoin, 1974.

Hiroshige, T., and Sato, T. Circadian rhythm and stress-induced changes in hypothalamic content of corticotropin-releasing activity during postnatal development in the rat. *Endocrinology,* 1970, *86,* 1184–1186.

Hiroshige, T., Abe, K., Wada, S., and Kaneko, M. Sex difference in circadian periodicity of CRF activity in the rat hypothalamus. *Neuroendocrinology,* 1973, *11,* 306–320.

Hoffman, K. Angeborene Tagesperiodik bei Eidechsen. *Naturwissenschaften,* 1957, *44,* 359–360.

Hoffman, K. Die Aktivitätsperiodik von im 18- und 36-Stunden-Tag erbrüteten Eidechsen. *Zeitschrift für Vergleichende Physiologie,* 1959, *42,* 422–432.

Honma, S., and Hiroshige, T. Pubertal manifestation of sex difference in circadian rhythm of corticotropin-releasing activity in the rat hypothalamus. *Acta Endocrinilogia,* 1977, *86,* 225–234.

Honova, E., Miller, S. A., Ehrenkranz, R. A., and Woo, A. Tyrosine transminase: Development of daily rhythm in liver of neonatal rat. *Science,* 1968, *162,* 999–1001.

Illnerova, H., and Skopkova, J. Regulation of the diurnal rhythm in rat serotonin-N-acetyltransferase activity and serotonin content during ontogenesis. *Journal of Neurochemistry,* 1976, *26,* 1051–1052.

Kapen, S., Boyar, R., Hellman, L., and Weitzman, E. Twenty-four-hour patterns of luteinizing hormone secretion in humans: ontogenetic and sexual considerations. *Progress in Brain Research,* 1975, *42,* 103–113.

Kleitman, N., and Englemann, T. G. Sleep characteristics of infants. *Journal of Applied Physiology,* 1953, *7,* 269–282.

Krieger, D. T. Circadian corticosteroid periodicity: Critical period for abolition by neonatal injection of corticosteroid. *Science,* 1972, *178,* 1205–1207.

Lanman, J. T., and Seidman, L. Length of gestation in mice under a 21-hour day. *Biology of Reproduction,* 1977, *17,* 224–227.

Lee, M. H. S., and Williams, D. I. A longitudinal study of mother–young interaction in the rat: The effects of infantile stimulation, diurnal rhythms, and pup maturation. *Behavior,* 1977, *63,* 241–261.

Lengvari, I., Branch, B. J., and Taylor, A. N. The effect of perinatal thyroxine treatment on the development of the plasma corticosterone diurnal rhythm. *Neuroendocrinology,* 1977, *24,* 65–73.

Lenn, N. J., Bruce, B., and Moore, R. Y. Postnatal development of suprachiasmatic hypothalamic nucleus of the rat. *Cell and Tissue Research,* 1977, *178,* 463–475.

Levin, R., and Levine, S. Development of circadian periodicity in base and stress levels of corticosterone. *American Journal of Physiology,* 1975, *229,* 1397–1399.

Levin, R., and Stern, E. Maternal influences on ontogeny of suckling and feeding rhythms in the rat. *Journal of Comparative and Physiological Psychology,* 1975, *89,* 711–721.

Levine, S. The pituitary–adrenal system and the developing brain. *Progress in Brain Research,* 1970, *32,* 79–85.

Lobban, M. C., and Tredre, B. E. Diurnal rhythms of renal excretion and of body temperature in aged subjects. *Journal of Physiology* (London), 1967, *188,* 48P–49P.

Lorenz, R. J., Branch, B. J., and Taylor, A. N. Ontogenesis of circadian pituitary–adrenal periodicity in rats affected by neonatal treatment with ACTH. *Proceedings of the Society for Experimental Biology and Medicine,* 1974, *145,* 528–532.

Machado, C. R. S., Machado, A. B. M., and Wragg, L. E. Circadian serotonin rhythm control: Sympathetic and nonsympathetic pathways in rat pineals of different ages. *Endocrinology,* 1969, *85,* 846–848.

Machado, C. R. S., Wragg, L. E., and Machado, A. B. M. Circadian rhythm of serotonin in the pineal body of immunosympathectomized rats. *Science,* 1969, *164,* 442–443.

Martin du Pan, R. Some clinical applications of our knowledge of the evolution of the circadian rhythm in infants. In L. E. Scheving, F. Halberg, and J. E. Pauly (Eds.), *Chronobiology.* Tokyo: Iguku Shoin, 1974.

Miles, L. E. M., Raynal, D. M., and Wilson, M. A. Blind man living in normal society has circadian rhythms of 24.9 hours. *Science,* 1977, *198,* 421–423.

Miyabo, S., and Hisada, T. Sex difference in ontogenesis of circadian adrenocortical rhythm in cortisone-primed rats. *Nature,* 1975, *256,* 590–592.

Mohan, C., and Radha, E. Circadian rhythm in acetylcholinesterase activity during aging of the central nervous system. *Life Sciences*, 1974, *15*, 231–237.

Mohan, C., and Radha, E. Circadian rhythms in the central cholinergic system in aging animals. In H. V. Samis, Jr., and S. Capobianco (Eds.), *Aging and Biological Rhythms*. New York and London: Plenum Press, 1978.

Moore, R. Y., and Eichler, V. B. Loss of an adrenal corticosterone rhythm following suprachiasmatic lesions in the rat. *Brain Research*, 1972, *42*, 201–206.

Mosko, S., and Moore, R. Y. Neonatal suprachiasmatic nucleus ablation: Absence of functional morphological plasticity. *Proceedings of the National Academy of Science, USA*, 1978, *75*, 6243–6247.

Moudgil, V. K., and Kanungo, M. S. Effect of age on the circadian rhythm of acetylcholinesterase of the brain of the rat. *Comparative and General Pharmacology*, 1973, *4*, 127–130.

Mullin, J. J. Development of the diurnal temperature and motility patterns in a baby. *American Journal of Physiology*, 1939, *126*, 589.

Nagamachi, N. The effects of ovariectomy on the nuclear sizes of the neurons of the hypothalamic nuclei and the sex differences in the nuclear sizes of the neurons of the hypothalamic nuclei in developing rats. *Shikoku Acta Medica*, 1977, *33*, 251–262.

Okada, F. The maturation of the circadian rhythm of brain serotonin in the rat. *Life Sciences*, 1971, *10*, 77–86.

Pittendrigh, C. S., and Daan, S. Circadian oscillations in rodents: A systematic increase of their frequency with age. *Science*, 1974, *186*, 548–550.

Pittendrigh, C. S., and Daan, S. A functional analysis of circadian pacemakers in nocturnal rodents. I. The stability and lability of spontaneous frequency. *Journal of Comparative Physiology*, 1976a, *106*, 223–252.

Pittendrigh, C. S., and Daan, S. A functional analysis of circadian pacemakers in nocturnal rodents. V. Pacemaker structure: A clock for all seasons. *Journal of Comparative Physiology*, 1976b, *106*, 1537–1539.

Pittendrigh, C. S., and Minis, D. H. Circadian systems: Longevity as a function of circadian resonance in *Drosophila melanogaster*. *Proceedings of the National Academy of Science, USA*, 1972, *69*, 1537–1539.

Quay, W. B. Pineal homeostatic regulation of shifts in the circadian activity rhythm during maturation and aging. *Transactions of the New York Academy of Sciences*, 1972, *34*, 239–254.

Ralph, C. L., Binkley, S., MacBride, S. E., and Klein, D. C. Regulation of pineal rhythms in chickens: Effects of blinding, constant light, constant dark, and superior cervical ganglionectomy. *Endocrinology*, 1975, *97*, 1373–1378.

Ramaley, J. A. Changes in daily serum corticosterone values in maturing male and female rats. *Steroids*, 1972, *20*, 185–197.

Ramaley, J. A. The effect of an acute light cycle change on adrenal rhythmicity in prepubertal rats. *Neuroendocrinology*, 1975, *19*, 126–136.

Ramaley, J. A. The adrenal rhythm and puberty onset in the female rat. *Life Sciences*, 1978, *23*, 2079–2088.

Richter, C. P. Inborn nature of the rat's 24-hour clock. *Journal of Comparative and Physiological Psychology*, 1971, *75*, 1–4.

Sacher, G. A., and Duffy, P. H. Age changes in rhythms of energy metabolism, activity, and body temperature in *Mus* and *Peromyscus*. In H. V. Samis, Jr., and S. Capobianco (Eds.), *Aging and Biological Rhythms*. New York and London: Plenum Press, 1978.

Saint Paul, U. von, and Aschoff, J. Longevity among blowflies *Phormia terraenovae* R. D. kept in non-24-hour light-dark cycles. *Journal of Comparative Physiology*, 1978, *127*, 191–195.

Samis, H. V. Aging: the loss of temporal organization. *Perspectives in Biology and Medicine*, 1968, *12*, 95–102.

Sander, L. W., Stechler, G., Burns, P., and Julia, H. L. Early mother–infant interaction and 24-hour patterns of activity and sleep. *Journal of the American Academy of Child Psychiatry*, 1970, *9*, 103–123.

Schild, M. Ontogeny of nocturnal feeding rhythm in rats and effect of prolonged diurnal feeding experience. In L. E. Scheving, F. Halberg, and J. E. Pauly (Eds.), *Chronobiology*. Tokyo: Iguku Shoin, 1974.

Selinger, M., and Levitz, M. Diurnal variation of total plasma estriol levels in late pregnancy. *Journal of Clinical Endocrinology and Metabolism*, 1969, *29*, 005–997.

Serio, M., Piolanti, P., Romano, S., De Magistris, L., and Guisti, G. The circadian rhythm of plasma cortisol in subjects over 70 years of age. *Journal of Gerontology*, 1970, *25*, 95–97.

Silver, J. Abnormal development of the suprachiasmatic nuclei of the hypothalamus in a strain of genetically anophthalmic mice. *Journal of Comparative Neurology*, 1977, *176*, 589–606.

Smolensky, M., Halberg, F., and Sargent, F., II. Chronobiology of the life sequence. In S. Itoh, K. Ogata, and H. Yoshimura (Eds.), *Advances in Climatic Physiology*. Tokyo: Iguku Shoin, 1972.

Stein, D. G., Rosen, J. J., and Butters, N. *Plasticity and Recovery of Function in the Central Nervous System*. New York: Academic Press, 1974.

Sterman, M. B. Relationship of intrauterine fetal activity to maternal sleep stage. *Experimental Neurology,* 1967, *Suppl. 4,* 98–106.

Takahashi, K., Hanada, K., Kobayashi, K., Hayafuji, C., Otani, S., and Takahashi, Y. Development of the circadian adrenocortical rhythm in rats: Studied by determination of 24- or 48-hour patterns of blood corticosterone levels in individual pups. *Endocrinology,* 1979, *104,* 954–961.

Taylor, A. N., and Lengvari, I. Effect of combined perinatal thyroxine and corticosterone treatment on the development of the diurnal pituitary–adrenal rhythm. *Neuroendocrinology,* 1977, *24,* 74–79.

ter Haar, M. B., MacKinnon, P. C. B., and Bulmer, M. G. Sexual differentiation in the phase of the circadian rhythm of [^{35} S] methionine incorporation into cerebral proteins, and of serum gonadotropin levels. *Journal of Endocrinology,* 1974, *62,* 254–265.

Ulrich, R. S., and Yuwiler, A. Adrenocortical influences on the development of the diurnal rhythm in hepatic tyrosine transaminase. *Endocrinology,* 1971, *89,* 936–942.

Webb, W. B. Sleep biological rhythms and aging. In H. V. Samis, Jr., and S. Capobianco (Eds.), *Aging and Biological Rhythms.* New York and London: Plenum Press, 1978.

Wenisch, H., and Hartwig, H. G. Karyometric investigations of the suprachiasmatic nucleus in blinded rats. *Zeitschrift für Zellforschung und Mikroskopische Anatomie,* 1973, *142,* 142–147.

Wever, R. Das Problem des Alterns unter den Bedingungen des Weltraumflugs. *Bundesministerium für Wissenschaftliche Forschung, Forschungsberichte,* 1968, *W68-30,* 328–333.

Wever, R. The meaning of circadian rhythmicity with regard to aging. *Verhandlungen der Deutschen Gesellschaft für Pathologie,* 1975, *59,* 160–180.

Yunis, E. J., Fernandes, G., Nelson, W., and Halberg, F. Circadian temperature rhythms and aging in rodents. In L. E. Scheving, F. Halberg, and J. E. Pauly (Eds.), *Chronobiology.* Tokyo: Iguku Shoin, 1974.

Yuwiler, A., Klein, D. C., Buda, M., and Weller, J. L. Adrenergic control of pineal *N*-acetyltransferase activity: Devlopmental aspects. *American Journal of Physiology,* 1977, *233,* E141–E146.

Zucker, I. Light–dark rhythms in rat eating and drinking behavior. *Physiology and Behavior,* 1971, *6,* 115–126.

15

Adaptive Daily Strategies in Behavior

SERGE DAAN

INTRODUCTION: SELECTION PRESSURES FOR DAILY RHYTHMS

For most animals, the environment is a complex of variables fluctuating with a distinct 24-hr periodicity. There are abiotic fluctuations as a direct consequence of the earth's rotation on its axis and of the periodic exposure of its surface to irradiation from the sun. Foremost among the physical factors with a distinct 24-hr pattern are light and temperature and, in addition, water vapor pressure and wind in the terrestrial milieu, oxygen pressure and turbulence in the aquatic milieu. Secondarily, there are biotic variations, due to organisms on other trophic levels, such as food species, predators, and parasites, or on the same trophic level: competitors and reproductive mates. By the creation of such daily patterns, the earth's rotation has profoundly affected the ecological complexity of animal communities. Only a few environments, such as deep caves and ocean abysses, are fairly constant throughout the day. Some are only temporarily constant, at least in some variables (e.g., when covered by insulating snow and ice), or are polar habitats at the summer and winter solstices.

Daily routines in the behavior of individual animals can be viewed as strategies to cope with the time structure of the environment. Such routines, like other elements of behavior, are rough products from the mold of natural selection, polished by individual experience. An analytical dissection of daily routines would distinguish, in the first place, an innate and relatively inflexible component, common to the species and independent of individual experience with environmental time patterns. As such a basic program, one may view for instance the circadian cycle of sleep–wakefulness that recurs in some species generation after generation in constant laboratory conditions (Aschoff, 1955). Second, there are contributions from individual experience with temporal variations in the environment.

SERGE DAAN   Zoology Department, Groningen State University, Haren, 9750 AA, The Netherlands.

Third, part of the daily pattern is evoked directly by changing environmental stimuli. The basic program and it modifications by individual experience create a daily pattern of changing motivational state. Any time of the animal's internal day is characterized by its own distribution of probabilities of the occurrence of both spontaneous behaviors and responses to stimuli. For instance, "death-feigning behavior," or tonic immobility, is a widely used antipredation device elicited by a predator's attack. It is a stimulus–response behavior, but the parameters of the system (e.g., duration of the response to a constant stimulus) vary with time of day (as in chickens; Rovee, Kaufman, Collier, and Kent, 1976). Daily changes in motivation to respond to a predator may be adaptively related to the daily distribution of predator attacks in the species's evolutionary history.

The basis of adaptive daily routines, fixed in the genetic makeup or due to learning or response to stimuli, is related to the predictability of the relevant environmental factors. If a certain environmental variation is unpredictable, a system adaptive to such variation can employ direct responses only. Internal temporal programs would be of no use. In contrast, a highly predictable cyclic variation—persisting for as long as an organism's lifetime, such as the cycle of light and darkness—would allow rigid circadian programming of behaviors as an adaptive strategy. Between these extremes, there is a wide area of more-or-less restricted predictabilities. An environmental cycle on any one day correlates to some extent with the next cycle but contains less information about temporal variations 10 or 20 cycles later. In this domain, there is little use for rigid preprogramming. Yet the correlations from day to day would allow the use of an innate circadian time structure combined with individual experience to optimally adjust the behavioral sequence to the temporal pattern of the environment. It is in this area, still hardly explored, that the major adaptive significance for innate circadian oscillators has been sought (Enright, 1970).

Apart from environmental predictability there are other constraints on fixed or changeable programs. Behavior, such as feeding, that occurs frequently in an organism's life is probably temporally more easily adjusted by individual experience than behavior that is rare or occurs only once. In insects, the time of day when emergence of the imago from nymph or pupa occurs is probably fixed by an innate circadian pacemaker in many species; there is no prior experience with the act of emergence to guide the pharate adult inside the pupa in choosing the appropriate time.

Even in the case of emergence, an insect can use environmental information to predict the optimal time for its single critical act. The chironomid midge, *Chironomus thummi*, typically emerges from cold water in the early afternoon and from warm water just after sunset (Figure 1). Dusk is generally the preferred emergence time, except when night air temperatures are below the critical minimum for chironomid flight activity. At low air temperatures, midges emerging during the day have better chances of reproduction than those emerging during the night; at higher air temperatures, night swarming is apparently successful. Water temperature is used by the larvae as a cue predicting the optimal time (Kureck, 1979).

In nearly all such cases, the significant parameters of the evolutionary process leading to the temporal adjustment of behaviors remain to be defined. Yet, the chironomid emergence behavior illustrates some general principles. In the individual, the timing of emergence is controlled by a response to several *proximate* factors in the environment. It is most likely "gated" by an endogenous pacemaker (see Chapter 5) synchronized by the daily cycle of light and darkness. Either of two daily gates is opened in response to water temperature.

Together, these responses form a strategy, maximizing the probability of contributing viable offspring to the next generation. *Ultimate* factors in the environment, such as predation and swarming conditions (air temperatures), favor the genetic material of those animals responding appropriately to the proximate cues. The use of a proximate factor is predicated on the condition that the ultimate factor either acts too late or escapes the organism's perception but correlates well with a factor perceived in time. The outstanding proximate factor in the circadian programming of behavior is the daily light–dark cycle. In many environments, the LD cycle is the most reliable time cue. Synchronization of a circadian behavioral program with the light–dark cycle usually guarantees maximal accuracy of timing.

This chapter considers the ultimate factors in circadian rhythms of behavior. Ultimate factors act by differentially affecting the survival of genes contributing to different circadian strategies. Such selection pressure can be exerted either directly on mortality or mating chance or by a long-term slow accumulation of effects on physiological well-being, leading eventually to variance in the expectation of progeny. The empirical establishment of variance in reproductive output related to circadian behavior is restricted to the direct effects on mortality and mating chance.

An example of differential mortality related to daily timing of behavior is in the jumping of guillemot *(Uria lomvia)* fledglings from their breeding cliffs (Figure 2). The young are three weeks old and still flightless when they join their parents out to sea by gliding down the cliffs. They suffer heavy predation. Where the colonies are located some distance inland, the young are especially vulnerable when dropping on the ground before reaching the safety of the sea. Fledging is typically restricted to the evening hours, even in the Arctic summer, when continuous daylight prevails. Predation on dropped guillemots by glaucous gulls *(Larus hyperboreus)* is slightly less severe in the daily peak of jumping activity (2000–2400) than in the tails of the distribution. The predators were more occupied and

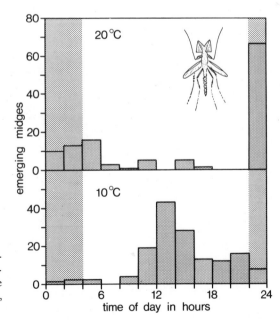

Fig. 1. The daily distribution of adult emergence in two populations of the midge *Chironomus thummi* in constant water temperature at 10°C and 20°C. (Modified from Kureck, 1979.)

satiated in the evening hours. They actively selected against those birds fledging before 2000 and after 2400 (Daan and Tinbergen, 1980). Hence, they apparently contributed to maintaining any genetic basis of the daily rhythm of juvenile jumping in the population, although it is not excluded that other, unknown benefits accrue from this rhythm. It is actually the behavior of an animal's conspecifics in the population that creates the daily variation in risk by affecting the predators' appetites. The colony is part of the individual's fluctuating environment. For any young bird, the optimal time of day to jump depends on when most of the other young jump.

In the guillemots, it is beneficial to the individual to conform to the behavior of the population majority. It is not necessarily the strategy that reduces total predation in the colony to the lowest possible levels. However, daily synchrony of vulnerable phases probably often *does* reduce risk to the population. Such a prey strategy of "swamping" is based on exploiting constraints of the predator. The latter's capacity to raise intake rate proportionally to prey availability is restricted by its "functional response." Its numerical response, on the other hand, is too slow to cope adequately with sudden food surges. The prey profits by synchronizing its vulnerable phases, either with respect to year (as in the emergence once every 13 or 17 years in periodical cicadas; Lloyd & Dybas, 1966), to time of year (e.g., sooty terns, *Sterna fuscata;* Ashmole, 1963) or to time of day as in the guillemot fledglings. The profit of population synchrony probably benefits all the many insects where emergence of the adults from the nymphal or pupal stages is a phase of increased vulnerability to predation. Daily rhythms of emergence are the rule rather than the exception in insects, but hypotheses on their functional significance have only rarely been substantiated (Remmert, 1962). Increased risk is presumably inherent in the emergence of many aquatic

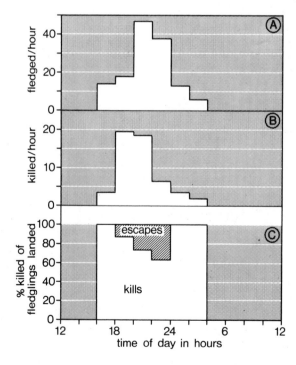

Fig. 2. (A) The daily distribution of jumping of young guillemots *(Uria lomvia)* from a cliff colony at Spitsbergen in continuous daylight. (B) The rhythm of predation on landed guillemot young by glaucous gulls *(Larus hyperboreus)*. (C) The fractions of killed and escaped young among those landed before reaching the sea. (Modified from Daan and Tinbergen, 1980.)

insects, such as Trichoptera (Morgan, 1956) and Odonata (Orians and Horn, 1969), and perhaps terrestrial forms as well. Benefits from population synchrony may, of course, be additional to other sources of differential selection in the course of the day, and often these are difficult to separate experimentally.

The second effect of allocation of behavior to times of day is directly on chances in the reproductive process. Daily synchronization of the sexes is important in animals in which sexual arousal or responsiveness lasts only a short time compared with a circadian cycle. Again, the emergence rhythm of many short-lived insect imagoes in which the adult stage serves only a reproductive function probably strongly promotes the chances of mating (Remmert, 1962). Mating success in two species of *Dacus* fruitflies was indeed related to the degree of emergence synchrony (Gee, 1969). In longer-lived species, sexual behavior may be restricted to specific times of day, allowing engagement in other activities at other times of day and yet ensuring optimal chances for mate finding and courtship success.

The third route of action of ultimate factors in the environment is that of gradual influences on the individual's well-being, slightly affecting its expectancy of life and hence of progeny. Such effects are difficult to establish. Nevertheless, they are conceptually in continuous operation, and their force in molding the genetic basis for optimal daily allocation of behaviors should not be underestimated. In maintenance behavior, food intake is optimal if minimal time and energy are spent for a given amount and quality of food. Concentration of feeding behavior at the times of day when food is most plentiful leaves most time for other vital activities.

Thus, the ultimate causes of circadian organization of behavior are numerous on a planet in rotation. Apart from physical variations in the environment and rhythmic changes in the availability of food and predators, the population in which the animal lives is a fluctuating part of its environment. Some of the evolutionary forces may be in the daily synchronization of reproductive mates or of vulnerable stages in the life cycle. The special use made of circadian rhythms in sun-compass orientation is treated elsewhere (see Chapter 16).

THE COMMUNITY: NOCTURNAL AND DIURNAL WAYS OF LIFE

The most general observation about an animal's daily distribution of behavior concerns the distinction between activity and rest. Animals are rarely continuously active, but times of activity alternate with periods of rest. Since day and night differ so dramatically in environmental parameters, activity is commonly concentrated in one or the other part of the cycle. Many species can be assigned to a *diurnal* or a *nocturnal* type. In addition, two other ecological types have been distinguished: *crepuscular* and *arrhythmic* species. The former are active during one or both of the twilight periods, around dawn and dusk. The latter distribute activity uniformly over night and day. Apparently, the species of a community have divided up the times of day among themselves as much as they have their space, food, and other resources. The ecologist would like to know what the benefits are that make any of these strategies a stable solution for a particular species. What are the behavioral, physiological, and morphological correlates of such ways of life? We shall concentrate on diurnalism and nocturnalism as the major strategies.

Serge Daan

The problems are different for aquatic and terrestrial habitats. Apart from the cycle in illumination, aquatic habitats are more stable and less affected by the earth's rotation than the more exposed terrestrial environment. Daily selective forces acting on animals in the water may more often be of biotic origin: daily fluctuations of surrounding trophic levels of the food web. In the terrestrial milieu, temperature and relative humidity are key factors varying with time of day. The first animals in evolutionary history who left the water to inhabit the terrestrial world must have faced the dangers of desiccation, especially in daytime. These early land forms were probably all nocturnal unless restricted to very humid habitats. Of the two major taxonomic groups that came to dominate the terrestrial scene, the pterygote insects and tetrapod vertebrates, the most primitive representatives today are nocturnal: ephemeropterans and plecopterans (Kennedy, 1928), as well as most terrestrial amphibians. Amphibians and primitive insects both have a thin integument making them vulnerable to dehydration. Later in the evolutionary history of the vertebrates, the energetic benefits of direct solar radiation were detected by both anurans and reptiles. In the latter group, which developed a heavy desiccation-proof integument, ectothermy and behavioral thermoregulation made diurnalism secondarily the fashionable way of life. By that time, around the Jurassic, insects also had evolved a waxy epicuticle as a shield against desiccation, and it is therefore conceivable that they filled the terrestrial landscapes also in daytime with a buzzing adaptive radiation. They must originally have formed a staple food supply for predators, setting the stage for the evolutionary boom of diurnal reptiles. Nocturnalism returned occasionally in many insect groups (Lewis and Taylor, 1964).

Diurnalism remained the rule in the birds, as it was in their ancestors. Some geckos and snakes are nocturnal and have evolved special adaptations to this way of life. Among birds, it is the owls and nightjars and a few other small groups that are nocturnal. Mammals, in contrast, assumed the nocturnal mode of life for at least the first 100 million years of their existence (McNab, 1978). Nocturnalism at that time probably offered wide opportunities. Many insect prey had escaped predatory pressure by reverting to night activity. Endothermy presumably put mammals at a competitive advantage above the nocturnal amphibians. Birds did not dominantly occupy the nocturnal niche, perhaps since flying made them dependent on vision as the major orienting sense, rather than on olfaction and hearing.

Temporal Specialization

Nocturnalism or diurnalism in many cases may turn out not to be a mandatory condition. A diurnal animal may be nocturnal at some stage of its life history; it may become nocturnal on a seasonal basis or in response to some outside pressure; or it may have specific activities that are performed at night. In spite of such flexibility, most animals can nonetheless be considered diurnal or nocturnal on the basis of primary adaptations, such as sensory specialization. While vision is the outstanding sense for animals with a diurnal lifestyle, it is of less importance to truly nocturnal animals. Many morphological differences in the vertebrate eye relate to its performance as a light receptor for nocturnal and diurnal animals (Walls, 1942). Truly keen vision we encounter especially among the diurnal birds. Mammals, in their occupation of the nocturnal niche, developed the acuity of other senses, such as hearing and smell. Nocturnal birds have also invested strongly in senses other than vision: owls have a refined hearing sense enabling them to localize noises made by their prey in pitch darkness. Nocturnal oilbirds exploit echolocation in much the same way as bats. The nocturnal and flightless kiwis are among the few birds with a well-developed olfactory apparatus; by such adaptations they were apparently able to fill the mammalian nocturnal niche in the absence of mammals in New Zealand. Among ducks and geese, the diving ducks (*Aythya* and related genera) find their food mainly by the tactile sense at the bottoms of lakes. They are predominantly nocturnal. Several groups of mammals have secondarily come to occupy the diurnal niche, and while color blindness is the rule among mammals, diurnal animals such as the primates and squirrels have redeveloped color vision.

Because the exploitation of vision and other sensory modalities is distributed unequally among nocturnal and diurnal animals, the signals given in animal communication differ accordingly. After the multitude of visual signals exchanged in the diurnal animal community, the nocturnal community typically reverts to noisy and aromatic ways of communication. Only a few groups of insects use luminescence and vision at night (see Chapter 8). In the majority, sex pheromones and calling songs advertise the sexual readiness of their bearers, much as visual courtship displays did during the day. Also, morphological adaptations affecting the conspicuousness of animals to their predators and prey are related to nocturnal and diurnal ways of life. The most elaborate forms of concealment coloration as a defense against predation are also found among nocturnal animals that pass the day in a motionless state (Cott, 1940). Well-known examples are the owls, the nightjars, and many kinds of moths with wing patterns resembling the bark of the trees they rest on during daylight. There are twiglike geometrid larvae and geckos in all sorts of disguising shapes and designs. Aposematic coloration, on the other hand, is characteristic of diurnal species. In the Cicadidae, a large insect family of generally nocturnal habits and cryptic coloration, one species *(Huechys sanguinea)* adapted to diurnal life is brilliantly colored in black and scarlet (Cott, 1940). This does not mean that aposematic warning is an exclusively diurnal affair. However, in the nocturnal forms combining some potent measure of defense with a conspicuous visual pattern, this nearly always is a pattern in black and white. Examples can be found in various mammalian groups, such as porcupines (Rodentia), skunks, badgers, and polecats (Carnivora), and hedgehogs (Insectivora). They possess black and white fur patterns, often with the white warning signals displayed on the upper parts of head and back (Cott, 1940).

TEMPORAL SEGREGATION

Thus, intricate specializations and adjustments accompanied the nocturnal or diurnal way of life in the course of evolution. Several authors have suggested that the separation of the animal community into a diurnal and a nocturnal part results in a reduction of competition for resources (Park, 1940). This is not an obvious consequence. The same food resource may be exploited by a diurnal and a nocturnal species in the community, alternately. The two species are likely to deprive each other of food even if they do not feed synchronously. The past decade has witnessed a surge in research interest in the analysis of ecological niches and resource utilization in animal communities. Such analysis has been directed at the description of the niche characteristics of groups of closely related, sympatric species.

Niche dimensions fall into three primary groups: food type, habitat or space, and time. In a thoughtful review, Schoener (1974) concluded that temporal segregation of activity among species is rare compared with segregation as to habitat or food type. However, such segregation may occur and complement otherwise incomplete spatial and food segregation. Use of the same perches by several species of Jamaican *Anolis* lizards is possible by different preferences for sun and shade combined with daily changes in such exposure of the perches (Schoener, 1970). Costa Rican butterfly species visit the same food source at different times of day (Young, 1972). The extent of segregation among species of a community with respect to a particular resource is related to the environmental heterogeneity in that resource. The possibility of food segregation is obviously limited if only a few food types are around. Likewise, the occurrence of temporal segregation on a daily basis is related to the extent of daily variation in the environment. Daily segregation is more frequently found among predators and among terrestrial poikilotherms than in other groups. Temporal heterogeneity in abiotic factors presumably affects terrestrial poikilotherms more than others. Similarly, temporal heterogeneity in food availability is generally larger for predators, faced with prey that itself has a rhythmic pattern of availability, than for herbivores, with their more permanent food source. Schoener (1974) also noted that the chances of temporal segregation rapidly deteriorate with an increasing number of competing species. More than food and space segregation, temporal segregation would imply a rapid reduction of activity time and thereby of energy intake. Thus, within diurnal and nocturnal communities, a great deal of temporal overlap is usual. The important segregation has been *between* day and night. Since major morphological, physiological, and behavioral adaptations often accompanied the specialization in nocturnal and diurnal ways of life, one rarely finds narrowly related species groups comprising both types.

This analysis of temporal segregation is not concerned with the mechanisms leading to the gross daily distribution of activity in a species community. Such mechanisms may be essentially evolutionary and genetic, or they may be based on individual behavioral responses. Accordingly, the distribution of daily activity of a species may be its position on the time axis of the Hutchinsonian "fundamental niche," or it may be the position realized in the presence of competing species. Whether competition can indeed lead to temporal restriction of activity should be established by experimental manipulation of the community's species composition.

Temporal Niche Shifts

Individual flexibility of the daily activity pattern is a prerequisite for temporal shifts in the occupied niche. More specifically, if animals can shift on the time axis of the niche in response to intraspecific competition as population density increases, they may do so in response to interspecific competition. So far, there is very little evidence of such shifts. In captive rodents, some temporal segregation in locomotor activity has been described as related to social rank in the group (Fujimoti, 1953; Bovet, 1972), but the effects of (artificial) density on this segregation are unconvincing. There are no field cases of animals changing their daily phase of activity in response to crowding. This is not to say that the innate temporal program of animals is generally too rigid to allow adjustments to pressure from their conspecifics. On the contrary, in many cases, circadian activity programs turn out to be more flexible than originally perceived. But in response to competition for food

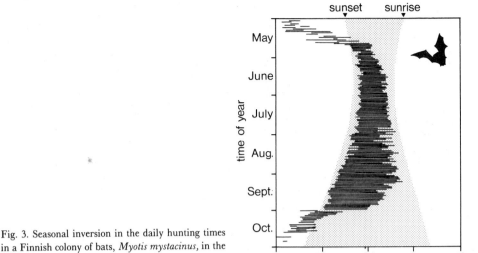

Fig. 3. Seasonal inversion in the daily hunting times in a Finnish colony of bats, *Myotis mystacinus,* in the course of the summer. (Modified from Nyholm, 1965.)

with increasing population density, animals are expected to extend their daily feeding period, allowing for even less temporal segregation than when their density is low. Rather, strong competition favors other means of segregation: by food type or habitat (Schoener, 1974).

Two phenomena are illustrative of adaptive changes of the daily activity time in response to other factors than competition: seasonal phase shifts and phase shifts in response to predation. Game animals have repeatedly been reported to have become nocturnal as a result of human hunting activity in daytime. This change was suggested, for instance, of European swine (*Sus scrofa;* Briedermann, 1971), and of the Nile crocodiles of Lake Victoria (*Crocodilus niloticus;* Corbet, 1960). The causal relationship has never been firmly established. More repeatably demonstrated although ecologically less understood are seasonal inversions of daily activity patterns. These cases usually involve inversion from nocturnalism in summer to diurnal life in winter, as is known, for example, from several vole species (e.g., Erkinaro, 1969) and bats (*Myotis mystacinus;* Nyholm 1965). In the latter case, the diurnal activity of normally nocturnal bats (Figure 3) was probably triggered by a predominance of daytime activity of insects in early spring and fall—perhaps related to the diurnal emergence of chironomid midges in cold spring water as discussed above. In several species of stream fishes feeding in the twilight on nocturnal invertebrate drift, activity may become truly nocturnal in summer at high latitudes where nights are light enough to permit visual hunting (Eriksson, 1973).

THE SPECIES: DAILY ALLOCATION OF TIME AND ENERGY

A species's typical daily repertoire consists of a sequence of behaviors, each occurring with varying frequency throughout the day. Such daily patterns can be assessed in natural circumstances in two ways, either by continuous monitoring of the behavior of single individuals over long time spans or by counting the frequencies of behaviors in which members of a population are engaged at any point in time. Figure 4 shows the daily program of a single male black grouse in springtime and of a wintering aggregation of teal, as examples. The activities distinguished obviously differ in the amounts of time they require. The time allocated to them varies considerably, of course, with the functional state of the organism and with environmental conditions. The theoretical principles governing the allocation of total time are beyond the scope of this chapter. We focus on the arrangement of behaviors within the 24 hrs of the environmental cycle. The eventual benefits of this arrangement are calculated by natural selection in the currency of genetic fitness, but the empirical analysis of such benefits has scarcely been begun. No complete analysis of a species's daily program has been made so far. We can, however, discuss some principles on the basis of foraging

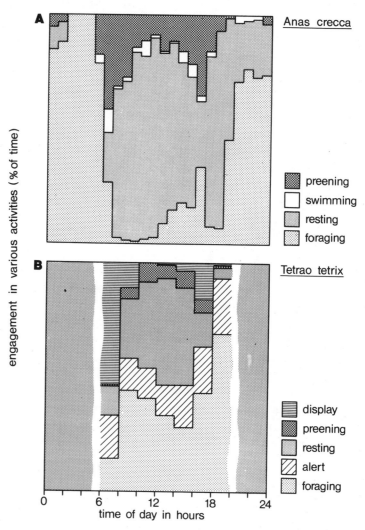

Fig. 4. Daily variation in the frequency of behavioral categories. (A) In a population of teal, *Anas crecca*, in September in the Camargue. (Modified from Tamisier, 1972.) (B) In a single male black grouse, *Tetrao tetrix*, at the time of lekking behavior, March 7–26. (Daytime observations, with activity scored every minute. Fochteloo, Netherlands; unpublished data by G. J. de Vos.)

behavior, where optimization is likely to be reflected in the balance of energy gained versus the time and energy spent.

Foraging and Food Intake

The temporal regulation of food intake is based conceptually on a balance between the energetic needs of the organism and the availability of food—between "deficit" and "incentive." To understand a species's daily pattern of feeding motivation, we have to be informed about both.

The metabolic demands of the species set some limits on the frequency with which food is taken, and thereby, they affect optimal timing. In animal feeding patterns, one can often distinguish meals (bouts of more-or-less continuous food intake) separated by non-feeding. The size of meals may be restricted, by gut capacity, for instance. The energetic content of the food, say s J/meal, is used in metabolism, at a rate of m J/hour. Energetic homeostasis (with no allowance for growth) then simply requires that meals are taken on average once every s/m hours. Variation around this average value may be restricted: the digestive process sets a lower limit on the interval between meals. Consequently, the maximum interval may also become short compared with the daily cycle. Limits on the duration of fasting become particularly severe when s/m is small. This effect holds, for instance, for small homeotherms with relatively high metabolic rates (m), or when s becomes small because of the low nutritious value of the food. The smallest species of birds and mammals, with body weights below 10 g, have solved this problem in various ways. Either they have daily strategies characterized by feeding activity spread evenly over day and night (e.g., shrews; Crowcroft, 1954), or they have evolved daily torpor to save metabolic energy in that part of the cycle where feeding would be dangerous or inefficient (e.g., hummingbirds, bats, small rodents; see Kayser and Heusner, 1967, for review). Such adaptations in the daily strategy are mandatory in spite of the highly nutritious food (large s) that these small homeotherms have specialized in. In other species, the daily feeding pattern can be adjusted to the caloric content of the meals and to metabolic needs. Voles *(Microtus)*, which are normally nocturnal, have increased daytime feeding when the nutritional content of the food is low (Hansson, 1971) or when the lactation of pups requires extra energy. Such options of extending feeding activity from night into day or vice versa are understandably open more to nonvisual feeders than to animals relying purely on vision. However, visually oriented diurnal predators may sometimes employ other hunting modes when conditions force them to extend foraging into the night. The oystercatcher *(Haemotopus ostralegus)* may visually search for cockles buried in mudflats in daytime, while at night, the bird finds its prey by "sewing," a low-yield technique of probing the mud with the bill for hidden bivalves (Hulscher, 1976).

Within the limits set by metabolic requirements to the temporal spacing of food intake over 24 hr, species have evolutionarily adjusted their daily foraging to times when optimal efficiency is predictable. In diurnal species, a pattern of two daily peaks of food intake, like the *bigeminus* ordinarily found in activity (Aschoff, 1962), is not uncommon (e.g., Zeigler, Green, and Lehrer, 1971). Sometimes these peaks are clearly related to the availability of prey animals. Stream fishes like trout and salmon tend to hunt especially in early morning and late evening, when the temporal extremes of nocturnal invertebrate drift, the "scouts" and the "stragglers," just come into daylight and are at the mercy of visual hunters (Elliott,

1970). For a diurnal animal, the afternoon feeding peak may be adaptive to storing an extra measure of reserves in anticipation of the nocturnal fast. The increased level of food intake in the morning has often been attributed to increased hunger as a consequence of nocturnal deprivation. This is not a simple causal sequence, however. Many species of diurnal songbirds typically start their day with singing. Foraging takes over only after rising light intensity has raised the efficiency of foraging above a reward threshold, as in the great tit, *Parus major* (Kacelnik, 1979).

The principles of optimal timing of feeding are best illustrated by those species that employ special behaviors to uncouple foraging and food intake. In most animals, a food item collected is eaten immediately, although swallowing is not always directly followed by digestion. Some species hoard food or cache it temporarily for later retrieval. Cricetine rodents like hamsters forage exclusively during the night, but part of the food may be hoarded and consumed in daytime (Toates, 1978). The cheek pouches and the hoarding habit may serve the purpose of *optimal meal timing,* with meals spread out over 24 hr, combined with *optimal foraging,* the collection of food at a time when risk due to predation is reduced by the absence of visually orienting raptors.

Food hoarding is not exclusively a herbivore's habit. It was also evolved by predators to exploit a surplus in unpredictable food supplies. Kestrels, diurnal raptors specializing in small mammal prey, tend to cache surplus prey in randomly chosen locations anywhere in their hunting area. Field observations revealed that caching occurs throughout the day, in both the American and the European kestrel. Prey cached are typically retrieved shortly before nightfall (Figure 5). By this system, the hunter is able to hunt at times of day that are optimal with respect to prey availability (Rijnsdorp, Daan, and Dijkstra, 1980). Meanwhile, meals can be postponed, since eating surplus rations in the morning would make the

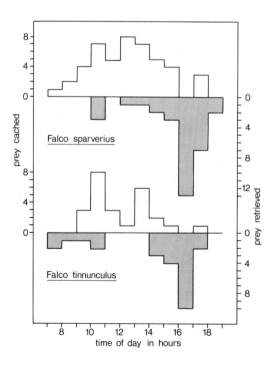

Fig. 5. Frequency of caching (open histogram) and retrieval of cached prey (crosshatched histogram) in kestrels. *Upper:* American kestrel, *Falco sparverius,* in California. (Modified from Collopy, 1977.) *Lower:* European kestrel, *Falco tinnunculus,* in the Netherlands. (Modified from Rijnsdorp *et al.,* 1981.)

bird unnecessarily heavy and would decrease the efficiency of further hunting. Eating "extra" prey just before retiring to the night roost seems appropriate to optimize the daily fluctuations of body weight. The exact cost–benefit functions of this sort of caching behavior remain to be calculated. They should involve some estimation of the risk of losing a cached prey to scavengers in addition to more detailed knowledge of hunting efficiency in relation to body weight. For the present purpose, this behavior nicely illustrates the two major principles governing optimal daily timing of feeding behaviors: optimalization with respect to the animal's metabolic requirements (deficit) and with respect to the fluctuations in food availability (incentive) in the world around.

In the future, the energy approach will lend itself to quantitative modeling as corresponding data on the natural behavior of animals become known. However, food intake concerns more than the acquisition of calories alone. Organisms are very well able to select among food items for special nutrients. Such selective feeding may again be dependent on time of day in an adaptive manner. Two examples are the rise in motivation for calcium intake in domestic fowl *(Gallus domesticus)* in the hours preceding ovulation (Hughes, 1972) and the tendency in rabbits *(Oryctolagus cuniculus)*, probably widespread among other rodents as well, to produce and immediately reingest soft fecal pellets. The latter type of food intake is restricted to the postdawn hours and is tightly coupled to an endogenous circadian rhythm (Hörnicke and Batsch, 1977). The pellets are rich in symbiotic microorganisms and are stored in a special chamber in the stomach. From there, they may inoculate new food taken in the next night. The programmed daily pattern of cecotrophy is likely to contribute to the efficiency of cellulose digestion with the help of the intestinal flora.

DAILY MOVEMENTS AND MIGRATION

The temporal allocation of activity to either night or day and of rest to the other half of the light–dark cycle for many species involves regular daily movements. Resting and sleeping are primarily adaptive behaviors, restricting energy expenditure and risk at times of day when activity would have a net negative effect on the chances of progeny (Meddis, 1975). While the location of active foraging is determined by the spatial distribution of food, resting sites are selected on the basis of criteria for energy and risk reduction. The ensuing spatial separation requires movements to and from the resting site at least twice daily. Such movements may be limited to daily excursions by lizards from the confines of their burrows to basking out in the sun (for an energetic discussion, see Porter, Mitchell, Beckman, and DeWitt, 1973). But in an extreme form, they may involve long-distance migration, as by starling flocks dispersing up to 50 miles from a communal winter roost. The energy spent on flying in the morning to such distant spots is presumably balanced by the birds against the positive effects of reducing competition on the periphery of the roost's feeding grounds (Hamilton and Gilbert, 1969). Also, the flight back to the roost in the evening may be paid off by an exchange of information about feeding areas (Ward and Zahavi, 1973) in addition to other flocking benefits.

Examples of such daily movements are easily observed by anyone interested in natural history. Again, the precise cost–benefit functions have not been defined for any such behavior. A generalized type of daily movements is the daily vertical migration of many animals in vertically stratified environments. Examples are the daily wanderings in mountainous

areas of wild goats (*Capra ibex;* Steinborn, 1973) and the vertical movements of invertebrates like ants and caterpillars (Kamran, 1968), as well as of whole bird communities
(Pearson, 1971) in tropical forests. These are only isolated instances compared with the
massive daily up-and-down movements of zooplankton in oceans and lakes all over our
planet. Numerous species from widely different taxonomic groups participate in this vertical migration. Essentially, it consists of an upward migration in the evening to the upper
water layers and a downward movement later in the night. Such movements may be based
on endogenous circadian rhythms (Enright and Hamner, 1967). For the herbivorous zoo-
plankters, food is continuously available in the feeding grounds in the upper water layers.
Their diurnal withdrawal to deep water therefore entails a temporary loss of food intake.
Apparently, some general benefit is conveyed by vertical migration to compensate for this
loss. A widely accepted hypothesis invokes the reduction of risk of being eaten by visually
hunting predators in the daylight zone. A recent hypothesis (Enright, 1977) stresses the
energetic savings to plankton organisms by withdrawing to colder water when the food
supply is suboptimal. If an appreciable increase of algal food takes place by photosynthesis
in the course of the day, the evening hours are obviously the best feeding time. The grazer
restricting feeding to this daily interval may be at an energetic advantage compared with
the continuous feeder, if it can drastically reduce metabolic expenditure during the remainder of the 24 hr. Nonfeeding and withdrawal to low temperature strata in the depth of the
ocean are proposed to effectuate this energy-saving policy. Several parameters in Enright's
model on the metabolic benefits of vertical migration remain to be measured. In any case,
the model predicts that the optimal feeding period should begin well (about 2 hr) before
sunset. In contrast, the predation hypothesis accounts for reduced risks only with decreasing
light intensity after sunset. In an attempt to distinguish experimentally between these predictions, Enright and Honegger (1977) established that the onset of feeding by the copepod
Calanus helgolandicus in the upper water layers sometimes begins well before sunset (Figure 6). There was considerable variation between life stages and between experiments at

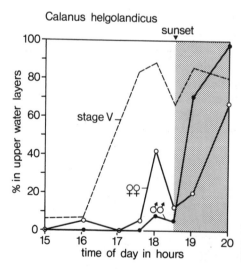

Fig. 6. The timing of upward migration in a marine
plankton organism *Calanus helgolandicus*. (From
Enright and Honegger, 1977.)

different seasons, though. The authors suggested that benefits from visual predator avoidance and metabolic advantages from vertical migration may accrue differentially to the life stages, and that the timing of upward migration is adjusted to these benefits.

Birds that, like the starlings discussed above, migrate daily between their feeding grounds and the night roost do so in full daylight. They sacrifice potential feeding time to arrive at the roost before darkness. Twice per year, however, they suddenly appear to be perfectly able to migrate over long distances during the night. This nocturnal activity is under endogenous circadian control, as demonstrated in the white-throated sparrow (*Zonotrichia albicollis;* McMillan, Gauthreaux, and Helms, 1970). It is displayed as daily *Zugunruhe* (see Chapter 3) in the confinement of lab cages just as well as in nature. It is further characterized by an endogenously programmed dark preference (Gwinner, 1975), by a special type of locomotor activity ("whirring"), and by absence of feeding (Gwinner, unpublished). Apparently, there is a tight internal program of nocturnal motivation for migratory activity and diurnal motivation for feeding. Nocturnal rest is clearly no necessity for the restoration of body resources from diurnal activity. When seasonal functions require, the organism is able to perform its alternating activities around the clock. Nocturnal migration is widespread among songbirds, and speculations about its functional significance have been manifold (Dorka, 1966). Reduced predation pressure during the night has often been advanced but has rarely been substantiated as a functional mechanism. There is no evidence that birds are more prone to predation when migrating than when foraging. Meteorological conditions prevailing during the night may be important for optimal energetic efficiency of migration. Nocturnal migration further leaves the daylight intervals for feeding and replenishing the energy reserves.

Reproduction and Life History

Many reproductive behaviors and developmental stages of animals are associated with specific times of day. An illuminating example is the dawn chorus. The territorial advertisement by male songbirds in the breeding season is usually concentrated in the hours around sunrise, commonly with a small secondary peak around sunset. The times of day when maximal food intake would be expected to compensate for the nocturnal fast are used for display. The significance of dawn territorial behavior apparently overrides the metabolic requirements. A study evaluating the adaptive meaning of the dawn chorus in the great tit *(Parus major)* indicates that, first, foraging efficiency is suppressed at dawn light intensities, while, second, the risk of intrusion of unadvertised territories is large in the first hours of the day (Kacelnik, 1979). Reduced foraging efficiency may indeed play a role in the darkness of woodlands. The risks of not advertising in the early morning are probably more general. Confirmation of territorial occupancy may also be functional, for instance, in the extended morning displays of black grouse *(Tetrao tetrix)* on their lek (Figure 4).

In cases like the dawn territorial and courtship displays of birds, the adaptiveness of timing for an individual evidently depends on the behavior of its conspecifics: the tendency of competing tits to intrude on an empty territory and of a female grouse to visit the lek and mate. This theme of adaptive circadian strategies' synchronizing individual behavior recurs throughout life histories. For instance, egg hatching and mammalian partus are quite generally events concentrated at specific times of day. In ravens *(Corvus corax)*, eggs hatch in daytime, allowing the parents to remove the chick from the eggshell and to clean it immediately (Gwinner, 1965). In many nidifugous birds, eggs hatch synchronously, permitting the whole clutch to leave the nest together. Nocturnal parturition is typical for most diurnal monkeys, so that the mother can keep up with the daily movements of her troop (Jolly, 1972). Further, mass synchronization of vulnerable stages may be one of the dominant adaptive functions of all the numerous insects having circadian timing of metamorphosis (see the first section).

The most conspicuous synchronizing function of circadian rhythms is the synchronization of sexes. The black grouse's strategy of restricting mating to specific times of day is shared by many insects. In very short-lived adult insects, like Ephemeroptera and Tipulida midges, synchronous activity of the sexes is commonly guaranteed by synchronous metamorphosis (Remmert, 1962). Longer-lived species have developed specific circadian synchronization mechanisms. Moth females generally attract males by releasing sex pheromones to which the males respond. Daily synchrony of female "calling" behavior and male responsiveness leads to optimal chances of mate finding (see Chapter 8). Closely related groups of moths often have identical sex pheromones. The allocation of mate attraction to different times of day in such cases can serve as an isolating mechanism (Wilson and Bossert, 1963). In fact, it is conceivable that the temporal isolation of individuals of a species copulating at different times of day has occasionally led to sympatric speciation. Perhaps, by such mechanisms, restricted species-specific flying times have developed in some insect

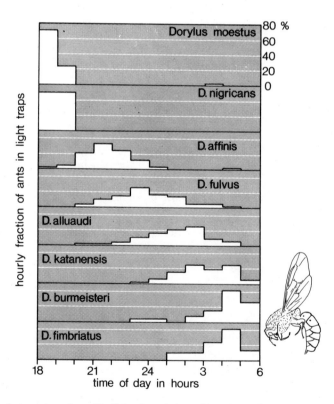

Fig. 7. Temporal staggering of specific flight times in sexually active male army ants in Uganda (genus *Dorylus*). (From Haddow *et al.*, 1966.)

groups, as exemplified by East African army ants (Figure 7). An example of reproductive isolation of related species by different daily emergence times has been described in the marine midges *Clunio marinus* and *C. balticus* (Heimbach, 1978).

THE INDIVIDUAL: DAILY HABITS

The genetic makeup of the species has set the stage for the individual daily routine. It has assigned part of the animal's circadian cycle to activity and another part to rest, depending on the ecological type: diurnal, nocturnal, crepuscular, or arrhythmic. Within this gross outline, it has allocated a specific part of the cycle to specific behaviors: daily movements, daily courtship, and territorial displays. The rough structure of an adaptive daily program in motivation for various behaviors and in physiological set points—such as in body weight and temperature—is what is probably fixed in the higher organism's internal day. But within this general program, adjustments can be made in response to the individual's experience with environmental time. Such adjustments not only attest to the plasticity of the circadian system; the fine tuning of behavior to daily fluctuations in the environment may be at the core of the functional meaning of circadian clocks (Enright, 1970)

TIME MEMORY IN HONEYBEES

What is involved in this tuning is most fully illustrated by the *Zeitgedächtnis* or time memory of the honeybee, *Apis mellifica*. Worker bees on a restricted food schedule return to their feeding dish around the time of day when sugar water was present the day before. Such feeding trips outside the hive are made also when no reward is given. Beling (1928) demonstrated this phenomenon in a series of elegant experiments, using individually marked bees, and taking care that no information about the presence or absence of food could reach the hive on test days. Wahl (1932) subsequently used two feeding dishes, located 30 m apart. He showed that on test days, the bees returned to the correct location in association with the prior feeding schedules (Figure 8). Also, honeybees easily learned to come to a feeding dish at the time of day when the sugar concentration was highest.

In many flowers visited by honeybees, nectar secretion and pollen presentation are subject to a daily rhythm. It is indeed advantageous for flowering plants to attract pollinating insects synchronously. The chances of cross-pollination are enhanced when the visits of an insect to two conspecific flowers follow each other closely. For the honeybee, it is efficient to concentrate on a flower species at the time of day of highest nectar production. In a buckwheat field, the efficient bee typically times its searching to the hours between 9 and 11 A.M., when buckwheat produces nectar at its highest rate. Indeed, careful measurements of the rates of nectar secretion and its sugar concentration have shown that the daily maximum in bee visits matches the time at which each food source is richest and sweetest (Kleber, 1935). With "pollen flowers," the bees prospect at times when the flowers are open and pollen is available. Such correlations do not prove that the bees indeed make use of Beling's *Zeitgedächtnis* to return to certain flowers at optimal times of day: some bees may always be prospecting randomly in the field and communicate rich food sources instantaneously to the hive. When Kleber (1935) presented open poppy flowers *(Papaver rhoeas)*

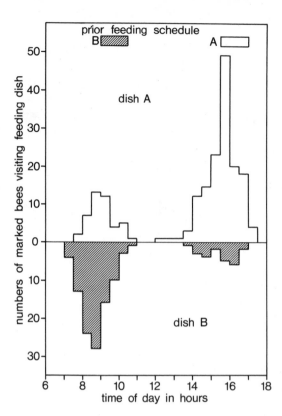

Fig. 8. Daily distribution of returns of marked worker honeybees, *Apis mellifica* to two dishes, spaced 30 m apart, at which bees had been trained to forage on previous days from 900 to 1030 (Dish B) and 1530 to 1700 (Dish A). (Based on data by Wahl, 1932.)

in a bed after 10 A.M. (i.e., the time of day when pollen presentation by poppies normally stops), she found that such flowers were indeed visited by many bees. However, those marked bees that had learned to visit the *Papaver* bed in the natural flowering period from 5:30 to 10 A.M. did not appear. They apparently relied on time memory rather than on information from other bees. Time-trained bees outside the training time, in fact, remain relatively inactive in remote parts of the hive, away from the "dance floor," where they otherwise would be informed of new food sources by other worker bees. Together with the individual fidelity of worker bees to certain plant species, these observations suggest that time memory is indeed used by honeybees in nature, as a means to minimize energy expenditure in search for food. Time memory facilitates especially the exploitation of the poorer food sources, since only rich sources are reported to the hive (Frisch, 1940).

The precision of the honeybee's daily clock involved in discrimination tasks considerably exceeds what was detectable in the early experiments. Bees correctly select between, for example, the scents of thyme and of geraniol, with the reward schedule alternating in daily sequence every 45 min (Koltermann, 1971). Such precision is not amazing, since the honeybee's time memory makes use of a truly circadian clock. It shows the usual circadian phenomena, like transient resetting following a phase shift in the LD cycle and a restricted range of entrainment between $T = 20$ and $T = 26$ hr (Renner, 1960; Beier and Lindauer, 1970). However, while the bee's time memory is based on an endogenous circadian program, only the periodicity can be innate. The details of the behavior pattern produced result from its experience with a temporal sequence of rewards offered by the environment.

Time memory has long been treated as a curiosity restricted to honeybees, or at least to animals that rely on specific periodic food sources. Beling (1935) herself suggested this after an unsuccessful attempt to train minnows *(Phoxinus phoxinus)* to discriminate between times of day. Indeed, the coevolution of plant and pollinator, in which the plant benefits from reproductive synchrony and the pollinator from more efficiently exploitable nectar sources due to temporal concentration, may have been particularly selective for precise timekeeping. There is now increasing evidence that the phenomenon may be more widespread. In the first place, a number of species, when kept on daily restricted food schedules, are known to exhibit increased activity shortly before the food is presented (e.g., rats—Richter, 1922; Bolles and Stokes, 1965; finches—Stein, 1951; killifish—Davis and Bardach, 1965). This "anticipatory" activity not only reflects a state of generally raised arousal but may be a real expression of increased feeding motivation; for example, caged starlings rewarded for key pecking during four 1-hr intervals per day show anticipatory key pecking (Adler, 1964). Such phases of increased feeding motivation at times of day at which food is available may be profitably used in situations where the efficiency of feeding varies predictably in the course of the day. Thus, kestrels *(Falco tinnunculus)* can concentrate their natural hunting activity at daily recurring times of high yield related to variations in vole availability (Rijnsdorp *et al.,* 1981).

In other situations, various sources of food vary in profitability in the course of the day, and their exploitation puts a premium on choosing at any time the most profitable source. Brewer's blackbirds *(Euphagus cyanocephalus;* Orians and Horn, 1969) and starlings *(Sturnus vulgaris;* Daan and Tinbergen, unpublished data) may visit particular parts of their feeding grounds in association with daily insect emergence peaks (dragonflies and tipulids, respectively). In such instances, it is not known if the birds did indeed make use of time memory as proposed in the honeybee. In the starling, at least, the capacity to discriminate between operant behaviors rewarded at different times of day is known to exist (Figure 9).

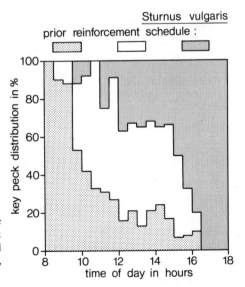

Fig. 9. Daily changes in distribution of pecks on three different keys in a starling, *Sturnus vulgaris,* on test days following training days with restricted reward schedules as indicated. (From Daan and Tinbergen, unpublished data.)

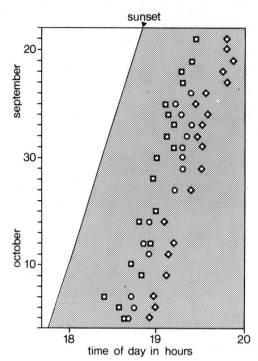

Fig. 10. Daily nursing times in three families (identified by different symbols) of hares, *Lepus europaeus*. (From Broekhuizen and Maaskamp, 1979.)

In some exceptional instances, time memory is further likely to be involved in the synchronization of individuals. In hares, the doe visits her young only once per day for 5–10 min. To suckle them, she returns to a particular area around the place of birth. Initially, the young stay at this spot also in daytime. While growing up, they tend to move further away. However, every night shortly after sunset, the family reunites for a few minutes and celebrates a suckling session. The exact time varies between families but is relatively constant from day to day (Rongstad and Tester, 1971; and see Figure 10). This behavior suggests that while motivation for suckling may generally be higher in the evening in hares, the coordinated return of a family to one particular spot makes use of individual fine tuning, creating a precise combination of behavior, time, and place, and guaranteeing optimal safety for the young.

THE STRATEGY OF HABITS

The unraveling of the mechanisms of time memory has only just begun. The individual adjustment of a daily routine to make use of prior experience obviously involves learning, memory, and motivational control. A significant step in the experimental analysis is the detection of periodicity in a learned task after single trainings; for example, rats trained in either appetitive or avoidance tasks showed significant peaks in performance 24, 48, and 72 hr after training (Holloway and Wansley, 1973; see also Chapter 11). Is memory retrieval tied to a circadian clock? If this proves to be the case, we may expect also that natural rewards of a behavior heighten the probability of recurrence of that behavior 24 hr later.

Whatever the concrete mechanism, its adaptive nature depends on the predictability of the temporal environment, that is, on the correlation from day to day in the timing of events. Another important factor is the opportunity for animals to collect the relevant information directly instead of relying on yesterday's experience. The stronger the emphasis on internal timing, the more we should expect individual daily habits to occur, that is, patterns of behavior repeated in organized temporal order day after day. Some anecdotal information on such habits has been collected (Hediger, 1946), but the phenomenon has not been consequently studied in animals in natural circumstances. This is not surprising. The detection of daily habits requires that animals be followed individually many days in a row, while their movements and behaviors are continuously monitored. With the advent of radio tracking, one may expect a surge of interest in long-term studies on individual animals. One recent example of daily habits in a European kestrel, *Falco tinnunculus,* is illustrated in Figure 11.

For a predator like the kestrel, the meaning of reliance on daily habits as an adaptive

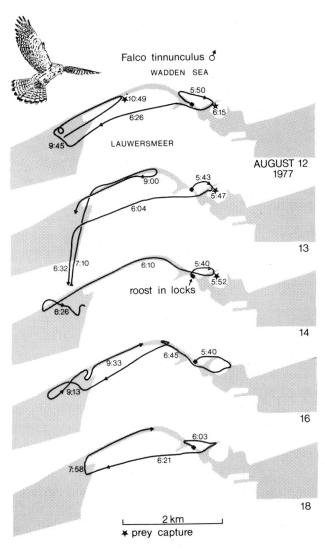

Fig. 11. Movements of a kestrel, *Falco tinnunculus,* on five mornings in August, 1977.
(From Rijnsdorp *et al.,* 1981.)

response to day-to-day correlations in prey availability is evident. Having found food at some time and place in its hunting area makes returning to that place at the same time next day an appropriate strategy, as Enright (1970, 1975) has pointed out. In the same vein, a negative experience would appropriately be answered by a change in schedule. The prey, on the other hand, should respond to a predator's attack with a change in schedule, since the attack implies that the old schedule may be hazardous. In the absence of such attacks, a prey would appropriately maintain its schedule of the previous day, other things being equal (Daan and Slopsema, 1978). Thus, sticking to daily habits may have survival value for both predator and prey as a basic behavior pattern that exploits the repetitiveness of events on a planet in rotation.

Individual daily habits have hardly been the subject of experimental analysis. Yet, they form a central theme in the discussion of the adaptiveness of circadian rhythms. Further analysis should concentrate on the extent to which what an animal does in the course of the day is an immediate response to stimuli outside, and what is preprogrammed, either coarsely fixed for the species or finely tuned to make use of individual learning and experience. Eventually, one may hope to know in quantitative detail how various degrees of environmental predictability and the presence of immediate cues for orientation in time have led to different degrees of flexibility in an animal's daily routines.

REFERENCES

Adler, H. E. Sensory factors in migration *Animal Behaviour,* 1964, *11,* 566–577.
Aschoff, J. Tagesperiodik bei Mäusestämmen unter konstanten Umgebungsbedingungen. *Pflügers Archiv,* 1955, *262,* 51–59.
Aschoff, J. Spontane lokomotorische Aktivität. *Handbuch der Zoologie,* 1962, *8,* 1–76.
Ashmole, N. P. The biology of the wideawake or sooty tern on Ascension Island. *The Ibis,* 1963, *103b,* 297–364.
Beier, W., and Lindauer, M. Der Sonnenstand als Zeitgeber für die Biene. *Apidologie,* 1970, *1,* 5–28.
Beling, I. Über das Zeitgedächtnis der Bienen *Zeitschrift für vergleichende Physiologie,* 1923, *9,* 259–338.
Beling, I. von Stein-. Über das Zeitgedächtnis bei Tieren. *Biological Reviews,* 1935, *10,* 18–41.
Bolles, R. C., and Stokes, L. W. The rat's anticipation of diurnal and adiurnal feeding. *Journal of Comparative Physiology and Psychology,* 1965, *60,* 290–294.
Bovet, J. On the social behavior in a stable group of long-tailed field mice *(Apodemus sylvaticus).* II. Its relations with distribution of daily activity. *Behaviour,* 1972, *41,* 55–67.
Briedermann, L. Ermittlungen zur Aktivitätsperiodik des mitteleuropäischen Wildschweines (*Sus s. scrofa* L.). *Zoologische Garten* (Leipzig), 1971, *40,* 302–327.
Broekhuizen, S., and Maaskamp, F. Behaviour of does and leverets of the European hare *(Lepus europaeus)* whilst nursing. *Journal of Zoology* (London), 1980, *191,* 487–501.
Collopy, M. W. Food caching by female American kestrels in winter. *The Condor,* 1977, *79,* 63–68.
Corbet, P. S. Discussion contribution. In A. Chovnick (Ed.), *Biological Clocks—Cold Spring Harbor Symposia on Quantitative Biology,* 1960, *25,* 354.
Cott, H. B. *Adaptive Coloration in Animals.* London: Methuen, 1940.
Crowcroft, P. The daily cycle of activity in British shrews. *Proceedings of the Zoological Society of London,* 1954, *123,* 713–729.
Daan, S., and Tinbergen, J. M. Young guillemots (Uria lomvia) leaving their Arctic breeding cliffs: A daily rhythm in numbers and risk. *Ardea,* 1980, *67,* 96–100.
Daan, S., and Slopsema, S. Short-term rhythms in foraging behaviour of the common vole, *Microtus arvalis. Journal of Comparative Physiology,* 1978, *127,* 215–227.
Davis, R. E., and Bardach, J. E. Time-coordinated pre-feeding activity in a fish. *Animal Behaviour,* 1965, *13,* 154–162.
Dorka, V. Das jahres- and tageszeitliche Zugmuster von Kurz- und Langstreckenziehern nach Beobachtungen auf den Alpenpässen Cou/Bretolet (Wallis). *Der Ornithologische Beobachter,* 1966, *63,* 165–223.

Elliott, J. M. Diel changes in invertebrate drift and the food of trout *Salmo trutta* L. *Journal of Fish Biology*, 1970, *2*, 161–165.

Enright, J. T. Ecological aspects of endogenous rhythmicity. *Annual Reviews of Ecology and Systematics*, 1970, *1*, 221–238.

Enright, J. T. The circadian tape recorder and its entrainment. In F. J. Vernberg (Ed.), *Physiological Adaptation to the Environment*. New York: Intext, 1975.

Enright, J. T. Diurnal vertical migration: Adaptive significance and timing. I. Selective advantage: A metabolic model. *Limnology and Oceanography*, 1977, *22*, 856–872.

Enright, J. T., and Hamner, W. M. Vertical diurnal migration and endogenous rhythmicity. *Science*, 1967, *157*, 937–941.

Enright, J. T., and Honegger, H. W. Diurnal vertical migration: Adaptive significance and timing. II. Test of the model: Details of timing. *Limnology and Oceanography*, 1977, *22*, 973–886.

Eriksson, L. O. Spring inversion of the diel rhythm of locomotor activity in young sea-going brown trout, *Salmo trutta trutta* L., and atlantic salmon, *Salmo salar* L. *Aquilo, Series Zoologica*, 1973, *14*, 68–79.

Erkinaro, E. Der Phasenwechsel der lokomotorischen Aktivität bei *Microtus agrestis* (L.), *M. arvalis* (Pall.) and *M. oeconomus* (Pall.). *Aquilo, Series Zoologica*, 1969, *8*, 1–31.

Frisch, K. von. Die Tänze und das Zeitgedächtnis der Bienen in Widerspruch. *Die Naturwissenschaften*, 1940, *28*, 5–69.

Fujimoto, K. [Diurnal activity of mice in relation to social order.] [*Physiology and Ecology*], Kyoto, 1953, *5*, 97–103.

Gee, J. H. Effect of daily synchronization of sexual activity on mating success in laboratory populations of two species of Dacus (Diptera: Tephritidae). *Australian Journal of Zoology*, 1969, *17*, 619–624.

Gwinner, E. Beobachtungen über Nestbau und Brutpflege des Kolkraben *(Corvus corax)* in Gefangenschaft. *Journal für Ornithologie*, 1965, *106*, 146–178.

Gwinner, E. Circadian and circannual rhythms in birds. In J. A. King and D. S. Farner (Eds.), *Avian Biology*. Vol. 5. New York: Academic Press, 1975.

Haddow, A. J., Yarrow, I. H. H., Lancaster, G. A., and Corbet, P. S. Nocturnal flight cycle in the males of African doryline ants (Hymenoptera: Formicidae). *Proceedings of the Royal Entomological Society, London (A)*, 1966, *41*, 103–106.

Hamilton, W. J., and Gilbert, W. M. Starling dispersal from a winter roost. *Ecology*, 1969, *50*, 886–898.

Hansson, L. Small rodent food, feeding and population dynamics. *Oikos*, 1971, *22*, 183–198.

Hediger, H. Bemerkungen zum Raum-Zeit-System der Tiere. *Schweizerische Zeitschrift für Psychologie*, 1946, *5*, 241–269.

Heimbach, F. Sympatric species, *Clunio marinus* Hal. and *Cl. balticus* n.sp. (Dipt., Chironomidae), isolated by differences in diel emergence time. *Oecologia*, 1978, *32*, 195–202.

Holloway, F. A., and Wansley, R. A. Multiple retention deficits at periodic intervals after active and passive avoidance learning. *Behavioral Biology*, 1973, *9*, 1–14.

Hörnicke, H., and Batsch, F. Coecotrophy in rabbits—A circadian function. *Journal of Mammalogy*, 1977, *58*, 240.

Hughes, B. O. A circadian rhythm of calcium intake in the domestic fowl. *British Poultry Science*, 1972, *13*, 485–493.

Hulscher, J. B. Localization of cockles (*Cardium edule* L.) by the oystercatcher (*Haematopus ostralegus* L.) in darkness and daylight. *Ardea*, 1976, *64*, 292–310.

Jolly, A. Hour of birth in primates and man. *Folia Primatologica*, 1972, *18*, 108–121.

Kacelnik, A. The foraging efficiency of great tits (*Parus major* L.) in relation to light intensity. *Animal Behaviour*, 1979, *27*, 237–241.

Kamran, N. A. Life history and behavior of *Polydesma umbricola* in Hawaii. *Annals of the Entomological Society of America*, 1968, *61*, 795–802.

Kayser, C., and Heusner, A. A. Le rhythme nycthéméral de la dépense d'énergie. *Journal de Physiologie*, 1967, *59*, 3–116.

Kennedy, C. H. Evolutionary level in relation to geographic, seasonal and diurnal distribution in insects. *Ecology*, 1928, *9*, 367–379.

Kleber, E. Hat das Zeitgedächtnis der Bienen biologische Bedeutung? *Zeitschrift für vergleichende Physiologie*, 1935, *22*, 221–262.

Koltermann, R. 24-Std-Periodik in der Langzeiterinnerung an Duft- und Farbsignalen bei der Honigbiene. *Zeitschrift für vergleichende Physiologie*, 1971, *75*, 49–68.

Kureck, A. Two circadian eclosion times in *Chironomus thummi* (Diptera), alternately selected with different temperatures. *Oecologia*, 1979, *40*, 311–323.

Lewis, T., and Taylor, L. R. Diurnal periodicity of flight by insects. *Transactions of the Royal Entomological Society, London*, 1964, *116*, 293–476.

Lloyd, M., and Dybas, H. S. The periodical circada problem. I,II. *Evolution,* 1966, *20,* 133–149, 466–505.

McMillan, J. P., Gauthreaux, S. A., and Helms, C. W. Spring migratory restlessness in caged birds: A circadian rhythm. *BioScience,* 1970, *20,* 1259–1260.

McNab, B. K. The evolution of endothermy in the phylogeny of mammals. *The American Naturalist,* 1978, *112,* 1–21.

Meddis, R. On the function of sleep. *Animal Behaviour,* 1975, *23,* 676–691.

Morgan, N. L. The biology of *Leptocerus aterrinus* Steph. with reference to its availability as food for trout. *Journal of Animal Ecology,* 1956, *25,* 349–365.

Nyholm, E. S. Zur Ökologie von *Myotis mystacinus* (Leisl.) und *M. daubentoni* (Leisl.) (Chiroptera). *Annales Zoologici Fennici,* 1965, *2,* 77–123.

Orians, G. H., and Horn, H. Overlap in foods and foraging of four species of blackbirds in the potholes of central Washington. *Ecology,* 1969, *50,* 930–938.

Park, O. Nocturnalism: The development of a problem. *Ecological Monographs,* 1940, *10,* 485.

Pearson, D. L. Vertical stratification of birds in a tropical dry forest. *The Condor,* 1971, *73,* 46–55.

Porter, W. P., Mitchell, J. W., Beckman, W. A., and DeWitt, C. B. Behavioral implications of mechanistic ecology: Thermal and behavioral modeling of desert ectotherms in their microenvironment. *Oecologia,* 1973, *13,* 1–54.

Remmert, H. *Der Schlüpfrhythmus der Insekten.* Wiesbaden: Steiner, 1962.

Renner, M. The contribution of the honey bee to the study of time sense and astronomical orientation. *Cold Spring Harbor Symposia of Quantitative Biology,* 1960, *25,* 361–367.

Richter, C. P. A behavioristic study of the activity of the rat. *Comparative Psychology Monographs,* 1922, *1,* 1–55.

Rijnsdorp, A., Daan, S., and Dijkstra, C. Hunting in the kestrel, *Falco tinnunculus,* and the adaptive significance of daily habits. *Oecologia,* 1981, in press.

Rongstad, O. J., and Tester, J. R. Behavior and maternal relations of young snowshoe hares. *Journal of Wildlife Management,* 1971, *35,* 338–346.

Rovee, C. K., Kaufman, L. W., Collier, G. H., and Kent, G. C. Periodicity of death feigning by domestic fowl in response to simulated predation. *Physiology and Behaviour,* 1976, *17,* 891–895.

Schoener, T. W. Nonsynchronous spatial overlap of lizards in patchy habitats. *Ecology,* 1970, *51,* 408–418.

Schoener, T. W. Resource partitioning in ecological communities. *Science,* 1974, *185,* 27–58.

Stein, H. Untersuchungen über den Zeitsinn bei Vögelin. *Zeitschrift für vergleichende Physiologie,* 1951, *33,* 387–403.

Steinborn, W. Beobachtungen zum Verhalten des Alpensteinbocks, *Capra ibex ibex* Linné, 1758. *Säugetierkundliche Mitteilungen,* 1973, *21,* 37–65.

Tamisier, A. Rhythmes nycthéméraux des sarcelles d'hiver pendant leur hivemage en Camargue. *Alauda,* 1972, *40,* 109–135, 235–256.

Toates, F. M. A circadian rhythm of hoarding in the hamster. *Animal Behaviour,* 1978, *26,* 631.

Wahl, O. Neue Untersuchungen über das Zeitgedächtnis der Bienen. *Zeitschrift für vergleichende Physiologie,* 1932, *16,* 529–589.

Walls, G. L. The vertebrate eye and its adaptive radiation. *Cranbrook Institute of Science Bulletin,* 1942, *19.*

Ward, P., and Zahavi, A. The importance of certain assemblages of birds as information centres for food finding. *The Ibis,* 1973, *115,* 517–534.

Wilson, E. O., and Bossert, W. H. Chemical communication among animals. *Recent Progress in Hormone Research,* 1963, *19,* 673–716.

Young, A. M. Community ecology of some tropical rain forest butterflies. *The American Midland Naturalist,* 1972, *87,* 146–157.

Zeigler, H. P., Green, H. L., and Lehrer, R. Patterns of feeding behavior in the pigeon. *Journal of Comparative and Physiological Psychology,* 1971, *76,* 468–477.

16

Clock-Controlled Orientation in Space

HANS G. WALLRAFF

INTRODUCTION

One of the most obvious expressions of rhythmicity in animal behavior is the periodic change in amount of locomotor activity. Locomotion, however, as a vectorial quantity, consists not only of amount (i.e., frequency of movements and velocity) but also of direction, and inevitably, it changes the relationship between the animal and its spatial environment. Thus, in some cases in which the amount of movement, and in all cases in which the direction of movement, is influenced by the periodically changing inner state of an organism, the underlying rhythm directly affects the animal's orientation in space. It will be shown here that influences of this kind exist and that they are of remarkable adaptive significance.

Most research on the subject of this chapter has been done in the 20 years following the discovery of the sun compass in 1950 by K. von Frisch (in bees) and G. Kramer (in birds). The topic has been more-or-less extensively treated by Hoffmann (1965, 1971) and, together with many other aspects of spatial orientation, by Jander (1963), Lindauer (1963), Frisch (1965/1967), Schmidt-Koenig (1965, 1975), Matthews (1968), Gwinner (1971), Keeton (1974), Wallraff (1974), and Emlen (1975).

BIOLOGICAL CLOCKS IN ASTRO-ORIENTATION

There are several reasons that the use of extraterrestrial cues for orientation in a terrestrial environment may be profitable. (1) The sun and the moon are very prominent

HANS G. WALLRAFF   Max-Planck-Institut für Verhaltensphysiologie, 8131 Seewiesen, West Germany.

"landmarks" that can easily be distinguished from all other environmental features and that can be localized without highly developed mechanisms of visual discrimination. (2) The uniqueness of celestial cues and the wide-range constancy of their appearance allow generalizations that would never be possible with respect to the manifold structures of the immediate environment. (3) The large distance of a celestial cue guarantees that maintaining a constant angle to it will result in a straight course and not in a spiral, as it would in most cases if the animal were to rely on an object in its close vicinity. (4) Theoretically, celestial bodies can be used not only for determining and maintaining directions but also for determining the observer's position on the earth.

These advantages of extraterrestrial cues, however, are accompanied by the disadvantage that their location in the sky varies, dependent on the daily rotation of the earth, on season, and on geographic latitude. As the time-dependent variability is strongly periodic, its effect can be compensated when an adequate chronometer is available. Thus, it has to be asked whether biological clocks are used for this purpose, and if so, how they are integrated in the orientational mechanisms, and where the limits of their applicability have to be considered.

THE SUN AS AN ORIENTATIONAL CUE

THE TIME-COMPENSATED SUN COMPASS. *Light compass reaction,* or *photomenotaxis* in a classical sense, means that an animal maintains, over a period of time, a constant course angle with respect to a light source (Fraenkel and Gunn, 1940/1961). This light source may be the sun, as can be tested in nature by means of a mirror (Santschi, 1911). The time-compensated sun compass, however, not only involves the use of the sun as an orientational cue but also takes into account its daily movement. In order to maintain a constant compass course, the animal has to change its menotactic light angle periodically in an appropriate manner. Sun-compass orientation, in this sense, has been found in many species of arthropods and vertebrates (for references, see Pardi, 1955; Jander, 1963; Lindauer, 1963; Schmidt-Koenig, 1975).

Ecological Context of Occurrence. In most cases, the adaptive value of the sun compass is obvious. The main fields of its application are as follows:

1. Animals living at borderlines between different environments (i.e., at the shore of the sea and at banks of rivers or lakes) show flight reactions toward the respective border when displaced either out to the water or inland. Such behavior is known in crustaceans, spiders, insects, and amphibians (e.g., Pardi and Papi, 1953; Pardi, 1955; Papi, Serretti, and Parrini, 1957; Ferguson, 1971).

2. Animals foraging at sites distant from their home territory have to find their way there and back. Certainly, there are several such cases in which the sun compass is used (e.g., Winn, Salmon, and Roberts, 1964), but the most famous and best-investigated example is that of the honeybee (Frisch, 1965/1967).

3. Migrating animals have to maintain constant directions over long distances. It seems probable that birds, fish, and insects make use of the sun compass during migration. In birds, it has been shown to be one of the components of their navigational system used for homing (Schmidt-Koenig, 1965, 1975; Keeton, 1974; Wallraff, 1974).

Dependence on Circadian Phase. Crustacean sandhoppers, when displaced from the shoreline to a dry place, try to escape toward the splash zone. They determine their direction as an angle with reference to the sun, and this angle changes continuously in the course of a day, varying by about 180° from morning to evening (Figure 1A). In this way, the animals keep their direction rather constant with respect to the terrestrial environment (Figure 1B).

In case this kind of orientation is based on a mechanism in which a daily rhythm of course orders (cf. Mittelstaedt, 1962) is controlled by a circadian oscillator, one should expect that the phase of this rhythm will depend on the LD cycle to which the animal is exposed (see Chapter 6). Thus, a phase shift in the LD cycle should result in a phase shift in the rhythm of orientation. If the animal is then confronted with the natural sun, it should deviate in a predictable manner from the normal compass course. Many of such clock-shift experiments with a variety of species have been conducted, and these expectations have always been met (for references, see Hoffmann, 1965, 1971; Schmidt-Koenig, 1975). Figure 2 demonstrates the effect in a riparian spider.

These results are in agreement with the assumption that the clock used for sun orientation is a circadian clock, but they do not definitely prove it. An hourglass mechanism, initiated by the onset of light, would still be sufficient. It has been shown, however, that the orientational rhythm is freerunning under constant conditions in synchrony with locomotor activity, and so it seems to possess all the properties that are typical of circadian periodicities (see Hoffmann, 1960, 1965, 1971).

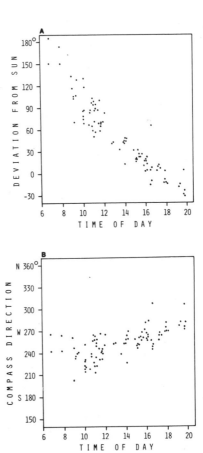

Fig. 1. Directions of attempts to escape in *Talitrus saltator* as a function of time of day. The same data are shown (A) as angles with respect to the sun azimuth (plus = sun at left), and (B) as compass directions. Each dot represents the mean of a single experiment in which animals were kept in a round vessel with visual landmarks shielded. (Redrawn from Pardi and Papi, 1953.)

The rhythm of orientation can be linked in various phase relations to the circadian clock, resulting in different compass directions toward which the animal tends to go. (A vertical shift of the LT curve in Figure 2A leads to a respective displacement of the LT line in Figure 2B.) The phase relation, and thus the intended compass direction, can be phylogenetically determined in a population-specific way, as is the case, according to Pardi (1960), in littoral amphipods. Usually, however, it is more flexible, since individuals have to adapt themselves to differently oriented banks of rivers, lakes, etc. (Papi and Tongiorgi,

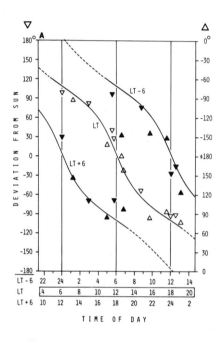

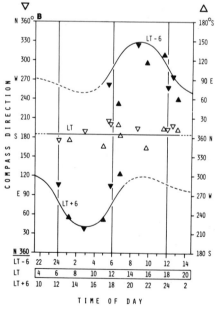

Fig. 2. Clock-shift experiments with wolf spiders, *Arctosa variana*. In May, specimens of two populations living at opposite sides of a river (about 44°N) were tested for their flight reactions on the surface of water in a round vessel. In nature, the direction from the water to the home bank was south (185°, left ordinates, triangles pointing downward) and north (5°, right ordinates, triangles upward). Three groups were exposed for several days to different LD cycles. In the controls (open symbols), the cycle was synchronized with the natural day, that is, with local time (LT). In the experimentals (solid symbols), the LD phase was either delayed or advanced by 6 hr (LT − 6 and LT + 6). Each symbol represents the mean direction of 6–10 individuals. The same data are shown (A) as angles with respect to the sun azimuth (plus = sun at left) and (B) as compass directions. The line LT corresponds to the direction toward the home bank. In (A), the curves LT − 6 and LT + 6 are displaced horizontally against LT by 6 hr. In (B), the resulting compass directions [cf. vertical distances in (A)] are shown. The curves are dashed during the respective night phase. (Redrawn from Papi *et al.*, 1957.)

1963; Ferguson and Landreth, 1966), or since they have to select rapidly changing directions to and from varying foraging sites or other places.

303

CLOCK-CONTROLLED
ORIENTATION IN
SPACE

The Shape of the Orientation Curve and Its Determinants. The curves representing
the daily rhythm of sun orientation can be very different, as is shown by some examples in
Figure 3. During daytime, they are usually more-or-less exact mirror images of the sun-
azimuth curve, which varies greatly as a function of geographic latitude and season (for
related graphs, see Braemer, 1960; Wallraff, 1974).

How do animals adapt their patterns of directional change to the different paths of
the sun? Lindauer (1960) concluded that each individual honeybee has to observe the sun's
path, or a part of it, to compensate for the sun's movement. Some birds, fish, and crustaceans, on the other hand, are reported to correct for this movement, at least in a rough
manner, without ever having seen the moving sun before (Hoffmann, 1953; Braemer, 1960;
Pardi, 1960; Papi and Tongiorgi, 1963). However, a mechanism ensuring more precise
adaptations of the rhythm pattern to the local and seasonal sun path seems necessary also
in some of these cases. Mittelstaedt (1962) has offered a hypothetical control system by
which a sun compass can work adequately in a global range. As inputs, it needs some
equivalents of the variables that we need for calculating the sun's azimuth: time of day
(hour angle of sun), time of year (declination of sun), and geographic latitude. For an
adequate setting of such a universal mechanism as well as for a method of curve fitting on
a more empirical basis, the animal has to evaluate external stimuli, possibly in connection
with circannual rhythmicity. The adaptation process could depend on such parameters as
(1) the photoperiod to which the animal is exposed; (2) sun-azimuth changes in relation to
some terrestrial reference; (3) sun altitude; and/or (4) direct perception of the apparent
motion of the sun. Influences of such kinds are indicated in some experiments (e.g.,
Schwassmann and Braemer, 1961; New and New, 1962; Schwassmann and Hasler, 1964;
Pardi and Ercolini, 1966). However, the whole complex has not yet been analyzed sufficiently, and in different taxa, different mechanisms are probably at work.

Such differences also become apparent in the mode of the sun-compass rhythm during
nighttime, which can be observed by means of either artificial light sources or clock-shifted
animals. It appears that both possible ways of coming back to the sunrise point are realized.
In the northern hemisphere, the "forward type" behaves as if the sun would continue its
clockwise movement from west over north to east (as the real sun in most latitudes does),
whereas the "backward type" behaves as if the virtual sun would return over the south.
Figures 3D and 3E show examples of the latter type, but under similar conditions, other
species (e.g., bees and fish) belong to the forward type (Lindauer, 1957; Braemer, 1960).

BICOORDINATE SUN NAVIGATION. After discovery of the sun compass, it was an
attractive idea to explain not only one-direction orientation but also the remarkable homing
capacities of birds by a navigational system that is based on observations of the sun, as has
been used by sailors for centuries. A variety of sun-navigation hypotheses have been presented that vary in detail but are all based on the same principles: the animal has to perceive
the sun's altitude and motion very precisely and to compare the observed data with some
remembered data of reference that are to be expected simultaneously at the home site. For
this comparison, the animal needs an adequate and precise time scale.

While sensory capabilities for sun localization appear to be highly developed in birds
(Pettigrew, 1978; Whiten, 1978), they do not seem to be used for determining the direction
toward home. The reason may be the incapability of living systems to solve related prob-

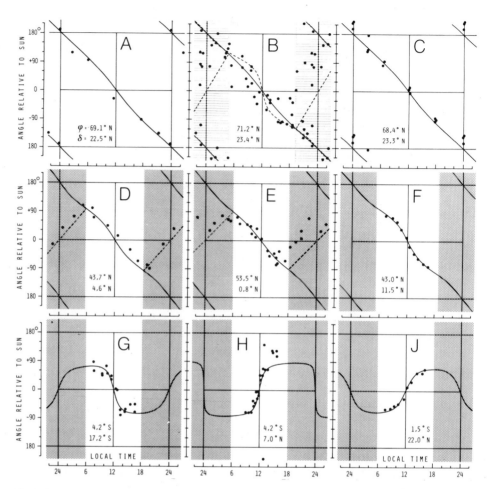

Fig. 3. Sun compass reactions of crustaceans (G, H), spiders (A, D), fish (F, J), and birds (B, C, E) in Arctic latitudes (A–C), in median latitudes (D–F), and in the equatorial zone (G–J). Dots represent mean directions of individuals or groups of animals. Curves show the expected directions as dependent on change of the sun's azimuth at the respective site (latitude, ϕ) and date (declination of sun, δ). Zero at the ordinate stands for the expected angle to the sun at noontime (+ is to the right, − to the left of this direction). Nighttime is marked by dotted areas. All experiments were conducted under the natural sun. Nighttime tests in D and E were done with clock-shifted animals. The parts outside of the frames are periodic repetitions of the same data. (A) Escape reactions of resident wolf spiders *(Lycosa fluviatilis)* in Finland (Papi and Syrjämäki, 1963). (B) Tests with three homing pigeons *(Columba domestica)* directionally trained at latitude 36.0°N. Experiments were done within 12 days after exposure to the permanent Arctic day. The dotted area indicates nighttime and the broken line the expected curve at the training site (Schmidt-Koenig, 1964). Note indicated transition from LD behavior (cf. E) to Arctic LL behavior (cf. C). (C) Directional choices of three starlings *(Sturnus vulgaris)* trained at latitudes 53.5°N and—only during "daytime" hours—at 68.4°N. Tests at "nighttime" were started about 15 days after exposure to the permanent Arctic day (Hoffmann, 1959). (D) Escape reactions of resident wolf spiders *(Arctosa variana)* in Italy (Tongiorgi, 1959). (E) Directional choices of one homing pigeon trained during daytime hours at the test site (Schmidt-Koenig, 1961). (F) Directional choices of six centrarchid fishes trained at the test site (Schwassmann and Hasler, 1964). (G) and (H) Escape reactions of resident amphipods *(Talorchestia martensi)* in Kenya from January 30 to February 3 (G) and September 3–6 (H) (Pardi and Ercolini, 1966). (J) Directional choices of six cichlid fishes trained at the test site (Braemer and Schwassmann, 1963). All figures are redrawn with precision dependent on the sources.

lems of chronometry that involve much greater demands on precision and rigidity than in the case of sun-compass orientation. Theoretical possibilities of complete or partial sun navigation as dependent on the time scales that the animal might be able to use, as well as deductions for experimental approach, have been outlined by Wallraff (1974). None of the conceivable expectations is met by the empirical data, of which many exist. Nevertheless, the sun is also used for homing. Obviously, however, it partakes only in the function of a compass, which is one of the components of a multiple-cue navigational system (for more details see Kramer, 1957; Hoffmann, 1965, 1971; Schmidt-Koenig, 1965, 1975; Matthews, 1968; Gwinner, 1971; Keeton, 1974; Wallraff, 1974; Benvenuti, 1976; Whiten, 1978). There is no indication that bird navigation uses any kind of time measurement different from biological rhythmicity as described in this volume.

THE MOON AS AN ORIENTATIONAL CUE

A time-compensated moon compass has been described for the above-mentioned crustacean sandhoppers (Papi and Pardi, 1959, 1963; Enright, 1972), and there are indications that it also exists in other arthropods (Pardi, 1954; Tongiorgi, 1970) and in amphibians (Ferguson and Landreth, 1966).

In the course of a night, the sandhoppers change their angle to the moon in a manner similar to their angle change with respect to the sun during the daytime. However, they cannot simply use their circadian clock, as in sun orientation, since the phase relation between the moon's azimuth and the LD cycle shifts every day by about 50 min or 12°. (The moon's velocity is 14.5°/h, that of the sun 15°/h.) There are at least three possible ways by which the moon's movement could adequately be taken into account:

1. In addition to, and independently of, their circa-solar-dian clock, the animals are provided with a circa-lunar-dian clock that is entrained to the 24.8-hr lunar day by some environmental factors as, for example, moonlight or tides.

2. The circa-solar-dian clock is used, and every day the calibration of the moon's azimuth is reset by 12°. Every 30 days (i.e., after a lunar cycle), nearly identical relationships are reestablished. In order to ensure this cycle and to avoid drift, the resetting mechanism should be controlled by a 30-day circalunar rhythm.

3. Similar to 2, however, recalibration is not done automatically, but in direct response to some environmental cues, for example, the shape of the moon, or the time of moonrise or moonset, or the moon's azimuth or altitude at time of sunset.

The last-mentioned possibility is experimentally excluded as far as an hourglass mechanism working for only a single night is concerned (Papi and Pardi, 1959, 1963; Pardi and Ercolini, 1965). There is also some indication that correct compensation for the moon's movement occurs even after 11–20 days of isolation from environmental cues in complete darkness (Papi and Pardi, 1959). However, the data do not completely rule out simple forms of fixed-angle orientation (cf. Enright, 1972). Thus, it appears that a type 3 mechanism, in which the last calibration persists for a few (less than 10) nights of isolation in darkness, is not definitely excluded. The hypothesis favored by Papi and Pardi and (with emphasized reluctance) also by Enright is an independent circa-lunar-dian clock according to type 1.

It is still unknown whether—and if so, in which way—the moon compass is linked to the complex of lunar and tidal rhythmicity that has been found in other functions of life (see Chapter 19).

HANS G. WALLRAFF

It is a well-established fact that birds, at least, are able to use the stellar sky for determining and maintaining compass directions (for references, see Emlen, 1975). Problems arising in this kind of nocturnal orientation are quite different from those of moon orientation. The small difference between stellar day and solar day (4 min) may be less important, although it is responsible for the seasonal change of the starry sky and thus complicates matters, too. The difference in the cues that are used may be more fundamental: instead of dealing with a single prominent object, as in sun and moon orientation, the animals are confronted with complex patterns of huge numbers of small spots. On the one hand, this possibility seems to make stellar orientation more difficult than single-cue orientation. On the other hand, however, once the problem of pattern recognition is solved, the related orientation mechanism need not make allowance for the time schedules of celestial movements. Each Boy Scout, necessarily looking at his watch to determine compass directions by means of the sun, is able to find the polestar without using his watch. His knowledge of some stellar configurations (e.g., the Great Dipper) and of their relation to the polar axis enables him to determine north no matter where in the sky the configurations are located, and thus no matter the time of day and year. A time-independent mechanism would be profitable in case of stellar orientation, since azimuth curves, being dependent on the different declinations of individual stars, are much more variable than those shown for the sun in Figure 3.

In the early planetarium experiments of Sauer (1957; Sauer and Sauer, 1960), some time-dependency was indicated. In all the subsequent experiments, however, clock shifts or equivalent planetarium settings did not influence the directional choices of the birds tested (Matthews, 1963; Emlen, 1967; Wallraff, 1968). Liepa (1978), on the other hand, observed time-dependent directional changes with respect to a single starlike light source. Thus, the role of circadian rhythms in stellar orientation is not yet definitely clarified, but it seems less important than in sun orientation.

Bicoordinate navigation based on observation of the stars has been claimed by Sauer (1957), but neither his nor later experiments convincingly support this hypothesis (Wallraff, 1960; Emlen, 1967, 1975).

OTHER ASPECTS OF PERIODIC CHANGE OF ORIENTED ACTIVITIES

In astro-orientation, the animals have to change their course orders periodically to keep their course constant with respect to the terrestrial environment. Periodic changes may also concern, however, the intended directions or distances within the terrestrial environment and thus lead to varying courses.

PERIODIC CHANGE OF DIRECTION

SWITCH OF SIGN. In many animals, preferences for certain habitats, and thus for certain directions leading toward them, alternate in synchrony with the day–night cycle. This alternation may result in commands as "go out" or "go home," or in changes between positive and negative phototaxis or geotaxis, etc. (e.g., Cloudsley-Thompson, 1961; Jander, 1963). In many cases, the behavior varies in direct response to environmental fluctuations and has nothing to do with time measurement. In other cases, however, there is some evidence that directional preferences switch from one state to another even in constant conditions and in a way typical of circadian periodicities (e.g., Birukow, 1964; Gwinner, 1966; Koch, 1967).

Similar changes of sign can occur in the course of a year. An example is the reversal of the direction of migration in fall and spring in birds. According to Emlen (1969), the change is influenced by the photoperiodic conditions. So far, it has not been shown to persist in circannual freerunning rhythm over several years.

GRADUAL CHANGE OF DIRECTION. Besides the rhythmic behavior in astro-orientation, little is known about regular changes of directions in the course of a day. Some smaller shifts (e.g., Figure 1B; Steidinger, 1968) may be interpreted as incomplete compensation for the movement of celestial cues. Gradual shifts of migratory directions in the course of weeks or months, however, appear to be adaptive and are interpreted as expressions of an endogenous time program (Groot, 1965; Gwinner and Wiltschko, 1978).

Some small directional changes in lower invertebrates and in homing pigeons are reported to be correlated with the lunar cycle (e.g., Brown, 1971; Larkin and Keeton, 1978). The biological context of these phenomena is not yet understood.

PERIODIC CHANGE OF LOCOMOTION

The daily pattern of activity—for instance, its bimodality (Chapter 11)—does not directly affect orientation as long as there is no systematic preference for a certain direction involved. In some instances, such preference may exist (see above), and then, how far the animal moves may depend on the level of activity.

More obvious are directional preferences in the annual cycle of migratory birds, and so the annual bimodality of migratory restlessness *(Zugunruhe)* may well be related to orientation in space. If all—or at least a defined percentage—of the locomotion is done toward the same direction, where the animal arrives depends on its amount. Gwinner (1977) concluded that first-year migrants may reach their wintering grounds on the basis of this kind of vector orientation (cf. Jander, 1963), in which the parameter distance is given as duration and intensity of *Zugunruhe*. Thus, there are indications that both components—distance as well as direction—are incorporated in an endogenous circannual program (see Chapter 21).

Acknowledgments

I am grateful to H. Kacher for drawing the figures, and I thank K. Hoffmann, H. Mittelstaedt, and F. Papi for their critical comments on the manuscript.

REFERENCES

Benvenuti, S. Homing pigeons with prism goggles: An experiment for testing the sun navigation hypothesis. *Monitore Zoologico Italiano (N.S.)*, 1976, *10*, 219–227.

Birukow, G. Aktivitäts- und Orientierungsrhythmik beim Kornkäfer (*Calandra granaria* L.). *Zeitschrift für Tierpsychologie*, 1964, *21*, 279–301.

Braemer, W. A critical review of the sun-azimuth hypothesis. *Cold Spring Harbor Symposia on Quantitative Biology*, 1960, *25*, 413–427.

Braemer, W., and Schwassmann, H. O. Vom Rhythmus der Sonnenorientierung am Äquator (bei Fischen). In H. Autrum *et al.* (Eds.), *Ergebnisse der Biologie.* Vol. 26. Berlin: Springer, 1963, pp. 182–201.

Brown, F. A., Jr. Some orientational influences of nonvisual, terrestrial electromagnetic fields. *Annals of the New York Academy of Sciences,* 1971, *188,* 224–241.

Cloudsley-Thompson, J. L. *Rhythmic Activity in Animal Physiology and Behaviour.* New York: Academic Press, 1961.

Emlen, S. T. Migratory orientation in the Indigo Bunting, *Passerina cyanea. Auk,* 1967, *84,* 309–342 and 463–489.

Emlen, S. T. Bird migration: Influence of physiological state upon celestial orientation. *Science,* 1969, *165,* 716–718.

Emlen, S. T. Migration: Orientation and navigation. In D. S. Farner and J. R. King (Eds.), *Avian Biology.* Vol. 5. New York: Academic Press, 1975, pp. 129–219.

Enright, J. T. When the beachhopper looks at the moon: The moon-compass hypothesis. In S. R. Galler *et al.* (Eds.), *Animal Orientation and Navigation.* Washington, D.C.: NASA SP-262, 1972, pp. 523–555.

Ferguson, D. E. The sensory basis of orientation in amphibians. *Annals of the New York Academy of Sciences,* 1971, *188,* 30–36.

Ferguson, D. E., and Landreth, H. F. Celestial orientation of Fowler's toad, *Bufo fowleri. Behaviour,* 1966, *26,* 105–123.

Fraenkel, G. S., and Gunn, D. L. *The orientation of animals.* Oxford: Oxford University Press, 1940. New edition: New York: Dover, 1961.

Frisch, K. von. *Tanzsprache und Orientierung der Bienen.* Berlin: Springer, 1965. [*The Dance Language and Orientation of Bees.*] Cambridge, Mass.: Harvard University Press, 1967.

Groot, C. On the orientation of young sockeye salmon *(Oncorhynchus nerka)* during their seaward migration out of lakes. *Behaviour,* 1965, *Suppl. 14,* 1–198.

Gwinner, E. Tagesperiodische Schwankungen der Vorzugshelligkeit bei Vögeln. *Zeitschrift für vergleichende Physiologie,* 1966, *52,* 370–379.

Gwinner, E. Orientierung. In E. Schüz, *Grundriss der Vogelzugskunde.* Berlin: Parey, 1971, pp. 299–348.

Gwinner, E. Circannual rhythms in bird migration. *Annual Review of Ecology and Systematics,* 1977, *8,* 381–405.

Gwinner, E., and Wiltschko, W. Endogenously controlled changes in migratory direction of the garden warbler, *Sylvia borin. Journal of Comparative Physiology,* 1978, *125,* 267–273.

Hoffmann, K. Die Einrechnung der Sonnenwanderung bei der Richtungsweisung des sonnenlos aufgezogenen Stares. *Naturwissenschaften,* 1953, *40,* 148.

Hoffmann, K. Die Richtungsorientierung von Staren unter der Mitternachtssonne. *Zeitschrift für vergleichende Physiologie,* 1959, *41,* 471–480.

Hoffmann, K. Experimental manipulation of the orientational clock in birds. *Cold Spring Harbor Symposia on Quantitative Biology,* 1960, *25,* 379–387.

Hoffmann, K. Clock-mechanisms in celestial orientation of animals. In J. Aschoff (Ed.), *Circadian Clocks.* Amsterdam: North-Holland, 1965, pp. 426–441.

Hoffmann, K. Biological clocks in animal orientation and in other functions. *Proceedings of the International Symposium on Circadian Rhythmicity,* Wageningen, 1971, 175–205.

Jander, R. Insect orientation. *Annual Review of Entomology,* 1963, *8,* 95–114.

Keeton, W. T. The orientational and navigational basis of homing in birds. *Advances in the Study of Behavior,* 1974, *5,* 47–132.

Koch, R. Tagesperiodik der Aktivität und der Orientierung nach Wald und Feld von *Drosophila subobscura* und *Drosophila obscura. Zeitschrift für vergleichende Physiologie,* 1967, *54,* 353–394.

Kramer, G. Experiments on bird orientation and their interpretation. *Ibis,* 1957, *99,* 196–227.

Larkin, T., and Keeton, W. T. An apparent lunar rhythm in the day-to-day variations in initial bearings of homing pigeons. In K. Schmidt-Koenig and W. T. Keeton (Eds.), *Animal Migration, Navigation, and Homing.* Berlin: Springer, 1978, pp. 92–106.

Liepa, V. [Orientation of European robin in circular cages under artificial light clues.] In H. Mihelsons, P. Blūms, and J. Baumanis (Eds.), *Orientatsija Ptits* [Bird Orientation]. Riga: Zinātne, 1978, pp. 77–179 (in Russian).

Lindauer, M. Sonnenorientierung der Bienen unter der Äquatorsonne und zur Nachtzeit. *Naturwissenschaften,* 1957, *44,* 1–6.

Lindauer, M. Time-compensated sun orientation in bees. *Cold Spring Harbor Symposia on Quantitative Biology,* 1960, *25,* 371–377.

Lindauer, M. Allgemeine Sinnesphysiologie: Orientierung im Raum. In H. Bauer (Ed.), *Fortschritte der Zoologie.* Vol. 16. Stuttgart: G. Fischer, 1963, pp. 58–140.

Matthews, G. V. T. The astronomical bases of "nonsense" orientation. *Proceedings XIIIth International Ornithological Congress,* Ithaca, N.Y., 1963, 415–429.

Matthews, G. V. T. *Bird Navigation* (2nd ed.). Cambridge, England: Cambridge University Press, 1968.

Mittelstaedt, H. Control systems of orientation in insects. *Annual Review of Entomology,* 1962, *7,* 177–198.

New, D. A. T., and New, J. K. The dances of honeybees at small zenith distances of the sun. *Journal of Experimental Biology,* 1962, *39,* 271–291.

Papi, F., and Pardi, L. Nuovi reperti sull'orientamento lunare di *Talitrus saltator* Montagu (Crustacea Amphipoda). *Zeitschrift für vergleichende Physiologie,* 1959, *41,* 583–596.

Papi, F., and Pardi, L. On the lunar orientation of sandhoppers. *Biological Bulletin,* 1963, *124,* 97–105.

Papi, F., and Syrjämäki, J. The sun-orientation rhythm of wolf spiders at different latitudes. *Archivio Italiano di Biologia,* 1963, *101,* 59–77.

Papi, F., and Tongiorgi, P. Innate and learned components in the astronomical orientation of wolf spiders. In H. Autrum *et al.* (Eds.), *Ergebnisse der Biologie.* Vol. 26. Berlin: Springer, 1963, pp. 259–280.

Papi, F., Serretti, L., and Parrini, S. Nuove ricerche sull' orientamento e il senso del tempo di *Arctosa perita* (Latr.) (Araneae Lycosidae). *Zeitschrift für vergleichende Physiologie,* 1957, *39,* 531–561.

Pardi, L. Über die Orientierung von *Tylos latreillii* Aud. and Sav. (Isopoda terrestria). *Zeitschrift für Tierpsychologie,* 1954, *11,* 175–181.

Pardi, L. Orientamento solare in un Tenebrionide alofilo: *Phaleria provincialis* Fauv. (Coleopt.). *Bollettino dell' Istituto e Museo di Zoologia dell' Università di Torino,* 1955, *5,* 1–39.

Pardi, L. Innate components in the solar orientation of littoral amphipods. *Cold Spring Harbor Symposia on Quantitative Biology,* 1960, *25,* 395–401.

Pardi, L., and Ercolini, A. Ricerche sull'orientamento astronomico di Anfipodi litorali della zona equatoriale. II. L'orientamento lunare in una popolazione somala di *Talorchestia martensii* Weber. *Zeitschrift für vergleichende Physiologie,* 1965, *50,* 225–249.

Pardi, L., and Ercolini, A. Ricerche sull'orientamento astronomico di Anfipodi litorali della zona equatoriale. III. L'orientamento solare in una popolazione di *Talorchestia martensii* Weber a Sud dell'Equatore (4° Lat. S). *Monitore Zoologico Italiano,* 1966, *64 Suppl.,* 80–101.

Pardi, L., and Papi, F. Ricerche sull'orientamento di *Talitrus saltator* (Montagu) (Crustacea-Amphipoda). I. L'orientamento durante il giorno in una popolazione del litorale tirrenico. *Zeitschrift für vergleichende Physiologie,* 1953, *35,* 459–489.

Pettigrew, J. D. A role for the avian pecten oculi in orientation to the sun? In K. Schmidt-Koenig and W. T. Keeton (Eds.), *Animal Migration, Navigation, and Homing.* Berlin: Springer, 1978, pp. 42–54.

Santschi, F. Observations et remarques critiques sur le méchanisme de l'orientation chez les fourmis. *Revue Suisse de Zoologie,* 1911, *19,* 303–338.

Sauer, E. G. F., and Sauer, E. M. Star navigation of nocturnal migrating birds: The 1958 planetarium experiments. *Cold Spring Harbor Symposia on Quantitative Biology,* 1960, *25,* 463–473.

Sauer, F. Die Sternenorientierung nächtlich ziehender Grasmücken *(Sylvia atricapilla, borin* und *curruca).* *Zeitschrift für Tierpsychologie,* 1957, *14,* 29–70.

Schmidt-Koenig, K. Die Sonnenorientierung richtungsdressierter Tauben in ihrer physiologischen Nacht. *Naturwissenschaften,* 1961, *48,* 110.

Schmidt-Koenig, K. Sun compass orientation of pigeons upon displacement north of the arctic circle. *Biological Bulletin,* 1964, *127,* 154–158.

Schmidt-Koenig, K. Current problems in bird orientation. *Advances in the Study of Behavior,* 1965, *1,* 217–278.

Schmidt-Koenig, K. *Migration and Homing in Animals.* Berlin: Springer, 1975.

Schwassmann, H. O., and Braemer, W. The effect of experimentally changed photoperiod on the sun-orientation rhythm of fish. *Physiological Zoology,* 1961, *34,* 273–286.

Schwassmann, H. O., and Hasler, A. D. The role of the sun's altitude in sun orientation of fish. *Physiological Zoology,* 1964, *37,* 163–178.

Steidinger, P. Radarbeobachtungen über die Richtung und deren Streuung beim nächtlichen Vogelzug im Schweizerischen Mittelland. *Der Ornithologische Beobachter,* 1968, *65,* 197–226.

Tongiorgi, P. Effects of the reversal of the rhythm of nycthemeral illumination on astronomical orientation and diurnal activity in *Arctosa variana* C. L. Koch (Araneae-Lycosidae). *Archivio Italiano di Biologia,* 1959, *97,* 251–265.

Tongiorgi, P. Evidence of a moon orientation in the wolf spider *Arctosa variana* C. L. Koch (Araneae, Lycosidae). *Bulletin du Muséum National d'Histoire Naturelle,* 2ᵉ Série, 1970, *41, Suppl. 1,* 243–249.

Wallraff, H. G. Does celestial navigation exist in animals? *Cold Spring Harbor Symposia on Quantitative Biology,* 1960, *25,* 451–461.

Wallraff, H. G. Direction training of birds under a planetarium sky. *Naturwissenschaften,* 1968, *55,* 235–236.

Wallraff, H. G. *Das Navigationssystem der Vögel.* München: Oldenbourg, 1974.

Whiten, A. Operant studies of pigeon orientation and navigation. *Animal Behaviour,* 1978, *26,* 571–610.

Winn, H. E., Salmon, M., and Roberts, N. Sun-compass orientation by parrot fishes. *Zeitschrift für Tierpsychologie,* 1964, *21,* 798–812.

17

The Circadian System of Man

JÜRGEN ASCHOFF AND RÜTGER WEVER

PATTERNS OF RHYTHMS: REPRODUCIBILITY AND DEPENDENCE ON CONDITIONS

As in other vertebrates, the human circadian system is characterized by a distinct temporal order of its components. This order is maintained by the coupling forces between various oscillators as well as by the entraining signals from the zeitgebers (see Chapter 12). There is hardly a tissue or function that has not been shown to have some 24-hr variation. As an example, Figure 1 presents results of an experiment in which six subjects were held in groups of two on the same rigorous schedule. Although there were considerable interindividual differences and also day-to-day variations, patterns like those shown in Figure 1 are satisfactorily reproducible. This reproducibility is again illustrated in Figure 2, which summarizes data on plasma cortisol collected in six laboratories. To account for possible phase-controlling effects of sleep (see below), the curves are normalized with regard to the various sleep times of the subjects. Despite the fact that cortisol, like many other hormones, is secreted in a highly variable sequence of episodes (see Chapter 12, Figure 1), a clear circadian pattern emerges in each curve, averaged from the data on n subjects, and there is perfect correspondence in phase and relative amplitude between the curves. It is noteworthy that two submaxima appear in all curves at about the same circadian phases. Presumably, they are not consequences of the usual meal timing but may represent a rhythm component interposed between the circadian domain and the episodes (cf. the discussion in Aschoff, 1979).

As another example, the rhythms of three psychomotor performances are reproduced in Figure 3. The curves differ slightly in pattern (e.g., in their ascending slopes), but they

JÜRGEN ASCHOFF AND RÜTGER WEVER   Max-Planck-Institut für Verhaltensphysiologie, 8131 Andechs, West Germany.

agree with regard to the range of oscillation, which amounts to only about 10–20% of the 24-hr mean, in strong contrast to the roughly 200% of plasma cortisol (Figure 2).

Circadian rhythms in physiological and psychological functions are influenced by the alternation of wakefulness and sleep (activity and rest), but they are not caused by it. They can be observed in subjects who observe strict bed rest, as well as during prolonged sleep deprivation. The three curves of rectal temperature reproduced in Figure 4 are averaged from data obtained in several laboratories; they can be considered representative of the various conditions. As compared with the "standard curve" from subjects who slept at night and pursued "normal" activities during daytime, the two experimentally altered curves have smaller ranges of oscillation—the curve for bed rest because of a decrease in the day values, and the curve for sleep deprivation because of an elevation in the night values. In

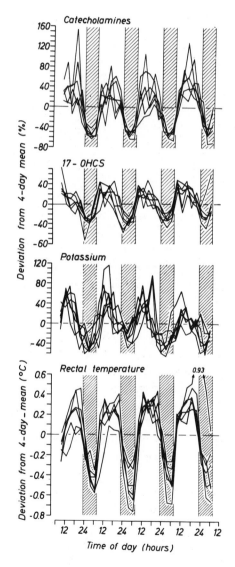

Fig. 1. Circadian rhythms of three urine constituents and of rectal temperature in six subjects on the same strict routine for 4 days. Shaded area: sleep in darkness. (From Aschoff: "Circadian Rhythms." In D. Krieger (Ed.), *Endocrine Rhythms,* © 1979, Raven Press, New York. Reprinted with permission.)

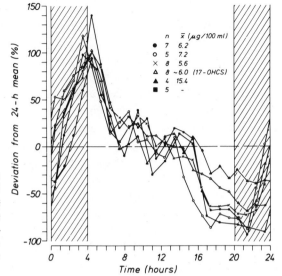

Fig. 2. Circadian rhythm of plasma cortisol in man. Each curve averaged from n subjects. $\bar{x}$ = 24-hr mean. Shaded area: approximate sleep time. (For reference sources, see Figure 27 in Aschoff, 1979.) (From Aschoff: "Circadian Rhythms." In D. Krieger (Ed.), *Endocrine Rhythms,* © 1979, Raven Press, New York. Reprinted with permission.)

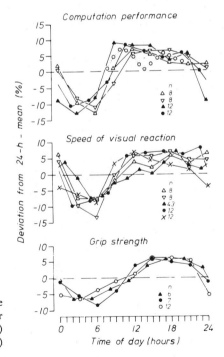

Fig. 3. Circadian rhythms in three performances. Each curve averaged from n subjects. Dotted line: schoolchildren. (For reference sources, see Figure 12 in Aschoff and Wever, 1980.) (Reprinted with permission of Springer-Verlag, Heidelberg.)

contrast to temperature and other physiological variables, rhythms in performance may show the same range on days with and without sleep (cf. Figure 3 in Aschoff, 1980a) or even a larger range during sleep deprivation, because of a decrease in the night values. On the other hand, there are variables such as some hormones whose secretion is largely "triggered" by sleep (e.g., growth hormone) and hence shows no rhythm during the first 24 hr of sleep deprivation (cf. Aschoff, 1979, pp. 35, 41).

Under normal conditions, all circadian rhythms maintain distinct phase-relationship to the sleep–wake cycle. Furthermore, a shift of sleep time is usually followed by a shift of other rhythms (for a review, see Aschoff, Hoffmann, Pohl, and Wever, 1975). From these two observations, it has often been concluded that sleep is a major phase determinant for the circadian system. Such a statement ought to be qualified for several reasons:

1. The environment normally contains a variety of zeitgebers, all of which may contribute to the entrainment of the circadian system. It is not yet clear to what extent various oscillating units within the organism can be reached independently by different zeitgebers (see Chapter 12), but there is evidence that, for example, the rhythm of body temperature can be entrained by a zeitgeber while at the same time the rhythm of wakefulness and sleep is freerunning ("partial entrainment," see Figure 13).

2. Each zeitgeber not only influences the primary oscillators (pacemakers) that basically constitute the circadian system but also affects the overt rhythms in a more direct way that has no (immediate) bearing on phase control but, rather, masks it (see Chapter 6, Figure 10).

3. Abrupt changes can be observed in rhythmic functions after waking up or falling asleep. Many of these effects resemble those of masking by a zeitgeber, for example, the decrease in body temperature whenever a subject falls asleep, and the increase whenever he becomes active. Hence, changes in posture or the change from wakefulness to sleep and vice versa can produce changes in the waveform of rhythms that do not reflect control of phase.

Phase control by sleep has been suggested as a result of the fact that interindividual variability in patterns decreases when the rhythms of several subjects are standardized with

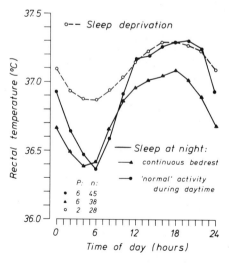

Fig. 4. Standard pattern of human rectal temperature in sleep-deprived subjects and in subjects with about 8 hr of sleep either kept in bed for 24 hr or pursuing "normal" activities during daytime. (From Aschoff, 1980a. Reprinted with permission of the editor and the publisher.)

reference to their various sleep times instead of local time (cf. Figure 6 in Aschoff, 1980a). This argument does not hold up completely because the same reduction in variability can probably be achieved by using the rhythm of temperature as a reference. Furthermore, a delay in the acrophases of autonomic rhythms seen during sleep deprivation (cf. Figures 7 and 8 in Aschoff, 1978a) does not necessarily indicate a true shift in phase because of changes in waveform that occur when the masking effects of sleep are excluded (Wever, 1979a, p. 225). Phase control by sleep, however, has been demonstrated by the shift of rhythms in subjects who reversed their sleep times in constant conditions with continuous illumination (Krieger, Kreuzer, and Rizzo, 1969).

By means of sleep displacement, some of the (masking) effects of sleep and activity can be shown to depend on the phase of the circadian system. This has been demonstrated for decreases in rectal temperature due to 4-hr naps at different times of day (Mills, Minors, and Waterhouse, 1978; cf. Figure 8 in Aschoff, 1980a). In view of these findings, and the effects of sleep on range of oscillation (see Figure 4) and phase, it has often been assumed that the interaction between the sleep–wake cycle and other components of the circadian system is unidirectional. It is, however, equally likely that the rhythms of autonomic functions may act on the sleep–wake cycle. This possibility is strikingly documented by the observation that duration of sleep depends on the phase of the temperature rhythm (see Figure 12). Similarly, it has been shown that the structure of sleep, monitored during arbitrarily placed naps, is a function of the time of day (see Chapter 26). In summary, then, there is increasing evidence that various components of the circadian system can affect each other mutually. It is this bidirectional interaction that complicates the analysis of the system (see Chapter 12).

Freerunning Rhythms

When isolated in soundproof experimental units and deprived of all time cues, human subjects usually show freerunning rhythms with periods somewhat longer than 24 hr. The interindividual variability is remarkably small. Within a sample of 147 subjects, the overall mean of the period, measured in the rhythm of rectal temperature, was found to be 25.0 hr with a standard deviation of only ±0.50 hr (Wever, 1979a). The period of a freerunning rhythm is furthermore quite independent of conditions, as illustrated in Figure 5. The left diagram shows results of a "standard experiment," with constant conditions throughout the 24 days. In the middle diagram, it can be seen that the rhythm remained unchanged when bright illumination of the unit was replaced by continuous darkness during the last 10 days. The right diagram demonstrates that a change from leisure activity (first 11 days) to heavy work on a bicycle ergometer (seven 20-min work sessions at 100 W daily) also had no effect on the period of the freerunning rhythm. There are still exceptions to those rules: a change in light intensity can either shorten or lengthen the period by small amounts (Wever, 1973), and ergometer work sometimes lengthens the period (Webb and Agnew, 1974; Wever, 1979b). Nevertheless, on the average, these factors have little if any effect on the period. Other conditions have been found to interfere with the freerunning rhythm in a systematic manner. The period was lengthened in subjects who had been given the chance to select for themselves a light–dark cycle (Wever, 1969) or a cycle of higher and lower room temperature (Wever, 1974). In addition, the period was shortened under the influence of a weak electric AC field of 10 Hz (Wever, 1971). Most of these changes remain within narrow limits, and the predominant impression one gets is that the system is extremely stable.

The internal temporal order of a freerunning circadian system differs from that of a system entrained to 24 hr. Under normal conditions, the maxima of rectal temperature occur in late afternoon, and the minima during the second half of sleep time. In the freerunning system, these two extrema are advanced relative to the sleep–wake cycle by several hours (see the position of the triangles within the first few cycles in each of the records in Figure 5). As a consequence, temperature mainly decreases during wakefulness and increases during sleep, in strong contrast to the pattern found in a normally entrained system. These changes in the internal phase-relationship, which are illustrated for a variety of functions in Figure 6, contradict the hypothesis of a simple cause-and-effect relationship between the activity rhythm and other rhythmic functions within the organism. They indicate rather that the various rhythms are coupled to (driven by) different circadian oscillators, which change their phase relationship according to the conditions.

Freerunning, internally synchronized rhythms are further characterized by a negative correlation between the duration of activity time (α) and rest time (ρ) (see Chapter 6, Figure 3). Such a negative correlation is not surprising under normal conditions where the time for getting up is usually fixed. A subject consequently gets less sleep after having stayed awake longer than usual. In a freerunning rhythm, under conditions of isolation without time cues, the negative correlation is not a necessary consequence of routine and needs to be explained. It disagrees with expectations based on the assumption that sleep is a restoring process whose duration is determined by the duration of prior wakefulness. A negative correlation between α and ρ is, however, compatible with and even demanded by a model in which onset of wakefulness and sleep are determined by the crossings of a basic circadian oscillation through a threshold (see Figure 7 in Aschoff, Gerecke, Kureck, Pohl, Rieger, Saint Paul, and Wever, 1971). It finally has to be mentioned that in freerunning rhythms, successive cycles of activity and rest or of body temperature are negatively correlated with each other, indicating that the overt rhythms are driven by self-sustaining oscillations of pacemakers (Wever, 1979a, p. 41).

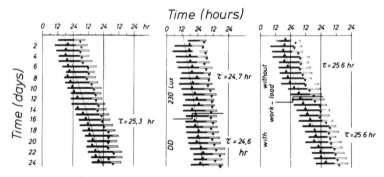

Fig. 5. Circadian rhythms of wakefulness and sleep (black and white bars) and of rectal temperature (triangles above bars for maxima, below bars for minima), recorded in three subjects, each of which lived alone in an isolation unit. *(Left)* constant conditions; *(middle)* change from continuous illumination to darkness (DD); *(right)* change from a leisurely routine to work 7 times daily on a bicycle ergometer. τ: circadian period. (From Aschoff, 1978a. Reprinted with permission of Taylor & Francis, Ltd., London, England.)

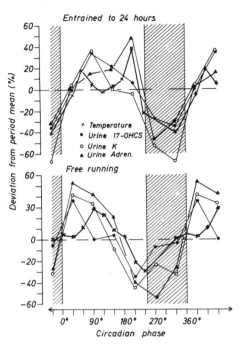

Fig. 6. Circadian rhythms of rectal temperature and of three urine constituents in an isolated subject during entrainment to 24 hr (above) and when freerunning with a period of 26 hr (below). Shaded area: sleep. (Data from Kriebel, 1974.)

ENTRAINMENT BY ARTIFICIAL ZEITGEBERS

In contrast to the majority of other organisms, human subjects are not readily entrained by light–dark cycles as long as they are in a choice situation, that is, not "immobilized" by total darkness when the main lights in the isolation unit are turned off (Wever, 1970). If they are allowed the use of small reading lamps, subjects seem to prefer a freerunning rhythm, crossing through the zeitgeber with a period longer than 24 hr despite the unpleasantness that on some days, they have to sleep in bright light and to stay awake in a dimly illuminated room (Figure 7A). Under such conditions, some effects of the (nonentraining) zeitgeber still remain, as indicated by the occurrence of relative coordination, that is, slight modulations of the mean period.

To make a light–dark cycle in the presence of reading lamps an effective zeitgeber, it suffices to provide an additional time structure, for example, by offering gong signals in regular intervals. The signals call the subject to collect his urine, and they are perceived by him, contrary to the light–dark cycle, as a more direct and "social" contact with the experimenter. By means of such zeitgebers, human circadian rhythms have been entrained also to periods other than 24 hr. The example given in Figure 7B shows entrainment to a 24-hr as well as to a 26.7-hr day and failure of entrainment to a 22.7-hr day. As was to be expected, the subject who was a "late riser" in the 24-hr day became an "early riser" in the lengthened day. Interestingly enough, he was not aware of the change in lighting conditions and of his change in habit up to Day 20, when, to his surprise, he woke up for the first time before the lights were turned on. It further should be noted that again, relative coordination became apparent at the end of the experiment when the rhythms lost entrainment and crossed through the zeitgeber.

JÜRGEN ASCHOFF
AND RÜTGER WEVER

In a series of experiments with such relatively weak zeitgebers, it has been found that the limits of the range of entrainment (see Chapter 6) are reached when the zeitgeber period approaches 23 or 27 hr. Within this range, all rhythms change their phase-angle difference, ψ, to the zeitgeber in a systematic manner. As indicated in Figure 8 by the two dashed lines, the change in ψ due to a 1-hr change in period is larger for the temperature rhythm than for the activity rhythm. In other words, there is a steady change in the internal phase-relationship between the two variables from short to long days, as indicated in Figure 8 by the solid lines. This observation supports again the hypothesis that the two overt rhythms are mainly driven by different pacemakers. From the difference in slope between the two dashed lines, it can be further assumed that the two rhythms (or the pacemakers to which they are coupled) differ in their range of entrainment (cf. Aschoff and Pohl, 1978). This conclusion is supported by the observation that in two of five subjects whose activity

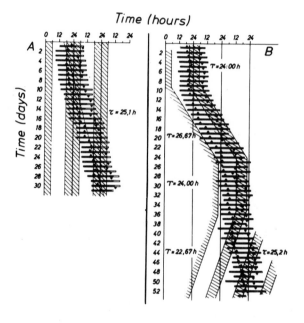

Fig. 7. Circadian rhythms of wakefulness and sleep (black and white bars) and of rectal temperature (triangles for maxima and minima) in two isolated subjects (A) and (B), who were exposed to light–dark cycles (LD; shaded area: darkness) but had reading lamps at their disposal. (A) only LD; (B) LD supplemented by regular gong signals. τ: circadian period. T: zeitgeber period. (For reference sources, see Figure 5 in Aschoff, 1978a.) (Reprinted with permission of Taylor & Francis, Ltd., London, England.)

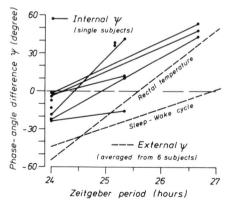

Fig. 8. Phase-angle differences between circadian rhythms and the zeitgeber (dashed lines), as well as between the two circadian rhythms (solid lines and closed circles), measured in six isolated subjects during entrainment to light–dark cycles (supplemented by gong signals) with periods varying between 24 and 26.6 hr.

rhythms remained entrained to a 26.7-hr day, the rhythms of rectal temperature were free-running. Similarly, entrainment to a 22.7-hr day could be achieved only for the activity rhythm and not for the temperature rhythm in one of the five subjects tested. These results demonstrate that the circadian system can be split into components that run with different frequencies, a state that is called *internal desynchronization*. In the cases just mentioned, internal desynchronization was associated with "partial entrainment," that is, with the entrainment of one rhythm while the other one was freerunning. These phenomena are discussed in more detail in the following section.

INTERNAL DESYNCHRONIZATION AND PARTIAL ENTRAINMENT

Entrainment to non-24-hr days by means of a weak zeitgeber as described above (light–dark cycle and gong signals, with additional reading lamps available) resulted in internal desynchronization only occasionally. It is, however, easy to enforce desynchronization in every subject by applying a "strong" zeitgeber, that is, by not providing reading lamps. Under such conditions, the subject can hardly do anything as long as the room is dark and hence is more-or-less forced to adjust his activity–rest cycle to the light–dark cycle. Consequently, it is possible to entrain the rhythm of wakefulness and sleep to periods of 28 and even up to 32 hr, as demonstrated in Figure 9. These periods are beyond the limits of entrainment for the rhythm of rectal temperature. As indicated in the top diagram of Figure 9 by the triangles, the temperature rhythm remained entrained only in the 24-hr day and freeran with a mean period of 24.8 hr in the 28-hr as well as in the 32-hr day. The simultaneously measured rhythm of computation speed (see the solid lines that connect acrophases) remained synchronized with the temperature rhythm in the 28-hr day, and with the activity rhythm in the 32-hr day. The period analysis of the time series (Figure 9, lower diagram) reveals that during internal desynchronization, the temperature rhythm contains two frequency components, a major one with $\tau = 24.8$ hr, and a minor one corresponding to the respective zeitgeber periods. In the performance rhythm, two frequencies are present in the 28-hr day, but only the zeitgeber period in the 32-hr day. Like others, these findings disagree with the often advanced hypothesis that performance rhythms are causally related to the body temperature (see Chapter 18).

If the period of a strong zeitgeber is lengthened steadily in small steps (e.g., by 10 min per day), various autonomic and performance rhythms do not become separated from the zeitgeber simultaneously. It is generally the rule rather than the exception that the rhythm of rectal temperature splits away first, and other rhythms only after a substantial further lengthening of the zeitgeber period. These observations support the idea that various rhythmic functions differ in their ranges of entrainment. Thus, forced "fractional" desynchronization may become one of the tools used to disentangle components of the circadian system (Wever, 1980a).

While internal desynchronization can always be enforced by means of a strong zeitgeber, it may also occur in freerunning rhythms spontaneously (Aschoff, 1965). As illustrated in Figure 10, this can happen by a sudden lengthening (above) or shortening (below) of the activity rhythm. These two types of internal desynchronization also differ in other respects. The system in which desynchronization occurs by a lengthening of the activity rhythm has, prior to desynchronization, a relatively long period, and its temperature rhythm is slightly shortened after desynchronization. The converse applies to the system in which the activity cycle suddenly shortens: when still synchronized with each other, the common period of the two rhythms is relatively short, and the period of the temperature rhythm is slightly lengthened after desynchronization. The mean values of such measures, derived from 26 experiments, are given in Table I. These findings suggest that two oscillators (two classes of oscillators) exist with different characteristics and of different importance for the overt rhythms (Wever, 1975). The oscillator that mainly controls the activity rhythm is highly variable in frequency, and the other one, which mainly controls the temperature rhythm, is hardly variable. When coupled to each other, the two oscillators have to compromise on a common period, which, because of the difference in variability, is much closer to that of the temperature rhythm than of the activity rhythm. Coupling is lost—and desynchronization occurs—when the activity rhythm lengthens or shortens its period beyond the limits of entrainability by the temperature rhythm.

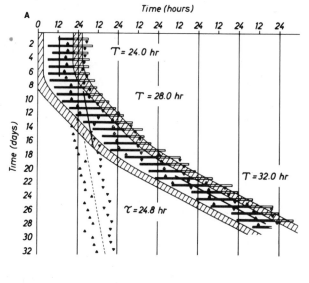

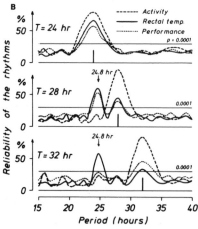

Fig. 9. (A) Circadian rhythms of wakefulness and sleep (black and white bars), of rectal temperature (triangles for maxima and minima), and of computation speed (solid line connecting the acrophases) in a subject exposed to a light–dark cycle (shaded area: darkness) without reading lamps. T: zeitgeber period. τ: circadian period. (B) Period analysis (reliability below 30%: random fluctuations). (From Wever, 1980b. Reprinted with permission of the editor and the publisher.)

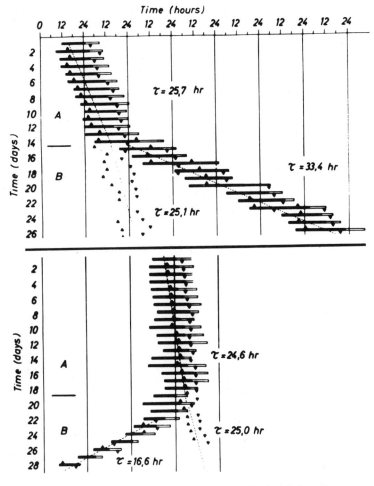

Fig. 10. Circadian rhythms of wakefulness and sleep (black and white bars), and of rectal temperature (triangles for maxima and minima) in two singly isolated subjects. (A) Internal synchronization. (B) Spontaneous internal desynchronization. τ: circadian period. (From Aschoff and Wever, 1976. Reprinted with permission of the Federation of American Societies for Experimental Biology.)

TABLE I. MEAN PERIODS FOR THE RHYTHMS OF ACTIVITY AND RECTAL TEMPERATURE BEFORE AND AFTER INTERNAL DESYNCHRONIZATION

	Desynchronization by shortening ($n = 11$)	Desynchronization by lengthening ($n = 15$)
Circadian period (hr):		
Before desynchronization		
Activity and temperature	24.47 ± 0.15	25.55 ± 0.46
After desynchronization		
Temperature	24.88 ± 0.13	24.85 ± 0.30
Activity	17.91 ± 1.00	34.04 ± 2.3

Two circadian oscillators that can entrain each other and that differ in the range of entrainment are normally entrained in a 1:1 ratio of their frequencies. Still, entrainment in 1:2 ratio should also be possible. Such "synchronization by demultiplication" has, in fact, been observed in a few instances (Aschoff, Gerecke, and Wever, 1967a). If during internal desynchronization the period of the activity rhythm reaches values that are close to half or twice that of the temperature rhythm, mutual entrainment can again occur. This state of "apparent desynchronization" (Wever, 1967) is of special interest for extremely long activity rhythms with a τ value of about 50 hr because such a "circa-bi-dian" period implies that on the average, the subject is awake continuously for 35 hr and asleep for 15 hr. An example is given in the lowermost diagram of Figure 11 with data from an experiment in which electroencephalographic recordings were made during sleep. The diagram clearly demonstrates that two cycles of the temperature rhythm coincide with each cycle of wakefulness and sleep. For comparison, Figure 11 also gives examples of the two other possible states of a freerunning rhythm: true internal desynchronization (middle) and internal synchronization (above).

The reasons for internal desynchronization are not yet understood. Within a sample of 159 subjects (44 females, 115 males) who were studied in constant conditions, true internal desynchronization has been observed in 24% and apparent internal desynchronization in 8%. There was no difference between the sexes (34% females, 31% males). On the other hand, the tendency toward true internal desynchronization seems to increase with age above 40 years: it occurred in 22% of the younger subjects (17 to 34 years old) and in 70% of the older ones (41 to 71 years old) (Wever, 1979a). Within the group of younger subjects, no dependence on age could be detected. There was, however, a significantly higher incidence

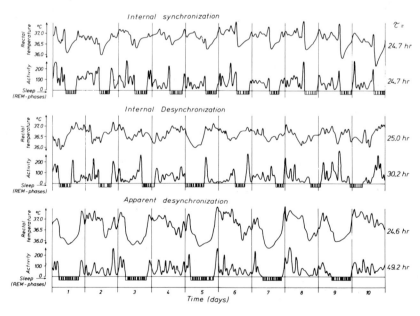

Fig. 11. Rhythms of rectal temperature and of activity, recorded (together with EEG during sleep) in three singly isolated subjects. τ: circadian period (circa-bi-dian in the lowermost activity record). (From Wever, 1979c. Reprinted with permission of Hoffman-La Roche, Grenzach-Wyhlen.)

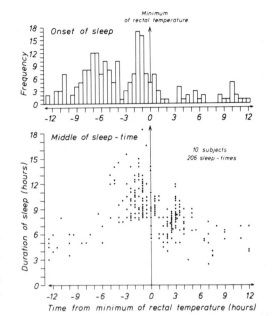

Fig. 12. Onset and duration of sleep, taken from 10 subjects who showed internal desynchronization during a freerun in isolation. The times for onset and middle of sleep, respectively, are drawn with reference to the phase of the rhythm of rectal temperature (zero at the abscissa = temperature minimum). (From Aschoff, 1980a. Reprinted with permission of the editor and the publisher.)

of true internal desynchronization among those who had relatively high scores in tests for neuroticism (Lund, 1974).

When internally desynchronized, the activity rhythm and the rhythm of rectal temperature cross through each other continuously. Consequently, sleep coincides on successive days with different phases of the temperature rhythm. This phenomenon enables one to analyze effects of temperature on sleep in a specific way. As shown in the lower half of Figure 12, duration of sleep strongly depends on the phase of the temperature rhythm: long sleep times coincide with decreasing temperatures (hours prior to the minimum of temperature), short sleep times with increasing and high temperatures. Equally striking is the nonrandom, bimodal distribution of sleep onsets. Of the two maxima in the frequency histogram (Figure 12, upper part), the first one coincides with a phase of the temperature rhythm (about 6–7 hr before the minimum) where onset of sleep is likely to occur in subjects synchronized to 24 hr (Aschoff, Gerecke, and Wever, 1967b). The second peak in the histogram coincides approximately with that phase of the temperature where it is most difficult to stay awake under normal conditions and at which it is likely that onset of sleep occurs in subjects whose rhythms are freerunning but remain internally synchronized (cf. Figure 6).

During internal desynchronization, the rhythms of autonomic functions usually show periods close to 25 hr in all subjects whose rhythms are freerunning in constant conditions. However, desynchronization may occur as well in the presence of a plain light–dark cycle, which seldom entrains a freerunning activity rhythm efficiently. In several such instances, it has been observed that the desynchronized rhythm of rectal temperature became entrained by the zeitgeber instead of freerunning. Three examples of such "partial entrainment" are provided in Figure 13. In each of the three individuals, the freerunning rhythms remained internally synchronized for 10–12 days (section A). After internal desynchronization had taken place by lengthening of the activity cycle (section B), the rhythm of rectal temperature locked onto the light–dark cycle, with the maxima occurring near lights-off and the minima around lights-on. In one of the subjects (lowermost diagram), entrainment of the temperature rhythms lasted for 10 days, after which the rhythm started to freerun with a period of 25.8 hr (section C). These findings demonstrate again that a light–dark cycle can be a powerful zeitgeber for parts of the system. They also indicate that a given zeitgeber differs in its effectiveness in entraining various components of the system. There are three possibilities for an interpretation of these results: (1) the light–dark cycle reaches the pacemaker that drives the temperature rhythm, but not the pacemaker driving the activity rhythm; (2) the pacemaker driving the activity rhythm is also reached by light but

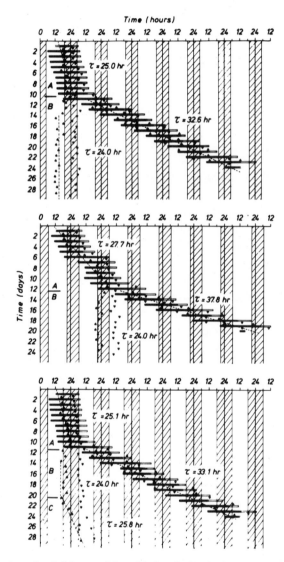

Fig. 13. Circadian rhythms of wakefulness and sleep (black and white bars) and of rectal temperature (triangles for maxima and minima) in three subjects, singly isolated and exposed to light–dark cycles (shaded area: darkness) with reading lamps available. Spontaneous change from internal synchronization (A) to desynchronization (B and C) τ: circadian period. (From Wever, 1980b. Reprinted with permission of the editor and the publisher.)

is less responsive than the pacemaker driving the temperature rhythm; and (3) both pacemakers are equally responsive to light, but the activity rhythm, because of its desynchronized long period, has gone out of the range of entrainment by light. More data are needed to differentiate among these possibilities.

SHIFT EXPERIMENTS AND FLIGHTS

Shifts of zeitgebers (see Chapter 6) and transmeridian flights provide an opportunity to study the kinetics of circadian systems in a transient state. Representative results from both types of experiments are reproduced in Figure 14. It shows rhythms of rectal temperature before and after 6-hr shifts of a light–dark cycle in the isolation unit (curves a and c) as well as before and after flights across six time zones (curves b and d). In each case, the abscissa represents local time before the shift or flight. To indicate the slow course of reentrainment, small downward arrows mark the minima of temperature as they occur in each cycle, and upward arrows the time at which the minima are expected to occur after the completion of entrainment. The effects of delays and advances differ mainly in one circadian parameter: the range of oscillation remains nearly unchanged after the delays (upper two curves) but is drastically reduced after the advances (lower two curves). On theoretical grounds it could be expected that the rate of reentrainment is correlated with changes in the range of oscillation: a larger reduction is likely to result in a faster shift (Wever, 1980a). This prediction is confirmed by both sets of data used for Figure 14, although in the case of the flights, the conclusion is less convincing because of difficulties in determining the exact rate of reentrainment in absolute time (cf. the discussion in Aschoff *et al.*, 1975, p. 69, and in Wever, 1980c).

Rates of reentrainment after shifts in different directions may safely be compared if the same technique is applied to the analysis of all data. Thus, daily acrophases were computed for each of the subjects whose average curves are displayed in Figure 14. Rates of

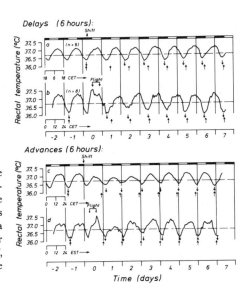

Fig. 14. Rhythms of rectal temperature measured before and after a 6-hr phase shift of the zeitgeber in an isolation unit (curves a and c; white and black bars for the light–dark cycle) and flights across six time zones (curves b and d). Arrows are drawn at the minima (downward) and where they are expected to occur after complete reentrainment (upward). (From Aschoff, 1980a. Reprinted with permission of the editor and the publisher.)

reentrainment were then estimated from the shift of acrophases. The results are reproduced in Figure 15. Both types of experiments reveal a positive correlation between the preflight range of oscillation in rectal temperature and the time needed for two-thirds reentrainment to occur; the correlation is stronger for advances than for delays. In accordance with these findings, a negative correlation has been seen in shift workers between the range of oscillation and the amount of shift after the first day of night work (Reinberg, Vieux, Ghata, Chaumont, and Laporte, 1978). The conclusion seems justified that the range of oscillation can be used as a measure of "oscillatory strength," that is, of the resistance of the oscillation against exogenous manipulations.

During reentrainment, all circadian rhythms may move in a direction that corresponds with that of the shift in zeitgebers or the flight. However, it can also happen that the circadian system is split into two components that move in opposite directions. This effect is illustrated in Figure 16 by the results from an experiment carried out in the isolation unit. After a 6-hr advance shift of the zeitgeber on Day 10, the rhythm of wakefulness and sleep was advanced by 6 hr, but the rhythm of temperature was delayed by 18 hr; the delay shift on Day 21 was followed by delays in both rhythms. In the right half of Figure 16, the period analysis from 7-day sections of the temperature record demonstrates that on Days 11–17 the period was substantially longer than 24 hr (Wever, 1980c). Such a "reentrainment by partition" (Aschoff, 1978b) seems to be more likely to occur after advance shifts (eastbound flights) than after delay shifts (westbound flights), and its probability increases with the extent of the shift (the number of time zones crossed). Mills and co-workers (1978a) tested 127 subjects in an isolation unit after 8-hr shifts; they observed reentrainment by partition in about 78% of the cases after advance shifts, but in only about 20% after delay shifts. (For a summary, see Figure 17 in Aschoff, 1980a.)

The transient state of reentrainment is always characterized by temporal disorder within the organism, either because different rhythms are shifted at a different rate or, more dramatically, because of partitioning. It is likely that this disorder contributes to performance decrements (cf. Figure 40 in Aschoff et al., 1975) and to indispositions observed

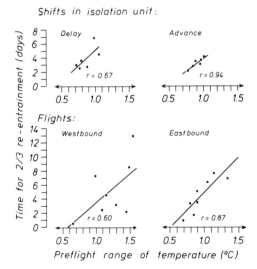

Fig. 15. Duration of two-thirds reentrainment after a 6-hr zeitgeber shift in the isolation unit or after flights across six time zones, drawn as a function of the range of oscillation measured in the rhythm of rectal temperature before shift or flight. (From Aschoff, 1980a. Reprinted with permission of the editor and the publisher.)

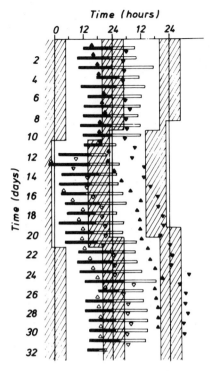
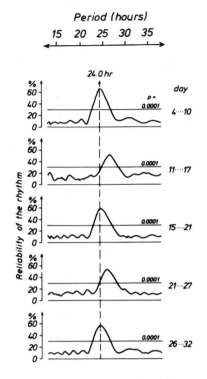

Fig. 16. Shift of circadian rhythms in a subject in an isolation unit exposed to a light–dark cycle (shaded area: darkness) and to gong signals, with reading lamps available. White and black bars for wakefulness and sleep, triangles for maxima and minima of temperature (open triangles: double plot). Period analysis of the temperature data for 7-day intervals (reliability below 30%: random fluctuations). (From Wever, 1980c. Reprinted with permission of Casa Editrice "Il Ponte," Milan.)

after flights. The question to what extent repeated shifts or flights may result in more harmful effects, remains to be answered (for effects in animals, see Chapter 6). The problem is related to those of shift workers who usually live in a situation of conflict between partially shifted and partially nonshifted zeitgebers. Therefore, their circadian system is seldom adjusted to the working hours, and it seems that changes seen in the waveform of overt rhythms reflect masking effects rather than true shifts (Aschoff, 1980a; see also additional recommended readings on p. 331).

APPLICATION TO PROBLEMS IN MEDICINE

Although of minor importance within the framework of behavioral neurobiology, brief mention should be made of two areas where the circadian time structure has become of special interest in medical practice. In recent years, a large body of data has been accumulated on this subject that can be treated in only a very selective way; for more detailed information, recommended readings are added to the list of references (p. 331).

The response of an organism to any stimulus usually depends on circadian phase in a systematic manner. In medicine, such rhythms of responsiveness are of relevance with regard to the action of drugs. Quite impressively, this was first demonstrated by Halberg and co-workers in 1959. The mortality of mice due to an intraperitoneal injection of *E. coli* endotoxin is 80% toward the end of the rest time of the animals, but below 20% in the middle of the activity time (Figure 17, left). Similarly, a given dose of ethyl alcohol kills 60% of the animals at the beginning of the activity time, but only about 20% at the beginning of the rest time (Figure 17, right). For man, phase-dependent differences in drug effectiveness are also well documented. As an example, Figure 18 shows the 24-hr variation in duration of anesthesia, and the threshold for pain reaction, measured in a tooth after the application of a cold or an electric stimulus, respectively. (NOTE: It seems preferable to go to the dentist after lunch rather than in the morning.) An increasing number of studies on rhythms of sensitivity to drugs has opened the new area of chronopharmacology (reviews in Reinberg and Halberg, 1971, and Scheving, Mayersbach, and Pauly, 1974), and chronotherapy may soon become of general usage after its start in endocrinology with the properly timed administration of corticosteroids (cf. Aschoff, Ceresa, and Halberg, 1974). Possibilities for chronotherapy in other fields (such as cancer) have been discussed, for example, in view of positive effects in the treatment of mouse leukemia with arabinosylcytosine according to a circadian protocol (Haus, Halberg, Scheving, and Simpson, 1979).

The circadian time structure also has to be taken into account for diagnostic purposes. Whenever reference values are used to differentiate between a normal and a pathological state, it must be assured that measurements are made at the same circadian phase at which reference values were taken. In many instances, it may also be appropriate to forget about reference values and instead to introduce the concept of circadian reference patterns (cf. Aschoff and Wever, 1980). The elaboration of circadian standard pattern, as they are now available (e.g., for some hormones; Aschoff, 1979), allows one to test whether certain diseases are characterized by distinct abnormalities in temporal order. In this context, internal desynchronization must be considered not only as a symptom but also as a possible cause of a diseased condition, especially in psychiatry (cf. Aschoff, 1980b). This whole area of symptomatic and ethological chronomedicine, though of potential importance, is still undeveloped.

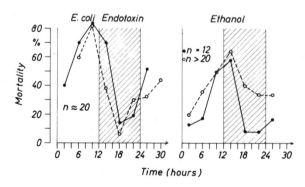

Fig. 17. Circadian rhythms of mortality in mice, kept in light–dark cycles (shaded area: darkness), due to an ip injection of *E. coli* endotoxin (100 μg/20 g body weight) or of ethanol (0.8 ml, 25% solution). Replicate experiments. (Data sources: left, Halberg *et al.*, 1960; right, Haus and Halberg, 1959.)

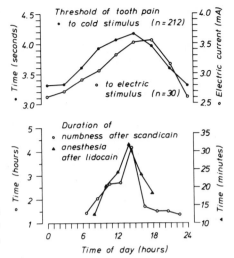

Fig. 18. Variation in the threshold of tooth pain and in the duration of local anesthesia in the jaw. (Data from: ▲ Reinberg and Reinberg, 1977; ● and ○ Pöllmann, 1977, and personal communication.)

Acknowledgment

This chapter is dedicated to Professor Dr. Detlov Ploog on the occasion of his 60th birthday.

REFERENCES

Aschoff, J. Circadian rhythms in man. *Science,* 1965, *148,* 1427–1432.

Aschoff, J. Features of circadian rhythms relevant for the design of shift schedules. *Ergonomics,* 1978a, *39,* 739–754.

Aschoff, J. Problems of re-entrainment of circadian rhythms: Asymmetry effect, dissociation and partition. In I. Assenmacher and D. Farner (Eds.), *Environmental Endocrinology.* Berlin–Heidelberg–New York: Springer-Verlag, 1978b, pp. 185–195.

Aschoff, J. Circadian rhythms: General features and endocrinological aspects. In D. Krieger (Ed.), *Endocrine Rhythms.* New York: Raven Press, 1979, pp. 1–61.

Aschoff, J. Circadian rhythms: Interference with and dependence on workrest schedules. In L. C. Johnson, D. I. Tepas, W. P. Colquhoun, and M. J. Colligan (Eds.), *The 24 Hour Workday. A Symposium on Variations in Work-Sleep Schedules.* Washington, D. C.: National Institute for Occupational Safety and Health, 1980a.

Aschoff, J. Wie gestört ist der circadiane Rhythmus bei Depressiven? In H. Heimann (Ed.), *Neue Strategien in der Depressionsforschung.* Symp. auf der Weitenburg, 1980b.

Aschoff, J., and Pohl, H. Phase relations between a circadian rhythm and its zeitgeber within the range of entrainment. *Naturwissenschaften,* 1978, *65,* 80–84.

Aschoff, J., and Wever, R. Human circadian rhythms: A multioscillator system. *Federation Proceedings,* 1976, *35,* 2326–2332.

Aschoff, J., and Wever, R. Über Reproduzierbarkeit circadianer Rhythmen beim Menschen. *Klinische Wochenschrift,* 1980.

Aschoff, J., Gerecke, U., and Wever, R. Desynchronization of human circadian rhythms. *Japanese Journal of Physiology,* 1967a, *17,* 450–457.

Aschoff, J., Gerecke, U., and Wever, R. Phasenbeziehungen zwischen den circadianen Perioden der Aktivität und der Kerntemperatur beim Menschen. *Pflügers Archiv,* 1967a, *295,* 173–183.

Aschoff, J., Gerecke, U., Kureck, A., Pohl, H., Rieger, P., Saint Paul, U. von, and Wever, R. Interdependent parameters of circadian activity rhythms in birds and man. In M. Menaker (Ed.), *Biochronometry.* Washington, D.C.: National Academy of Sciences, 1971, pp. 3–27.

Aschoff, J., Ceresa, F., and Halberg, F. (Eds.). Chronobiological aspects of endocrinology. *Chronobiologia*, 1974, *1* (Supplement 1).

Aschoff, J., Hoffmann, K., Pohl, H., and Wever, R. Re-entrainment of circadian rhythms after phase shifts of the zeitgeber. *Chronobiologia*, 1975, *2*, 23–78.

Halberg, F., Johnson, E. A., Brown, B. W., and Bittner, J. J. Susceptibility rhythm to *E. coli* endotoxin and bioassay. *Proceedings of the Society for Experimental Biology and Medicine*, 1960, *103*, 142–144.

Haus, E., and Halberg, F. 24-Hour rhythm in susceptibility of C mice to a toxic dose of ethanol. *Journal of Applied Physiology*, 1959, *14*, 878–880.

Haus, E., Halberg, F., Scheving, L. E., and Simpson, H. International cancer research workshop on Chronotherapy of cancer—A critical evaluation. *International Journal of Chronobiology*, 1979, *6*, 67–107.

Kriebel, J. Changes in internal phase relationships during isolation. In L. E. Scheving, F. Halberg, and J. E. Pauly (Eds.), *Chronobiology*. Stuttgart: Georg Thieme Verlag, 1974, pp. 451–459.

Krieger, D. T., Kreuzer, J., and Rizzo, F. A. Constant light: Effect on circadian pattern and phase reserval of steroid and electrolyte levels in man. *Journal of Clinical Endocrinology and Metabolism*, 1969, *29*, 1634–1638.

Lund, R. Personality factors and desynchronization of circadian rhythms. *Psychosomatic Medicine*, 1974, *36*, 224–228.

Mills, J. N., Minors, D. S., and Waterhouse, J. M. Adaptation to abrupt time shifts of the oscillators controlling human circadian rhythms. *Journal of Physiology*, 1978a, *285*, 455–470.

Mills, J. N., Minors, D. S., and Waterhouse, J. M. The effect of sleep upon human circadian rhythms. *Chronobiologia*, 1978b, *5*, 14–27.

Pöllmann, L. Über spontan-rhythmische Schwankungen der Schmerzschwelle. *Deutsche zahnärztliche Zeitschrift*, 1977, *32*, 180–182.

Reinberg, A., and Halberg. F. Circadian chronopharmacology. *Annual Review of Pharmacology*, 1971, *11*, 455–492.

Reinberg, A., and Reinberg, M. A. Circadian changes of the duration of action of local anaesthetic agents. *Naunyn-Schmiedeberg's Archiv für Pharmakologie*, 1977, *297*, 149–152.

Reinberg, A., Vieux, N., Ghata, J., Chaumont, A. J., and Laporte, A. Is the rhythm amplitude related to the ability to phase-shift circadian rhythms of shift-workers? *Journal de Physiologie Paris*, 1978, *74*, 405–409.

Scheving, L. E., Mayersbach, H. von, and Pauly, J. E. An overview of chronopharmacology. *Journal Européen de Toxicologie*, 1974, *7*, 203–227.

Webb, W. B., and Agnew, H. W. Sleep and waking in a time-free environment. *Aerospace Medicine*, 1974, *45*, 617–622.

Wever, R. Über die Beeinflussung der circadianen Periodik des Menschen durch schwache elektromagnetische Felder. *Zeitschrift für vergleichende Physiologie*, 1967, *56*, 111–128.

Wever, R. Autonome circadiane Periodik des Menschen unter dem Einfluss verschiedener Beleuchtungs-Bedingungen. *Pflügers Archiv*, 1969, *306*, 71–91.

Wever, R. Zur Zeitgeber-Stärke eines Licht-Dunkel-Wechsels für die circadiane Periodik des Menschen. *Pflügers Archiv*, 1970, *321*, 133–142.

Wever, R. Influence of electric fields on some parameters of circadian rhythms in man. In M. Menaker (Ed.), *Biochronometry*. Washington, D.C.: National Academy of Sciences, 1971, pp. 117–133.

Wever, R. Der Einfluss des Lichtes auf die circadiane Periodik des Menschen. I. Teil. Einfluss auf die autonome Periodik. *Zeitschrift für Physikalische Medizin*, 1973, *3*, 121–134.

Wever, R. The influence of self-controlled changes in ambient temperature on autonomous circadian rhythms in man. *Pflügers Archiv*, 1974, *352*, 257–266.

Wever, R. The circadian multi-oscillator system of man. *International Journal of Chronobiology*, 1975, *3*, 19–55.

Wever, R. *The Circadian System of Man*. Berlin–Heidelberg–New York: Springer Verlag, 1979a.

Wever, R. Influence of physical work load on freerunning circadian rhythms in man. *Pflügers Archiv*, 1979b, *381*, 119–126.

Wever, R. Schlaf und circadiane Rhythmik. In G. Harrer and V. Leutner (Eds.), *Schlaf und Pharmakon*. Stuttgart–New York: F. K. Schattauer Verlag, 1979c, pp. 29–62.

Wever, R. Fractional desynchronization as a method for evaluating functional interdependencies. *Proceedings of the XIV International Conference of the International Society of Chronobiology*. Hannover (1979), 1980a.

Wever, R. On varying work–sleep schedules: The biological rhythm perspective. Symposium on *"Variations in Work–Sleep Schedules: Effects on Health and Performance,"* San Diego, Calif. (1979), 1980b.

Wever, R. Phase shifts of human circadian rhythms due to shifts of artificial zeitgebers. *Chronobiologia*, 1980c.

Colquhoun, P., Folkhard, S., Knauth, P., and Rutenfranz, J. (Eds.). *Experimental Studies of Shiftwork.* For-
schungsberichte des Landes Nordrhein-Westfalen, Nr. 2513. Opladen, Westdeutscher Verlag, 1975.
Conroy, R. T. W. L., and Mills, J. N. *Human Circadian Rhythms.* London: J. & A. Churchill, 1970.
Czeisler, C. A. *Human circadian physiology: Internal organization of temperature, sleep–wake, and neuroen-
docrine rhythms monotored in an environment free of time cues.* Ph.D. thesis, Stanford University, 1978.
Hildebrandt, G. *Biologische Rhythmen und Arbeit.* Wien–New York: Springer-Verlag, 1976.
McGovern, J. P., Smolensky, M. H., and Reinberg, A. (Eds.). *Chronobiology in Allergy and Immunology.*
Springfield, Ill.: Charles C. Thomas, 1977.
Richter, C. P. *Biological Clocks in Medicine and Psychiatry.* Springfield, Ill.: Charles C. Thomas, 1965.

18

Rhythms in Performance

PETER COLQUHOUN

INTRODUCTION: THE MEASUREMENT OF PERFORMANCE RHYTHMS

In this chapter, we consider the evidence for circadian periodicity in that class of behavior designated as *performance*. By this we mean, essentially, measures or scores of efficiency at various tasks that require the use of cerebral processes in responding to specified sensory information by appropriate motor actions.

The complexity of both the sensory and the motor components of a task may vary, as may the difficulty of performing it; however, in general, the tasks so far studied for evidence of circadian periodicity have been relatively simple ones. But it must be admitted at the outset that even the most apparently simple task is, in truth, extraordinarily complex, and that we are not at all certain what particular underlying mental process is in fact being indirectly measured by the scores we obtain. It is also necessary to point out that the investigation of possible circadian periodicity in human performance is beset by a number of problems that do not exist in corresponding investigations of physiological processes. Perhaps the most obvious of these problems is that task performance is a voluntary activity. Thus, any apparent periodicity in performance at a particular task may, to some extent (or even entirely), be merely a reflection of fluctuations in motivation, rather than an indication of true changes in efficiency.

A second problem is fatigue arising from carrying out the task itself. It is difficult for even the most constantly motivated subject to keep up his performance for any length of time. The usual solution to this problem is to restrict the length of any test session, as well as the total number of such sessions. Unfortunately, this limitation, in turn, imposes constraints on the type of task that can be used and also the frequency with which performance

PETER COLQUHOUN   Medical Research Council Perceptual and Cognitive Performance Unit, University of Sussex, Brighton, BN1 9QG England.

at it can be assessed; the latter raises further problems when it comes to analysis, which is discussed below.

Whereas fatigue degrades performance at a task, repeated practice, on the other hand, enhances it. Practice effects of this kind occur in even the most apparently familiar kinds of activity, when these are incorporated into a test situation. Although these effects can (in theory) be removed by the complex procedure of "detrending" the data, the problem is more usually tackled by taking one of two approaches. The first of these is to administer a sufficient number of tests before the start of the experimental series to ensure that any residual practice effects during the latter will be small enough to allow them to be ignored. The disadvantage of this technique is the formidable difficulty of maintaining motivation (or avoiding fatigue) over the extended length of the observation period that it normally entails.

The second approach is to control for practice effects by an appropriate experimental design. Thus, time of day may be considered the treatment in, for example, a cyclical Latin square in which individual subjects start their sequence of test sessions at different times. Although such a design has the advantage that the number of occasions on which any one person has to perform need be no greater than the number of times of day for which a measure is desired, it is, of course, not possible to make intersubject comparisons, and the basic outcome of an experiment of this kind is a mean rhythm for the whole group only. Certain assumptions have also to be made concerning the independence of practice effects and treatment order; even when these have been shown to be valid, it is still the case that the observed (mean) rhythm represents only that present in the performance of a "novel" task. This rhythm may not necessarily have the same characteristics as the one that would be seen in a fully practiced situation.

Practice effects can, of course, be avoided altogether by testing each subject once only. In this case, a between-subject design is used, in which a separate group of subjects is tested at each of the times of day for which an assessment of (mean) performance level is sought. However, the problem of matching these groups (e.g., for ability and personality) usually makes this approach an impracticable one.

Finally, although it may be obvious, it is often forgotten that performance is by definition a function only of the waking subject. Sleeping people do not perform; thus, one-third of any rhythm being looked for must be absent in the results of any experiment, whatever procedure is adopted. Although it is possible to fill in the missing portion, either by waking subjects up at intervals during their sleep, or by keeping them awake for the whole 24 hr, the test performances then recorded are inevitably confounded by the masking effects of the resulting sleep interruption or sleep deprivation and thus cannot strictly be considered true data points in the cycle. It follows that in the analysis of typical performance data for circadian periodicity, we are necessarily dealing with a partially sampled function. Bearing in mind the fact that even this partial sampling can rarely, for the reasons discussed above, be other than relatively sparse, it is not surprising that the methods of time-series analysis are not usually found to be appropriate for detecting periodicity of the circadian order in human performance, and that obtained test scores are normally analyzed by more conventional techniques (such as analysis of variance, or t tests) to determine the statistical significance of changes in mean level during the waking day. Such changes are perhaps more appropriately described by the label "time-of-(waking)-day effects"; it is with such effects that we are concerned below.

Fluctuations in mental efficiency during the waking day have been studied for at least the last 100 years. Thus, Ebbinghaus (1885/1964) reported a consistent tendency for learning (of nonsense syllables) to be more rapid in the morning, an effect that he assumed to occur because "in the later hours of the day mental vigour and receptivity are less." On the other hand, Bechterew (1893) maintained that "the speed of the psychic processes is retarded in the morning and accelerated in the evening. The lowest speed occurred in the afternoon." This afternoon trough was also commented on by Kraeplin (1893), who related it to the midday meal. Kraeplin, who conducted extensive research on the "work-curve," also mentioned a "warm-up" period in the morning and concluded, in apparent contradiction of Ebbinghaus, that the decrements (and associated phenomena) that he observed were "no indication of [work] fatigue," since they "disappear after 2–3 hours, even when work is continued."

Thus, even in this earliest work, there are suggestions of two differing overall time-of-day trends and also of a "postlunch" effect. Fatigue was clearly accepted as being of importance, but its precise temporal manifestations appeared to be a matter of dispute. Gates (1916), whose work was addressed primarily to the question of school timetabling, concluded that "as far as the morning is concerned [the curves of efficiency] are identical" (i.e., performance improves up to about noon). But in the afternoon, "certain characteristic differences were found," namely, that "more strictly mental" processes reached their maximum in the later forenoon and showed a greater postlunch decrement, whereas the more "motor" functions showed "a continuous increase in efficiency during the [school] day." He noted that his work confirmed the earlier conclusions of Winch (e.g., Winch, 1913) in this respect; the findings on motor tasks are also similar to those of Hollingworth (1914), who maintained, in addition, that the timing of the peak in such tasks is partly dependent on the subject's customary hours of work.

Laird (1925) was highly critical of previous laboratory studies, attributing the disagreement among them to a "lack of experimental insight" (Laird himself found an almost continuous fall over the day in performance at tests of several different mental functions, including memory, given to college students in a carefully controlled experiment). Laird's criticisms would appear a little unfair, though Freeman and Hovland (1934), in their review of the area, would seem to be in agreement with them, since their conclusion that all four possible basic shapes of diurnal efficiency curves (a continuous rise; a continuous fall; a rise followed by a fall; and a fall followed by a rise) had been shown by different workers is tantamount to saying that there is no consistent pattern whatsoever. However, it seems more likely that different kinds of task give rise to different diurnal trends, as had already been shown by Gates (1916).

In a series of carefully controlled studies by himself and his colleagues, Kleitman (1963) found that all the curves they obtained were of the third shape distinguished by Freeman and Hovland (1934), with a peak of performance in the middle of the waking period (i.e. somewhere during the afternoon). He concluded that "most of the curves of performance can be brought into line with the known 24-hour body-temperature curves, allowing for individual skewing of the curves towards an earlier or later, rather than a mid-afternoon, peak." On the basis of this observed parallelism, Kleitman (1963) hypothesized a causal connection between temperature and performance. But of course, mere correlation can never "prove" a causal relationship. In any case, the close parallelism obtained by Kleitman (1963) is rarely seen in other studies. For instance, in an investigation by Ruten-franz and Hellbrügge (1957) of simple computation by schoolchildren, two clear perfor-mance peaks were found (one before lunch and one in the late afternoon), strikingly con-firming early observations by Baade (1907) and clearly showing a curve that is incompatible with the parallelism argument.

In the experiments by Blake (1967b), conducted on young servicemen, the highest scores in a number of what Hockey and Colquhoun (1972) described as "immediate infor-mation-processing tasks" were seen at 2100 hr (see Figure 1), although an earlier, morning peak was also observed in the majority of cases. Blake's studies represent one of the best recent examples of carefully controlled experimentation in this area, but it is possible that the "late peaking" observed by him was due to an exceptionally large end effect (a last-test-of-the-day effect) specific to the particular subject population he used. This suggestion might seem a little farfetched, were it not for the fact that it is only in such military groups (e.g., Colquhoun, Blake, and Edwards, 1969; Adam, Brown, Colquhoun, Hamilton, Ors-born, Thomas, and Worsley, 1972) that it appears ever to be seen. On the other hand, Blake's finding that performance on the only truly "cognitive" test that showed significant variation in his series ("digit span," a test of short-term memory) reached its *lowest* level at 2100 hr (see Figure 1) could be argued to militate against this end-effect interpretation; the trend of performance at this test is in fact in line with that found by some of the earlier

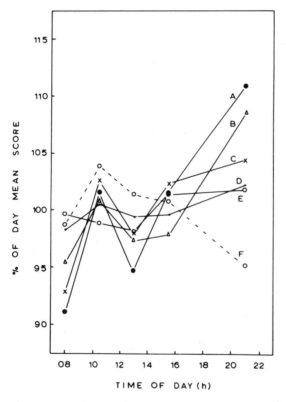

Fig. 1. Variation in performance over the waking day. (A) Signal detection efficiency at a vigilance task. (B), (C), (D), (E) Rate of work at tests of calculations, letter cancel-lation, card sorting, and serial choice reac-tion, respectively. (F) Digit span. $N = 25$ or 30 in each case. (Based on data in Blake, 1967b.)

observers of mental function already mentioned, namely, a morning rise, followed by a continuous fall thereafter.

The deterioration in short-term memory efficiency in the afternoon observed by Blake (1967b) has been confirmed in subsequent studies (Baddeley, Hatter, Scott, and Snashall, 1970; Hockey, Davies, and Gray, 1972; Folkard and Monk, 1978), and the prediction that tasks involving both immediate information-processing *and* short-term memory will show a compromise time-of-day function has been confirmed by Folkard (1975) for tests of simple logical reasoning. These sorts of effect have been interpreted in terms of the hypothesis that arousal increases over the day (see Kleitman, 1963; Colquhoun, 1971), and the possible effects of fatigue that concerned the earlier workers have tended to be played down. Arousal theory has also been invoked as an explanation of the discovery (Folkard, Monk, Bradbury, and Rosenthall, 1977) that in contrast to short-term memory, long-term retention is better for material originally presented in the *afternoon* than in the morning (a finding that has implications for educational timetabling that conflict with the earlier conclusions of Gates, 1916).

Most of the tasks used in the studies mentioned above have a minimal motor component. There are relatively few recent investigations of motor tasks, but those that have been carried out tend to confirm the conclusions of the earlier workers that this type of performance peaks later in the day. Of course, the "purer" the motor task, the more a score from it becomes a *physiological* measure rather than one of true performance and, therefore, the more experiments using it become irrelevant to the question of rhythmicity in *mental* processes. It is true that tasks such as the psychomotor Kugeltest (Klein, Herrmann, Kuklinski, and Wegmann, 1977), nut-and-bolt assembly (Hughes and Folkard, 1976), and rifle aiming (Halberg, 1970), all of which show the later peak, have a clear perceptual component; but the degree to which higher cerebral processes are involved in such tasks is typically small and is virtually zero in the case of tests of grip strength, and tapping speed, as used by Aschoff, Giedke, Pöppel, and Wever (1972) in their studies of circadian rhythms in a zeitgeber-controlled situation. This is unfortunate, since a question of key importance is whether performance rhythms are truly endogenous, as has been shown to be the case for physiological processes, or whether they are partly, or even wholly, determined by exogenous factors. However, Aschoff *et al.* (1972) showed in these same studies that at least time-of-day effects in the clearly mental tasks of simple computation and time estimation are indeed endogenous, since they persisted (with an increased "period" length) when all zeitgebers were removed.

In sum, there is ample evidence of the existence of time-of-day effects on performance in a wide range of tasks, varying both in complexity, and in the degree of involvement of motor processes. It would appear that the majority of these time-of-day effects fall into three types: an overall rise in efficiency over most of the day; an initial rise followed by an overall fall; and a double-peak, or postlunch dip, type. The extent to which fatigue influences the observed curves is at present unclear, as is whether they represent segments of actual circadian rhythms or, rather, daily variations in waking efficiency caused by the action of factors that may or may not themselves be periodic. One thing is certain, however: the effects are not ephemeral, since they have been shown in several large-scale studies (e.g., Colquhoun, Blake, and Edwards, 1968b) to persist unabated over periods of testing as long as 12 days, and recently (in unpublished studies by the author and his colleagues) for even longer times, thus confirming the results obtained by the earlier pioneer workers who doggedly tested (only) themselves day after day for months at a time.

ROUND-THE-CLOCK STUDIES

As was mentioned in the introduction, it is impossible to obtain measures of performance during night hours that are unconfounded either by sleep deprivation or by the effects of sudden awakening. Nevertheless, a number of round-the-clock studies have been carried out, since from a purely practical (applied) point of view, it is clearly often necessary to know whether or not performance efficiency at a particular type of task is degraded at night, regardless of the fact that theoreticians may have difficulties in proving that any observed changes are true reflections of an underlying oscillatory system.

Much of the support for these studies has come from military sources, since in defense systems it is clearly of the utmost importance to ensure that a high degree of operational readiness is maintained at all times. Thus, Kleitman and Jackson (1950) and Colquhoun, Blake, and Edwards (1968a) investigated the efficiency of naval ratings on a range of tasks, some of which simulated the men's actual duties, under the rapidly rotating watch-keeping schedules commonly followed by personnel on warships. The results confirmed the general prediction from laboratory-experimental waking-day studies (more especially those in which enlisted men served as subjects) that performance levels on those tasks involving immediate information-processing would be higher during watches held in the afternoon-evening hours than during those held in the morning. They also provided the additional information that during watches held in night hours (either before delayed night sleep or after a reduced period of such sleep), efficiency at such tasks was degraded and reaction

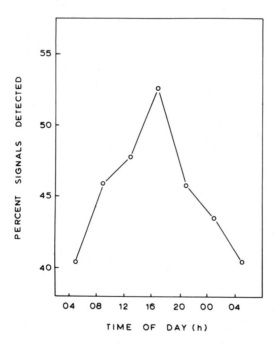

Fig. 2. Mean signal-detection efficiency in 2-hr sessions at a simulated sonar task, held during the first half of 4-hr watches commencing at 00, 0400, 0800, 1200, 1600, or 2000 hr, scheduled in a cycle that was repeated four times during 12 days of observation. $N = 12$ enlisted men. (After Colquhoun *et al.*, 1968a.)

times increased (see also Rutenfranz, Aschoff, and Mann, 1972). When the mean watch scores obtained in such studies are plotted on a single 24-hr time scale, the suggestion of a circadian rhythm is very strong (see Figure 2).

A similar strong suggestion of the existence of circadian rhythmicity is provided by the results of other studies in which subjects have either been kept awake or been awakened at intervals for testing during night hours. Thus, Klein *et al.* (1977) measured performance on psychomotor, cancellation, and addition tasks and also on a flight simulator, in various experiments conducted over the complete 24-hr period, and found that the points they obtained in night hours fitted those from daytime testing in such a way as to indicate a pattern of efficiency changes that appeared very clearly as a rhythm. Similar patterns were reported by Aschoff *et al.* (1972) for their motor tasks when an artificial (but "normal") light–dark cycle was imposed on subjects living in a bunker. Other workers who have shown 24-hr variation in performance by including night tests in their series include Jansen, Rutenfranz, and Singer (1966) for calculation rate and speed at a simultaneously performed tracking task, Voigt, Engel, and Klein (1968) for auditory reaction time, and Fort and Mills (1972) for short tests of cancellation, simple aiming, and syllogistic reasoning.

Aside from the military, changes in performance efficiency round the clock are, in the real world, most relevant to organizations employing shift workers. Such people (in contrast to subjects in laboratory studies) have to work more-or-less continuously for 8 or more hours, on night as well as on day shifts; from the results of the experiments described above, it would be predicted that their efficiency in the former case would be lower than in the latter. The classic study by Bjerner, Holm, and Swensson (1955) of errors made by shift-working meter readers following a three-shift system at a gasworks showed that performance on a real-life industrial task is indeed poorer at night, and that the overall pattern displayed by the data, when collated from all shifts, appears to be one of continuous and fairly substantial variation round the clock (see also Browne, 1949). However, the maximum extent of this variation may be masked in the reported results from such shift-work studies by the occurrence of partial adaptation to the altered sleep–waking cycle during the extended period of night working over which the readings are normally summed. Closer estimates of the "true" magnitude of the circadian changes might thus be expected to be obtained in situations where such adaptation had not occurred (e.g. in rapidly rotating shift systems where only, say, two night shifts are worked in succession). In a recent investigation of such a rapidly rotating (2–2–2) system, Folkard, Knauth, Monk, and Rutenfranz (1976) found a very large (40% peak–trough) 24-hr variation in efficiency at an interpolated immediate information-processing task, approximately of the form predicted from waking-day studies, when the readings taken on each of the three shifts were collated into a single time series. However, the addition of a considerable memory load to the task altered the phase of the apparent rhythm by about 8 hr (see Figure 3); this differing (though less marked) trend, with high-memory-loaded performance being better at night, would, of course, be predicted from the waking-day studies of memory tasks reviewed earlier, but it is particularly pleasing to see the prediction confirmed so clearly.[1]

The overwhelming impression given by round-the-clock studies is thus of systematic

---

[1]Note that the memory involved in this task was of the short-term variety. Long-term memory would be expected to be worse for material presented at night (see previous section), and this prediction has been confirmed (Monk and Folkard, 1978).

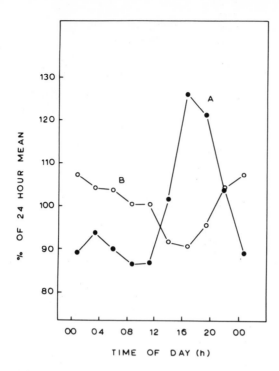

Fig. 3. Round-the-clock variation in rate of work at a visual search task in a rapidly rotating three-shift system. (A) Immediate-processing version (minimal memory load). (B) High-memory-load version. $N = 2$. (Based on data in Folkard *et al.*, 1976.)

24-hourly variations in performance that appear to reflect circadian rhythms in mental processes similar to those exhibited in physiological functions. However, many of the studies have, of necessity, been conducted in conditions (such as sleep deprivation or shift working) that may themselves be producing the very rhythmicity that is being looked for. The question is not whether circadian (round-the-clock) variations in performance occur, since clearly they do, but whether these variations (or, indeed, those observed within the waking day only) represent a truly endogenous periodicity in the underlying process or processes responsible for them. Such a question is very difficult to answer, but study of the ways in which performance rhythms alter in response to changes in the zeitgeber schedule throws a little more light on the problem. These alterations are discussed in the next section.

EFFECTS OF PHASE SHIFTS OF THE ZEITGEBER

One of the tests used to determine whether an observed physiological rhythm is endogenous is whether it fails to change its phase immediately after an abrupt shift in the phase of the zeitgeber. Several studies have provided evidence on this point in the case of performance rhythms. Some of these studies have been conducted in isolation chambers, where phase shifts are induced by altering the time on a clock; others have been conducted in "normal" conditions, where changes are imposed on the sleep–waking cycle without any alterations in clock time; and a few have observed performance rhythms before and after flights involving the crossing of several time zones.

Mills and Fort (1975) tested performance on cancellation and aiming tasks before and after a phase advance or a phase retard of 8 hr, achieved by altering the clock time in an isolation chamber. They found that the phase adjustment of performance was faster after

the advance shift than after the retard, and also that the time required to adjust the performance rhythm was longer when sleep occurred between 0800 hr and 1600 hr (as is
usual for workers on a night shift) than when it was taken between 1600 hr and midnight.
In the former case, the normal sequence of sleep, work, and leisure time is, of course,
changed, and thus the rhythm has to adjust to this change as well as to the phase shift in
clock time.

Experiments such as these raise the question of what the effective zeitgebers are for
human rhythms, including performance rhythms (Aschoff *et al.*, 1972). Whether or not the
light–dark cycle is a critical zeitgeber for man, the fact that social factors seem to be important would lead one to expect that when a phase-shifted routine is forced on a group of
subjects, requiring them to work at night and sleep during the day in an otherwise normal
environment, there will be a conflict between the social zeitgebers produced by the life of
the surrounding population and those arising from the activities of the group itself. Thus,
the rate of rhythm adjustment to such a phase shift should be faster in socially isolated
circumstances than in a typical urban community. However, Hughes and Folkard (1976)
found that even in a group completely cut off from contact with the outside world (but not
from the normal physical zeitgeber), not all the performance rhythms that they tested had
fully phase-adjusted to an 8-hr shift in the sleep–waking cycle after 10 days. On the other
hand, the degree of adjustment that did occur was generally considerably greater than that
observed over a similar period in the experimental night-shift study of Colquhoun *et al.*
(1968b), conducted in the context of a normal community. In fact, on the one task that was
common to both studies—namely, simple calculations—adjustment was complete in the
isolated-group investigation but was apparently only partial in the night-shift experiment.

Some results of this night-shift experiment are illustrated in Figure 4. This figure

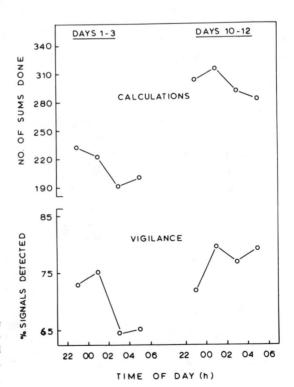

Fig. 4. On-shift performance trends at the
beginning and end of a 12-day period of consecutive night shifts, for two tasks alternated
at approximately 1-hour intervals. *N* = 10.
(After Colquhoun *et al.*, 1968b.)

demonstrates a further, most important point: the rate of adjustment of performance rhythms to phase shifts is typically found to be different for different tasks. In this experiment, an alteration in the sleep–waking cycle of some 8 hr evidently resulted in a considerably greater degree of phase adjustment (as assessed by the change in the shape of the on-shift trend) in the rhythm of signal-detection ability than in that of calculation rate. (NOTE: The increases in the *mean levels* exhibited by both scores are of the order to be expected from practice effects alone and do not reflect rhythm adjustment.) Task differences in degree of phase adjustment were also observed in the Hughes and Folkard socially-isolated-group study; in this case, tasks of calculations and logical reasoning showed greater adjustment of performance rhythms than those requiring manual dexterity or visual search. More recently, Monk, Knauth, Folkard, and Rutenfranz (1978) have obtained evidence that rate of adjustment is at least partially dependent on the memory load of a task, even when this is manipulated within a single test.

Although the results of these studies appear to conflict in certain respects, they each indicate that the concept of a single rate of adjustment for all rhythms of performance appears to be as unacceptable as the proposition that such rhythms all have the same basic phase.

When people arrive in a different country after crossing several time zones in the course of a rapid jet flight, *all* zeitgebers (whether physical or social) are phase-shifted simultaneously, and by the same amount. Thus, this would seem the ideal situation in which to demonstrate the endogenous nature of a rhythm and, indeed, has been used for just this purpose in the case of various physiological functions. Studies of performance rhythms in this context are, however, few, and there are only two in which the number of subjects tested has been sufficiently large to allow reasonably firm conclusions to be drawn.

The first of these is the series by Klein and his colleagues (see Klein *et al.*, 1977), in which it was found that in general, complete phase adjustment of performance rhythms took up to five days or more. A faster mean adjustment rate was found with westbound (i.e., phase retard) than with eastbound (i.e., phase advance) flights. This finding is in apparent contradiction of the results obtained in experimental studies with shifted artificial light–dark cycles, but Klein *et al.* (1977) noted that, on eastward flights, some subjects apparently (in terms of their temperature rhythm) adjusted "backwards," that is, by a phase *delay,* so that, for example, when crossing eight time zones, they were, in fact, having to adjust to a phase shift of 16 hr.

In agreement with the experimental shift-work findings discussed above, Klein *et al.* (1977) observed that the rhythms of different performance functions adjusted at different rates to the flight-imposed phase shifts; they suggested that the complexity of the task is an important variable here, and they also advanced the hypothesis that the rate of adjustment of a performance rhythm in this situation is in part dependent on its basic stability in the preflight phase; that is, the more pronounced the rhythm, the longer it takes to adjust.

In contrast to these results, Adam *et al.* (1972) found that the mean performance rhythms of detection efficiency and response time in a vigilance task, and of rate of work on a calculation test, all appeared to adjust virtually instantaneously after an 8-hr eastward time-zone change. Although in this experiment only time-of-day effects were measured, the results were sufficiently striking, and sufficiently different from those of Klein *et al.* (1977), to suggest that the picture is not yet by any means clear, and that further experimentation is required to determine whether, by this jet-lag test, performance rhythms can be said to be truly endogenous. Particular attention should be paid to possible masking factors in this situation. For example, in the Adam *et al.* (1972) study, the subjects were exposed not only to a phase shift of the zeitgeber but to a marked change in the climate as well; and in the Klein *et al.* (1977) series, sleep deprivation resulting from night testing must presumably have been occurring.

Phase shifts of the zeitgeber obviously result in major changes in the rhythms of performance functions. However, changes can also be produced by other factors, not so far mentioned, that can affect the amplitude, and even to some extent the phase, of a performance rhythm (or a time-of-day effect), even when the zeitgebers are held constant. These factors are discussed in the next section.

Motivation, Situational Factors, and Individual Differences

The basic problem of controlling motivation in experiments on rhythms in human performance has been mentioned in the introduction. The substantial effect of variations in this psychological state is clearly shown by the results of studies in which it has been deliberately manipulated. These studies have been premised either on the simple proposition that "If you try hard enough you can overcome anything" (in this case, presumably, the assumed adverse effects of lowered physiological activation at the trough of the circadian cycle), or on the (perhaps) slightly more sophisticated hypothesis that the level of arousal, itself suggested as largely determining observed performance, can be influenced by psychological as well as physiological factors.

Such theories are notably lacking in quantitative predictions, and there are few indications as to possible mediating mechanisms for the postulated effects. However, this fact does not in any way detract from the importance of the results of the studies themselves, not least for their implications for the conduct of all experiments in the performance-rhythm area. Equally important are the observations on the influence of personality on rhythm characteristics, for which adequate explanations are at present similarly lacking, but which, like the motivational effects, are of obvious relevance to our eventual understanding of the phenomena considered in this chapter.

The suggestion that an end effect may have been responsible for the late peaking observed by Blake in his time-of-day experiments described earlier implies that motivation was affecting the nature of the diurnal variation he found. Blake himself considered motivation a possible factor and, in a subsequent experiment (Blake, 1971), was able to demonstrate that alterations in motivation could indeed exert a substantial influence on the amplitude of the time-of-day effect seen in an immediate processing task (letter cancellation). Taking advantage of the fact that his subjects were well known to each other, he increased motivation by announcing each individual's score immediately after each test session, in the presence of all the members of the group. This supplying of knowledge of results (KR) in a social context produced a strong spirit of competition in the subjects and reduced the extent of the mean time-of-day variation to a nonsignificant level. The results of this study are shown in Figure 5, from which it will be seen that the effect of the increased motivation was most marked at times of day when performance was relatively poor (early morning and after lunch), but barely noticeable at the "best" time (2100 hr).

In further analyses of these results, Blake (1971) found that the effects of increased motivation were far more marked in "extravert" subjects than in "introverts." This complex interaction of personality, motivation, and time of day has been interpreted by Blake and Corcoran (1972) in terms of an inverted-U model of the effects of arousal on performance (see Corcoran, 1962); however, these authors admitted that when other data on the effects of personality are taken into account, this model has some difficulty in accounting for all the results.

Chiles, Alluisi, and Adams (1968) also demonstrated the "dampening" effect of raised levels of motivation on the amplitude of circadian performance variation, in their studies of the effects on performance efficiency of various work–rest schedules followed by different groups during prolonged confinement to a simulated aerospace-vehicle crew compartment. In these studies, daily variations were observed in several of the performance measures taken; however, this variation was not significant in a group who were shown the cyclical curves obtained from earlier groups and "were requested to put forth extra effort whenever they sensed any drop in their 'sharpness.' Thus, they were asked to attempt to prevent the appearance of the low points (or cycling in their performance curves)." The fact that the subjects were able to do what was asked of them points up the importance of taking the whole test situation into account when considering the results of any particular experiment and also provides a warning of the dangers of generalizing from one subject population to a different one.

Mention has already been made of the influence of the introversion–extraversion dimension of personality in determining the effects of raised motivation on time-of-day effects. But even without any such deliberate manipulation of motivational state, it would appear that introverts, in any case, differ from extraverts in terms of the phase of the time-

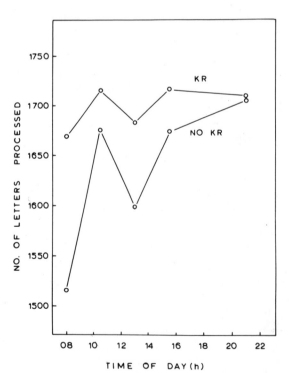

Fig. 5. Variation over the waking day in rate of work at a simple letter cancellation task. KR: With "knowledge of results" incentive (see text). NO KR: Without incentive. N = 30 and 25, respectively. (From Blake: "Temperament and Time of Day." In W. P. Colquhoun [Ed.], *Biological Rhythms and Human Performance.* Copyright, 1971, Academic Press Inc. [London] Ltd. Reprinted with permission.)

of-day curves they show when performing immediate processing tasks. Thus, Colquhoun (1960) observed a consistent positive correlation between scores of introversion and of detection rate on a visual inspection task within groups of subjects tested in the early forenoon, but either no correlation, or a tendency toward a *negative* one, within other groups tested later in the day. This morning superiority of introverts was later confirmed by Colquhoun and Corcoran (1964) on a simple cancellation task, but only when the subjects were tested in isolation (as they had been in Colquhoun's series); group testing abolished the difference between the two personality types—further evidence of the importance of situational factors. Blake (1971), using the same task, was able to show, within a single subject group, not only the expected positive correlation between performance and introversion in the morning, but also a negative one in the evening; again, the individual members of the group were tested in isolation.

Further relationships have been found to exist between personality factors and certain *physiological* rhythms (notably body temperature). Thus a reanalysis of Blake's data by Colquhoun and Folkard (1978) has revealed that the phase difference in the temperature rhythm reported by him (Blake, 1967a) to exist between introverts and extraverts is considerably more marked in "neurotic" than in "stable" subjects. Colquhoun and Folkard (1978) further showed that although small, these personality differences can result in quite substantial variations in the extent to which the rhythm adjusts to a phase shift. After a flight across eight time zones, for example, not only was there a significant difference between introverts and extraverts, but the rhythm of neurotic introverts was found to have adjusted hardly at all at a time when that of neurotic extraverts was showing almost complete adjustment. Again, night nurses of the neurotic introvert type were shown to exhibit considerably less rhythm adjustment on the first day of a night-shift period than those rated as neurotic extraverts.

These findings, along with the observation that the temperature readings of extraverts are more variable from day to day than those of introverts, led Colquhoun and Folkard to advance the hypothesis that the rhythmic system of at least neurotic extraverts may have an underlying periodicity greater than 24 hr. Partial support for this hypothesis could be said to have been provided by Lund (1974), who showed that a greater desynchrony of rhythms occurred in neurotic subjects in a prolonged sojourn in a zeitgeber-free environment. An alternative suggestion (Colquhoun, 1978) is that neurotic and/or introverted people are less labile, physiologically (as well as psychologically) speaking, and that their rhythms are thus less likely to respond to changes in the external event structure, whether familiar or not (see below).

In the case of another physiological rhythm, resting pulse rate, Colquhoun and Folkard (in an unpublished study from the author's laboratory) have shown, in an analysis of data originally collected by Blake, that the postprandial rise in this index after a heavy midday meal is significantly smaller in introverts than in extraverts and is apparently virtually absent altogether in neurotic introverts. It has also been observed (Colquhoun, 1978) that people of the latter type show the least postlunch decrement in a task of simple calculations; however, owing to the small numbers of subjects so far tested, the statistical reliability of these physiological and performance differences between neurotic introverts and others cannot yet be taken as established. This is also true of the greater degree of postflight decrement at the calculations task found to be shown by this type of subject compared with others in the time-zone experiment referred to above (Colquhoun, unpublished).

Thus, at present, the differential effects of various situational factors on the *performance* rhythms of people of different personality type are, on the whole, more suggestive than proven, but the findings on physiological rhythms are clearer, and there is a sufficient degree of consistency between the two to warrant the conclusion that there are important links here, which future experimentation will eventually substantiate and, hopefully, explain.

CONCLUDING REMARKS

The conclusion from the evidence presented in this chapter is that performance on a wide range of tasks varies considerably at different times within the waking day, and that measures on such tasks taken at times when the subject would normally have been sleeping fit in with those taken in waking hours in such a way as to strongly suggest the presence of an underlying circadian rhythm in the process or processes underlying the performance. However, it is also clear that the phase, the amplitude, and the detailed shape of these circadian variations can be affected to a greater or lesser extent by a number of factors, acting either alone or in combination. These factors include the degree of memory load involved in the task, the taking of meals, the level of motivation, the personality type of the individual subject, and the general test situation. It would also appear that fatigue may affect the nature of the observed trends, though in what particular ways is somewhat obscure.

It is a somewhat depressing fact that, despite a considerable amount of experimentation, little progress in our understanding of these phenomena has been achieved over the last 100 years. Most of the recent findings have simply confirmed (though sometimes on a more reliable basis) those made by the pioneer workers at the turn of the century. It is true that laboratory investigations using special facilities such as zeitgeber-controlled chambers, as well as field studies of phase shifts induced by rapid time-zone transitions, have provided fairly strong support for the hypothesis that performance rhythms, like those in physiological processes, are basically endogenous, but it cannot really be said that we are significantly nearer to identifying the underlying "mental" processes responsible for these endogenous variations nor, indeed, to determining their connection with any particular cyclical physiological state or states.

One factor that may partly account for this lack of progress is that experimenters are continuing to use tasks or tests that are essentially the same as those that were used in the earliest studies of time-of-day effects, and that what exactly it is that these tests are measuring is still not understood. Really significant advances are therefore perhaps unlikely to be made until new and more sophisticated methods for assessing cerebral functioning have been developed. In the meantime, the best hope of progress would seem to lie in the refinement of our existing measuring instruments. One way in which this refinement could be achieved is through studies of the manner in which particular manipulations affect the readings given by standard tests at different times of day. Thus, for example, in the area of short-term memory, recent research in the author's laboratory by Folkard and Monk (1979) has revealed that the normal morning superiority in an accepted test of this ability is abolished by preventing subvocal rehearsal of the material, suggesting that time-of-day variations in tasks involving storage and encoding may be mediated by strategy changes in the use of the articulatory loop. It is by experiments such as this that we can expect to get closer to the actual mechanisms underlying the scores of performance that exhibit rhythmic variation. We will then be able to devise new, direct tests of the operation of these mechanisms themselves.

References

Adam, J., Brown, T., Colquhoun, P., Hamilton, P., Orsborn, J., Thomas, I., and Worsley, D. Nycthemeral rhythms and air trooping: Some preliminary results from "Exercise Medex." In W. P. Colquhoun (Ed.), *Aspects of Human Efficiency: Diurnal Rhythm and Loss of Sleep.* London: English Universities Press, 1972.

Aschoff, J., Giedke, H., Pöppel, E., and Wever, R. The influence of sleep-interruption and of sleep deprivation on circadian rhythms in human performance. In W. P. Colquhoun (Ed.), *Aspects of Human Efficiency: Diurnal Rhythm and Loss of Sleep.* London: English Universities Press, 1972.

Baade, W. Experimentelle und kritische Beiträge zur Frage nach den sekundären Wirkungen des Unterrichts insbesondere auf die Empfänglichkeit des Schülers. *Pädagogische Monographien,* Band III, Leipzig, 1907.

Baddeley, A. D., Hatter, J. E., Scott, D., and Snashall, A. Memory and time of day. *Quarterly Journal of Experimental Psychology,* 1970, *22,* 605–609.

Bechterew, W. von. Über die Geschwindigkeitsveränderungen der psychischen Prozesse zu verschiedenen Tageszeiten. *Neurologisches Zentralblatt,* 1893, *12,* 290–292.

Bjerner, B., Holm, A., and Swensson, A. Diurnal variation in mental performance: A study of three-shift workers. *British Journal of Industrial Medicine,* 1955, *12,* 103–110.

Blake, M. J. F. Relationship between circadian rhythm of body temperature and introversion-extraversion. *Nature,* 1967a, *215,* 896–897.

Blake, M. J. F. Time of day effects on performance in a range of tasks. *Psychonomic Science,* 1967b, *9,* 349–350.

Blake, M. J. F. Temperament and time of day. In W. P. Colquhoun (Ed.), *Biological Rhythms and Human Performance.* London: Academic Press, 1971.

Blake, M. J. F., and Corcoran, D. W. J. Introversion–extraversion and circadian rhythms. In W. P. Colquhoun (Ed.), *Aspects of Human Efficiency: Diurnal Rhythm and Loss of Sleep.* London: English Universities Press, 1972.

Browne, R. C. The day and night performance of teleprinter switchboard operators. *Occupational Psychology,* 1949, *23,* 1–6.

Chiles, W. D., Alluisi, E. A., and Adams, O. Work schedules and performance during confinement. *Human Factors,* 1968, *10,* 143–196.

Colquhoun, W. P. Temperament, inspection efficiency, and time of day. *Ergonomics,* 1960, *3,* 377–378.

Colquhoun, W. P. Circadian variations in mental efficiency. In W. P. Colquhoun (Ed.), *Biological Rhythms and Human Performance.* London: Academic Press, 1971.

Colquhoun, W. P. Working efficiency, personality, and body rhythms. *Department of Employment Gazette,* 1978, *86,* 682–685.

Colquhoun, W. P., and Corcoran, D. W. J. The effects of time of day and social isolation on the relationship between temperament and performance. *British Journal of Social and Clinical Psychology,* 1964, *3,* 226–231.

Colquhoun, W. P., and Folkard, S. Personality differences in body-temperature rhythm, and their relation to its adjustment to night work. *Ergonomics,* 1978, *21,* 811–817.

Colquhoun, W. P., Blake, M. J. F., and Edwards, R. S. Experimental studies of shift work. I. A comparison of "rotating" and "stabilized" 4-hour shift systems. *Ergonomics,* 1968a, *11,* 437–453.

Colquhoun, W. P., Blake, M. J. F., and Edwards, R. S. Experimental studies of shift work. II. Stabilized 8-hour shift systems. *Ergonomics,* 1968b, *11,* 527–546.

Colquhoun, W. P., Blake, M. J. F., and Edwards, R. S. Experimental studies of shift work. III. Stabilized 12-hour shift systems. *Ergonomics,* 1969, *12,* 865–882.

Corcoran, D. W. J. *Individual Differences in Performance after Loss of Sleep.* Unpublished Ph.D. thesis, University of Cambridge, England, 1962.

Ebbinghaus, H. *Memory.* 1885. Republished in translation. New York: Dover Publications, 1964.

Folkard, S. Diurnal variation in logical reasoning. *British Journal of Psychology,* 1975, *66,* 1–8.

Folkard, S., and Monk, T. H. Time of day effects in immediate and delayed memory. In M. M. Gruneberg, P. E. Morris, and R. N. Sykes (Eds.), *Practical Aspects of Memory*. London: Academic Press, 1978.

Folkard, S., and Monk, T. H. Time of day and processing in free recall. *Quarterly Journal of Experimental Psychology*, 1979, *31*, 461–475.

Folkard, S., Knauth, P., Monk, T. H., and Rutenfranz, J. The effect of memory load on the circadian variation in performance efficiency under a rapidly rotating shift system. *Ergonomics*, 1976, *19*, 479–488.

Folkard, S., Monk, T. H., Bradbury, R., and Rosenthall, J. Time of day effects in school children's immediate and delayed recall of meaningful material. *British Journal of Psychology*, 1977, *68*, 45–50.

Fort, A., and Mills, J. N. Influence of sleep, lack of sleep and circadian rhythm on short psychometric tests. In W. P. Colquhoun (Ed.), *Aspects of Human Efficiency: Diurnal Rhythm and Loss of Sleep*. London: English Universities Press, 1972.

Freeman, G. L., and Hovland, C. I. Diurnal variations in performance and related physiological processes. *Psychological Bulletin*, 1934, *31*, 777–799.

Gates, A. I. Variations in efficiency during the day, together with practise effects, sex differences, and correlations. *University of California Publications in Psychology*, 1916, *2*, 1–156.

Halberg, F. A study of possible variation in rifle marksmanship as a function of circadian system phase. *Air Force Contract F29600-69-C-0011: Report No. 1*. Minneapolis: University of Minnesota, 1970.

Hockey, G. R. J., and Colquhoun, W. P. Diurnal variation in human performance: A review. In W. P. Colquhoun (Ed.), *Aspects of Human Efficiency: Diurnal Rhythm and Loss of Sleep*. London: English Universities Press, 1972.

Hockey, G. R. J., Davies, S., and Gray, M. M. Forgetting as a function of sleep at different times of day. *Quarterly Journal of Experimental Psychology*, 1972, *24*, 386–393.

Hollingworth, H. L. Variations in efficiency during the working day. *Psychological Review*, 1914, *21*, 473–491.

Hughes, D. G., and Folkard, S. Adaptation to an 8-h shift in living routine by members of a socially isolated community. *Nature*, 1976, *264*, 432–434.

Jansen, G., Rutenfranz, J., and Singer, R. Über eine circadiane Rhythmik sensumotorischer Leistungen. *Internationale Zeitschrift für angewandte Physiologie einschliesslich Arbeitsphysiologie*, 1966, *22*, 65–83.

Klein, K. E., Herrmann, R., Kuklinski, P., and Wegmann, H. M. Circadian performance rhythms: Experimental studies in air operations. In R. R. Mackie (Ed.), *Vigilance: Theory, Operational Performance, and Physiological Correlates*. New York: Plenum Press, 1977.

Kleitman, N. *Sleep and Wakefulness*. Chicago: University of Chicago Press, 1963.

Kleitman, N., and Jackson, D. P. Body temperature and performance under different routines. *American Journal of Applied Physiology*, 1950, *3*, 309–328.

Kraeplin, E. Über psychische Dispositionen. *Archiv für Psychiatrie und Nervenkrankheiten*, 1893, *25*, 593.

Laird, D. A. Relative performance of college students as conditioned by time of day and day of week. *Journal of Experimental Psychology*, 1925, *8*, 50–63.

Lund, R. Personality factors and desynchronization of circadian rhythms. *Psychosomatic Medicine*, 1974, *36*, 224–228.

Mills, J. N., and Fort, A. Relative effects of sleep disturbance and persistent endogenous rhythm after experimental phase shift. In P. Colquhoun, S. Folkard, P. Knauth, and J. Rutenfranz (Eds.), *Experimental Studies of Shiftwork*. Opladen: Westdeutscher Verlag, 1975.

Monk, T. H., and Folkard, S. Concealed inefficiency of late-night study. *Nature*, 1978, *273*, 296–297.

Monk, T. H., Knauth, P., Folkard, S., and Rutenfranz, J. Memory based performance measures in studies of shiftwork. *Ergonomics*, 1978, *21*, 819–826.

Rutenfranz, J., and Hellbrügge, T. Über Tagesschwankungen der Rechengeschwindigkeit bei 11-jährigen Kindern. *Zeitschrift für Kinderheilkunde*, 1957, *80*, 65–82.

Rutenfranz, J., Aschoff, J., and Mann, H. The effects of a cumulative sleep deficit, duration of preceding sleep period, and body-temperature on multiple-choice reaction time. In W. P. Colquhoun (Ed.), *Aspects of Human Efficiency: Diurnal Rhythm and Loss of Sleep*. London: English Universities Press, 1972.

Voigt, E. D., Engel, P., and Klein, H. Über den Tagesgang der körperlichen Leistungsfähigkeit. *Internationale Zeitschrift für angewandte Physiologie einschliesslich Arbeitsphysiologie*, 1968, *25*, 1–12.

Winch, W. H. Mental adaptation during the school day, as measured by arithmetical reasoning. *Journal of Educational Psychology*, 1913, *4*, 17–28, 71–84.

PART III

Tidal, Lunar, and Annual Rhythms

19

Tidal and Lunar Rhythms

Dietrich Neumann

Biological rhythms of locomotor activity, reproduction and other aspects of behavior can be observed in synchrony not only with daily and seasonal variations of environmental conditions but also with the tides and the lunar cycle. In the intertidal zone, animals are confronted with rising and falling water levels and, on some coasts, with the high amplitudes of spring tides recurring twice every lunar month. In terrestrial surroundings and in shallow fresh water, night-active species may be subjected to periodic changes in the brightness of moonlight, so that some of them synchronize their activities with the lunar day of 24.8 hr or even with specific phases of the lunar month. As a result of these influences of tides and moonlight, a variety of tidal and lunar rhythms have evolved. Interest in experimental studies of these rhythms has considerably increased during the last 20 years (for summaries, see DeCoursey, 1976; Enright, 1975; Naylor, 1976; Neumann, 1969, 1976c; Palmer, 1973). This chapter aims at compiling the results in the following aspects: (1) the adaptive significance of these rhythms in relation to environmental fluctuations; (2) the variety of timing mechanisms that synchronize the organism to specific characteristics of tides or moonlight; and (3) the combination of two different timing mechanisms resulting in a complex temporal program.

TIDAL RHYTHMS

ENVIRONMENTAL CONDITIONS BETWEEN TIDEMARKS

The tide-generating forces result from gravitational and centrifugal forces determined by the earth, the moon, and the sun, and their orbital motions. Although the magnitude and the temporal variation of these forces are well known for all parts of the world, it is

Dietrich Neumann   Zoologisches Institut der Universität Köln, 5000 Köln 41, West Germany.

extremely difficult to calculate their action even in a small marine water-basin and to pre-dict from this calculation the resulting tides along coastlines. The reason is that several topographical and physical influences, such as the size and the depth of the oceanic basins, as well as the extent and the direction of oceanic and tidal currents, both deflected by Cor-iolis forces, come into play. Hence, the actual tides reveal a complex temporal structure differing along coastlines all over the world. However, by accurate long-term registrations of local tides and appropriate Fourier analysis, more than 100 harmonic constituents have been identified so that hydrographers can reliably predict any tidal situation in nearly all parts of the world, formulated for each year in the tide tables. In general, three main types of tides have been observed (Defant, 1961; Barnwell, 1976).

The *semidiurnal tides* predominate on the coasts of the Atlantic Ocean, the North Sea, and parts of the Indian Ocean. Their period is about 12.4 hr, generally ebbing and flowing twice a day with an approximately equal amplitude. The resulting pattern of emersion and submersion, as experienced by organisms living at midtide level, is illustrated in Figure 1. The amplitude of these tides varies during the synodic month (the interval between one new moon and the following one, a period of 29.53 days) because the tide-generating forces reach maximum values during the syzygies when the earth, the moon, and the sun move into conjunction (new moon) or opposition (full moon); minimum values occur when the sun comes into a rectangular position with relation to the earth and the moon (quarters of the moon). Thus, the amplitude varies in a semimonthly (synonyms: *semilunar, semisy-nodic*) cycle of spring and neap tides in parallel with the changes of the moon. The spring tides are characterized by both extreme high levels of high water and extreme low levels of low water recurring every 14 or 15 days (mean 14.76 days) at about 1–2 days after full and new moons. On the other hand, the neap tides, with relatively small amplitudes, occur at about the quarters of the moon.

The *diurnal tides* are characterized by only one high tide and one low tide per day

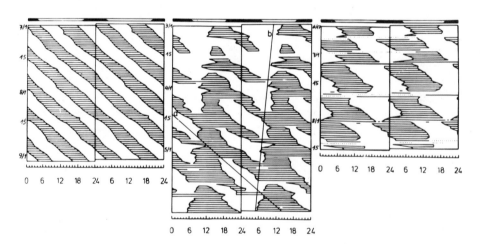

Fig. 1. Different tidal patterns at midtide level (ordinate: successive days of at least two months; abscissa: time of day, duplicated plotting; times of inundation are indicated by horizontal lines, times of exposure by gaps). *(Left)* Semidiurnal tides at New Port, Rhode Island. *(Middle)* Mixed tides, mainly semidiurnal, at Saint Petersburg, Florida (lines a and b indicate different shifts in the tidal pattern). *(Right)* Diurnal tides at Ocean Springs, Mississippi. (After Barnwell, 1976. Reprinted with permission of the author.)

during times with high tidal amplitude. Their periods are mainly determined by two constituents of the tide-generating forces, one of 25.8 hr and another of 23.9 hr. Diurnal tides are distributed along the Gulf of Mexico and in Southeast Asia and New Guinea. As in the case of the Gulf of Mexico (Figure 1), the pattern of emersion and submersion differs quite strikingly from that of semidiurnal tides by phase shifts of 180° (together with low tidal heights) that recur in intervals of about 13–14 days (mean 13.66 days). This period is correlated with the declinational cycle of the moon (synonym: *tropical month,* 27.32 days) depending on the declination of the moon's orbit and on the interval of 13.66 days between two successive transits of the moon over the equator. Within the same period, a cycle of "spring" and "neap" tides is generated in diurnal tides differing from any coincidence with the synodic month and the changes of the moon.

The *mixed tides* occur along most parts of the coastlines of the Pacific Ocean, on most Australian coasts, and in the regions of the Caribbean Sea and the Arabian Sea. The properties of this tidal type are obvious inequalities in the height as well as in the interval of two succeeding tides, resulting in a complex pattern of emersion and submersion at midtide level (Figure 1, middle). Thus, there exists a wide geographical and seasonal variation in the mixed tides.

The ebbing and flowing of the tides influence the distribution of organisms within the *littoral zone* because the frequency and the duration of exposures, increasing from the sublittoral to the supralittoral, are differentially well tolerated. The resulting vertical zonation of algae and of sessile animals can be correlated on most coasts with the four main tidemarks (see Newell, 1970, for review). The mean high- and low-water levels of neap tides (MHWN, MLWN) define the midlittoral zone, where exposures and submersions occur on each day. The mean low-water level of spring tides (MLWS) limits the sublittoral fringe of the midlittoral, which in its lower range is exposed only every two weeks, while the mean high-water level of spring tides (MHWS) fixes the supralittoral fringe of the midlittoral, which may be exposed up to nearly two weeks in its higher range.

A wide variety of *environmental factors* fluctuate simultaneously with the rise and fall of the tides: exposure and submersion, wave agitation (correlated with water turbulence, underwater sound and bottom vibrations, all of them stronger during flood tide than during ebb tide), hydrostatic pressure (0.1 atm per meter of the water column), temperature (correlated with differences between shallow and deep waters on sheltered shores, or between atmosphere and water modified by both seasonal and day–night differences), the intensity of light and its spectral composition, salinity changes as well as differences in chemical constituents between incoming and outgoing currents in estuary areas, and, lastly, predation.

Temporal Adaptations of Behavior to Intertidal Conditions

The littoral fauna between tidemarks reveals a high diversity of gradations between an aquatic way of life and a terrestrial one. The majority of the species are of marine origin, with representatives from most marine phyla (Green, 1968; Newell, 1970). A small but respectable number of species are of terrestrial origin, such as marine insects, arachnids, and centipedes living within intertidal crevices, in rock pools, or in substrates as far down as the sublittoral (Cheng, 1976; Green, 1968); during low tide, birds and even some reptiles may come from the nearby land to forage in the intertidal zone (Fricke, 1970). Most species of the intertidal resident fauna are benthic animals. Much less information is available on the plankton and nekton of the littoral, and, last but not least, on the planktonic larval stages of many benthic animals because quantitative observations in tidal currents are extremely difficult.

In the context of this chapter, it is most important that intertidal animals be generally specialized in their particular behavioral adaptations to either the aquatic situation during inundation or the terrestrial situation during exposure. Thus, a reliable synchronization of distinct behavioral activities with the tides can be of high selective importance. The following compilation of adaptations may demonstrate the range of possibilities.

LOCOMOTOR ACTIVITIES. Table I summarizes some species that have been extensively analyzed during recent years in nature as well as in the laboratory. Most of the observed activities are concerned mainly with feeding. In the case of the swimming crustaceans, most authors mention that the tidal timing of locomotor activity prevents the animals from being stranded in an unfavorable intertidal range or from being driven out to the sea by the ebbing tide. In some walking amphipods *(Talitrus, Orchestia)* and in carabid beetles *(Thallassostrechus)*, which are active on the exposed shore, the activities are additionally restricted to the night time, which might be an adaptation to the impact of predators (birds) or other environmental factors (light, temperature). Even in guillemots, while breeding on cliff ledges and feeding close inshore, the foraging activities may fluctuate parallel to the tides, probably as a consequence of the changing availability of fish in tidal streams (Slater, 1976). However, it should be mentioned that tide-related activities may also be concerned with territorial activities, with local exploration behavior, and with mating as, for example, in fiddler crabs.

MIGRATIONS. Upshore and downshore migrations within shallow waters in conjunction with the tides have been observed in young plaice and other, less abundant fish (Gibson, 1973), in sand crabs (Cubit, 1970), and in the brown shrimp (Al-Adhub and Naylor, 1975). Besides the correct timing of swimming during oncoming and ebbing tides and of burrowing during low tide, one has to postulate oriented responses to the direction and the velocities of the ingoing and outgoing streams.

Orientation efforts correlated with tidal streams can also be observed in migrating fish while they are passing an estuary toward inland waters, such as in *Lampetra fluviatillis* and *Lota lota* on its ways to the spawning grounds (Tesch, 1967). In the upstream migration of elvers *(Anguilla vulgaris)*, there is evidence that the young fish can discriminate between the ingoing flood stream and the outgoing ebb by odor. In combination with rheotactic responses, they are passively transported to inland waters by the flood stream (negative rheotactic response), and they go to the bottom of the river during the ebbing tide (positive rheotactic response) (Creutzberg, 1963). A critical situation arises in the upper tidal region of the river, where the tides are transmitted to the freshwater area, hindering the olfactory discrimination. It has been suggested that elvers can pass this critical area (e.g., with a length of 70 km in the river Elbe) by an endogenous tidal timing of their positive and negative rheotactic responses (Tesch, 1965). In postlarval pink shrimps, such endogenous tidal timing was established during continuous recording of swimming directions in current chambers, while in nature this larval stage migrates from offshore spawning sites to inshore nursery areas (Hughes, 1972).

The tide-related drift of plankton within tidal creeks and rivers of flat salt-marsh areas has been carefully observed in calanoid copepods. During flood tide, these animals concentrate near the bottom of the tidal current, where the dense oceanic water flows faster under the lighter water of the sound. The adaptive significance of this orientation behavior guarantees an upstream drift and hinders dispersal into the widespread marsh by surface water (Jacobs, 1968). Among the benthos, vertical migrations correlated with the tides have been known for over 70 years from the green flatworm *Convoluta roscoffensis,* which emerges from its intertidal interstices to the surface of the sediment during daytime low tides (for review, see Palmer 1973, p. 365).

HOMING. Excellent homing abilities of individuals in correlation with tidal locomotory behavior were observed in limpets. In *Patella* species, it has been shown by laboratory

TABLE. I. EXAMPLES OF TIDAL RHYTHMS IN LOCOMOTORY BEHAVIOR[a]

Species with behavioral tidal rhythms	Behavior in nature			Experiments on rhythmic behavior		
	Activity	Phase relationship to tides	Tidal type	Freerunning (d = days)	Zeitgeber for reinitiation of the rhythm	Authors
Gastropoda						
Melanerita atramentosa	loc, f	HT and thereafter	2	Circatidal (4–6 d)	Chilling	Zann, 1973
Decapoda						
Crangon crangon	em, sw, up-m	HT and thereafter	1	Circatidal (3 d)	l, suggested hp + wm	Al-Adhub and Naylor, 1975
Palaemon elegans	em, sw	Ebb tide	1	Circatidal (3 d)	l	Rodriguez and Naylor, 1972
Carcinus maenas	loc, f	About HT	1	Circatidal (>3 d)	hp,wm,sal,wc (seasonal restricted effectivities)	Naylor, 1976; Taylor and Naylor, 1977
Uca minax, Long Island	loc, f	About LT	1	Circatidal (> 30 d)	Not analyzed	Barnwell, 1966
Uca crenulata, California	loc, f	About LT	2	Mostly diffuse	wm	Honegger, 1976
Uca urvillei, Kenya	loc, f	About LT	1	Arrhythmic	wm	Lehmann, Neumann, and Kaiser, 1974
Isopoda						
Eurydice pulchra	sw	Flood tide	1	Circatidal	wm, hp, chilling	Jones and Naylor, 1970
Excirolana chiltoni	em, sw	About HT	2	Circatidal (>60 d)	wm	Enright, 1965a; Klapow, 1972b
Amphipoda						
Synchelidium sp.	em, sw	HT and thereafter	2	Circatidal	Probably wm	Enright, 1963
Corophium pugilator	sw	HT and thereafter	1	Circatidal (3 d)	hp	Morgan, 1965
Acari						
Bdella interrupta	loc	About LT on days with covering tides	1	(Probably circatidal)	Not analyzed	Foster, Treherne, and Ruscoe, 1979
Coleoptera						
Thallassostrechus barbarae	loc	LT during night	2	Circadian (7 d) + Circatidal (3 d)	Not analyzed	Evans, 1976
Diptera						
Clunio marinus, Arctic population	em, reproduction	Exposure of substrate	1	Only 1 cycle	temp. rise	Pflüger, 1973
Teleostei						
Blennius pholis	loc, f	About HT	1	Circatidal (4 d)	chilling, hp	Gibson, 1971
Pleuronectes platessa	up-m, down-m	Flood + ebb tide	1	Circatidal (1–3 d)	Not analyzed	Gibson, 1973

[a]Behavior: em = emergence from sand or mud; f = feeding; loc = locomotion on substrate; sw = swimming; up-m or down-m = upshore or downshore migration. Tides: HT = high tide, time about high water; LT = low tide. Type of tide: (1) semidiurnal; (2) mixed; (3) diurnal. Zeitgebers: hp = hydrostatic pressure changes; l = light reduction correlated with the tidal amplitude or with turbid water during high tide; sal = salinity changes; wc = tidal temperature cycles of warmer and colder water; wm = water movement correlated with mechanical disturbances of water.

experiments that during the ebbing tide, they return to their home site on tracks marked by chemical substances, with a tidal timing of migration (Funke, 1968). Another well-documented example is the intertidal lizard *Cryptoblepharus* on Madagascar, which migrates between its supralittoral resting place and distinct intertidal feeding areas during daytime low tides. The lizards are able to find their individual home range even when experimentally translocated over a distance of about 200 m (Fricke, 1970).

COLOR CHANGE. The dispersion and concentration of pigments in the chromatophores of many intertidal marine organisms may undergo a daily rhythm, being dispersed during the daytime and concentrated at night, as has been extensively observed in fiddler crabs (see Palmer, 1973, for review). As Brown, Fingermann, Sandeen, and Webb, (1953) reported on fiddler crabs, such daily rhythms may be modified during the daytime in synchrony with the rise and fall of the tides, even in constant laboratory conditions.

REPRODUCTION. Finally, it should be mentioned that the sexual and reproductive activities of intertidal organisms have to be well synchronized with the tides, not only in the simple sense that these activities are most often correlated with extensive locomotory activities, but also as a consequence of the adaptation of the reproduction time to specific tidal situations (p. 371).

CIRCATIDAL RHYTHMS

INTRODUCTORY REMARKS. Tidal rhythms of locomotory activity have been experimentally analysed in a sufficiently great number of intertidal species from different taxonomic classes by observing either single individuals or small groups (Table I). In many of these cases, freerunning rhythms with periods close to those of the tides have been recorded over a few days or even longer. These freerunning rhythms were undoubtedly interpreted by most authors as the output of an endogenous, oscillatory timing mechanism, uncoupled from tidal as well as from daily environmental cycles. Thus, the rhythms were named in analogy to "circadian" rhythms as *circatidal rhythms,* meaning endogenously controlled rhythms with peak activities about 12.4 hr apart that can be entrained by tides. Most of these circatidal rhythms lack the persistence and the degree of precision that is apparent in many circadian rhythms. Thus, there often exist difficulties in calculating their precise period as well as in planning subtle experiments in order to decide whether freerunning circatidal rhythms are based on an endogenous oscillator with a period of about 12.4 hr or of about 25 hr. With regard to problems in the properties of the underlying timing mechanism, the interpretation of circatidal rhythms is still open for discussions and further experimentation (p. 361).

Another interpretation of the freerunning tidal rhythms has been maintained in relation to unknown and subtle geophysical factors forcing the rhythms in constant conditions (Brown, 1972). The details may be omitted in the context of this chapter because the hypothesis has been shown to be untestable (for detailed discussions, see Enright, 1965b, 1975).

REGISTRATION. Several recording devices have been applied in order to record automatically the temporal pattern of activity bouts and rest under controlled laboratory conditions. The tipping of boxes or of lattices, both caused by the movement of test animals, is restricted to benthic organisms of sufficient size. The interruption of a dim red light beam impinging on a photosensitive resistor can be used for the registration of smaller animals.

Thermistor techniques for detecting slight changes in the heat conductance of an aquatic environment can be chosen in measuring the swimming activities of single isopods and prawns (Heusner and Enright, 1966). The swimming activities of amphipods and isopods were also successfully recorded by time-lapse photography (Enright, 1963). In intertidal beetles, the changes of the capitance of an electric field were correlated with the runs within a circular arena (Evans, 1976). A Geiger-counter technique was used in fiddler crabs measuring individuals tagged with a 60 Co-wire by means of two rate meters indicating the movement or rest of the animal (Lehmann, Neumann, and Kaiser, 1974). The last method can even be applied within tanks of 1-m height or more with simulated tidal rise and fall.

PERSISTENCE IN CONSTANT, NONTIDAL CONDITIONS. Persistent tidal rhythms have been observed during recent years in an increasing number of intertidal animal species, of which a selected number are presented in Table I. The first well-documented example was the fiddler crab *Uca pugnax,* revealing periods that were slightly longer than the tidal cycle on the seashore (see Bennett, Shriner, and Brown, 1957, for a reanalysis of the data in Enright 1965b). The best examples of long-term recordings were found in some *Uca* species from eastern North America (Figure 2; Barnwell, 1966), and in the isopod *Excirolana chiltoni* from the Pacific coast of California (Heusner and Enright, 1966; Enright, 1972). Both had periods clearly deviating from the actual tides near the laboratory (Figure 4). However, in most of the other species analyzed, the circatidal rhythms faded out within a few days, as opposed to the majority of circadian rhythmicities, which run for weeks or even months.

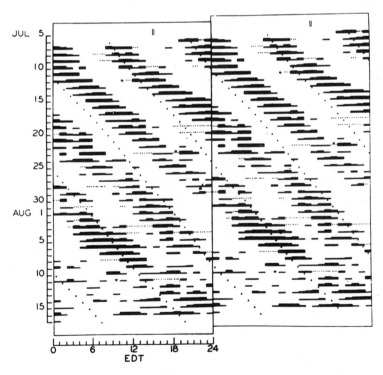

Fig. 2. Freerunning tidal rhythm of locomotory behavior in *Uca minax* in LL (<10 lux). The small points indicate the times of high tide at the collection site near the Woods Hole laboratory. (After Barnwell, 1966. Reprinted with permission of the author.)

Up to now, it has not been possible to analyze whether the damping of the rhythms (or their change to irregular activity bouts) resulted from inadequate laboratory conditions in the registration boxes (e.g., unnatural substrate conditions for feeding and hiding, artificial constant light conditions) or whether it was symptomatic of many tidal behavioral rhythms. Good arguments might exist for the latter alternative, indicating a physiological flexibility in the coupling of the overt behavioral rhythm with the endogenous oscillator and some additional sensory input. This flexibility would be an advantageous adaptation to intertidal environments and their frequent modification by nontidal weather conditions. However, in some fiddler crab species, it has been demonstrated that weak rhythmicities or even nonrhythmic behavior in constant conditions represent a special type of behavioral timing well adapted to fluctuating tidal conditions (p. 364).

Records of species collected on shores with *semidiurnal tides* (see Table I, Type 1) have in most cases produced data with two similar activity peaks per day and a freerunning period near to that of the actual tides (Figure 2). Species living on shores with *mixed tides* (p. 353) have resulted in more complex records with two activity peaks of different heights per day, and with asymmetrical intervals (Figure 3). Because the intervals and the heights of the tides change during a lunar month, Enright (1963) was able to compare the freerunning period of groups collected on days with different tidal patterns. He demonstrated that the intervals of the freerunning rhythms of freshly collected *Synchelidium* always corresponded with the pattern of the preceding tides on the day of collection. Thus, the freerunning rhythm could be best described by double tidal periods of about 26 hr, according to the sequence of repeated asymmetrical intervals. Identical results were found in the isopod *Excirolana* from the same beach area (Klapow, 1972b; Enright, 1976). The only records of animals from shores with *diurnal tides* demonstrated diffuse patterns (*Uca minax,* Barnwell, 1968; p. 363).

The freerunning period was relatively independent of the level of temperature in the green crab (range 10–25°C; Naylor, 1963); it could be manipulated by chemicals (D_2O, ethanol) in *Excirolana* (Enright, 1971). Both results on circatidal rhythms correspond well with the known properties of the circadian oscillator. The range of the freerunning period can be modified to some extent by some preceding conditions (Figure 4).

ZEITGEBER EXPERIMENTS. Intertidal organisms are exposed to a complex pattern of fluctuating physical factors concomitant with the rise and fall of the tides (p. 353). Reviewing the literature on zeitgebers (Table I), one can determine that (1) mechanical stimulation by increased wave agitation seems to be of major importance; and (2) more than one factor

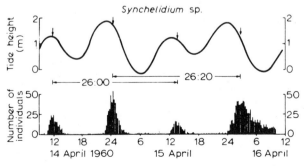

Fig. 3. Freerunning tidal rhythm (constant dim light) in conjunction with the shape of the actual tides on the seashore where the animals had been collected just before the start of the recordings. (After Enright, 1975. Reprinted with permission of John Wiley & Sons, Ltd.)

can act as an entraining stimulus (a fact corresponding with the multiple-zeitgeber concept of circadian rhythms).

First evidence for the effectiveness of mechanical disturbance was demonstrated by treating groups of the isopod *Excirolana* with an intermittent swirling of water and sand for a period of 6 hr, cycling with 6 hr of undisturbed water over a total of 2.5 days (Enright, 1965a). In other species, cycling changes of hydrostatic pressure were a zeitgeber, as demonstrated by the resynchronization of arrhythmic individuals of the isopod *Eurydice* after increases of 0.5 atm for 30 min at 12-hr intervals over a period of 5 days (Jones and Naylor, 1970). Some synchronization effects could be also produced by chilling, but these experiments are of minor relevance to the zeitgeber conditions in nature. However, temperature cycles have to be regarded as potentially weak zeitgebers, at least in the green crab (Naylor, 1976), while no apparent temperature influences could be established in *Synchelidium* (Enright, 1963) and in *Blennius* (Gibson, 1971). To a great extent, these zeitgeber experiments presented only qualitative kinds of evidence for the effectiveness of tidal factors. Further experiments are still lacking on the range of entrainment, the influence of the intensity of zeitgebers, and the stronger or weaker effectiveness of factors in relation to the phase relationship between the zeitgeber and the biological rhythm.

The discussion on influences of 24-hr light–dark cycles has been controversial. Barnwell (1966) suggested a zeitgeber influence on a 12.4-hr rhythm under tideless conditions, but further evidence—for example, from phase-shift experiments—was not ascertained. On the other hand, modifications of the amplitude of tidal activity rhythms in connection with day and night have been observed by several authors (p. 366).

When simultaneously exposed to several tidal factors fluctuating in a tidal machine, individual fiddler crabs responded with a different phase relationship to the tidal regime (Lehmann *et al.*, 1974). This individual variety in the response may indicate that some intertidal animals with highly evolved behavioral capacities can change the phase of their tidal rhythm in a complex pattern of environmental time cues, perhaps dependent on pretreatment or on adaptation to instantaneous experiences.

PULSE EXPERIMENTS AND THE PROBLEM OF THE BASIC OSCILLATOR. When comparing the variability of persisting circatidal rhythms, one has to ask whether the basis of the endogenous timing mechanism is an oscillator with an innate period close to 12.4 hr or 24.8 hr, or whether both possibilities can be verified. The freerunning rhythms of *Synchelidium* and *Excirolana*, which depend on the heights and intervals of the preceding mixed tides, indicate a double tidal period, but this interpretation implies two possibilities.

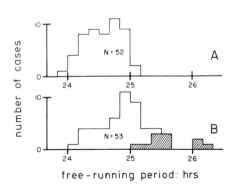

Fig. 4. Range of freerunning period values in *Excirolana chiltoni*, from three sets of freshly collected individuals in 1972 (A) and 1975 (B). (After Enright, 1976. Reprinted with permission of Springer-Verlag, Heidelberg.)

The temporal pattern of the specific peak heights and their asymmetrical intervals may be based (1) on a single double-tidal oscillator with a modifiable bimodal pattern of its peaks; or (2) on two double-tidal oscillators, each unimodal, with one peak per day, but held in some flexible antiphase relationship with each other (Enright, 1963). Any further progress on these problems of the basic mechanisms in circatidal rhythms can result only from pinpointed experiments.

Important steps in the current analysis of circatidal rhythms have been made in *Excirolana* by means of pulse experiments in which groups or single individuals were subjected to a "wave simulator" for turbulence pulses of a few hours while kept under tideless conditions in constant dim light. A single pulse on a previously desynchronized group resulted in a clear "circadian" rhythm, or, in the vocabulary of this chapter, in an obvious circatidal rhythm with a double-tidal period of about 25 hr. By subjecting arrhythmic groups to two stimuli or to a semidiurnal tidal pattern of repeated stimuli simulating the impact of water turbulence on the beach, freerunning rhythms with two peaks per day could be evoked, corresponding to the freerunning rhythms of freshly collected *Excirolana* (Klapow, 1972b). From these results it seems evident that in *Excirolana,* the natural period of the circatidal oscillator approximates the double-tidal period of 24.8 hr rather than the tidal period of 12.4 hr. But with regard to the one- or two-oscillator hypotheses, the experiments are not conclusive.

Further information can be drawn from another series of pulse experiments in *Excirolana* resulting in a phase-response curve (Figure 5). The points on the curve have been calculated by the observed advances or delays in the freerunning rhythm of individuals when subjected to a single 2-hr pulse during different phases of their locomotor cycle. The shape of a phase-response curve mirrors the sensitivity of the oscillator system to phase-shifting zeitgeber stimuli and offers a physiological basis for the entrainment of the oscillator to environmental cycles (see Chapter 7). In the case of *Excirolana*, the curve reflects the sensitivity to a tidal stimulus within the double-tidal period. Its shape is unique in the family of response curves: it is bimodal instead of unimodal as in true circadian rhythms. That means it has two peaks for advance shifts and two peaks for delay shifts during the 25-hr period, whereby both types alternate at intervals of about 6 hr. From an ecological point of view, this kind of phase-response curve guarantees a reliable stability of the entrained double-tidal oscillator by the zeitgeber pattern of the mixed tides in which the higher of the two daily high tides occurs during the first half of the day over one fortnight

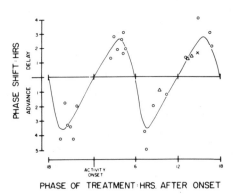

Fig. 5. Phase-response curve of *Excirolana chiltoni*. (After Enright, 1976. Reprinted with permission of Springer-Verlag, Heidelberg.)

and during the second half of the day over the next. Thus, during the entire lunar month, an adequate sensitivity to entraining stimuli ensures the entrainment of the system. However, the simplest interpretation of the bimodal phase-response curve favors the hypothesis of a double-tidal oscillator instead of an oscillator with tidal period because the behavioral pattern of this isopod repeats itself at about 25-hr intervals (Enright, 1976).

Laboratory-reared green crabs that had never experienced environmental rhythms of 12.4-hr periodicity demonstrated a circadian rhythmicity. When these crabs were subjected to one 15-hr chilling period of 4°C, a rhythmicity of about 12.4 hr was evoked. One might suggest that in this species from coasts with semidiurnal tides, the period of the basic oscillator corresponds with the tidal period (Williams and Naylor, 1967).

Summing up all the experimental results on circatidal rhythms, it might be concluded that a circatidal timing mechanism represents nothing other than a tidally synchronized circadian oscillator with a period of about 25 hr. But it has to be considered (1) that the analysis of the crustaceans from shores with mixed tides has demonstrated particularly adaptive properties unknown in circadian rhythms (modifiable interval and height between consecutive peaks of the overt rhythm, bimodal phase-response curves) and (2) that both types of oscillator period might be verified in different species, perhaps as a result of a genetic adaptation to the pattern of local tides. Therefore, one should continue to use the term *circatidal* (instead of *circadian* and *semicircadian*) for freerunning tidal rhythms representing a specific type of biological rhythms related to circadian rhythms, but with distinct, adaptive qualities.

OTHER MECHANISMS FOR TIDAL TIMING

DIRECT RESPONSE TO TIDAL STIMULI. In some intertidal species with well-adapted tidal activity rhythms in the field, no persisting tidal rhythms were present in constant laboratory conditions. One may suggest that in these species, the behavior is controlled directly by the submersion and emersion of the habitat. In the sea anemone *Actinia equina*, the spreading of the tentacles was directly induced by light influences under submerged laboratory conditions in the range between LD 12:12 and LD 2:2, where the individuals expanded during the dark time and contracted during the light time (diMilia and Geppetti, 1964). Barnacles showed similar results (Sommer, 1972). Even the filtering activity of the mussels *Mytilus edulis* and *M. californicus* seems to be mainly controlled by external factors, as has been stated in Pickens's reanalysis of the findings of Rao on persisting tidal rhythms (cited in Enright, 1963). In all of these species, an increased sensitivity to some external variable and a constant preparedness for immediate response seems to be a reliable and economic adaptation to the fluctuating intertidal environment. It may be supposed that this "direct-response" type is restricted to benthic animals with relatively simple behavioral performance.

STOCHASTIC PRINCIPLES OF TEMPORAL CONTROL OF ACTIVITY. In most discussions on the temporal control of intertidal behavior, the interpretations are dominated by two main alternatives: an endogenous timing via self-sustained oscillators with a phase-dependent control by external time cues or a direct control by environmental factors only. This restriction implies a simplification of the manifoldness of possible tidal mechanisms because further principles of temporal control can be identified.

In the two fiddler crab species, *Uca annulipes* and *U. urvillei,* from an East African shore with semidiurnal tides, the bursts of locomotor activity and the duration of rests could be continuously registered by means of a radioactive marker technique (p. 357). Under the influence of artificial tides, a clear-cut tidal rhythm resulted in most individuals, with no daily modulation of the activity's amplitude, when a 24-hr light–dark cycle was additionally present (Figure 6). Switched from the tides to constant conditions without any further disturbances of the individuals, the specimens generally demonstrated noncircatidal bursts of activity during the following weeks (top of Figure 7). Because the crabs were kept under natural-like conditions, it is reasonable to assume that the arrhythmic pattern might be an undisturbed and species-specific response.

A detailed periodogram analysis of the actograms yielded randomized and controversial data, even when a "circadian" front of activities on consecutive days could be occasionally discerned. In order to look for any other arrangements in the freerunning patterns of the crabs, a new approach to a quantitative analysis of actograms was applied, measuring the duration of each activity bout (A) and each rest (R) separately, and then plotting their frequency distribution. On this basis, one can easily quantify the arrangement of temporal patterns, independent of any preconception of underlying oscillatory timing mechanisms.

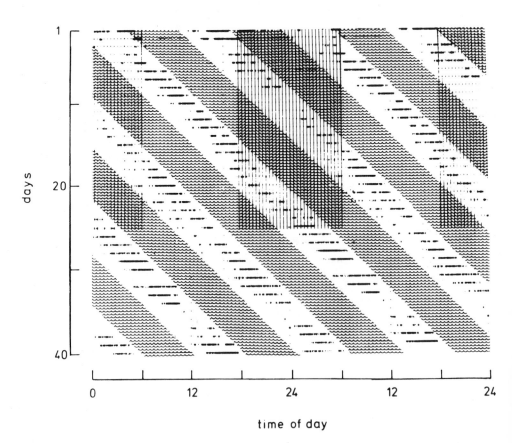

time of day

Fig. 6. Entrained tidal rhythm of locomotory behavior in *Uca urvillei* in LD 12:12 (Days 1–25) and in LL (Days 26–40). Horizontal hatching: times of inundation of the artificial 12.5-hr tides. Vertical hatching: times of darkness. (After Lehmann *et al.,* 1974. Reprinted with permission of Springer-Verlag, Heidelberg.)

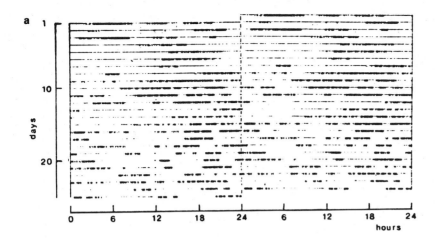

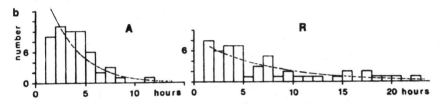

Fig. 7. (a) Actogram of the freerunning activity of an East African *Uca* in DD on the days before the crab was entrained to artificial tides as in Figure 7b. (b) Frequency histograms of the duration of the activity bouts (A) and the rests (R). The columns represent the observed frequency values; the broken lines represent the fitted exponential functions. (After Kaiser and Lehmann, 1975. Reprinted with permission of Springer-Verlag, Heidelberg.)

In the case of a circadian actogram, one would expect peaked frequency distributions of preferred durations in A and R summing up to about 24 hr. For circatidal rhythms, the preferred A and R should be shorter, totaling together 12–13 hr. However, most of the individual fiddler crabs in question demonstrated neither preferred durations of A or R nor any equidistribution of the intervals observed, but the frequency distributions could be fitted by negative exponential frequency functions (bottom of Figure 7). In addition, no significant correlation was found between the duration of A and the following R or any other series of these events. Thus, both exponential curves quantify an important property of the arrhythmic actograms: the duration of each activity bout and each rest is determined by a time-independent probability value for the transition from one state to the other. The transition probability was influenced neither by the duration of the present state nor by the duration of the preceding state; that is, the sequence of events in these patterns resulted from stochastic decisions.

This "freerunning" stochastic pattern was markedly changed in tidal conditions (Figure 8, left side) where the tidal factors obviously controlled the duration of the resting period only, while the duration of activity was stochastically determined as under constant conditions (Lehmann *et al.*, 1974). In relation to these results, a stochastic model was described (Figure 8, right side) and its applicability tested by computer simulations with data from the crabs (Kaiser and Lehmann, 1975; Lehmann, 1976). The model demonstrates a relatively simple physiological mechanism for a somewhat flexible, but nevertheless reliable timing of a tidal behavioral pattern. Attention should be focused on the fact that an exogenously induced, preferred duration of only the resting period can generate appropriate patterns of tidal rhythmicity, while an autonomous control of stochastically shorter activity bouts guarantees some potential flexibility in the sequence of A to R. In the upper intertidal range, where the next onset of submersion or emersion can be changed by spring tides, winds, and storms, this kind of tidal timing may have some advantages. It enables the crabs to react immediately to unexpected situations without any phase-shifting consequences on the following activity time, as it would occur in the case of control by a strong oscillator.

Similar arrhythmic patterns of freerunning locomotor activity have also been observed in other *Uca* populations (*Uca minax* from a location with diurnal tides—Barnwell, 1968; *Uca pugnax*—Palmer, 1973; *Uca crenulata* from a location with mixed tides—Honegger, 1976), and probably in several other cases that have never been published because of their diffuse and nontidal appearance.

TIDAL HOURGLASS TIMING. A third modus of tidal timing without oscillatory processes has been demonstrated in an Arctic population of the intertidal midge *Clunio marinus*. During midsummer, the intertidal populations reproduce twice a day parallel to the tidal cycle, starting when the range of the habitat becomes exposed (top of Figure 9). No persisting tidal rhythm existed in cultures kept under constant conditions. With a single simulation of the slight temperature rise that, in nature, is associated with each exposure, the emergence of the short-lived midges became synchronized during the next 18 hr (Figure 9, middle). Some midges emerged just after the temperature rise (direct response of old pupae prepared for direct emergence); others emerged about 11–13 hr later (single pro-

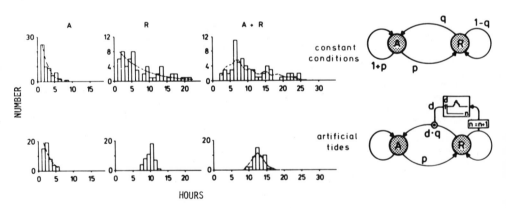

Fig. 8. *(Left)* Frequency histograms of the duration of activity bouts (A), rests (R), and the sum of A and consecutive R (A + R) in two specimens of East African *Uca* (above: constant conditions as in Figure 8; below: artificial tides in LL as in Figure 7). The curves in A and R represent fitted exponential functions, the curves for A + R are computed by random combination of A and R in relation to the frequency histograms. *(Right)* Stochastic models for the simulation of the activity behavior: A and R symbolize the alternating states "activity" and "rest," p describes the transition probability from activity to rest, q the transition probability from rest to activity, both p and q being time-independent; dq describes the modified q when there is a time-dependent influence of the tides on a preferred time of rest (e.g., between 7 and 13 hr). (Combined after Kaiser and Lehmann, 1975, and Lehmann et al., 1974.)

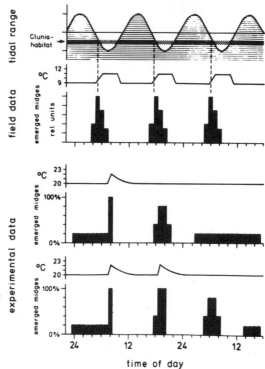

Fig. 9. Tidal rhythm of emergence in an Arctic population of *Clunio marinus* in nature and in experiments demonstrating direct responses and hourglass processes. (Schematically after Pflüger, 1973, from Neumann, 1976c.) (Reprinted with permission of the author.)

gramming of somewhat younger pupae). Any earlier pupal stage remained unsynchronized, so that after some time, the overaged pupae were again spontaneously emerging (distributed equally in the model population of continuous age composition). Temperature pulses repeated every 12.4 hr, as in the intertidal environment, resulted in a strong tidal emergence rhythm by the coincidence of the single programming and the direct response (demonstrated for the case of two pulses in bottom of Figure 9). The single programming must be based on a single endogenous timing process comparable with the hourglass principle. Its Q_{10} was about 1.2 in the range between 10 and 20°C (Pflüger, 1973).

Another hourglass reaction of a few hours has been observed in the timing of the vertical migrations of the turbellarian *Convoluta roscoffensis*, which contrasts with some earlier laboratory observations (cited by Palmer, 1973). This reaction, in combination with a direct response to bottom vibrations, ensures the up and down migrations correlated with the tidal submersion on the high beach (Neumann, 1976c). An hourglass mechanism was also hypothesized for some individuals of the "arrhythmic" fiddler crab population (p. 363), which produced resting periods of 7–11 hr or even up to 20 hr, with a higher probability than expected by chance (Lehmann *et al.*, 1974). In combination with the stochastic processes controlling the activity bouts, both mechanisms result in a higher degree of probability for a "circatidal" pattern during several consecutive days, as has been confirmed by computer-simulated patterns using the stochastic model (Kaiser and Lehmann, 1975). It seems very promising to analyze such examples of flexible tidal activity rhythms and their variety more extensively, with respect to ecological adaptations as well as to the generation of the underlying processes by the nervous system.

DIETRICH NEUMANN

The amplitude of tidal rhythms can be modified in conjunction with the daily illumination and the semimonthly inequalities in the height of the tides. Good indications have been found that in at least a few species, these modifications are based on an endogenous control, either by the combination of circatidal and circadian processes or by the combination of circadian and endogenous monthly ones.

DAILY MODULATION. In the grapsoid crab *Sesarma reticulatum,* a simultaneous persistence of both circadian and circatidal rhythms was evident when, over a period of 2 months, five groups of crabs (10 individuals each) were replaced at intervals of about 2 weeks and when, additionally, the data were summarized and filtered out for minor fluctuations in order to demonstrate the major trends (Palmer, 1967). The intertidal beetle *Thalassostrechus* is strictly nocturnal and forages on the high beach during low water; under constant conditions, a circadian rhythm of locomotion persisted for a week and a vague circatidal component for about 3 days (Evans, 1976). Also, the sandhopper *Talorchestia* emerges from the sand only during the night for feeding within the exposed upper tidal range; in DD, a clear circadian activity rhythm was observed for several weeks, together with a slight circatidal period of inhibited activity during the first days. A new circatidal component was induced by 2-hr pulses of water movement, so that a circatidal clock was postulated in addition to the dominating circadian clock (Benson and Lewis, 1976). Under tideless laboratory conditions with natural illumination, persisting circatidal rhythms with a higher amount of activity, mostly during the night, have been recorded in fiddler crabs (Barnwell, 1966), amphipods (Fincham, 1970), isopods (Fish and Fish, 1972), snails (Zann, 1973), and fish (Gibson, 1971). In green crabs, the higher "nocturnal" peaks even occurred in constant dim light conditions as would have been expected if a circatidal rhythm were superimposed on a circadian rhythm (Naylor, 1958). However, strong evidence of the coexistence of both circatidal and circadian clock mechanisms and their simultaneous influence on locomotor output is still required, because so far, in none of the intertidal species cited have the experimenters as yet succeeded in long-term registrations for single individuals with unequivocal results. Phase-shifting experiments with different zeitgebers for both clocks would probably be most conclusive. For the present, additional interpretations should not be excluded as, for example, some kind of aftereffect in the shape of only one clock system and, at least in some cases, a direct response to natural illumination.

SEMILUNAR MODULATIONS. Examples exist demonstrating an important adaptive significance of these long-term modulations. The isopod *Eurydice pulchra* emerges from the sand during flood in the range of the wave wash about mean high-tide level. In conjunction with the semimonthly cycle of the tide's amplitude, the populations are displaced up and down the beach. When specimens were collected every two days, the migrations on the shore were correlated with different amount of activity during the next few days under laboratory conditions, being less during days with neap tides and greater during spring tides; an endogenous semilunar component was indicated by two long-term registrations under neutral LD (Fish and Fish, 1972; Alheit and Naylor, 1976). In the amphipod *Marinogammarus,* the semilunar modulation of swimming activities was reversed, probably in relation to increased sexual activities during the days of neap tides (Fincham, 1972). In spite of the suggested interpretation of the examples by two endogenous clocks (circatidal and circasemilunar), it cannot be absolutely excluded that the semilunar modulation may also be based on an exogenously induced modification, determining the general amount of activity for some days in pretreatment effects. However, an endogenously controlled long-term modulation of a circatidal rhythm was obvious in the "virtuoso" isopod *Excirolana chiltoni,* persisting for two months in constant dim light conditions with freerunning periods between about 26 and 33 days. By superimposition of the circatidal and the circasemilunar rhythm, the individuals recapitulated regular fluctuations of the mixed, mainly semidiurnal tides of the Californian beach (Enright, 1972). The coexistence of both endogenous rhythms seems to be a successful ecological adaption in programming the activity pattern to complex, but regularly fluctuating environments.

LUNAR RHYTHMS

ENVIRONMENTAL CONDITIONS RELATED TO THE PHASES OF THE MOON

There exist two remarkable influences of the moon on environmental conditions: the illuminant influence during the night, predominantly about the time of full moon, and the gravitational influence on the tides. Both moonlight and tides can affect behavioral as well as developmental performances, resulting in important and species-specific adaptations to nocturnal or tidal environments. Other weak influences of the moon on geophysical factors—for example, atmospheric pressure and magnetic field—have been discussed by a few authors in combination with vague correlations between some animal performances and the phases of the moon; however, these correlations remain outside of the topics of the present compilation because the evidence of lunar adaptation is uncertain and, additionally, because the evaluation of the raw data would require detailed inspection.

MOONLIGHT AND TIDES. The visible moonlight is sunlight reflected from the lunar surface, with nearly the same spectral composition, but with a shift of its intensities somewhat toward the red (Kopal, 1969). The relatively low amount of illumination (0.2 lux and less) varies with the phases of the moon, the length of time that the moon is above the horizon, the moon's height, and the weather (Bowden, 1973). The nocturnal light climate distributed by the moon during a synodic month is relatively constant at tropical latitudes (Figure 10), with only slight seasonal changes in the times of moonrise and moonset. At higher latitudes, there exist complex seasonal changes with relation to the elevation of the moon and the sequence of times of moonrise and moonset. In general, the full moon culminates above the horizon at about the height that the sun had reached half a year before (for further details, see Werner, 1960).

As has already been described (p. 352), the tide-generating forces and their relation to the phases of the moon result in a semimonthly modulation of the tidal amplitude on those seashores that are exposed to semidiurnal or mixed tides.

LUNAR TERMINOLOGY. The term *lunar rhythm* may be used, on one hand, as a category of all kinds of biological rhythms related to the moon: (1) the *lunar-day* rhythm (synonym: *lunadian, bitidal*) corresponding with the 24.8-hr period between two consecutive culminations of the moon; (2) the *lunar-semimonthly* or *semilunar* rhythm (synonym: *syzygic*) corresponding with the 14.76-hr period between successive spring low waters or,

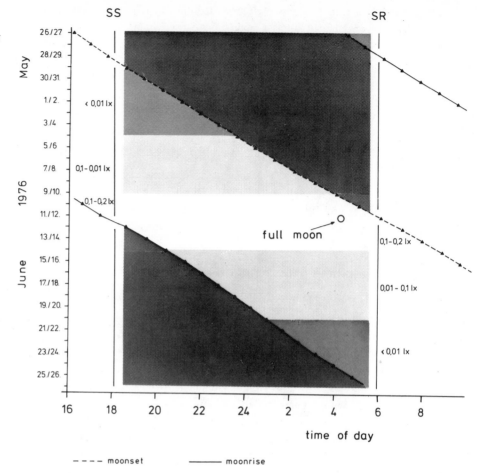

Fig. 10. Times of moonrise and moonset, and the approximate intensities of illumination during a synodic month near the equator. The precise illumination values of the crepuscular light and of the period between moonrise (or moonset) and the moon's elevation above 45° (with undiminished light, interval of about 3 hr) have been neglected. The starlight during the period of no moon amounts to 0.0009 lux. (Calculated after Astronomical-Ephemeris and Danthanarayana, 1976.)

in relation to the moon, between successive syzygies of the moon (p. 352); and (3) the *lunar-monthly* cycle (synonym: *lunar, synodic*) related to the 29.53-hr period of the synodic month (p. 352). On the other hand, the word *lunar* may be often restricted to the monthly rhythms only. In order to avoid any misunderstandings in the following chapters, the predefined terms are used because these are directly understandable to everyone.

LUNAR-RHYTHMIC ADAPTATIONS OF BEHAVIOR

LUNAR-DAY RHYTHMS IN TERRESTRIAL ANIMALS. The possible influence of moonlight on the nocturnal activities of terrestrial animals suggested by several occasional observations can be demonstrated best when individuals are maintained for months in registration cages under natural illumination. In this way, it was established that the nocturnal restlessness of robins and redstarts was increased during the migratory season in conjunction with the nocturnal illumination from the moon (Gwinner, 1967). Evidence of clear-cut lunar-day rhythms corresponding well with the periods of illuminated night have been shown in nocturnal mammals of the tropics (Figure 11). In the night monkey *Aotus trivigatus,* the nocturnal activities increased with relation to the dim lunar light; they decreased in the phyllostomatic bat *Artibeus literatus;* and in other bat species, transitional forms of both activity types existed. On the basis of records under laboratory conditions, it can be suggested that the activity pattern of these tropical animals is predominantly determined by a circadian timing that is *exogenously* modulated by a species-specific direct response to moonlight, exaggerating or suppressing the activity output (Erkert, 1974).

Indications of an *endogenously* controlled lunar-day rhythm have been presented in the case of the nocturnal activities of the ant lion *Myrmeleon obscurus,* revealing a lunar-monthly rhythm of its pit volume that was large during the full moon period and small during the new moon period. The pit volume corresponded with the pit-building activities, which had a clear peak 4 hr after moonrise, indicating a lunar-day rhythm of locomotor activity. Because the activities were additionally restricted to the night period, the combination of both lunar-day rhythm and daily rhythm resulted in the observation of a lunar-monthly rhythm. The monthly rhythm persisted in the laboratory under constant dark conditions (for two cycles) and was phase-shifted for half a month under a reversed LD 14:10. The latter observation suggests that the phase-shifted daily rhythm was pushed into

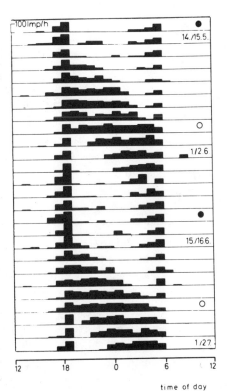

Fig. 11. Actogram of the Columbian night monkey *Aotus trivigatus* under natural light conditions. O: full moon, ●: new moon. (After Erkert, 1974.)

time of day

a new phase relationship with the freerunning lunar-day rhythm (Youthed and Moran, 1969).

A moonlight-related activity modulation may be widely distributed among nocturnal animals (for example, kangaroo rats—Lockard and Owings, 1974; migrating silver eels—Hain, 1975; nocturnal bees—Kerfoot, 1967; and other crepuscular and nocturnal insects mentioned in the next section).

LUNAR-MONTHLY RHYTHMS IN INSECT POPULATIONS. Light-trap catches have revealed lunar fluctuations in the flight activities and in the abundance of a number of insect species of Plecoptera, Ephemeroptera, Trichoptera, Diptera (especially Chironomidae), and Lepidoptera, most of them at tropical latitudes in Africa, but some others also at higher latitudes, such as in Australia and Florida (summarized literature in Danthanarayana, 1976; Fryer, 1959). The possible interpretation of these fluctuations as an artifact resulting from a change in the relative brightness of the trap with relation to the background illumination from the moon was carefully evaluated and had to be refused, at least in certain species (Bowden and Church, 1973). This was also confirmed by the observation of Corbet (1958) that out of 37 species studied in the area of Lake Victoria, only 4 species were obviously rhythmic. It has been suggested that the lunar-monthly rhythm of at least some populations is caused by a lunar rhythm of emergence and reproduction (p. 371) because several species have relatively short-lived imagoes of a few days or even less, such as the mayfly *Povilla adusta*. This ephemeropteran insect (Lake Victoria and Lake Albert) emerges and swarms within 5 days of the full moon when the early moonrise lengthens the dim light of dusk so that the mating and egg laying of this short-lived crepuscular insect are guaranteed in spite of the short tropical twilight period of only 30 min. The lunar timing of emergence persisted in the laboratory after the nymphs had been kept in the dark for 10 days and in two individuals for even 6 weeks, so that an endogenous lunar-monthly component may be supposed (Hartland-Rowe, 1955).

LUNAR-MONTHLY RHYTHMS IN THE SENSITIVITY TO LIGHT. When the small freshwater fish *Lebistes reticulatus* is illuminated under constant dark conditions by a point source of light from one side, the fish orients his dorsal–ventral axis according to the resultant angle between light and gravitational stimulus (dorsal light reaction). The angle reflects the momentary subjective sensitivity to light stimuli. In long-term registrations of the angle displayed, Lang (for summary, 1977) detected obvious fluctuations in the angle, corresponding to changes in the subjective sensitivity of the fish. In the course of years, these fluctuations were correlated during some periods with the lunar month (maximum sensitivity to yellow light about the time of the full moon, and minimum values about the time of the new moon), while during other periods, a reversed phase relationship or no regular modulation occurred. In additional short-term registrations, only a circadian rhythm but not a lunar-day rhythm was found, so that the lunar-month rhythm was not caused by a combination of both circadian and lunar-day components. It was suggested by Lang that the lunar sensitivity rhythm mirrors an exogenous control by some unknown influences of the moon, whereby the influences of moonlight, gravity, atmospheric pressure, and magnetic field are excluded. Further registrations under constant as well as experimentally modified conditions have to be conducted to determine whether these obvious long-term fluctuations are definitely dependent on an exogenous influence of the moon or whether they are endogenously determined (thus comparable to the menstruation cycle of women), being from time to time randomly synchronous with the lunar month.

EXAMPLES FROM THE SEASHORE AND TROPICAL LAKES. In several intertidal organisms inhabiting coasts with semidiurnal tides or with mixed tides (p. 352), both lunar-semimonthly and lunar-monthly rhythms of reproduction have been observed in conjunction with the cycles of spring and neap tides. Despite the daily delay of the tides, it is important to recognize that in both tidal types, any semidiurnal phase of the tides coincides every 14–15 days with about the same time of day, and this goes on throughout the year, because a daily delay of 0.84 hr results in a 12.4-hr delay during the 14.76-day cycle. Thus, any specific situation of the local tides recurs in relation to the time of day every 2 weeks. For example, the mean time of the afternoon low water on days with spring tides during several years differed on Helgoland in the North Sea according to the prediction of the tide tables by only 2 min (Neumann, 1978). Intertidal species with semimonthly or monthly rhythms of developmental and behavioral performances related to reproduction have adapted to tidal situations of such kinds. As is shown by the field data for the six best-observed animal species, the biological long-term rhythms guarantee not only a concentration of the mating partners, but also a distinct tidal situation that is advantageous for the release of eggs or early larval stages.

The atherinid fish *Leuresthes tenuis,* the grunion, spawns high on the beaches of Southern California and Mexico during the spring and summer months, and this every 15 days at about midnight during the high tide of spring tides; the fertilized eggs are buried in the sand at about the MHWS tidemark (p. 353). The larvae hatch 8–12 days later, when the next series of stronger high tides wash the upper beach (Walker, 1949). The imagoes of the short-lived marine insect *Clunio marinus* (European coast of the Atlantic Ocean and North Sea) emerge every 15 days shortly before the afternoon low water of spring tides; after a mating flight on the water surfaces and exposed substrates, the sticky egg masses are fixed 0.5–2 hr later to unsubmerged substrates around the MLWS tidemark, where they cannot be washed away by the next flood. In different *Clunio* species and their local populations, a variety of temporal adaptations of the semimonthly rhythm exists in relation to the local tidal conditions (see Neumann, 1976a, for review; Heimbach, 1978).

The land crabs, *Sesarma haemotocheir* and *S. intermedium* release their zoea–larvae in a freshwater river (1.5 km from the ocean) just after sunset every 15 days about the time of the new and full moons so that the down-drifting larvae will arrive at the sea during the ebbing tides (Saigusa and Hidaka, 1978). In the fiddler crab, *Uca pugilator* (western Florida), females mate once each month, either 4–5 days before the spring tides of the full moon or 15 days later; the release of the zoea–larvae occurs about 13 days later, that is, about 7 days before each spring tide during the ebb (Christy, 1978).

The famous example of the Palolo worm, *Eunice viridis,* of the South Pacific Ocean is characterized by an extreme seasonal restriction of the lunar timing; the synchronous swarming of the epitokous segments and the release of the gametes into the open sea occur during the last quarter of the moon in late October or early November, mainly during only one night (at Tutuila, Samoa, between midnight and 2 A. M.) (Caspers, 1961; Hauenschild, Fischer, and Hoffmann, 1968). The nuptial dances of the mature form of the polychaete *Platynereis dumerilii* take place in a lunar-monthly rhythm from March to October, as has been observed by Ranzi in a population of the European Mediterranean Sea (characterized by weak tides). The peak activity was, on an average, on the third day after full moon during the early night (cited by Korringa, 1947). Similar results on lunar rhythms have been collected in a wide variety of marine organisms of the intertidal environments and the sublittoral (for review of the older literature, see Korringa, 1947; isopods—Klapow, 1972a; sea urchins—Pearse, 1972).

Examples from tropical lakes are connected with the lunar-monthly rhythms described on p. 370.

BREEDING EXPERIMENTS. Evidence of the interaction of both endogenous components and exogenous time cues can be expected only from breeding experiments under controlled laboratory conditions. Hauenschild (1960) was the first to succeed. He evoked a lunar-monthly rhythm of swarming in the polychaete *Platynereis dumerilii,* independent of the phases of the moon, by simulating moonlight in artificial 24-hr light–dark cycles every 30 days during a few consecutive nights. With the same method, lunar-semimonthly rhythms were induced in the brown algae *Dictyota dichotoma* (synchronous release of the gametes; Bünning, 1973) and in the chironomid midge *Clunio marinus* (Neumann, 1966). The control of a semimonthly rhythm by monthly time cues demonstrates the existence of an important endogenous component determining the period of the rhythm. Considering the developmental processes that are related to the lunar rhythms (ripening of gametes, metamorphosis to the "heteronereis" in *Platynereis,* and to a pupa 3–5 days before the day of swarming in *Clunio*), one may *a priori* exclude in both lunar-semimonthly and lunar-monthly rhythms any direct response to the influence of artificial moonlight.

PERSISTING LUNAR RHYTHMS. Evidence of the existence of endogenous clock mechanisms with a period in the range of the natural reproductive rhythm was demonstrated in two sets of experiments under uniform conditions (Figure 12; release of synchronized cultures; exposure of asynchronous cultures only once to the synchronizing stimulus, that is, with no information on the lunar period). From the freerunning rhythms of the populations, one may conclude that the population rhythm reflects an endogenous long-term rhythm in an individual. This endogenous clock mechanism enables the start of metamorphosis and reproduction only at lunar-semimonthly or lunar-monthly intervals. The freerunning period is a population-specific property (Figure 12), in *Platynereis* about 30 days

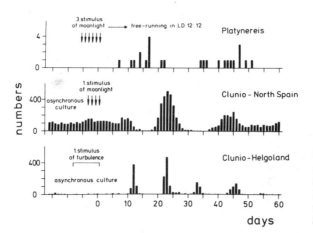

Fig. 12. Freerunning lunar-monthly and lunar-semimonthly rhythms. (*Platynereis:* Hauenschild 1960; *Clunio:* Neumann, 1966, 1976b.) (Reprinted with permission of Fischer-Verlag, Stuttgart.)

and in *Clunio* about 22 days (stock North Spain), 11 days (stock Helgoland), or 15 days (stock Normandy, not in figure). Thus, in correspondence to circadian phenomena, the period of the endogenous, freerunning rhythm has been named *circalunar* (in the case of lunar-monthly rhythms) and *circasemilunar* (in the case of lunar-semimonthly rhythms).

In *Platynereis*, the freerunning period was influenced by the periodicity of the preceding illumination program (artificial moonlight every 28–30 days, successive τ about 33 days; moonlight every 21 days, successive τ about 25 days; Hauenschild 1960). Also in *Clunio*, a wide range of entrainment was demonstrated (North Spain population: moonlight cycles of 24 and 36 days), but the successive sequence of freerunning peaks was uniformly independent of the cycles, so that the period of this species seems to be an innate property of the rhythm (Neumann, 1976b).

THE BASIC PERIOD OF THE CLOCK. It can be tested whether the periods of the freerunning rhythms are based on an interaction between a circadian oscillator and a circatidal one ($\tau \sim 12.4$ hr or 25 hr). They would reinforce each other about every 15 or 30 days when both oscillators came into a state of physiological coincidence to control the lunar-semimonthly or lunar-monthly events ("beat" hypothesis or two-oscillator hypothesis). If this were true, one could expect a changed period of the recurring coincidence and the resulting rhythm when the cultures are entrained by an abnormal daily zeitgeber period. One would further expect a phase shift of the lunar freerunning rhythm if the circadian-oscillator component were phase-shifted by a single phase jump of the LD cycle. When *Platynereis* cultures were subjected to a 23.25-hr day and a 30-day moonlight cycle (expectation according to the beat hypothesis: daily shifting between both oscillators of about 1.5 hr instead of 0.8 hr, totaling to a 24-hr shifting with recurring coincidence after 15 days instead of 30 days), the lunar rhythm of swarming was still 30 days (Hauenschild, 1960). *Clunio* cultures were exposed to false days as well as to phase jumps of the LD cycle, likewise with no consequences in the semimonthly rhythm of emergence (Neumann, 1976b). Thus, no support for the two-oscillator hypothesis has been produced. It has to be concluded that the semimonthly and monthly rhythms of these animals are based on a truly endogenous long-term rhythm.

ZEITGEBER EXPERIMENTS. It has been demonstrated that moonlight is not the only zeitgeber for lunar-semimonthly rhythms. In *Clunio* populations from northern Europe, moonlight was nearly ineffective in the breeding experiments (Neumann, 1966; Neumann and Heimbach, 1979). Good entrainment was produced by artificial tidal cycles in combination with a 24-hr LD cycle, whose phase relationships were identical every 15 days. The effective tidal zeitgeber was the mechanical disturbance of the water, simulated by frequencies of mainly 50–200 cps above the background noise level, which is in the range of the increased underwater sound during flood tide (Neumann, 1978). In the laboratory, some populations situated farther south responded to both moonlight and tides as zeitgebers (Figure 13), while some southern European populations were synchronized only by moonlight. Comparing the quality of entrainment by artificial tides with respect to the geographical latitude of the locations of several *Clunio* stocks, it was established that in the northern populations above 49°N, the tidal factors are strong zeitgebers resulting in adequate phase relationships between the emergence peak and the tidal zeitgeber program (Neumann and Heimbach, 1979). This can be interpreted as a successful geographic adaptation of lunar-semimonthly rhythms to the conditions of the northern fringe of temperate latitudes, where

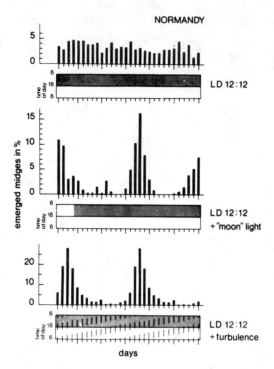

Fig. 13. Zeitgeber experiments in the semilunar emergence rhythm of *Clunio marinus* (mean distribution of entrained cultures and their control). The zeitgeber conditions are shown schematically. *(Above)* Control; *(Middle)* 12 hr of 0.4-lux dim light every 30 days on 4 consecutive nights (light gray bar); *(Below)* 12.4-hr rhythm of mechanical disturbance (vertical line time of mean distribution). (After Neumann, 1976b.)

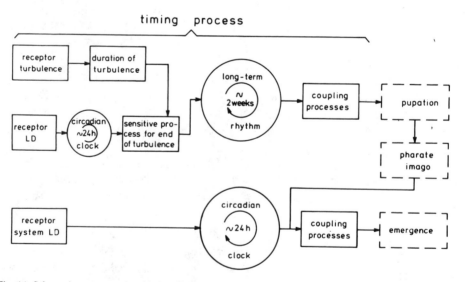

Fig. 14. Schematic representation of the physiological components of the internal timing mechanisms in the semilunar emergence rhythm of *Clunio marinus* (Helgoland population). The upper half represents the semilunar timing of pupation, the lower half the circadian timing of emergence after a pupal stage of 3–5 days during summer (15–20°C). The daily emergence is adapted to a specific environmental situation (time of local afternoon low water of spring tides). (After Neumann, 1976c.)

moonlight is an unreliable environmental factor during summer (because of the low height of the full moon, long crepuscular periods, and above 55°N a short or even no interval of total darkness about the time of the new moon).

PERCEPTION OF THE TIDAL ZEITGEBER FOR LUNAR-SEMIMONTHLY RHYTHMS. The astonishing result of the foregoing experiments is that a semilunar rhythm can be entrained by a tidal factor occurring twice each day but with shifting phase relationships from day to day. In experiments with modified zeitgeber cycles, the period of the induced "semi-monthly" rhythm was correlated with the periodic return of identical phase relationships between the artificial tides and the LD cycle; for example, the period was 12 days in a 12.5-hr tidal cycle and LD 12:12 (the daily shift between both was 1 hr, totaling 12 hr and equal phases every 12 days). Thus, both the tides and the LD cycle are the requisite zeit-gebers, and a distinct phase relationship between them apparently offers the decisive stimulus for the entrainment of the circasemilunar clock mechanism (Neumann, 1968).

In the next step, the main physiological components of the circasemilunar timing mechanism for the perception of this recurring tidal phase relationship have been unraveled in a series of experiments (Figure 14, upper half). First, the tidal zeitgeber was effective only if the mechanical disturbance lasted for 6 hr or more (comparable with the raised intensity of turbulence during flood tide). Second, it was concluded that the change between the tidal stimulus and calm is a further component of the system. The most simple hypothesis for the perception of a distinct phase relationship between the end of a turbulence stimulus and the time of day was a sensitive daily phase of a circadian clock system. Following this suggestion in a third series of experiments with a modified 15-day pattern of tidal stimuli, a sensitive daily phase was obviously indicated (in the Helgoland stock: turbulences from 600 to 1200 and from 1800 to 2400 hr). In a last series, it could be demonstrated that the perception of the tidal factor during a daily sensitive phase is a circadian function. The cultures were subjected to a 48-hr LD cycle (LD 12:36), while the tidal stimulus was given only every second day during the dark time of the last 24 hr of the LD cycle. The successful entrainment in this abnormal LD cycle indicates that the sensitive daily phase recurred during the prolonged dark period as only an endogenous circadian rhythm would do. The results are summarized in the schematic model of Figure 14, combining an endogenous semilunar pacemaker with a circadian clock system for measuring a distinct phase relationship between the tides and the time of day.

This schedule of semilunar pupation control in *Clunio* resembles the photoperiod control of seasonal development in other insects, in that a circadian clock is involved, determining a photosensitive time of day for the initiation of diapause (Bünning, 1973). Additionally, it might be supposed that the perception of moonlight as an entraining photoperiodic stimulus of lunar rhythms is based on similar components.

THE COMBINATION WITH A CIRCADIAN TIMING. As has been mentioned on the basis of the field observations (p. 371), semimonthly and monthly lunar rhythms of reproductive behavior are characterized by timing to both a few days of the lunar month and a specific time of day. In *Clunio marinus*, this complex adaptation to a regularly recurring situation of the intertidal environment is put into effect by the combination of two physiological timing mechanisms, a circasemilunar timing system and an additional circadian system, both controlling successive developmental steps of the metamorphosis to the adult and sexually mature insect (Figure 14). The circadian clock has been established by freerunning experiments in LL as well as by the effect of single light pulses on asynchronous LL-cultures, resulting in freerunning circadian rhythms; it is entrained by the 24-hr LD cycle (Neumann, 1966) and corresponds in its properties to the known insect eclosion clock (Pittendrigh, 1960). The phase of the entrained circadian rhythm of *Clunio* is correlated with a time of day when in nature the intertidal habitat is exposed on days of emergence (Figure 15). In correlation with the time displacement of the tides along the coasts, the phase of the circadian clock is genetically adapted to that time of day when the low-water time recurs every 15 days, as has been demonstrated by crossbreeding between stocks of different locations. Thus, gene-controlled parameters of the timing mechanisms can be identified by the comparison of local geographic races (Neumann, 1966). If we look at all the experimental results from *Clunio,* the lunar-semimonthly rhythms reveal a multioscillatory organization used in a complex temporal programming. The question of whether a similar combination of components is also verified in the lunar rhythms of other organisms must be analyzed in the future.

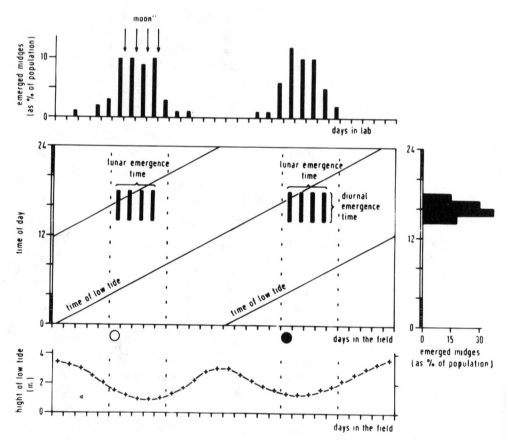

Fig. 15. Adaptation of semilunar and daily reproduction to tidal conditions in *Clunio marinus* (population from Normandy, France); comparison of field observations and laboratory results. *(Below)* Change of the height of low water during one lunar month. *(Middle)* Time of low water during one lunar month (schematically) and emergence times in nature. *(Above)* Semilunar emergence times in experiments under LD 16:8 and artificial moonlight (4 nights with 0.4 lux every 30 days). *(Right)* Diurnal emergence times on the days of semilunar emergence (L from 400 to 2000 hr). (After Neumann, 1967. Reprinted with permission of Biologische Anstalt Helgoland, Hamburg.)

Al-Adhub, A. H. Y., and Naylor, E. Emergence rhythms and tidal migrations in the brown shrimp *Crangon crangon* (L.). *Journal of the Marine Biological Association of the United Kingdom*, 1975, *55*, 801–810.

Alheit, J., and Naylor, E. Behavioral basis of intertidal zonation in *Eurydice pulchra* Leach. *Journal of Experimental Marine Biology and Ecology*, 1976, *23*, 135–144.

Barnwell, F. H. Daily and tidal patterns of activity in individual fiddler crabs (genus *Uca*) from the Woods Hole region. *Biological Bulletin*, 1966, *130*, 1–17.

Barnwell, F. H. The role of rhythmic system in the adaptation of fiddler crabs to the intertidal zone. *American Zoologist*, 1968, *8*, 569–583.

Barnwell, F. H. Variation in the form of the tide and some problems it poses for biological timing systems. In P. J. DeCoursey (Ed.), *Biological Rhythms in the Marine Environment*. Columbia: University of South Carolina Press, 1976.

Bennett, M. F., Shriner, J., and Brown, R. A. Persistent tidal cycles of spontaneous motor activity in the fiddler crab, *Uca pugnax*. *Biological Bulletin*, 1957, *112*, 267–275.

Benson, J. A., and Lewis, R. D. An analysis of the activity rhythm of the sand beach amphipod, *Talorchestia quoyana*. *Journal of Comparative Physiology*, 1976, *105*, 339–352.

Bowden, J. The influence of moonlight on catches of insects in light-traps in Africa. I. The moon and moonlight. *Bulletin of Entomological Research*, 1973, *63*, 113–128.

Bowden, J., and Church, B. M. The influence of moonlight on catches of insects in light-traps in Africa. II. The effect of moon phase on light-trap catches. *Bulletin of Entomological Research*, 1973, *63*, 129–142.

Brown, F. A., Jr. The "clocks" timing biological rhythms. *American Scientist*, 1972, *60*, 756–766.

Brown, F. A., Jr., Fingermann, M., Sandeen, M., and Webb, H. M. Persistent diurnal and tidal rhythms of colour change in the fiddler crab, *Uca pugnax*. *Journal of Experimental Zoology*, 1953, *123*, 29–60.

Bünning, E. *The Physiological Clock*. Berlin–Heidelberg–New York: Springer, 1973.

Caspers, H. Beobachtungen über Lebensraum und Schwärmperiodizität des Palolowurmes *Eunice viridis*. *Internationale Revue der gesamten Hydrobiologie*, 1961, *46*, 175–183.

Cheng, L. (Ed.). *Marine Insects*. Amsterdam: North-Holland, 1976.

Christy, J. H. Adaptative significance of reproductive cycles in the fiddler crab *Uca pugilator:* A hypothesis. *Science*, 1978, *199*, 453–455.

Corbet, P. S. Lunar periodicity of aquatic insects in Lake Victoria. *Nature* (Lond.), 1958, *182*, 330–331.

Creutzberg, F. The role of tidal streams in the navigation of migrating elvers (*Anguilla vulgaris* Turt.). *Ergebnisse der Biologie*, 1963, *26*, 118–127.

Cubit, J. Behavior and physical factors causing migration and aggregation of the sand crab *Emerita analoga* (Stimpson). *Ecology*, 1970, *50*, 118–123.

Danthanarayana, W. Diel and lunar flight periodicities in the light brown apple moth, *Epiphyas postvittana* (Walker) (Tortricidae) and their possible adaptive significance. *Australian Journal of Zoology*, 1976, *24*, 65–73.

DeCoursey, P. J. (Ed.). *Biological Rhythms in the Marine Environment*. Columbia: University of South Carolina Press, 1976.

Defant, A. *Physical Oceanography*. Vol. 2. New York: Pergamon Press, 1961.

di Milia, A., and Geppetti, L. On the expansion–contraction rhythm of the sea anemone, *Actinia equina* L. *Experientia* (Basel), 1964, *20*, 571–572.

Enright, J. T. The tidal rhythms of activity of a sandbeach amphipod. *Zeitschrift für vergleichende Physiologie*, 1963, *46*, 276–313.

Enright, J. T. Entrainment of a tidal rhythm. *Science*, 1965a, *147*, 864–867.

Enright, J. T. The search for rhythmicity in biological time series. *Journal Theoretical Biology*, 1965b, *8*, 426–468.

Enright, J. T. The internal clock of drunken isopods. *Journal of Comparative Physiology*, 1971, *75*, 332–346.

Enright, J. T. A virtuoso isopod: Circa-lunar rhythms and their tidal fine structure. *Journal of Comparative Physiology*, 1972, *77*, 141–162.

Enright, J. T. Orientation in time: endogenous clocks. In O. Kinne (Ed.), *Marine Ecology. Vol. II. Physiological Mechanisms* (Part 2). London: Wiley, 1975.

Enright, J. T. Plasticity in an isopods clockworks: Shaking shapes form and affects phase and frequency. *Journal of Comparative Physiology*, 1976, *107*, 13–37.

Erkert, H. G. Der Einfluss des Mondlichts auf die Aktivitätsperiodik nachtaktiver Säugetiere. *Oecologia* (Berl.), 1974, *14*, 269–287.

Evans, W. G. Circadian and circatidal locomotory rhythms in the intertidal beetle *Thalassostrechus barbarae* (Horn): Carabidae. *Journal of Experimental Marine Biology and Ecology*, 1976, *22*, 79–90.

Fincham, A. A. Rhythmic behaviour of the intertidal amphipod *Bathyporeia pelagica*. *Journal of the Marine Biological Association of the United Kingdom*, 1970, *50*, 1057–1068.

Fincham, A. A. Rhythmic swimming and rheotropism in the amphipod *Marinogammarus marinus*. *Journal of Experimental Marine Biology and Ecology*, 1972, *8*, 19–26.

Fish, J. D., and Fish, S. The swimming rhythm of *Eurydice pulchra* Leach and a possible explanation of intertidal migration. *Journal of Experimental Marine Biology and Ecology*, 1972, *8*, 195–200.

Foster, W. A., Treherne, J. E., and Ruscoe, C. N. E. Short-term changes in activity rhythms in an intertidal arthropod (Acarina: *Bdella interrupta* Evans). *Oecologia* (Berl.), 1979, *38*, 291–301.

Fricke, H. W. Die ökologische Spezialisierung der Eidechse *Cryptoblepharus boutoni cognatus* (Boettger) auf das Leben in der Gezeitenzone (Reptilia, Skinkidae). *Oecologia* (Berl.), 1970, *5*, 380–391.

Fryer, G. Lunar rhythm of emergence, differential behavior of the sexes, and other phenomena in the African midge, *Chironomus brevibucca* (Kief.). *Bulletin of Entomological Research*, 1959, *50*, 1–8.

Funke, W. Heimfindevermögen und Ortstreue bei *Patella* L. (Gastropoda, Prosobranchia). *Oecologia* (Berl.), 1968, *2*, 19–142.

Gibson, R. N. Factors affecting the rhythmic activity of *Blennius phobis* L. (Teleostei). *Animal Behavior*, 1971, *19*, 336–343.

Gibson, R. N. Tidal and circadian activity rhythms in juvenile plaice, *Pleuronectes platessa*. *Marine Biology*, 1973, *22*, 379–386.

Green, J. *The Biology of Estuarine Animals*. London: Sidgwick and Jackson, 1968.

Gwinner, E. Die Wirkung des Mondlichtes auf die Nachtaktivität von Zugvögeln.—Lotsenversuch an Rotkehlchen *(Erithacus rubecula)* und Gartenrotschwänzchen *(Phoenicurus phoenicurus)*. *Experientia* (Basel), 1967, *23*, 227.

Hain, J. H. W. The behaviour of migratory eels, *Anguilla rostrata*, in response to current, salinity and lunar period. *Helgoländer wissenschaftliche Meeresuntersuchungen*, 1975, *27*, 211–233.

Hardtland-Rowe, R. Lunar rhythm in the emergence of an ephemeropteran. *Nature* (Lond.), 1955, *176*, 657.

Hauenschild, C. Lunar periodicity. *Cold Spring Harbor Symposia on Quantitative Biology*, 1960, *25*, 491–497.

Hauenschild, C., Fischer, A., and Hoffmann, D. K. Untersuchungen am pazifischen *Palolowurm Eunice viridis* (Polychaeta) in Samoa. *Helgoländer wissenschaftliche Meeresuntersuchungen*, 1968, *18*, 254–295.

Heimbach, F. Emergence times of the intertidal midge *Clunio marinus* (Chironomidae) at places with abnormal tides. In D. S. McLusky and A. J. Berry (Ed.), *Physiology and Behavior of Marine Organisms*. Oxford and New York: Pergamon Press, 1978.

Heusner, A. A., and Enright, J. T. Longterm activity recording in small aquatic animals. *Science*, 1966, *154*, 532–533.

Honegger, H. W. Locomotor activity in *Uca crenulata*, and the response to two zeitgebers, light–dark and tides. In P. J. DeCoursey (Ed.), *Biological Rhythms in the Marine Environment*. Columbia: University of South Carolina Press, 1976.

Hughes, D. A. On the endogenous control of tide-associated displacements of pink shrimp, *Penaeus duorarum* Burkenroad. *Biological Bulletin*, 1972, *142*, 271–280.

Jacobs, J. Animal behavior and water movement as co-determinants of plancton distribution in a tidal system. *Sarsia*, 1968, *34*, 355–370.

Jones, D. A., and Naylor, E. The swimming rhythm of the sand beach isopod *Eurydice pulchra*. *Journal of Experimental Marine Biology and Ecology*, 1970, *4*, 188–199.

Kaiser, H., and Lehmann, U. Tidal and spontaneous activity patterns in fiddler crabs. II. Stochastic models and simulations. *Journal of Comparative Physiology*, 1975, *96*, 1–26.

Kerfoot, W. B. The lunar periodicity of *Sphecodogastra texana*, a nocturnal bee (Hymenoptera: Halictidae). *Animal Behavior*, 1967, *15*, 479–486.

Klapow, L. A. Fortnightly molting and reproductive cycles in the sandbeach isopod, *Excirolana chiltoni*. *Biological Bulletin*, 1972a, *143*, 568–591.

Klapow, L. A. Natural and artificial rephasing of a tidal rhythm. *Journal of Comparative Physiology*, 1972b, *79*, 233–258.

Kopal, Z. *The Moon*. Dordrecht, Holland: D. Reidel, 1969.

Korringa, P. Relations between the moon and periodicity in the breeding of marine animals. *Ecological Monographs*, 1947, *17*, 349–381.

Lang, H. J. Lunar periodicity of colour sense of fish. *Journal of Interdisciplinary Cycle Research*, 1977, *8*, 317–321.

Lehmann, U. Interpretation of entrained and free-running locomotor activity patterns of *Uca*. In P. J. DeCoursey (Ed.), *Biological Rhythms in the Marine Environment*. Columbia: University of South Carolina Press, 1976.

Lehmann, U., Neumann, D., and Kaiser, H. Gezeitenrhythmische und spontane Aktivitätsmuster von Winkerkrabben—ein neuer Ansatz zur quantitativen Analyse von Lokomotionsrhythmen. *Journal of Comparative Physiology,* 1974, *91,* 187–221.

Lockard, R. B., and Owings, D. H. Moon-related surface activity of bannertail *(Dipodomys spectabilis)* and Fresno *(D. nitratoides)* kangaroo rats. *Animal Behavior,* 1974, *22,* 262–273.

Morgan, E. The activity rhythm of the amphipod *Corophium volutator* (Pallas) and its possible relationship to changes in hydrostatic pressure associated with the tides. *Journal of Animal Ecology,* 1965, *34,* 731–746.

Naylor, E. Tidal and diurnal rhythm of locomotory activity in *Carcinus maenas* (L.). *The Journal of Experimental Biology,* 1958, *35,* 602–610.

Naylor, E. Temperature relationships of the locomotor rhythm of *Carcinus. The Journal of Experimental Biology,* 1963, *40,* 669–679.

Naylor, E. Rhythmic behavior and reproduction in marine animals. In R. C. Newell, *Adaptation to the Environment: Essays on the Physiology of Marine Animals.* London, Boston: Butterworths, 1976.

Neumann, D. Die lunare and tägliche Schlüpfperiodik der Mücke *Clunio:* Steuerung und Abstimmung auf die Gezeitenperiodik. *Zeitschrift für vergleichende Physiologie,* 1966, *53,* 1–61.

Neumann, D. Genetic adaptation in the emergence time of *Clunio* populations to different tidal conditions. *Helgoländer wissenschaftliche Meeresuntersuchungen,* 1967, *15,* 163–171.

Neumann, D. Die Steuerung einer semilunaren Schlüpfperiodik mit Hilfe eines künstlichen Gezeitenzyklus. *Zeitschrift für vergleichende Physiologie,* 1968, *60,* 63–78.

Neumann, D. Die Kombination verschiedener endogener Rhythmen bei der zeitlichen Programmierung von Entwicklung und Verhalten. *Oecologia* (Berl.), 1969, *3,* 166–183.

Neumann, D. Adaptations of chironomids to intertidal environments. *Annual Review of Entomology,* 1976a, *21,* 387–414.

Neumann, D. Entrainment of a semilunar rhythm. In P. J. DeCoursey (Ed.), *Biological Rhythms in the Marine Environment.* Columbia: University of South Carolina Press, 1976b.

Neumann, D. Mechanismen für die zeitliche Anpassung von Verhaltens und Entwicklungsleistungen an den Gezeitenzyklus. *Verhandlungen der Deutschen Zoologischen Gesellschaft,* 1976c, 9–28.

Neumann, D. Entrainment of a semilunar rhythm by simulated tidal cycles of mechanical disturbance. *Journal of Experimental Marine Biology and Ecology,* 1978, *35,* 73–85.

Neumann, D., and Heimbach, F. Time cues for semilunar reproduction rhythms in European populations of *Clunio.* I. The influence of tidal cycles of mechanical disturbance. In E. Naylor (Ed.), *Cyclical Phenomena in Marine Plants and Animals.* Oxford: Pergamon Press, 1979.

Newell, R. C. *Biology of Intertidal Animals.* London: Logos Press, 1970.

Palmer, J. D. Daily and tidal components in the persistent rhythmic activity of the crab, *Sesarma. Nature* (Lond.), 1967, *215,* 64–66.

Palmer, J. D. Tidal rhythms: The clock control of the rhythmic physiology of marine organisms. *Biological Review,* 1973, *48,* 377–418.

Pearse, J. S. A monthly reproductive rhythm in the diadematid sea urchin *Centrostephanus coronatus* Verrill. *Journal of Experimental Marine Biology and Ecology,* 1972, *8,* 167–186.

Pflüger, W. Die Sanduhrsteuerung der gezeitensynchronen Schlüpfrhythmik der Mücke *Clunio marinus* im arktischen Mittsommer. *Oecologia* (Berl.), 1973, *11,* 113–150.

Pittendrigh, C. S. Circadian rhythms and the circadian organization of living systems. *Cold Spring Harbor Symposia on Quantitative Biology,* 1960, *25,* 159–182.

Rodriguez, G., and Naylor, E. Behavioral rhythms in littoral prawns. *Journal of the Marine Biological Association of the United Kingdom,* 1972, *52,* 81–95.

Saigusa, M., and Hidaka, T. Semilunar rhythm in the zoea-release activity of the land crab *Sesarma. Oecologia* (Berl.), 1978, *37,* 163–176.

Slater, P. J. B. Tidal rhythm in a seabird. *Nature* (Lond.), 1976, *264,* 636–637.

Sommer, H. H. Endogene und exogene Periodik in der Aktivität eines niederen Krebses *(Balanus balanus* L.). *Zeitschrift für vergleichende Physiologie,* 1972, *76,* 177–192.

Taylor, A. C., and Naylor, E. Entrainment of the locomotory rhythm of *Carcinus* by cycles of salinity changes. *Journal of the Marine Biological Association of the United Kingdom,* 1977, *57,* 273–277.

Tesch, F.-W. Verhalten der Glasaale *(Anguilla anguilla)* bei ihrer Wanderung in den Ästuarien deutscher Nordseeflüsse. *Helgoländer wissenschaftliche Meeresuntersuchungen,* 1965, *12,* 404–419.

Tesch, F.-W. Aktivität und Verhalten wandernder *Lampetra fluviatilis, Lota lota* und *Anguilla anguilla* im Tidegebiet der Elbe. *Helgoländer wissenschaftliche Meeresuntersuchungen,* 1967, *16,* 92–111.

Walker, B. W. *Periodicity of spawning by the grunion, Leuresthes tenuis, an atherine fish.* Ph.D. thesis, University of California at Los Angeles, 1949, 166 pp.

Werner, H. *Vom Polarstern bis zum Kreuz des Südens*. Stuttgart: Gustav Fischer, 1960.

Williams, B. G., and Naylor, E. Spontaneously induced rhythm of tidal periodicity in laboratory-reared *Carcinus*. *The Journal of Experimental Biology*, 1967, *47*, 229–234.

Youthed, G. J., and Moran, V. C. The lunar-day activity rhythm of myrmeleontid larvae. *Journal of Insect Physiology*, 1969, *15*, 1259–1271.

Zann, L. P. Interactions of the circadian and circatidal rhythms of the littoral gastropod *Melanerita atramentosa* Reeve. *Journal of Experimental Marine Biology and Ecology*, 1973, *11*, 249–261.

20

Annual Rhythms: Perspective

EBERHARD GWINNER

THE PHENOMENON OF SEASONALITY

The habitats of most organisms are subject to pronounced seasonal fluctuations. Literally all physical environmental factors important to an organism—like temperature, day length, and rainfall—vary with season to such an extent that most plants and animals could not escape the necessity of developing adaptational strategies to cope with them. The most obvious expression of this necessity is that many biological activities are concentrated or restricted to the times of the year when they are most likely to be successful. This is true, for instance, of reproduction, which is timed in such a way that the growth of the offspring occurs when environmental conditions are most favorable, that is, late spring and summer. Other seasonally restricted activities include behavioral, physiological, and morphological processes by which organisms overcome or avoid severe winter or extreme summer conditions, that is, dormancy, diapause, hibernation, and migration. Developmental processes like molt of skins, furs, and plumages are often inserted between reproduction and the processes occurring in winter. In addition, numerous physiological functions like basal metabolism or growth rate change continuously with the time of year as a direct or indirect consequence of environmental seasonal variations (for reviews, see, e.g., Immelmann, 1963b, 1967, 1971; Aschoff, 1955; Lack, 1950; Murton and Westwood, 1977; Farner and Follett, 1979).

Since seasonal differences in environmental conditions normally increase with increasing latitude, annual rhythmicity is most clearly expressed in organisms inhabiting temperate and arctic zones. Good examples can be found among the annual cycles of reproduction. Figure 1 shows the distribution of reproductive seasons in birds at various latitudes. In regions close to the equator, incubating birds are found throughout the year without any obvious preferences for certain seasons. On the other hand, in northern and southern

EBERHARD GWINNER   Max-Planck-Institut für Verhaltensphysiologie, D-7760 Radolfzell-Möggingen, West Germany.

regions beyond about 30°, reproduction is concentrated in the favorable spring and summer months. Moreover, the reproductive season in both hemispheres begins later and becomes more sharply defined as latitude increases, corresponding with the later onset and shorter duration of optimal spring and summer conditions (Baker, 1938b).

The general trends illustrated in Figure 1 for temperate and arctic environments are representative not only of birds in general (and many other animals) but also of most of the individual orders, families, and even species of birds. On the other hand, the situation in the tropics is obscured by the pooling of data from birds of different systematic and ecological categories. Even though Figure 1 indicates a continuous reproductive season for tropical birds in general, individual species very often breed with an annual rhythmicity. However, different ecological groups may breed at different times, and geographical variation is usually much greater than in the temperate and arctic zones, resulting in the spreading out of the overall breeding season as indicated in Figure 1 (for general reviews, see Baker, 1938a,b; Aschoff, 1955; Miller, 1960; Immelmann, 1967, 1971).

In the tropics, avian reproduction usually bears a clear relationship to the seasonal distribution of rainfall. As a rule, birds inhabiting tropical rain forests with very heavy rains show a tendency to breed in the dryer months. Inhabitants of regions with one rainy and one dry season reproduce during the rainy season, whereas in areas with two dry and two wet seasons, some species breed only during one, others during both rainy seasons. Among the latter are species in which two separate populations breed at different times, as well as species in which even an individual bird may come into reproductive condition twice a year, thus exhibiting a 6-month cycle. It is important to note that all these generalizations are very tentative. The actual situation is far more complex because of many exceptions to these overall trends. For instance, although many birds nest around the rainy season, there are some ecological groups that prefer the dry season, for example, raptors and some fish-eating birds (see Immelmann, 1963b, 1971, for reviews).

Although in most tropical regions avian reproduction is organized on the basis of an annual (or semiannual) rhythmicity, there are a few species with reproductive cycles that bear no relationship to annual environmental rhythmicities. A classic example is the sooty tern *(Sterna fuscata)* on Ascension Island that breeds regularly at 10-month intervals (Chapin and Wing, 1959). Similar breeding cycles with periods shorter than 1 year have

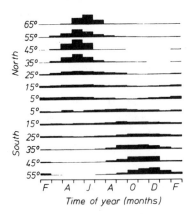

Fig. 1. Distribution of avian breeding seasons as a function of latitude. Diagrams show the relative numbers of times that fresh or incubated eggs have been found in each 10° of latitude, the means of which are given in the left-hand margin. (After Baker, 1938b.)

been found among other tropical sea birds (see Immelmann, 1971, for a review) and in two passerine birds inhabiting the tropical rain forests of Borneo (Fogden, 1972).

The only areas for which truly arrhythmic reproductive patterns have been reported are some arid regions, especially the Central Australian deserts. Here, many species of water and passerine birds breed only after the highly unpredictable rainfalls (e.g., Keast and Marshall, 1954; Keast, 1959; Immelmann, 1963a). A similar, although less pronounced, situation is found in the dry parts of Southwest Africa (Maclean, 1971).

Although annual reproduction (here illustrated by avian breeding cycles) is perhaps the most conspicuous seasonal phenomenon demonstrating the diversity of patterns and their geographical variations, there are numerous other activities that show the same general trends, for example, migratory behavior, hibernation, and diapause. As a whole, these seasonal functions within an individual constitute annual phase maps comparable to the circadian phase maps described in Chapters 12 and 17. Obviously, some of these activities are necessarily mutually exclusive because they are temporally or ergonomically incompatible with each other (e.g., reproduction and migration); others are dependent on each other (e.g., migration and fattening). It is clear then that any evolutionary strategy for seasonal adaptation must take into account not only the differential environmental demands of these various activities but also their mutual interdependencies. The overall overt seasonal patterns, therefore, always entail complex compromises between a great variety of different selection pressures.

ULTIMATE FACTORS CONTROLLING ANNUAL RHYTHMS

Although it is difficult to elucidate the various external and internal dependencies that determine the overall annual cycles of an organism, it is probably safe to assume that natural selection favors the gene complexes of those individuals that carry out a particular seasonal activity when environmental conditions are most propitious. Those environmental variables that, in the course of evolution, have exerted selection pressure to restrict an activity to a particular time of the year were called "ultimate causes" by Baker (1938a). This term was slightly altered into "ultimate factors" by Thomson (1950). Ultimate factors differ greatly, depending on the species and the seasonal activity, and even a particular seasonal activity may be controlled by more than one ultimate factor.

A large food supply, sufficient for raising the offspring and for covering the extra energy costs of the parents, is assumed to be a major ultimate factor of reproduction (e.g., Lack, 1950). This idea is supported by the fact that in all species studied, the reproductive season coincides with the maximal abundance of their preferred food items. This coincidence is most conspicuous in food specialists inhabiting extreme environments, such as the red-backed sandpiper *(Calidris alpina)* in Alaska, whose young hatch exactly when adult Diptera, the major food item of the chicks, emerge. If they miss that time, they suffer high mortality (Holmes, 1966). That food is an important ultimate factor of reproduction is also indicated by those few temperate-zone bird species that do not breed in spring; they are all specialized on food items that are available at other seasons. For instance, Elleonara's falcon *(Falco eleonorae)*, which inhabits small Mediterranean islands, breeds mainly in August and September. It feeds its young almost exclusively on small passerine birds that cross the

Mediterranean Sea in large numbers at that time of the year on their fall migration (Walter, 1968).

Although food is the dominating ultimate factor of reproduction, it is certainly not the only one. In several bird species, the availability of appropriate nest sites contributes to determining the actual time of reproduction. An example is the grass-nesting birds that tend to begin nest building relatively late in the wet season, that is, after the grass has grown long enough to provide cover. In the tropics, birds that nest in river banks (swallows, bee-eaters, kingfishers) often breed late in the dry season, when water levels are low and, hence, more potential nesting sites are available. In many Arctic birds, breeding appears to be timed, at least in part, relative to the melting of snow and ice. Other ultimate factors of reproduction comprise environmental variables related to predation, competition, etc. (see Immelmann, 1971, for a review).

PROXIMATE FACTORS CONTROLLING ANNUAL RHYTHMS

Most seasonal activities cannot be initiated instantaneously when the ultimate factors reach critical values; they need instead relatively long periods to develop. This effect is most conspicuous in reproduction, where, as mentioned before, the main ultimate factor (i.e., food supply for raising the offspring) operates during the end of the reproductive season. To guarantee that the young are born in the optimal season, the preceding processes of gonadal development, courtship, nest building, and gestation or incubation must be initiated long in advance and often at a time of suboptimal living conditions. Similarly, the migrations of many organisms require thorough preparation, as sufficient energy reserves must be stored up to cope with the extra energy demands of migration. From these examples, it is evident that in many instances, the ultimate factors—or rather, the critical values of the ultimate factors to which a seasonal activity is timed—are not suitable stimuli for the acute control of these processes because they occur too late. It can be assumed that the fitness of individuals is increased if they are capable of obtaining information about the season to come well in advance. It is understandable, therefore, that many organisms have developed strategies for using reliable forewarning stimuli—which vary in close relation to the ultimate factors—to time their seasonal events. Baker (1938a) called cues of this kind, which actually control the annual cycles by affecting physiological processes, "proximate causes," as opposed to the ultimate causes, which exert their effects during evolution by changing gene frequencies. Thomson (1950) again proposed later the use of "proximate factors" instead of "proximate causes."

The extent to which an organism has been able to select forewarning proximate factors differing from the ultimate ones depends on its special ecological requirements, on the properties of the environment in which it lives, and on the function to be timed. It is possible to arrange many of the known phenomena along a scale extending from cases in which the proximate factors are identical with or very closely related to the ultimate factors, to cases in which the proximate factors are qualitatively different and temporally separated from the ultimate factors by many months. In the most extreme situation, the control mechanisms have become partly incorporated as endogenous time-programs into the organism's own internal organization.

A direct control of seasonal functions by environmental factors of this kind is found in situations where the separation of proximate and ultimate factors is either not necessary or not possible. The first category comprises activities that can be initiated within a relatively short period of time and, hence, do not require long preparation times. The seasonal colony foundation of African earth-dwelling termites provides a good example. It is accomplished by the simultaneous swarming of winged reproductive males and females from existing colonies. In many species, the swarming behavior and the preceding final stages of sexual development are triggered by rainfall occurring after dry periods. Rain is not only the major proximate factor but also the dominating ultimate factor for that behavior, since rain softens the ground and thereby enables the termites to dig a new burrow (Owen, 1961).

In some tropical areas that are characterized by extended periods of favorable conditions, even seasonal activities that *do* require long preparation times may be controlled by ultimate factors or by stimuli that are temporally closely related to them. Although thorough investigations are lacking, there is some evidence suggesting that in such areas, avian breeding activities are primarily controlled by the changing food supply itself. These birds can *afford* to waste some time in waiting for optimal conditions because the optimal conditions last long enough for them to complete one or several broods (see Immelmann, 1971, for examples).

In areas where environmental conditions vary in an irregular and unpredictable manner, animals are often *forced* to time their activities by stimuli that are closely related to the ultimate factors, because in such aseasonal environments, reliable sources of predictive information are simply not available. This situation applies especially to organisms inhabiting the central and western Australian deserts, where life depends to a high degree on the very irregular rainfalls. In contrast to the tropical areas mentioned earlier, favorable conditions following rainfalls are usually short, and hence, animals have to respond quickly in order to take advantage of them. Many birds inhabiting these areas have evolved highly sophisticated strategies to cope with this difficult situation (e.g., Marshall, 1959; Immelmann, 1963a,b; Serventy, 1971; Keast and Marshall, 1954; Keast, 1959). One of them is to keep the reproductive systems permanently at a relatively high state of development; an additional adaptation allows them to respond almost instantaneously to stimuli related to rainfall. This is true of the zebra finch *(Taeniopygia guttata)* whose gonads are almost always partially developed. It begins intense courtship and nest building with the first showers, even if the preceding drought period has lasted for many months or even years (Immelmann, 1963a,b). Egg laying may begin as early as two weeks after the first rainfalls. Obviously, stimuli related directly to the rains provide the proximate factors. It has been proposed that the sight or the noise of the falling rains may be of significance, or changes in the osmotic state of the birds, but experimental evidence is lacking. Recently, Priedkalns and Bennett (1978) demonstrated experimentally that testicular growth can be initiated by increasing the relative humidity, a finding that is consistent with field observations indicating that nest building may begin even before it actually begins to rain.

Opportunistic breeders of the kind just described are not restricted only to arid areas but occur in limited numbers even in temperate zones. Among birds, the most prominent representative is the crossbill *(Loxia curvirostra)*, a species that feeds and raises its young almost exclusively with the seeds of firs and—to a lesser extent—other conifers. In any particular area fructification of firs occurs at about 2- to 4-year intervals, at different times of the year in different areas depending on the microclimate. Correspondingly, breeding crossbills have been found at almost any time of the year, but always in close temporal relationship with the abundance of cones (Newton, 1972). The major proximate factors controlling reproduction in this species have not yet been identified, but they are almost certainly linked closely to the availability of cones.

Proximate Factors Temporally Separated from Ultimate Factors

In contrast to the exceptional case of the crossbill mentioned above (and a few other species), most other organisms inhabiting higher latitudes have selected as major proximate factors environmental stimuli that are only indirectly related to the ultimate causes but that still bear a rigid temporal relationship to them. This selection, in turn, allows the animals to prepare long in advance for the times when the ultimate factors will reach critical values, and it ensures that even long-lasting developmental processes (like reproductive maturation, incubation, or gestation) will be completed at the appropriate times. The evolution of such mechanisms has become possible in higher latitudes because in these areas, many environmental variables change both very regularly and also with a characteristic and relatively constant temporal relationship. As a consequence, almost any environmental variable contains predictive information about the other factors and hence can be exploited as a forewarning control factor.

Ideal proximate factors are obviously such environmental variables that show regular and consistent seasonal changes. Temperature fulfills this criterion, at least partly, and indeed does play a considerable role in many mid- and high-latitude species, especially poikilotherms (e.g., Danilevskii, 1965; Hoar, 1969; Lofts, 1974). However, a much better-suited cue is photoperiod, the light fraction of the 24-hr day, which among all obvious environmental variables constitutes the most reliable indicator of season. It is not surprising, therefore, that in numerous temperate-zone plants and animals, photoperiod is involved in one way or another in the control of seasonal activities. In fact, "there is no other environmental factor in any climatic region that is of comparable importance for the immediate control of annual cycles" (Immelmann, 1973). The functions that are controlled by photoperiod comprise essentially all classes of activities known to show seasonal variation. The diversity of activities that are under photoperiodic control is matched by the diversity of mechanisms used to measure photoperiod and transform its information into the appropriate physiological or behavioral response. Photoperiodic control systems are dealt with in great detail in Chapters 22 and 23.

Circannual Rhythms

The evolution of photoperiodic response systems in organisms of temperate and higher latitudes had long been thought to represent the final stage in the process of becoming independent from the direct control of seasonal activities by ultimate factors. Only recently has it become clear that at least in some species, this process of emancipation has gone even further insofar as they have incorporated a great deal of the seasonal timing machinery into their own endogenous organization. This is most conspicuously so in species whose annual cycles have been preprogrammed into an endogenous circannual rhythmicity that can persist even under constant environmental conditions.

The advantages of circannual control systems, as opposed to systems that depend exclusively on external proximate factors, is by no means clear. Since circannual rhythms can fulfill their functions only in connection with external seasonal zeitgebers that synchronize them with the natural year, the question arises whether these external factors alone could not do the same job quite as well. As with circadian rhythms (Enright, 1970), there appears to be no convincing general answer to this question as yet, although there are several findings suggesting one or another adaptive function in a few groups of organisms (see Chapter 15). A major general function of circannual rhythms may be to improve the timing precision of seasonal activities in organisms that inhabit environments with pronounced seasonal changes, at least for part of the year. If these organisms relied entirely on external cues, a considerable year-to-year variability in the timing of their seasonal activities would be expected as a result of the variability in weather conditions. Even photoperiod, the most reliable of the known external cues, is not free from variations, and the seasonal information provided by it can be considerably falsified, for example, by cloud conditions. At high latitudes, overcast can reduce the effective day length by several hours. It seems likely that a circannual rhythmicity, by virtue of its inherent inertia and/or as a result of the specific mechanisms of entrainment, might buffer the control system against such environmental noise. If this were true, then circannual mechanisms would be most necessary for organisms that are extremely dependent on the precise timing of their seasonal activities. This prediction appears to hold up under experimental investigation (see Chapter 21).

Hierarchical Organization of Proximate Factors

In the previous sections, an attempt was made to arrange the known proximate control mechanisms of seasonal activities according to their degree of remoteness from the ultimate factors and to relate the patterns of control to the ecological requirements of the individual species. To simplify matters, attention was focused on those proximate factors that provide the dominating time cues. However, as with ultimate factors, seasonal functions are usually under the control of more than one proximate factor, and the most important of these, the primary factors, are normally enhanced by a variety of secondary stimulatory or inhibitory cues. This holds true especially where the dominating proximate factors are widely separated from the ultimate ones and for species equipped with a circannual rhythmicity. Here, the dominating proximate causes are often responsible for preparing the organism only partially for a particular seasonal activity, whereas the fine tuning is achieved by stimuli that are more closely related to the ultimate factors (for reviews, see Immelmann, 1971; Farner and Follett, 1979). Examples are found among migratory birds in which a circannual rhythmicity and/or photoperiod determines the times at which animals come into general migratory condition, but the immediate stimuli for migration are provided by the weather situation or food conditions (Farner, 1950; Berthold, 1975). Similarly, in many female birds of higher latitudes, photoperiodic stimulation leads to only a partial development of the ovary, whereas vitellogenesis and the final follicular development require supplementary information from the environment, for example, stimulation by a territorial male and the availability of adequate food (Immelmann, 1973; Murton and Westwood, 1977; Farner and Follett, 1979).

Acknowledgment

This chapter and the following chapter are dedicated to Professor Dr. Konrad Lorenz on the occasion of his 75th birthday.

REFERENCES

Aschoff, J. Jahresperiodik der Fortpflanzung bei Warmblütern. *Studium Generale*, 1955, *8*, 742–776.

Baker, J. R. The evolution of breeding seasons. In. G. R. de Beer (Ed.), *Evolution: Essays on Aspects of Evolutionary Biology*. Oxford: Oxford University Press, 1938a, pp. 161–177.

Baker, J. R. The relation between latitude and breeding seasons in birds. *Proceedings of the Zoological Society London*, 1938b, *108A*, 557–582.

Berthold, P. Migration: Control and metabolic physiology. In D. S. Farner and J. R. King (Ed.), *Avian Biology*. Vol. 5. New York, San Francisco, London: Academic Press, 1975, pp. 77–128.

Chapin, J. P., and Wing, L. W. The wideawake calendar, 1953 to 1958. *The Auk*, 1959, *76*, 152–158.

Danilevskii, A. S. *Photoperiodism and Seasonal Development of Insects*. Edinburgh and London: Oliver and Boyd, 1965.

Enright, J. T. Ecological aspects of endogenous rhythmicity. *Annual Review of Ecology and Systematics*, 1970, *1*, 221–238.

Farner, D. S. The annual stimulus for migration. *Condor*, 1950, *52*, 104–122.

Farner, D. S., and Follett, B. K. Reproductive periodicity in birds. In E. J. W. Barrington (Ed.), *Hormones and Evolution*. London: Academic Press, 1979.

Fogden, M. P. The seasonality and population dynamics of equatorial forest birds in Sarawak. *Ibis*, 1972, *114*, 307–343.

Hoar, W. S. Reproduction. In W. S. Hoar and D. H. Randall (Eds.), *Fish Physiology*. Vol. 3. New York: Academic Press, 1969, pp. 1–72.

Holmes, R. T. Breeding ecology and annual cycle adaptations of the red-backed sandpiper (*Calidris alpina*) in northern Alaska. *Condor*, 1966, *68*, 3–46.

Immelmann, K. Drought adaptations in Australian desert birds. *Proceedings 12th International Ornithological Congress*, 1963a, 649–657.

Immelmann, K. Tierische Jahresperiodik in ökologischer Sicht. *Zoologische Jahrbücher (Systematik)*, 1963b, *91*, 91–100.

Immelmann, K. Periodische Vorgänge in der Fortpflanzung tierischer Organismen. *Studium Generale*, 1967, *20*, 15–33.

Immelmann, K. Ecological aspects of periodic reproduction. In D. S. Farner and J. R. King (Eds.), *Avian Biology*. Vol. 1. New York, San Francisco, London: Academic Press, 1971, pp. 341–389.

Immelmann, K. Role of the environment in reproduction as source of "predictive" information. In D. S. Farner (Ed.), *Breeding Biology of Birds*. Washington, D.C.: National Academy of Sciences, 1973, pp. 121–147.

Keast, A. Australian birds: Their zoogeography and adaptations to an arid environment. In A. Keast, R. L. Crocher, and C. S. Christian (Eds.), *Biogeography and Ecology in Australia*. The Hague: Junk Publishers, 1959, pp. 89–114.

Keast, J. A., and Marshall, A. J. The influence of drought and rain-fall on reproduction in Australian desert birds. *Proceedings of the Zoological Society London*, 1954, *124*, 493–499.

Lack, D. The breeding seasons of European birds. *Ibis*, 1950, *92*, 288–316.

Lofts, B. Reproduction. In B. Lofts (Ed.), *Physiology of the Amphibia*. Vol. 20. New York, San Francisco, London: Academic Press, 1974, pp. 107–218.

Maclean, G. L. The breeding seasons of birds in the southwestern Kalahari. *Proceedings of the 3rd Pan-African Ornithological Congress*, 1971, 179–192.

Marshall, A. J. Internal and environmental control of breeding. *Ibis*, 1959, *101*, 456–478.

Miller, A. H. Adaptation of breeding schedule to latitude. *Proceediings of the 12th International Ornithological Congress*, 1960, 513–522.

Murton, R. K., and Westwood, N. J. *Avian Breeding Cycles.* Oxford: Clarendon Press, 1977.

Newton, J. *Finches.* Glasgow: Collins, 1972.

Owen, D. F. *Animal Ecology in Tropical Africa.* Edinburgh and London: Oliver and Boyd, 1961.

Priedkalns, J., and Bennett, R. K. Environmental factors regulating gonadal growth in the zebra finch, *Taeniopygia guttata* castanotis. *General and Comparative Endocrinology,* 1978, *34,* 80.

Serventy, D. L. Biology of desert birds. In D. S. Farner and J. R. King (Eds.), *Avian Biology.* Vol. 1. New York, San Francisco, and London: Academic Press, 1971, pp. 287–339.

Thomson, A. L. Factors determining the breeding seasons of birds: an introductory review. *Ibis,* 1950, *92,* 173–184.

Walter, H. Zur Abhängigkeit des Eleonorenfalken (*Falco eleonorae*) vom mediterranen Vogelzug. *Journal für Ornithologie,* 1968, *109,* 323–365.

21

Circannual Systems

EBERHARD GWINNER

INTRODUCTION

The existence of circannual rhythms was first postulated for such organisms as exhibit pronounced seasonal cycles in their physiology and behavior despite their exposure to either relatively constant or unpredictable and highly complex environmental conditions. In the first category are a variety of tropical organisms that inhabit areas with little seasonal variability but still show conspicuous seasonality in various activities, like flowering in plants or reproduction in animals. It seemed reasonable to assume that these functions were primarily independent of external factors and rather were controlled by an endogenous annual clock (e.g., Moreau, 1931; Chapin, 1932; Baker, 1938; Aschoff, 1955; Marshall, 1960; Immelmann, 1973). The second category comprises, among other organisms, many migratory birds that experience peculiar seasonal patterns in photoperiod, temperature, and other factors as a consequence of their migrations across large ranges of latitude and longitude. Baron von Pernau speculated back in 1702 that such birds were "driven by a hidden urge" to commence migration at the appropriate time, and that environmental factors like food and temperature were of minor significance. Much later, the concept of an endogenous annual rhythmicity involved in the control of annual functions in such birds was proposed more explicitly by Rowan (1926), Chapin (1932), Marshall (1960), and others.

Early evidence of circannual rhythms came, in fact, primarily from studies carried out on tropical organisms and migratory birds, which were found to continue exhibiting normal seasonal variations, at least for some months in constant environmental conditions (e.g., Zimmerman, 1966; Merkel, 1963; Marshall and Serventy, 1959; Lofts, 1964). However, true progress in the field was made only after the early 1950s, when circadian rhythm research had defined the criteria required for the demonstration of an endogenous rhythmicity. Since then, a number of rigidly controlled experimental studies have been carried

EBERHARD GWINNER   Max-Planck-Institut für Verhaltensphysiologie, D-7760 Radolfzell-Möggingen, West Germany.

out. From these, the existence of circannual rhythms has been convincingly documented not only for members of the ecological groups mentioned above but also for a variety of other organisms.

DEMONSTRATION AND DISTRIBUTION OF CIRCANNUAL RHYTHMS

Circannual rhythms were first rigorously demonstrated by Pengelley and Fisher (1957, 1963) in the golden-mantled ground squirrel *(Citellus lateralis)*, by Blake (1959) in the carpet beetle *(Anthrenus verbasci)*, and by Segal (1960) in the slug *(Limax flavus)*. An example from the work of Pengelley, Asmundson, Barnes, and Aloia (1976) is presented in Figure 1, where the occurrence of hibernation in five groups of ground squirrels is plotted. The animals were kept in constant DD, LL, or LD 12:12. Hibernation occurred for all the animals about once a year throughout the experiment. The period of the rhythm, however, deviated from exactly 12 months. This deviation is more conspicuous in Figure 1B, in which symbols connected by lines indicate the mean dates on which animals of the five experimental groups commenced hibernation in successive years. It is clear that most animals entered hibernation earlier each year than the previous year, indicating that the period of the annual hibernation cycle was shorter than 12 months. In other words, the squirrels' subjective year deviated from the true, objective year in these conditions: their circannual clocks ran fast.

The results summarized in Figure 2 document circannual rhythms in an avian species, the garden warbler, *Sylvia borin* (Berthold, Gwinner, and Klein, 1972). As long-distance migrants, these birds exhibit intense nocturnal migratory restlessness *(Zugunruhe)* during the migratory seasons in spring and autumn, which is accompanied by an increase in body weight due to fat deposition. A molt is carried out in summer and winter. Figure 2 shows

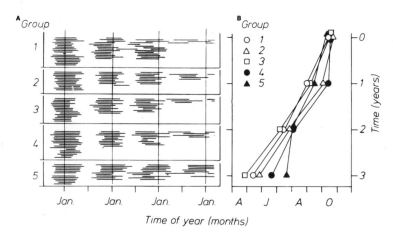

Fig. 1. Circannual rhythms of hibernation in golden-mantled ground squirrels, *Citellus lateralis,* kept for 47 months under constant conditions of photoperiod and temperature. Group 1: DD, 3°C, animals surgically blinded. Group 2: LL (500 lux), 3°C. Group 3: LL (500 lux), 3°C, animals surgically blinded. Group 4: LL (20 lux), 3°C. Group 5: LD 12:12 (200:0 lux), 3°C. (A) Black bars arranged in horizonal rows represent periods of hibernation of individual animals. (B) Symbols connected by lines indicate mean dates at which the animals of the various groups entered hibernation in successive years of the experiment. (After Pengelley *et al.,* 1976.)

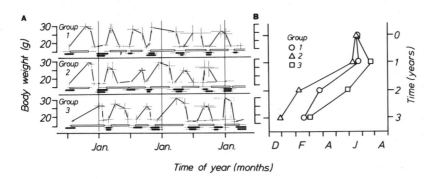

Time of year (months)

Fig. 2. Circannual rhythms of migratory restlessness, body weight, and molt in garden warblers, *Sylvia borin*, kept for 33 months under constant conditions of photoperiod and temperature. Group 1: LD 10:14 (400:0.01 lux). Group 2: LD 12:12 (400:0.01 lux). Group 3: LD 16:8 (400:0.01 lux). Temperature for all groups: 20 ± 1.5°C. Each group consisted of six to eight birds. (A) Curves show changes in body weight. Open bars indicate times during which the birds showed migratory restlessness. Solid bars show periods of molt (upper row: molt of body feathers; lower row: molt of the flight and tail feathers). Horizontal lines at the bars and horizontal and vertical lines at the curve points: standard deviations. (B) Symbols connected by lines indicate mean dates at which the birds of the three groups initiated summer molt in successive years of the experiment. (After Berthold *et al.*, 1972.)

that the rhythms of *Zugunruhe*, body weight, and molt in three groups of garden warblers maintained under a constant LD 10:14, LD 12:12, or LD 16:8 continued for at least 3½ years. Again, the period of these rhythms deviated from 12 months, as is shown on the right-hand diagram for the rhythm of summer molt. In some warblers, the circannual molt rhythms could be followed over an extended period of time. The data shown in Figure 3 are from a garden warbler and a blackcap *(Sylvia atricapilla)* that were kept in a constant LD 10:14 for 9 years (Berthold, 1978). Both birds had a circannual molt rhythm with a period of about 10 months throughout the experiment; by the end of the experiment, they had run through nine cycles within 8 years.

Circannual rhythms persisting under constant environmental conditions for at least two cycles with periods deviating from 12 months have now been demonstrated in at least 29 animal species comprising mollusks, arthropods, reptiles, birds, and mammals. Functions as diverse as locomotor activity, hibernation, migratory behavior, milk production, and plasma hormonal levels have been found to be under circannual control. In addition,

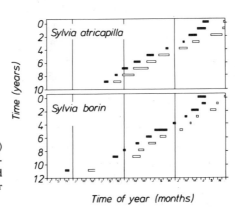

Fig. 3. Circannual rhythms of summer molt (black bars) and winter molt (open bars) in a blackcap *(Sylvia atricapilla)* and a garden warbler *(S. borin)* kept for 8 and 10 years, respectively, under a constant LD 10:14. (After Berthold, 1978.)

Time of year (months)

there are at least 16 other species in which the participation of a circannual rhythmicity is likely. In these cases, the evidence is not considered convincing, either because the experiments lasted less than 2 years or because the period of the rhythms was indistinguishable from 12 months, so that their exogenous origin could not be excluded with certainty. Finally, there are at least 3 species that under constant environmental conditions did show persisting rhythms but their periods deviated to such an extent from 12 months (e.g., 4 months) that it is not clear whether they should be called circannual (see Gwinner, 1971, for a review).

In view of all this evidence, it may appear as though circannual rhythms are fairly widespread among animals. It is clear that circannual rhythms are not restricted to tropical organisms and long-distance migrating birds. Instead, circannual rhythms have been found in animals from a large range of geographical latitudes, including regions close to the Arctic circle (e.g., *Citellus lateralis*), as well as in extremely sedentary bird species (e.g., *Parus cristatus*). On the other hand, there is a considerable amount of evidence suggesting that circannual rhythms are by far not as ubiquitous as circadian rhythms. One reason is that circannual rhythms would primarily be expected only among the small percentage of animals that have life spans of at least one year. Moreover, animals that are sufficiently long-lived for a circannual rhythmicity to be of potential significance have evolved relatively recently and independently in various groups of organisms (e.g., Farner, 1970). It is to be expected, then, that circannual rhythms are of heterogeneous origin. As a result, one has to be wary of generalizations about common features of circannual rhythms; formal similarities do not necessarily indicate identical mechanisms.

PROPERTIES OF CIRCANNUAL RHYTHMS UNDER CONSTANT ENVIRONMENTAL CONDITIONS

PERSISTENCE OF CIRCANNUAL RHYTHMS

As indicated in the previous section, circannual rhythms may differ widely among species with regard to their degree of persistence. The annual cycles of hibernation in golden-mantled ground squirrels and of molt in garden warblers and blackcaps have been found to continue for at least five and nine cycles, respectively, that is, essentially for the whole life of these animals (Pengelley and Asmundson, 1969; Berthold, 1978). In many other cases circannual rhythms have shown tendencies to disappear with time (e.g., Pengelley and Kelly, 1966; Heller and Poulsen, 1970; Zimmerman, 1966; Gwinner, 1971). In several species, such as the blackcap, the annual rhythms of some functions have been found to persist over many cycles (e.g., *Zugunruhe* and molt), whereas others (e.g., body weight) ceased after the first year (Berthold *et al.*, 1972). Even in animals with long-lasting circannual rhythms, the range of conditions under which these rhythms are expressed is rather narrow. For instance, European starlings *(Sturnus vulgaris)* showed a well-defined annual rhythm of testicular size when kept in constant LD 12:12 but not when kept in photoperiods of 11 hr or less, and 13 hr or more (Schwab, 1971). On the other hand, in the sika deer, *Cervus nippon,* antlers were shed with a circannual rhythmicity in animals exposed to constant light or to a constant 16- or 8-hr photoperiod, but these rhythms disappeared in a 12-hr photoperiod (Goss, 1969b).

These and other similar observations (Gwinner, 1971) indicate that the conditions that permit the expression of circannual rhythms are limited and may eventually be of significance in the search for the underlying physiological mechanisms, but so far no convincing interpretations of any of these findings are available. At the same time, these observations clearly indicate that animals must be tested in various environmental conditions before it can be concluded that a particular species is not equipped with a circannual clock.

RANGE OF CIRCANNUAL PERIOD LENGTHS: TRANSIENTS

Circannual rhythms investigated in constant conditions sometimes go through one or two transient cycles before they reach an apparent steady state (compare Figures 2 and 3). Unfortunately, in most studies, only a few cycles have been measured. Many of the conclusions drawn about circannual rhythms under constant conditions should therefore be treated with caution because it is not always clear that they refer to the steady-state properties of these rhythms.

The period τ of freerunning circannual rhythms is usually found to be shorter than 1 year, although occasionally periods slightly longer than 12 months have been measured. Compared with circadian rhythms, the overall range of freerunning periods is relatively large. The extreme values are about 7 months and 15 months (i.e., deviations from 1 year of -40% and $+25\%$, respectively). Even within an individual species, τ may vary considerably in animals maintained under identical constant conditions (e.g., between about 9 and 14 months in golden-mantled ground squirrels; Pengelley et al., 1976). This wide range of freerunning periods of circannual rhythms corresponds with their large range of entrainment (see the section below on zeitgebers).

DEPENDENCE OF τ ON EXTERNAL CONDITIONS

There are only a few studies in which the effects of external conditions on freerunning circannual rhythms have been investigated. In most of these studies, only one or two cycles were recorded, so the rhythms were perhaps not in steady state. The little evidence that is available from long-term experiments suggests that once in steady state, the freerunning circannual τ is often remarkably invariant with respect to external conditions.

TEMPERATURE. In golden-mantled ground squirrels kept in LD 12:12 and under 3°C and 12°C, the first period of the circannual hibernation rhythm tended to be slightly longer in the animals living in the lower temperature ($\tau_{3°} = 361$ days, $\tau_{12°} = 333$ days, Pengelley and Kelly, 1966; $\tau_{3°} = 366$ days, $\tau_{12°} = 337$ days, Pengelley and Asmundson, 1969). In both studies, the differences were at the border of statistical significance. However, this difference disappeared during later cycles. If a mean τ is calculated for the second and third cycles from the data presented by Pengelley and Asmundson (1969), the respective values are $\tau_{3°} = 328$ days and $\tau_{12°} = 331$ days. These findings are remarkable because these hibernators spend many months each year in deep torpor, with body temperature lowered by many degrees. They suggest that the period of circannual rhythms may be temperature-compensated, like circadian rhythms.

PHOTOPERIOD. Effects of photoperiod, like those of temperature, have mainly been found during the first cycle (literature in Gwinner, 1971, 1975a), whereas in steady state, the period appeared to be little affected or not affected by photoperiodic conditions. For example, no consistent differences could be detected between the circannual rhythms of *Zugunruhe*, body weight, and molt of garden warblers and blackcaps maintained in LD 10:14, LD 12:12, or LD 16:8 (Berthold *et al.*, 1972). Only the data published by Pengelley *et al.* (1976) contain a few references to a possible photoperiodic effect on the steady-state period of the circannual hibernation rhythm in golden-mantled ground squirrels. Here, the second and third period tended to be longer in both animals maintained in either DD or LD 12:12 than in those in LL of either 500 lux or 20 lux. Again, these differences are only at the border of statistical significance. The meaning of such differences, if they do in fact exist, is obscure.

INNATENESS OF CIRCANNUAL RHYTHMS

Although evidence is again scarce, there are a few results indicating that a circannual rhythmicity may occur in animals that have never been exposed to annual environmental variations. Golden-mantled ground squirrels born in a constant 12-hr photoperiod exhibited a circannual rhythm in hibernation indistinguishable from that of conspecifics caught in the wild (Pengelley and Asmundson, 1970; Heller and Poulson, 1970). Similarly, ewes raised from birth under various constant photoperiods showed a circannual rhythm in reproductive activity throughout the 2½-year experiment (Ducker, Bowman, and Temple, 1973), and three species of warblers *(Phylloscopus trochilus, Sylvia borin,* and *S. atricapilla)* showed freerunning circannual rhythms in various functions when transferred to seasonally constant conditions at the age of 10 weeks or even only 1 week (Gwinner, 1971; Berthold, *et al.*, 1972). It appears, then, that these circannual rhythms do not become imprinted on the animals during ontogeny by external annual variations but represent an innate characteristic of the organism.

RELATIONSHIP BETWEEN VARIOUS CIRCANNUAL FUNCTIONS WITHIN AN INDIVIDUAL ORGANISM

In golden-mantled ground squirrels the rhythms of hibernation, body weight, food consumption, and reproductive condition have all been shown to persist simultaneously in a constant 12-hr photoperiod (see Pengelley and Asmundson, 1974, for a review). Similarly, in garden warblers, the annual cycles of *Zugunruhe*, body weight, food preference, and gonadal size in individual birds are controlled by a circannual rhythm (for a review, see Berthold, 1974; Gwinner, 1971). On the basis of these observations, the question arises to what extent these various overt circannual functions within an organism are mutually dependent on each other, as part of one clock system; or whether they are basically independent of each other, that is, the expression of separate circannual clocks.

The rigid temporal sequence in which the various events normally occur within an organism appears to favor the first alternative. In fact, some of the functions mentioned above must, at least to some extent, be causally dependent on each other (e.g., body weight and food consumption). On the other hand, there are at least three types of evidence indicating that various circannual functions can be independent of each other.

This independence is suggested by results indicating that under certain experimental conditions, the annual rhythms of some functions may continue while others damp out. This effect has been observed in several species of birds and mammals. For instance, in blackcaps kept in LD 10:14, LD 12:12, and LD 16:8, the rhythms of *Zugunruhe* and molt continued while the body weight rhythm disappeared (Berthold *et al.,* 1972).

The independence of various seasonal activities has also been shown in studies where one seasonal activity could be experimentally manipulated without affecting other functions. Thus, in the golden-mantled ground squirrel, castration did not affect the circannual hibernation rhythm (Pengelley and Asmundson, 1970). In the same species, suppression of the increase in body weight that normally precedes hibernation had no effect on the timing of hibernation (Pengelley, 1968). Similarly, the onset and end of fall *Zugunruhe,* as well as the following onset of winter molt, in garden warblers is not influenced by suppressing the body weight increase that normally accompanies *Zugunruhe.* In addition, suppression of fall *Zugunruhe* for two months did not affect the timing of winter molt (see Gwinner, 1977a, for review).

Perhaps the strongest evidence of the existence of more than one circannual clock can be seen in cases where the different rhythms within an organism may drastically alter their internal phase relationship to each other, depending on the photoperiodic conditions. This phenomenon has been documented for warblers in which, under constant photoperiodic conditions, the circannual rhythms of testicular size, molt, body weight, and migratory restlessness may shift relative to each other by several months (Gwinner and Dorka, 1976). In starlings, the temporal relationship between various circannual functions differs among animals synchronized by zeitgebers with different properties (Aschoff,1980; compare Figure 6). These results are consistent with the idea that different functions may be primarily independent of each other and possibly controlled by separate circannual oscillators that, depending on conditions, may alter their mutual internal phase relationship.

Synchronization of Circannual Rhythms

Zeitgebers

The action of circannual zeitgebers is illustrated by the results of a displacement experiment with woodchucks *(Marmota monax)* shown in Figure 4 (Davis and Finnie, 1975). If kept in a constant LD 16:8 and under a constant temperature of 20°C or 6°C, this species performs a circannual rhythm of body weight that persists for at least two cycles. When animals maintained under natural photoperiodic conditions were displaced from the northern hemisphere to the southern hemisphere, their body weight rhythms resynchronized with the inverted zeitgeber conditions within about three years (Figure 4).

Circannual zeitgebers have only rarely been identified so far, but it is now clear that the annual cycle of photoperiod can synchronize circannual rhythms in some species. This effect is illustrated in Figure 5 for the circannual rhythm of testis size of the European starling (Gwinner, 1977b). Groups of 8–12 starlings were exposed to sinusoidal changes in photoperiod simulating in amplitude and general shape the seasonal photoperiodic alterations at 40° latitude. The period T of this photoperiodic cycle, however, varied from 1 cycle per year (T = 12 months, upper panel) to 4 cycles per year (T = 3 months, lowest panel), as indicated in the right-hand margin. It is clear that the rhythm of testis size followed the photoperiodic rhythm in all instances.

In this study with starlings, the limits of the range of entrainment were not reached. On the other hand, in an experiment with the sika deer *(Cervus nippon),* some of the

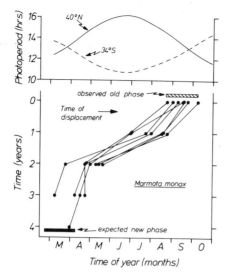

Fig. 4. Resynchronization of the circannual rhythms of body weight in seven woodchucks *(Marmota monax)* after displacement from the northern hemisphere (Pennsylvania, USA, about 40°N) to the southern hemisphere (Sydney, Australia, about 34°S). At both locations, the animals were exposed to natural conditions of photoperiod and temperature. *Upper* diagram indicates the photoperiodic variations to which the animals were exposed before (solid curve) and after (dashed curve) displacement. In *lower* diagram, symbols connected by lines indicate the dates at which the animals attained maximal body weights before (Year 0) and after (Years 1–4) displacement. (After Davis and Finnie, 1975.)

photoperiodic cycles employed were obviously beyond these limits. In this species, the antlers are normally replaced once a year. Goss (1969a) demonstrated that this annual rhythm of antler shedding and regrowth represents a circannual rhythm that persists for at least four cycles under various constant photoperiodic regimes. When exposed to sinusoidal changes in photoperiod with periods of $T = 12$ months, 6 months, or 4 months, the circannual rhythm became readily entrained. However, if the period of the photoperiodic cycle was $T = 3$ months, some of the cycles were omitted, and under $T = 2$ months, the deer replaced their antlers only every sixth photoperiodic cycle, thereby falling back to a

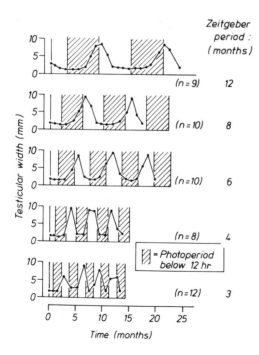

Fig. 5. Rhythm of testicular width in five groups of European starlings *(Sturnus vulgaris)* kept in light–dark cycles with periodically varying photoperiods. Duration of the photoperiodic cycles is indicated in the right-hand margin. Each curve represents the mean of *n* animals. Shaded area: photoperiod below 12 hr. White area: photoperiod above 12 hr. (From Aschoff, 1980; after Gwinner, 1977b.)

rhythm with a period close to its natural period of about 1 year. At the other end of the range of entrainment, a photoperiodic cycle with a period of 24 months was followed by the rhythms in three out of five animals, whereas the other two replaced their antlers every 12 months (twice a cycle), thereby indicating entrainment to a submultiple of the photoperiodic rhythm (Goss, 1969a). The experiments show, once again, that the annual rhythm in photoperiod is a zeitgeber of this circannual rhythm, and moreover, they indicate that the range of entrainment extends from about $T = 4$ months to $T = 24$ months.

Apart from the European starling and the sika deer, the annual rhythm of photoperiod has been demonstrated to be a zeitgeber for circannual rhythms in another bird species, the garden warbler, and three species of mammals (see Gwinner, 1971, for a review). Since photoperiod is commonly involved as a proximate factor in the control of annual rhythms (see Chapter 23), it is very likely that photoperiod is rather generally involved as a zeitgeber for circannual rhythms. Data supporting this idea have been discussed elsewhere (Gwinner, 1971, 1973; Aschoff, 1980). Zeitgebers other than photoperiod have not yet been demonstrated. However, a few findings in the carpet beetle suggest that temperature cycles might be effective in that species (Blake, 1960). In addition, some data from golden-mantled ground squirrels indicate that social stimuli may have zeitgeber qualities (Pengelley and Asmundson, 1970).

BEHAVIOR WITHIN THE RANGE OF ENTRAINMENT

The results presented in Figure 5 suggest that within the range of entrainment the phase relationship between circannual rhythms and their zeitgebers changes as a function of the zeitgeber period. This effect can be seen more clearly in Figure 6, which is based on

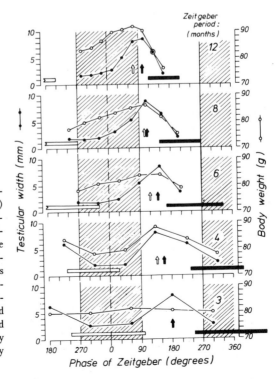

Fig. 6. Rhythms of testicular width (closed circles), body weight (open circles), and molt (bars) in five groups of European starlings *(S. vulgaris)* kept in light–dark cycles with periodically varying photoperiods. The duration of the photoperiodic cycle is indicated in the right-hand margin. The mean pattern of several cycles is drawn with reference to the phase of the zeitgeber (0° = shortest day). Shaded area: photoperiod below 12 hr. White area: photoperiod above 12 hr. Arrows: centers of gravity around the maxima of testicular width (black) and body weight (white). (From Aschoff, 1980; partly after Gwinner, 1977b.)

the results on starling testicular size from Figure 5 and contains some additional data on body weight changes and molt from the same birds. Unlike in Figure 5, the time course of all three functions is drawn on an abscissa showing relative zeitgeber time; that is, the data have been normalized in relation to the period of the photoperiodic cycle, so that its period represents 360° regardless of its actual value (in hours). Zero degrees represent the phase of the shortest day (photoperiodic midwinter). It is clear that with decreasing zeitgeber period, the maxima of testicular size and body weight as well as molt move progressively to the right (i.e., to later phases of the zeitgeber rhythm), indicating a steady decrease of the phase-angle difference between the exogenous and the endogenous rhythm. Such a decrease in phase-angle difference with decreasing zeitgeber period has been found in all studies in which circannual rhythms have been entrained to zeitgeber cycles of varying period. It is predicted by the general oscillator theory and has been confirmed in many studies of circadian rhythms as well (see Chapter 6).

Mechanisms of Circannual Rhythms

General Remarks

As has been shown in the previous sections, the annual rhythms of biological functions may continue for some time under seasonally constant conditions, and like circadian rhythms, these circannual rhythms behave in many respects like oscillators in a technical sense. Because of these (and only these) general features, the properties of both circadian and circannual rhythms are often described with the terminology of general oscillator theory. This descriptive approach is not primarily directed toward the analysis of the mechanisms of circannual rhythms and, hence, does not expound on any of the possible underlying processes generating them. This point is emphasized here because there has been some discussion in the literature about whether a circannual rhythmicity should be called a rhythm (or even an oscillator) if any one of the concrete underlying mechanisms that are discussed in this section actually exist (e.g., King, 1968; Mrosovsky, 1970, 1977; Hamner, 1971; Sansum and King, 1976). In fact, some of the models presented have been proposed as "alternatives" to the endogenous rhythm concept, whereas, in reality, they are hypotheses about the concrete underlying mechanisms.

The following account presents some of the models that have been discussed so far. Several of these hypotheses are not necessarily mutually exclusive but refer to possible mechanisms at different levels of the control systems. The presentation is necessarily condensed.

Circadian Rhythms as Possible Components of Circannual Rhythms

It is well established that in many organisms, circadian rhythms are involved in the control of annual rhythms by participating in the mechanism of photoperiodic time measurement (see Chapters 22 and 23). It is not surprising, therefore, that attention has been focused on the possibility that circannual rhythms may in some way be derived from circadian rhythms. Three classes of hypotheses can be distinguished.

FREQUENCY DEMULTIPLICATION OF CIRCADIAN RHYTHMS. There are physical
devices that generate low-frequency rhythms out of high-frequency rhythms by frequency
demultiplication. The electrical clock that produces a 24-hr rhythm by dividing the 50 or
60 cycles/sec frequency of the commerical electrical current provides an example. In an
analogous manner, organisms might transform circadian frequencies into circannual
rhythms. This hypothesis makes the unambiguous prediction that the period of the circannual rhythm should depend on the precise value of the period of the circadian rhythm.
Unpublished data obtained from European starlings disagree with this prediction. In these
experiments, one group of starlings was kept for about 3½ years in a constant LD cycle
with a period $T = 22$ hrs (LD 11:11) and another one for the same time in an LD cycle
with a period $T = 24$ hrs (LD 12:12). It turned out that the 22-hr birds tended to have
periods of their circannual rhythms of testis size and molt similar to or even slightly longer
than the 24-hr birds. The frequency-demultiplication hypothesis would have predicted a
shorter circannual period in the birds maintained under $T = 22$ hrs.

Apart from this direct experimental evidence against it, there are several phenomena
that are extremely difficult to reconcile with this model. For instance, it is hard to see how
it copes with the fact that (1) individual animals exposed to the same constant LD cycles
can show very different circannual τ values (Figure 1); (2) the circannual τ during the first
cycle is often different from the τ values in steady state (Figure 2); (2) the circannual τ
may be compressed to up to one-fourth its spontaneous value by exposing animals to photoperiodic cycles with periods shorter than one year (Figure 5); and (4) circannual rhythms
can be phase-shifted by exposing animals to phase-shifted zeitgeber cycles (Figure 4).

CIRCANNUAL RHYTHM OF A CIRCADIAN "BÜNNING" OSCILLATOR. According to the
"external coincidence" model proposed by Bünning (1936) and refined by Pittendrigh and
Minis (e.g., 1964), photoperiodic reactions depend on the coincidence of light with a particular phase of the circadian oscillation (see Chapter 22). Under natural conditions, the
annual cycles of overt functions result from this circadian phase's becoming periodically
exposed to light as a consequence of the seasonal variations in photoperiod. However, such
a periodic illumination of a photosensitive phase could take place even under constant photoperiodic conditions if one assumes that the phase relationship between the circadian
rhythm and the LD cycle to which it is entrained is subject to circannual variations. A
simplified version of this model is shown in Figure 7A. During the bird's subjective autumn
and winter, the phase relationship between circadian rhythm and the light–dark cycle is
such (ψ_w) that light never falls on the photosensitive phase that is indicated by the black
block. However, as the bird's subjective spring approaches, the circadian rhythm changes
its phase relationship spontaneously in such a way (ψ_s) that the photosensitive phase eventually becomes illuminated. As a consequence the photoperiodic response occurs. Later on,
the initial phase-relationship is reestablished. Hence, in this model, a circannual rhythmicity in overt functions (e.g., that of testis growth and regression) results from circannual
variations in the phase relationship between a circadian rhythm in photosensitivity and its
entraining light–dark cycle.

This model is appealing as it might explain several peculiarities of circannual rhythms
(for a discussion, see Gwinner, 1973). Moreover, changes in the circadian system related
to circannual phase have, indeed, been observed (e.g., Gwinner, 1973). Nevertheless, there
is clear evidence against it in several species: the model proposes that the overt circannual
rhythm depends on the alternate exposure of a particular phase to light and darkness, and

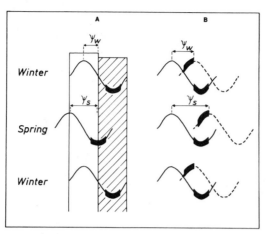

Fig. 7. Schematic representation of two models that derive circannual rhythms from spontaneous variations in the circadian system. (A) Overt circannual rhythm resulting from changes in the phase-angle difference (ψ) between a circadian rhythm and its entraining light–dark cycle; (B) from changes in the phase-angle difference between two circadian rhythms. (After Gwinner, 1973.)

hence, no circannual rhythmicity should develop in animals maintained in continuous light or darkness. However, clear circannual rhythms have been found under these conditions in at least six species of animals. Hence, although this model may apply to some organisms, it certainly does not apply to species where a circannual rhythm has been observed in the absence of daily light–dark cycles.

CIRCANNUAL VARIATIONS IN THE INTERNAL CIRCADIAN SYSTEM. Instead of postulating circannual changes in the external phase relationship between a circadian rhythm and its entraining LD cycle, one could assume a circannual rhythm in the internal phase-relationship between two or more circadian oscillations. This hypothesis is based on the "internal coincidence" model proposed by Pittendrigh (e.g., 1972) and others (see Chapter 22) to explain photoperiodic reactions. Figure 7B illustrates this version of the model. Here, each sine curve symbolizes a circadian oscillator, and on each one, a particular phase is delimited by a black marking. It is assumed (1) that the phase relationship between these two oscillators exhibits periodic variations, with the effect that the two phases coincide in spring (ψ_s) but do not coincide at other times of the year (ψ_w); and (2) that the photoperiodic response is initiated when these two phases are coincident. Hence, in this type of model, circannual rhythms in overt functions would eventually result from a circannual rhythm in the phase relationship between circadian oscillators.

There is evidence that seasonal variations in biological functions are indeed associated with changes in the circadian system that could be interpreted as changes in the phase relationship between circadian oscillators. For instance, it has been observed that testicular growth in spring is paralleled by an increase in circadian activity time α (Gwinner, 1975b). This increase in α is sometimes associated with a "splitting" of activity time, thus suggesting changes in the coupling between two, or two groups of, circadian oscillators (Gwinner, 1974). Even during long-term exposure to constant light, circannual variations in testicular size may be accompanied by circannual variations in circadian α (Gwinner, 1973). Unfortunately, in most of these studies, the causal relationship of these correlations is not clear. It seems possible that the variations in activity time reflect variations in the circadian system, which in turn cause the observed variations in testicular function. Alternatively, changes in testicular function may be responsible for alterations in α (see Gwinner, 1980, for a discussion).

So far, almost all of the available data support the second possibility. The most compelling evidence comes from experiments with male starlings in which it was found that an increase in α and the occurrence of splitting could be prevented by castration and induced again in the same birds by injecting testosterone (Gwinner, 1974, 1975b). These results obviously render it less likely that variations in the circadian system are responsible for the correlation between the circadian and the circannual parameters, although such a possibility is not entirely excluded.

In a more direct approach, A. Meier and his group have studied relationships between the circadian rhythms in the production and secretion of various hormones—especially prolactin and corticosterone—and annual cycles in the white-throated sparrow *(Zonotrichia albicollis)*. They proposed that changes in the phase-relationship between these two hormones are responsible for seasonal variations of annual functions like testicular activity, migratory disposition, and even migratory orientation (see Meier, 1976, for a review). Meier (1976) suggested that such a mechanism might also be the basis of circannual rhythms, but in the white-throated sparrow a circannual rhythmicity has apparently not yet been demonstrated. Nevertheless, Meier's hypothesis certainly suggests an interesting possibility that should be tested further.

CONCLUSIONS. From what has been said in the previous sections, it is obvious that none of the hypotheses suggesting the involvement of circadian rhythms in generating circannual rhythms have received convincing experimental support. Yet, it should be kept in mind that only a few investigations have been carried out to test these models so far, and there may be other more appropriate "circadian" hypothesis for circannual rhythms that have not yet been considered. On the other hand, it is quite possible that circannual rhythms originate independently of circadian rhythms and that circadian rhythms are of significance only in connection with the process of synchronization (e.g., in "photoperiodic time measurement"), which may be a separate physiological phenomenon. This latter view is perhaps supported by the fact that in some species (e.g., *Citellus lateralis*), circannual rhythms persist in continuous bright light; under such conditions, circadian rhythmicity is usually heavily disturbed or abolished (see Chapter 6).

A SEQUENCE OF STAGES? IF SO, AT WHAT LEVEL?

There has been some discussion in the literature about the possibility that circannual rhythms may not be "true" rhythms but only "a sequence of linked stages, each one taking a given amount of time to complete and then leading into the next, with the last stage linked back to the first again" (Mrosovsky, 1970). Such a possibility was first proposed as an alternative to the circannual rhythm concept, but Menaker (1974) has made it quite clear that "of course, both circadian and circannual rhythms must consist of sequences of interdependent steps" and that the question is what the steps are and at what level of organization they occur (see also Enright, 1970).

An attempt to identify the various stages in the chain of events and the way in which they interact appears to be the most promising strategy for analyzing the mechanisms of circannual rhythms. It has been pointed out repeatedly that in this respect, the analysis of circannual rhythms provides great prospective advantages over circadian rhythm analysis because of the long time constants involved and because components of the system are already known or can at least be reasonably speculated about.

The almost invariant temporal sequence in which various overt annual events occur may at first sight favor the hypothesis that these events themselves or the physiological processes directly controlling them comprise the stages from which the circannual cycle is built. For instance, in a migratory bird, the termination of the reproductive cycle (or the neuroendocrine events terminating it) may trigger postnuptial molt, the termination of which then initiates fall migratory disposition, etc. Indeed, the early proponents of the "sequence-of-stages" idea appear to have favored the possibility of interactions at such a peripheral level. For instance, in hibernators, the attainment of a heavy body weight due to fattening that normally precedes hibernation has been suggested as being "a prerequisite and perhaps a trigger to the onset of hibernation" (Pengelley, 1968). However, experiments carried out with ground squirrels clearly contradict this hypothesis. They indicate that in animals that were prevented from becoming fat, the onset of hibernation occurred at about the same time as in controls. Many of the findings presented in the section on circannual functions in individuals (above, p. 396) also suggest a high degree of independence among various circannual functions, even within individual animals.

In pursuing the sequence-of-stages approach, it might therefore be more fruitful to consider the various overt functions as circannual clocks that are primarily independent of each other, and to try to manipulate particular stages of these individual cycles. Taking the circannual reproductive cycle as an example, a possible way of doing this would be to alter the duration of that portion of the cycle in which gonads are active. If the processes responsible for active gonads do indeed constitute a "stage" of the whole cycle, then such an alteration should change the period of the circannual rhythm. Such attempts have apparently not yet been made. (For a more detailed discussion of these problems, see, e.g., Menaker, 1974; Mrosovsky, 1977).

Adaptive Significance of Circannual Rhythms

Timing of Seasonal Activities

As proposed previously (Chapter 20), circannual rhythms may improve the timing precision in seasonal activities by providing inertia that buffers the physiological control systems against noise in the seasonal environment. If this were the main function of circannual rhythms, they might be expected to be most rigorously involved in the control of seasonal activities in species heavily dependent on precise seasonal timing. This prediction is indeed supported by the results of a few comparative studies on closely related species.

In ground squirrels of the genus *Citellus* the annual rhythms of body weight and hibernation are most rigidly endogenously controlled in the obligatory hibernator *C. lateralis,* which inhabits the boreal life zone. Under constant conditions of photoperiod and temperature, these rhythms persist undamped for at least five cycles. Other related species inhabiting more arid environments depend to a lesser degree on such an endogenous rhythm. In constant conditions, their body weight and hibernation rhythms show tendencies to damp (e.g., *C. mohavenis*) or even disappear during the first cycle (e.g., *C. tereticaudus*). Pengelley and Kelly (1966) emphasized that a circannual rhythm is an excellent adaptation for *C. lateralis,* which inhabits a severe and regularly changing environment "where each event in the animal's life cycle must occur at an exact time in order for it to survive." The rhythm enables the animals to prepare for a changing environment long in advance. For the other species of *Citellus,* it seems to be more advantageous to be readily adaptable to the less predictable seasonal environmental fluctuations, hence the weaker expression of a circannual rhythmicity in these animals. Similar relationships between the rigidity of endogenous control and the predictability of the environment have also been found in four species of chipmunks of the genus *Eutamias* (Heller and Poulson, 1970).

Comparative studies on migratory birds revealed a very rigid circannual control of annual functions in long-distance migrants wintering at or close to the equator. Examples are provided by the willow warbler and the garden warbler, in which the rhythms of *Zugunruhe,* body weight, and molt have been found to persist for several cycles under constant environmental conditions (Gwinner, 1968, 1971; Berthold *et al.,* 1972). When close relatives of these species were investigated—the chiffchaff *(Phylloscopus collybita)* and the blackcap *(Sylvia atricapilla)* —less rigid circannual rhythms were found (Gwinner, 1971; Berthold *et al.,* 1972). The latter species are short-distance migrants that spend the winter in the Mediterranean area and in northern Africa. Under constant conditions, their body weight rhythms disappeared, and, at least in the chiffchaff, the rhythms of *Zugunruhe* and molt showed tendencies to damp out. It seems likely that the more rigid endogenous control of these activities in the two long-distance migrants is related to their annual time schedule's being much tighter because of the long migrations, which require a more precise timing. Indeed, there are reasons to believe that in the short-distance migrants, a more flexible control system allowing for modifying exogenous influences may be advantageous (Gwinner, 1971).

It remains to be seen whether this interpretation of the differences found between various species of squirrels or warblers is correct. It is based on correlations between the rigidity of their circannual control system and only one aspect of their ecology: the suspected need for precise timing. There are certainly other correlations, which may turn out to be more relevant. For instance, in the migratory warblers mentioned above, the rigidity of the endogenous control system is also correlated with the degree of the unpredictability or inaccuracy of seasonal variations in their winter quarters. In fact, it has been speculated that the rigorous endogenous control of seasonal activities in long-distance migrants may result from these birds' living for about six months of the year, from October to March, in a tropical environment where seasonal environmental changes are highly variable. A circannual clock is then obviously helpful for the timing of seasonal activities (Gwinner, 1968). The short-distance migrants, on the other hand, spend the winter in areas where seasonal changes in photoperiod and other factors are quite marked; hence, there may be less need for endogenous timing factors in these species.

There is currently no way of testing which one of these (or any other) alternatives is the more likely interpretation, and the two hypotheses are, of course, not necessarily mutually exclusive. In any case, the results and considerations presented in this section rather strongly suggest that the degree to which a circannual rhythmicity is involved in the control of seasonal activities may be radically different for different species, even in a genus. Furthermore, they point to the possibility that the selection pressures that have led to the evolution of circannual rhythms may have been very different in various groups of organisms. Hence, circannual rhythms might have to be considered special mechanisms that evolved not only independently (see section on demonstration and distribution, p. 392) but also for different purposes in various groups of organisms.

PROGRAMMING OF TEMPORAL PATTERNS

The point of view that circannual rhythms may owe their existence to various selection pressures is supported by results indicating that even in an individual species, circannual rhythms may fulfill rather different functions. This seems to hold true for warblers of the genera *Phylloscopus* and *Sylvia,* in which circannual rhythms are not of significance only in the appropriate timing of seasonal events in relation to the environmental seasonal cycles. They also appear to be part of the strategy by which first-year birds determine the temporal and spatial course, as well as the distance of migrations (see Gwinner, 1977a, for a review).

If first-year *Phylloscopus* or *Sylvia* warblers are maintained under a constant 12-hr photoperiod or under photoperiodic conditions similar to those they would experience in nature, the intensity of their fall migratory restlessness shows seasonal changes similar to the changes in migratory speed observed in free-living conspecifics during their actual migration. In the long-distance migrants, the most intense nocturnal activity is exhibited during the time when free-living birds cross the Mediterranean and the Sahara at their highest migratory speed. Later on, the migratory restlessness of the caged birds slowly declines, just as free-living birds also reduce their migratory speed. This coincidence has suggested that the temporal course of the first fall migration of these birds is determined, at least in part, by an endogenous time program that is part of a circannual rhythmicity.

There is evidence from comparative investigations that such a time program may even determine the distance covered by a bird during its first fall migration and, hence, that a circannual clock may be involved in their navigational performance. When various species of warblers were maintained under similar constant environmental conditions, drastic differences were found in the overall amount of migratory restlessness developed during the first fall migratory season. These differences were clearly related to the distance normally

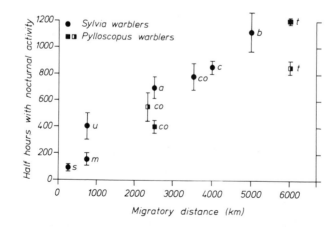

Fig. 8. Relationship between the distance covered during migration by free-living birds and the total time spent in fall migratory restlessness by caged conspecifics, in eight warbler species: a = *Sylvia atricapilla;* b = *S. borin;* c = *S. cantillans;* m = *S. melanocephala;* s = *S. sarda;* u = *S. undata;* co = *Phylloscopus collybita;* t = *P. trochilus.* Each symbol shows the mean duration (with standard errors) of migratory restlessness (expressed as the total number of half-hour intervals with nocturnal activity) of a group of six to nine caged birds. ●, ■ = results from birds kept under the photoperiodic conditions of their breeding grounds. ◨ = results from birds transferred by the end of September from the photoperiodic conditions of their breeding grounds to a constant 12-hr photoperiod. (From Gwinner, 1977a; after several sources.)

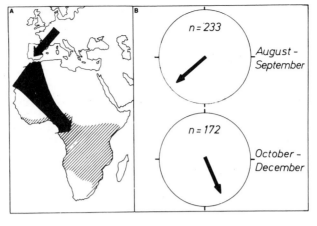

Fig. 9. (A) Schematic of changes in migratory direction of garden warblers on fall migration. (B) Average direction of migratory restlessness of garden warblers tested in circular orientation cages in August and September *(upper)* and in October through December *(lower)*. Numbers in the circular diagrams refer to the number of individual test nights during which the birds exhibited migratory restlessness. The mean direction of each of these nights was used as the statistical unit for further analysis. The mean direction preferred in August–September and that preferred in October–December are significantly different ($p < 0.001$, Watson and William test). (After Gwinner and Wiltschko, 1978.)

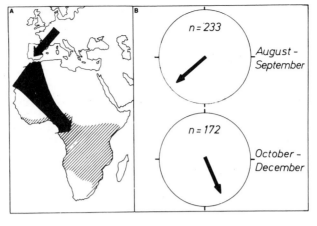

covered by these birds on their actual migrations (Figure 8): the longer the distance between breeding grounds and winter quarters, the more migratory restlessness was observed under cage conditions. Other results and considerations suggest that at least in the long-distance migrants, the proposed time program was, indeed, quantitatively organized in such a way as to produce, during the migratory season, the number of hours with migratory restlessness necessary to reach the species-specific winter quarters. Hence, it appears that these birds are able to find their winter quarters without having the capability of true bicoordinate navigation, namely, by flying in a particular direction for a particular number of hours (see Gwinner, 1977a, for a review).

Not only the temporal but also the directional component of migration appears to be affected by the circannual system. This effect is suggested by results obtained from garden warblers. This species reaches its African winter quarters by first flying in a southwesterly direction and later changing its migratory direction to south or southeast. This directional change in migratory direction has also been found in captive garden warblers that were tested in orientation cages (Gwinner and Wiltschko, 1978). These birds were maintained throughout the fall migratory season under a constant 12-hr photoperiod and were repeatedly tested in circular cages in which the mean direction of their perch-hopping activity was continuously recorded. During the tests, the birds had no access to celestial cues but were exposed to the natural magnetic field of the earth, which is known to be a directional cue for migratory orientation in that species. Figure 9 shows that under these conditions, the birds preferred a southwesterly orientation in August and September, when free-living birds also migrate southwest, but that they changed to southeast later on, just like their conspecifics in the wild, which also prefer more southeasterly directions during that stage of fall migration. Additional results suggest that the reversal from the grossly southerly migratory direction in autumn to the grossly northerly direction in spring is also endogenously preprogrammed (Gwinner and Wiltschko, 1980).

The mechanisms proposed here certainly require further and more rigorous testing. The interpretation of many of the results is impeded by the fact that the proposed annual time program, like circannual rhythmicity as a whole, is heavily affected by photoperiod and possibly other environmental variables. The final evaluation of the question of to what extent a circannual clock controls bird migration will depend on further information about its dependence on environmental cues.

REFERENCES

Aschoff, J. Jahresperiodik der Fortpflanzung bei Warmblütern. *Studium Generale,* 1955, *8,* 742–776.

Aschoff, J. Biological clocks in birds. *Proceedings of the 17th International Ornithological Congress,* 1980.

Baker, J. R. The evolution of breeding seasons. In G. R. de Beer (Ed.), *Evolution: Essays on Aspects of Evolutionary Biology.* Oxford: Oxford University Press, 1938, pp. 161–177.

Berthold, P. Circannual rhythms in birds with different migratory habits. In E. T. Pengelley (Ed.), *Circannual Clocks.* New York: Academic Press, 1974, pp. 55–94.

Berthold, P. Circannuale Rhythmik: Freilaufende selbsterregte Periodik mit lebenslanger Wirksamkeit bei Vögeln. *Naturwissenschaften,* 1978, p. 651.

Berthold, P., Gwinner, E., and Klein, H. Circannuale Periodik bei Grasmücken. I. Periodik des Körpergewichts, der Mauser und der Nachtunruhe bei *Sylvia atricapilla* und *S. borin* unter verschiedenen konstanten Bedingungen. *Journal für Ornithologie,* 1972, *113,* 170–190.

Blake, G. M. Diapause and the regulation of development in *Anthrenus verbasci* (L.) (Col., Dermestidae). *Bulletin of Entomological Research,* 1959, *49,* 751–757.

Blake, G. M. Decreasing photoperiod inhibiting metamorphosis in an insect. *Nature,* 1960, *188,* 168–169.

Bünning, E. Die endogene Tagesperiodik als Grundlage der photoperiodischen Reaktion. *Berichte der Deutschen Botanischen Gesellschaft,* 1936, *54,* 590–607.

Chapin, J. P. The birds of the Belgian Congo, Vol. 1. *Bulletin of the American Museum of National History,* 1932, *65,* 1–756.

Davis, D. E., and Finnie, E. P. Entrainment of circannual rhythm in weight of woodchucks. *Journal of Mammalogy,* 1975, *56,* 199–203.

Ducker, M. J., Bowman, J. C., and Temple, A. The effect of constant photoperiod on the expression of estrus in the ewe. *Journal of Reproduction and Fertility,* 1973, *19,* 143–150.

Enright, J. T. Ecological aspects of endogenous rhythmicity. *Annual Review of Ecology and Systematics,* 1970, *1,* 221–238.

Farner, D. S. Predictive functions in the control of annual cycles. *Environmental Research,* 1970, *3,* 119–131.

Goss, R. J. Photoperiodic control of antler cycles in deer. I. Phase shift and frequency changes. *Journal of Experimental Zoology,* 1969a, *170,* 311–324.

Goss, R. J. Photoperiodic control of antler cycles in deer. II. Alternations in amplitude. *Journal of Experimental Zoology,* 1969b, *171,* 223–234.

Gwinner, E. Circannuale Periodik als Grundlage des jahreszeitlichen Funktionswandels bei Zugvögeln. Untersuchungen am Fitis *(Phylloscopus trochilus)* und am Waldlaubsänger *(Ph. sibilatrix).* *Journal für Ornithologie,* 1968, *109,* 70–95.

Gwinner, E. A comparative study of circannual rhythms in warblers. In M. Menaker (Ed.), *Biochronometry.* Washington, D.C.: National Academy of Sciences, 1971, pp. 405–427.

Gwinner, E. Circannual rhythms in birds: Their interaction with circadian rhythms and environmental photoperiod. *Journal of Reproduction and Fertility,* 1973, *Supplement 19,* 51–65.

Gwinner, E. Testosterone induces "splitting" of circadian locomotor activity rhythms in birds. *Science,* 1974, *185,* 72–74.

Gwinner, E. Circadian and circannual rhythms in birds. In D. S. Farner and J. A. King (Eds.), *Avian Biology.* Vol. 5. New York, San Francisco, London: Academic Press, 1975a, pp. 221–285.

Gwinner, E. Effects of season and external testosterone on the freerunning circadian activity rhythm of European starlings *(Sturnus vulgaris).* *Journal of Comparative Physiology,* 1975b, *103,* 315–328.

Gwinner, E. Circannual rhythms in bird migration. *Annual Reviews of Ecology and Systematics,* 1977a, *8,* 381–405.

Gwinner, E. Photoperiodic synchronization of circannual rhythms in the European starling *(Sturnus vulgaris).* *Naturwissenschaften,* 1977b, *64,* 44.

Gwinner, E. Relationship between circadian activity patterns and gonadal function: Evidence for internal coincidence? *Proceedings of the 17th International Ornithological Congress,* 1980, in press.

Gwinner, E. Circannuale Rhythmen bei Tieren und ihre photoperiodische Synchronisation. *Naturwissenschaften,* 1981, *68,* in press.

Gwinner, E., and Dorka, V. Endogenous control of annual reproductive rhythms in birds. *Proceedings of the 16th International Ornithological Congress*, 1976, pp. 223–234.

Gwinner, E., and Wiltschko, W. Endogenously controlled changes in migratory direction of the garden warbler, *Sylvia borin. Journal of Comparative Physiology*, 1978, *125*, 267–273.

Gwinner, E., and Wiltschko, W. Circannual changes in migratory orientation in the garden warbler, *Sylvia borin. Behavioral Ecology and Sociobiology*, 1980, *7*, 73–78.

Hamner, W. M. On seeking an alternative to the endogenous reproductive rhythm hypothesis in birds. In M. Menaker (Ed.), *Biochronometry*. Washington, D.C.: National Academy of Sciences, 1971, pp. 448–462.

Heller, H. C., and Poulson, T. L. Circannian rhythms. II. Endogenous and exogenous factors controlling reproduction and hibernation in chipmunks *(Eutamias)* and ground squirrels *(Spermophilus)*. *Comparative Biochemistry and Physiology*, 1970, *33*, 357–383.

Immelmann, K. Role of the environment in reproduction as source of "predictive" information. In D. S. Farner (Ed.), *Breeding Biology of Birds*. Washington, D.C.: National Academy of Sciences, 1973, pp. 121–147.

King, J. Cycles of fat deposition and molt in white-crowned sparrows in constant environmental conditions. *Comparative Biochemistry and Physiology*, 1968, *24*, 827–837.

Lofts, B. Evidence of an autonomous reproductive rhythm in an equatorial bird *(Quelea quelea)*. *Nature*, 1964, *201*, 523–524.

Marshall, A. J. The role of the internal rhythm of reproduction in the timing of avian breeding seasons, including migration. *Proceedings of the 12th International Ornithological Congress*, 1960, pp. 475–482.

Marshall, A. J., and Serventy, D. L. Experimental demonstration of an internal rhythm of reproduction in a trans-equatorial migrant (the short-tailed shearwater Puffinus tenuirostris). *Nature*, 1959, *184*, 1704–1705.

Meier, A. H. Chronoendocrinology of the white-throated sparrow. *Proceedings of the 16th International Ornithological Congress*, 1976, pp. 355–368.

Menaker, M. Circannual rhythms in circadian perspective. In E. T. Pengelley (Ed.), *Circannual Clocks*. New York, San Francisco, London: Academic Press, 1974, pp. 507–520.

Merkel, F. W. Long term effects of constant photoperiods on European robins and whitethroats. *Proceedings of the 13th International Ornithological Congress*, 1963, pp. 950–959.

Moreau, R. E. Equatorial reflections on periodism in birds. *Ibis*, 1931, *1*, 553–570.

Mrosovsky, N. Mechanism of hibernation cycles in ground squirrels: Circannian rhythm or sequence of stages. *Pennsylvania Academy of Science*, 1970, *44*, 172–175.

Mrosovsky, N. Circannual cycles in hibernators. In L. Wang and J. W. Hudson (Eds.), *Strategies in Cold: Natural Torpidity and Thermogenesis*. New York: Academic Press, 1977, pp. 21–65.

Pengelley, E. T. Interrelationships of circannian rhythms in the ground squirrel, *Citellus lateralis. Comparative Biochemistry Physiology*, 1968, *24*, 915–919.

Pengelley, E. T., and Asmundson, S. M. Freerunning periods of endogenous circannian rhythms in the golden mantled ground squirrel, *Citellus lateralis. Comparative Biochemistry and Physiology*, 1969, *30*, 177–183.

Pengelley, E. T., and Asmundson, S. J. Free-running periods of endogenous circannian rhythms in the golden mantled ground squirrel, *Citellus lateralis. Comparative Biochemistry and Physiology*, 1970, *32*, 155–160.

Pengelley, E. T., and Asmundson, S. J. Circannual rhythmicity in hibernating mammals. In E. T. Pengelley (Ed.), *Circannual Clocks*. New York, San Francisco, London: Academic Press, 1974, pp. 95–160.

Pengelley, E. T., and Fisher, K. C. Onset and cessation of hibernation under constant temperature and light in the golden-mantled ground squirrel, *Citellus lateralis. Nature*, 1957, *180*, 1371–1372.

Pengelley, E. T., and Fisher, K. C. The effect of temperature and photoperiod on the yearly hibernating behavior of captive golden-mantled ground squirrels *(Citellus lateralis tescorum)*. *Canadian Journal of Zoology*, 1963, *41*, 1103–1120.

Pengelley, E. T., and Kelly, K. H. A "circannian" rhythm in hibernating species of the genus *Citellus* with observations on their physiological evolution. *Comparative Biochemistry and Physiology*, 1966, *19*, 603–617.

Pengelley, E. T., Asmundson, S. J., Barnes, B., and Aloia, R. C. Relationship of light intensity and photoperiod to circannual rhythmicity in the hibernating ground squirrel, *Citellus lateralis. Comparative Biochemistry and Physiology*, 1976, *53A*, 273–277.

Pernau, F. A. von. *Unterricht. Was mit dem lieblichen Geschöpff, denen Vögeln, auch ausser dem Fang, nur durch die Ergründung deren Eigenschafften und Zahmmachung oder anderer Abrichtung man sich vor Lust und Zeitvertreib machen könne*. Nürnberg: 1702.

Pittendrigh, C. S. Circadian surfaces and the diversity of possible roles of circadian organization in photoperiodic induction. *Proceedings of the National Academy of Sciences*, 1972, *69*, 2734–2737.

Pittendrigh, C. S., and Minis, D. H. The entrainment of circadian oscillations by light and their role as photoperiodic clocks. *American Naturalist,* 1964, *43,* 261–294.

Rowan, W. On photoperiodism, reproductive periodicity, and the annual migrations of birds and certain fishes. *Proceedings of the Boston Society of Natural History,* 1926, *38,* 147–189.

Sansum, E. L., and King, J. R. Long-term effects of constant photoperiods on testicular cycles of white-crowned sparrows *(Zonotrichia leucophrys gambelii). Physiological Zoology,* 1976, *49,* 407–416.

Schwab, R. G. Circannian testicular periodicity in the European starling in the absence of photoperiodic change. In M. Menaker (Ed.), *Biochronometry.* Washington, D.C.: National Academy of Sciences, 1971, pp. 428–447.

Segal, E. Discussion to the paper of A. J. Marshall. *Cold Spring Harbor Symposium on Quantitative Biology,* 1960, *25,* 504–505.

Zimmerman, J. L. Effects of extended tropical photoperiod and temperature on the dickcissel. *The Condor,* 1966, *68,* 377–387.

22

Insect Photoperiodism

D. S. SAUNDERS

INTRODUCTION

Insects, like several other major groups of organisms (flowering plants, birds, and mammals, for example), may use the number of hours of day or night to regulate seasonal cycles of activity, morphology, reproduction, or development. Such regulation is called *photoperiodic induction*. The use of day length (or photoperiod) to provide information on calendar time is advantageous to the organism because this geophysical variable is reliable, is relatively "noise-free," and changes with a mathematical accuracy with both season and latitude. At least in natural diel cycles, photoperiodic induction involves a response to the number of hours of light (or dark) per day, which the organism apparently compares with an inbuilt standard, or critical day length (or night length). It differs, therefore, from a circannual rhythm, which is known in at least one insect, the beetle *Anthrenus verbasci* (Blake, 1959), and which comprises an endogenous biological rhythm with a near annual periodicity *entrained by* the seasonal changes in day length (see Chapter 21).

Among the insects, photoperiod is known to control physiological events as diverse as the induction of diapause (Kogure, 1933), the termination of diapause (Baker, 1935), the appearance of seasonal morphs (Marcovitch, 1923), growth rates (Saunders, 1972), migration (Dingle, 1974), coloration (MacLeod, 1967), sexual behavior (Perez, Verdier, and Pener, 1971), sex ratio (Hoelscher and Vinson, 1971), fecundity (Atwal, 1955), insecticide sensitivity (Fernandez and Randolph, 1966), and recovery from heat stress (Pittendrigh, 1961). Control of seasonal morphs is known from the Orthoptera, Homoptera, Heteroptera, Thysanoptera, Neuroptera, and Lepidoptera. Control of larval growth rate has been recorded in the Orthoptera, Lepidoptera and Diptera. However, by far the most information is available on the photoperiodic induction of diapause: at the last "count," such regulation was known in over 200 insect species from about 12 orders (Saunders, 1976a).

D. S. SAUNDERS Department of Zoology, University of Edinburgh, Edinburgh EH9 3JT, Scotland.

Consequently, much of this chapter is concerned with this phenomenon. Furthermore—and in keeping with a volume entitled *Biological Rhythms*—most attention is directed at the nature of the biological clock involved in photoperiodic time measurement and, in particular, its relationship to the circadian system.

THE PHOTOPERIODIC RESPONSE

Photoperiodic induction in insects is a mechanism involving two interrelated processes: (1) the "measurement" of day or night length (or perhaps both); and (2) the summation and integration of successive photoperiodic cycles, either long or short, to a point at which induction is "complete." The first is accomplished by a mechanism hereafter referred to as the *clock;* the second by the photoperiodic *counter.* Time measurement by the clock is regulated by *periodic* aspects of the environment (particularly cycles of light and temperature), while a variety of environmental factors (temperature, diet, etc.) are known to affect the "expression" of the clock via the counting mechanism (Saunders, 1971, 1975a).

PHOTOPERIODIC RESPONSE CURVES

The reaction to day length and the properties of the clock are best described by photoperiodic response curves, which usually plot the incidence of diapause (or of a particular morph, etc.) in populations of insects exposed to a range of stationary photoperiods (Figure 1). Most insects are "long-day" species, which produce actively developing or reproducing individuals in the summer months when days are long but enter diapause or produce a winter morph when the hours of light fall below an often well-defined critical day length. A frequent feature of such curves is a decline in diapause incidence at ultrashort day lengths (< 6 hr), which rarely, if ever, occurs in the insect's natural environment, but nevertheless requires a physiological "explanation." In other species, there may also be a rise in diapause incidence in very long photoperiods. The often very abrupt change in the response at the critical day length is both physiologically and ecologically the most important feature of the curve; it shows the photoperiod at which one developmental or metabolic pathway gives way to the other, and it is the basis for assuming that the organism possesses some sort of time-measuring ability.

Short-day insects show an opposite reaction to day length, with long days inducing a high incidence of diapause and short days leading to "active" development. Most examples of short-day species are active in the autumn or winter months but spend the summer in an estival diapause (e.g., *Abraxas miranda,* Masaki, 1958). In the commercial silkmoth, *Bombyx mori,* on the other hand, the short-day response is associated with the fact that the diapause stage is in the egg, but the stages *sensitive* to photoperiod occur in the eggs and young larvae of the *maternal* generation. Thus, long days perceived during the summer give rise to moths' laying diapause eggs in the autumn, while short days (i.e., in the spring) give rise to moths' laying nondiapause eggs (Kogure, 1933).

Most of this chapter is concerned with the photoperiodic mechanism in long-day insects, because these are by far the most frequent. However, just to underline the variability of the response, the following should also be noted. In some insects, such as the Colorado potato beetle, *Leptinotarsa decemlineata,* diapause is induced in all photoperiods except a narrow range of long days (de Wilde, 1958). These species clearly show a tendency toward a univoltine life cycle, which, in an extreme example, shows an obligate diapause in every individual regardless of photoperiod. The tendency toward univoltinism and obligate diapause often increases towards the northern parts of an insect's distribution. At the opposite extreme are insects that appear to lack either a diapause or any true photoperiodic control of development and are thus said to be day-neutral. An example is the house fly, *Musca domestica,* which, being commensal, occurs wherever man lives, from the tropics to the polar regions. Some insects respond to the direction of change in day length, rather than to "absolute" day lengths, by determining a sequence of photoperiods, either short to long or long to short, at different stages of development (Norris, 1959). Still other insects appear capable of responding to photoperiods increasing or decreasing at a natural rate (Tauber and Tauber, 1973).

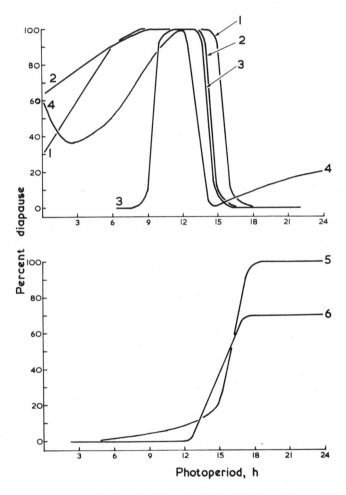

Fig. 1. Photoperiodic response curves for long-day *(upper)* and short-day *(lower)* insects. (1) *Acronycta rumicis* (Danilevskii, 1965); (2) *Sarcophaga argyrostoma* (Saunders, 1971); (3) *Ostrinia nubilalis* (Beck, 1962a); (4) *Pectinophora gossypiella* (Pittendrigh and Minis, 1971); (5) *Stenocranus minutus* (Müller, 1958); (6) *Bombyx mori* (Kogure, 1933).

D. S. SAUNDERS

The stages of the life cycle sensitive to photoperiod and the instars that enter diapause may or may not be temporally distinct. In some species, such as *Metriocnemus knabi* (Paris and Jenner, 1959), *Antheraea pernyi* (Williams and Adkisson, 1964), and *Pectinophora gossypiella* (Bell and Adkisson, 1964), the sensitive period extends to include the resultant diapause, so that the diapausing stages retain a photoperiodic sensitivity, and diapause termination, as well as induction, is under day-length control. Such insects are examples of Müller's (1970) "oligopause." In *A. pernyi* (Williams and Adkisson, 1964) and the pitcher plant mosquito, *Wyeomyia smithii* (Bradshaw, 1976), the critical day lengths for diapause induction and diapause termination are identical; presumably, the same "clock" mechanism is involved in both. Most insect species, however, show a photoperiodic sensitivity in instars that *precede* the diapause stage, and the latter is insensitive to day length. Such reactions have been called "delayed photoperiodic responses" (de Wilde, 1962). Reactivation in these species usually follows an accumulated experience of low winter temperatures, which brings them to a state of competence for renewed development when temperatures rise in the spring. An example of this type, called "eudiapause" by Müller (1970), is the flesh fly, *Sarcophaga argyrostoma*, which is maximally sensitive as embryos within the maternal uterus (Denlinger, 1972) and as young larvae (Saunders, 1971) but becomes insensitive to the diapause-inducing effects of short days by the time the larvae round up to form puparia. The diapause stage is the pupa. Although diapause reversal by long days cannot be achieved by these species in the diapause stage itself, it is reversible during the prior sensitive stage.

The most extreme examples of a delayed photoperiodic response are to be found in those species in which the sensitive stage occurs in one generation and the resultant diapause in the next. Examples of such maternally operating photoperiods include the "classic" example of *Bombyx mori* (Kogure, 1933), the parasitic wasp *Nasonia vitripennis* (Saunders, 1965), the braconid *Coeloides brunneri* (Ryan, 1965), and several species of Diptera (Ring, 1967; Vinogradova and Zinovjeva, 1972). In aphids, photoperiods experienced by the wingless, viviparous summer forms (virginoparae) may determine the morph (virginopara or ovipara) of her offspring and, in short days, the diapause state of the eggs deposited by her oviparous daughters (Lees, 1959). In this sense, therefore, photoperiodic sensitivity and the resulting diapause may span three generations. In at least some of these species (*N. vitripennis*, for example), the effects of photoperiod are transmitted from one generation to the next via the undifferentiated ovarian egg. This raises interesting and important questions about the nature of this transovarian mechanism, in particular whether it is nuclear or cytoplasmic.

Most insects seem to need to experience a *number* of sequential light cycles, the effects of which are accumulated during the sensitive period (Dickson, 1949; Williams and Adkisson, 1964; Beck, Cloutier, and McLeod, 1962). The number of cycles required for the full expression of the response, however, varies from species to species. In *S. argyrostoma*, for example, larvae require at least 13–14 short-day cycles for the induction of pupal diapause (Saunders, 1971), and *A. rumicis* (Belgorod strain) requires about 10–11 (Tyshchenko, Goryshin, and Azaryan, 1972). The mechanism for this summation has been called the photoperiodic "counter" (Saunders, 1976b). Frequently, the diapause-inhibiting or -reactivating effects of long days are "stronger" than the diapause-inducing or -maintaining effects of short days (Beck, 1968; Tyshchenko *et al.*, 1972). Diapausing larvae of *Chaoborus americanus,* for example, require only a single long day cycle (LD 17:7) for the reactivation of 30%–35% of the population (Bradshaw, 1969), although more are required for a full return to development.

THE EFFECTS OF TEMPERATURE ON THE PHOTOPERIODIC RESPONSE

Temperature may affect the photoperiodic response in a variety of ways, depending on the manner in which it is "offered," that is, as constant temperature, stepwise changes, cycles, or hot and cold pulses. Periodic changes in temperature (daily cycles and pulses) appear to exert their effect directly on the clock mechanism; constant temperature, on the other hand, may alter the proportion of the population entering diapause by more superficial means.

Daily temperature cycles (or thermoperiods) have been offered either with concurrent light cycles or in continuous darkness. In the former case, it is usually found that the high point of the daily temperature cycle acts as "day" and the low point as "night," and that nighttime temperature is more important than that during the day (Lees, 1953; Beck, 1962a; Goryshin, 1964; Pittendrigh and Minis, 1971). At a superficial level, this result is hardly surprising because the night is cooler than the day in natural conditions. It may also, however, suggest that night-length measurement is more "important" in terms of photoperiodic time measurement (see the section below on time measurement in photoperiodism).

Probably of a similar nature are the various experiments using short daily pulses of low or high temperature, which may produce often spectacular reversals of the photoperiodic response. In the knot grass moth, *Acronycta rumicis*, for example, Danilevskii (1965) showed that chilling at 5°C for 3 hr daily at the beginning or the end (but not the middle) of the light period in LD 17:7 converted the response from that of a long day to a short day. In the parasitic wasp *Nasonia vitripennis,* 4-hr periods of chilling (2°) or heating (35°) applied during the dark of an LD 14:10 cycle converted the response to that of a long day (short night), whereas a similar period of chilling or heating in the light of an LD 16:8 cycle converted the response from a long day to that of a short day. These reversals in photoperiodic response were attributed to effects on the clock mechanism itself (Saunders, 1967).

Thermoperiods may also have an inductive effect in the *absence* of a light cycle, thus indicating that temperature cycles are inductive in their own right. In the European corn borer, *Ostrinia nubilalis* (Beck, 1962b), and the pink bollworm moth, *Pectinophora gossypiella* (Menaker and Gross, 1965), for example, a "short-day" thermoperiod (about 11–12 hr at a raised temperature per day) resulted in more diapause than a constant temperature, and in *A. rumicis* and a number of other lepidopterous species, Goryshin and Kozlova (1967) demonstrated that a "short-day" thermoperiod (12 hr at 26–32° per day) induced more diapause than a "long-day" thermoperiod (18 hr at 25–29° per day). More extensive observations of this type, however, have been made for *N. vitripennis.* Females of this species were raised from the egg in continuous darkness, and then exposed as adults to a range of "square-wave" thermoperiods (13/23°C) with the higher temperature (= "day") occupying a different number of hours per 24. In "short-day" thermoperiods (between 6 and 10 hr at 23° per day), almost all of the wasps produced diapausing larvae. On the other hand, when the adult females were exposed to more than 14 hr per day at the higher temperature, almost all of their progeny were produced as developing larvae. The "critical thermoperiod" at about 13 hr at 23° per day was almost as "sharp" as the corresponding critical day length (Saunders, 1973b). A well-defined critical thermoperiod has also been observed for *Pieris brassicae* (Dumortier and Brunnarius, 1977). These observations may be important in considering the nature of the clock mechanism involved.

In long-day species, high constant temperatures tend to reduce or eliminate the effect of a short day length, while low temperatures enhance it. In *P. brassicae,* for example, a short-day regime (LD 12:12) is fully inductive up to about 25°; the incidence of diapause then drops as the temperature rises, being almost eliminated at 30° (Danilevskii, 1965). In *S. argyrostoma,* LD 10:14 induces a high incidence of pupal diapause at 15–18°, less at 20°, and almost none at 25° (Saunders, 1971). In several species, it has been noted that diapause supervenes even at long day length if the temperature is low enough (Danilevskii, 1965; Way and Hopkins, 1950). Thus, in long-day species, low constant temperatures and short days act together to induce diapause, whereas high temperatures and long days act together to avert it. In short-day species, however, the opposite may be true: in *B. mori* (Kogure, 1933) and *A. miranda* (Masaki, 1958), for example, high temperature promotes diapause and low temperature reduces it.

The effect of constant temperature on the critical day length is variable. Some species, such as *P. brassicae,* appear to be almost perfectly temperature-compensated in this respect over the entire ecological range (up to 25°C). In *M. viciae* and *O. nubilalis,* however, the critical day length shortens by about 15 min for each 5°C rise in temperature (Lees, 1963; Beck and Hanec, 1960), while in *A. rumicis,* the reduction is about 1½ hr for the same incremental change (Goryshin, 1955). In still other species, the effects may be greater.

In at least four insect species (*N. vitripennis, A. rumicis, S. argyrostoma,* and *Aëdes atropalpus;* Beach, 1978) these effects of constant temperature have been attributed to an interaction between the summation of light cycles and the length of the sensitive period, the former (or photoperiodic "counter") being temperature-compensated, the latter not (Saunders, 1966a, 1971; Goryshin and Tyshchenko, 1970). Reference to *S. argyrostoma* will suffice to illustrate this mechanism.

Cultures of *S. argyrostoma* larvae were raised at short day length (LD 10:14) and at temperatures between 16 and 26°C. The puparia were collected daily from these cultures as they formed, incubated in the dark for 10–14 days, then opened to ascertain the diapause status of the pupae within them. The length of larval development, between larviposition and puparium formation (which signifies the end of the larval sensitive period) was temperature-dependent: at 26° it was about 9 days, at 16° about 23 days, a Q_{10} of about 2.7. On the other hand, the number of short-day cycles required to raise the proportion of a day's batch of pupae to 50% diapause (the required day number—RDN) was found to be about 13–14, and temperature-compensated ($Q_{10} = 1.4$). At high temperature (26 and 24°C), therefore, all the larvae had pupated *before* they had experienced a sufficient number of short-day cycles, and diapause incidence was very low. At low temperature (18 and 16°C), on the other hand, a sufficient number of short-day cycles had been "seen" by the larvae before puparium formation, and diapause incidence was high (Figure 2). This mechanism accounts for the association between temperature and diapause so characteristic of the majority of insect species.

This model for diapause incidence was further tested in *S. argyrostoma* by manipulating the length of the larval sensitive period by means other than temperature (Saunders, 1975a). It was found that overcrowding larvae within a limited amount of food, or extracting them manually from their food before they had finished feeding, led to early pupation (and hence, a shortened sensitive period) and a reduction of pupal diapause. Conversely, allowing the larvae to wander in wet sawdust after leaving their food protracted larval development and raised the incidence of diapause. It is likely that this mechanism is widespread among the insects and is affected by many of the environmental variables. The availability of food, or the type of food, for example, can slow or accelerate development during the sensitive period, thereby altering the proportion of the population entering diapause (Saunders, 1966b; Clay and Venard, 1972).

The fourth recognized effect of temperature is that of temperature steps, either up or down (Gibbs, 1975). For example, larvae of *S. argyrostoma* reared at LD 10:14, 16°C, were split into two groups at puparium formation, one (the control) kept at the same temperature, the other transferred to a higher temperature (22, 24, 26, or 28°C). A temperature step-up at this point was found to reduce the incidence of pupal diapause, the degree of reduction being greater at higher temperatures. Conversely, a temperature step-down (22–16°C) at this point increased the subsequent incidence of diapause. Puparia were found to be maximally sensitive to such temperature shifts during the first 2 days after puparium formation, at a time when they had already lost their photoperiodic sensitivity. It was concluded that temperature changes at this stage must affect the "stored information" within the brain.

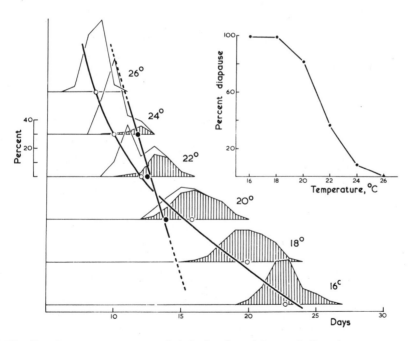

Fig. 2. The effect of constant temperature on the induction of pupal diapause in *Sarcophaga argyrostoma* at LD 10:14, showing the interaction between the temperature-dependent sensitive period, SP (length of larval development, open circles), and the temperature-compensated required day number, RDN (closed circles). See text for details. (After Saunders, 1971. Reprinted with permission of Pergamon Press, Ltd., Oxford.)

Natural day lengths contain "information" about latitude as well as season. Days at more northerly latitudes, for example, not only increase at a greater rate after the vernal equinox than in areas further south but also reach a longer absolute day length at the midsummer solstice. At higher latitudes, however, the summer "growing season" is generally shorter. Consequently, northerly populations of insects frequently produce fewer generations per year and enter diapause earlier at a longer critical day length. In Russian populations of the knot grass moth, *A. rumicis,* for example, the critical day length at Sukhumi (43°N) was found to be about 14½ hr/24, at Belgorod (50°N) 16½ hr/24, at Vitebsk (55°N) 18 hr/24, and at Leningrad (60°N) about 19½ hr/24 (Danilevskii, 1965). This species thus shows about a 1½-hr change in the critical day length for every 5° of latitude. The Leningrad population also shows the marked tendency toward univoltinism and an obligate diapause mentioned earlier. Geographical clines with respect to phenological characteristics are now known in a large number of insects. In *P. brassicae,* however, there may be two distinct races in the Soviet Union. Populations from Leningrad (60°N) to Belgorod (50°N) all showed a critical day length of about 15 hr/24, whereas populations from the Black Sea coast (43°N) showed a value of 10 hr/24.

Longitude is usually of less significance unless populations from widely differing climatic zones are compared. For example, the small cabbage white butterfly, *Pieris rapae,* accomplishes about six generations per year on the Black Sea coast and shows a critical day length of about 12 hr/24, whereas at Vladivostok, almost at the same latitude but with a much harsher climate, it shows only three generations per year and a critical day length of about 14½ hr/24 (Danilevskii, 1965). Altitude, however, is much more important. Populations at high altitude, because of the shorter growing season, frequently show fewer generations per year and a longer critical day length. The green-veined white butterfly, *Pieris napi,* for example, shows distinct races below *(meridionalis)* and above *(bryoniae)* about 1,500–1,600 m in the Caucasus. The former is multivoltine, with a critical day length of about 13 hr/24; the latter is almost univoltine, with only a rudimentary photoperiodic response at high temperature (Danilevskii, 1965). Bradshaw (1976) has recently produced data on the effect of altitude on the diapause characteristics of the pitcher plant mosquito, *Wyeomyia smithii.* Critical day lengths determined for 22 natural populations collected over 19° of latitude, 20° of longitude, and 1,200 m of altitude showed a range from 12 to 16 hr/24. Critical day lengths were closely correlated with latitude and altitude, but not with longitude. They were also closely correlated with the growing season (mean number of freeze-free days). Bradshaw calculated that latitude accounted for 80.5% of the variation, and altitude for about 15.5%. In the mosquito *Aëdes atropalpus,* differences between geographical strains have been attributed to differences in the required day number (RDN) as well as to the critical day lengths (Beach, 1978). For example, in a population from 14°N (El Salvador), nine or more cycles shorter than the critical value (about 12 hr/24) were required for diapause induction, whereas in a population from 45°N (Ontario), only four cycles of 15 hr/24 or less were required.

The diapause and photoperiodic characteristics of these geographical populations are genetically determined. Danilevskii (1965), for example, crossed *A. rumicis* from Leningrad (critical day length 19 hr/24) with those from Sukhumi (15 hr/24) and obtained F_1

hybrids with a critical day length of about 17 hr/24. Inbred hybrids (F_2) also showed an intermediate response, as did backcrosses with either parental type. The absence of any segregation in these results suggested that the genetic control was polygenic. The results also suggested the occurrence of a continuous gradient of gene frequencies with latitude. Other evidence of the genetic control of the photoperiodic response is derived from selection experiments in which almost diapause-free lines may be bred from those individuals that fail to diapause at short day length (Barry and Adkisson, 1966), or almost obligately diapausing strains from those few individuals that become dormant in long days (Tanaka, 1951).

The Physiology of Photoperiodic Induction

The foregoing sections demonstrate the complexity of the photoperiodic response, with interactions between external (environmental) and internal (genetic) factors. From the simplest point of view, however, the *minimal* requirements for the response are (1) a photoreceptor; (2) a mechanism for measuring the length of the night or day (the "clock") and, concurrently, for integrating successive photoperiodic cycles (the "counter"); and (3) an effector system. The last, which is outside the scope of the present chapter, is clearly known only for diapause induction and termination, and only then in very few species. In larval and pupal diapause, neurosecretory cells in the brain fail, under the appropriate photoperiodic influence, to release the brain or prothoracotrophic hormone; thus, the prothoracic glands remain inactive, and in the absence of ecdysone, growth and development stop (Williams, 1952; Novak, 1966). In adult (ovarian) diapause, inactivation of brain neurosecretory cells controlling the corpora allata leads to an absence of juvenile hormone and consequent suppression of the ovaries, often at the point where yolk deposition should have begun (de Wilde, Duintjer, and Mook, 1959). Other endocrine mechanisms for diapause control also exist, including that in *B. mori,* in which the egg diapause is controlled by a "diapause hormone" secreted by the maternal subesophageal ganglion (Fukuda, 1963). In this chapter, we consider the properties and location of the photoreceptor and the clocks involved in photoperiodism, and we merely note that the earliest known effects of photoperiodic induction are on the brain neurosecretory cells.

Photoreception and Spectral Sensitivity of the Photoperiodic Response

Studies on photoreception have included investigations of the properties of the photoreceptors involved (e.g., spectral sensitivity and intensity thresholds) and of their anatomical location.

Some insects, such as *B. mori* (Kogure, 1933), the oriental fruit moth *Grapholitha molesta* (Dickson, 1949), *P. brassicae* (Geispitz, 1957), *A. pernyi* (Williams, Adkisson, and Walcott, 1965), the codling moth *Carpocapsa pomonella* (Norris, Howell, Hayes, Adler, Sullivan, and Schechter, 1969), and the aphid *Megoura viciae* (Lees, 1971), are maximally sensitive to light in the blue-green and almost insensitive to red. In his study of *M. viciae,* Lees (1971) exposed test virginoparae to 1-hr or 0.5-hr pulses of near-monochromatic light of various intensities, placed either 1.5 hr after "dusk" (i.e., LD 13½:1½:1:8) or 2.5 hr before "dawn" (i.e., LD 13½:7½:½:2½), these positions being the most light-sensitive parts of the night (see p. 425). The results for early "night interruptions" showed a maximum sensitivity of about 450–470 nm and a sharp cutoff above about 500 nm. The insects were almost entirely insensitive to longer wavelengths. For late night interruptions, a similar curve was obtained but with a somewhat greater sensitivity to red. The threshold intensity (for a 50%) response at 450–470 nm was about 0.2 μW cm^{-2}.

In other species, such as *A. rumicis* (Geispitz, 1957), the Colorado potato beetle *Leptinotarsa decemlineata* (de Wilde and Bonga, 1958), *P. gossypiella* (Pittendrigh, Eichhorn, Minis, and Bruce, 1970), and *N. vitripennis* (Saunders, 1975c), there is a marked sensitivity to red light. In *N. vitripennis,* for example, maximum sensitivity for the "dawn" transition was at 554–586 nm, with considerable response to 617 nm, but a cutoff above 650 nm. At peak sensitivity, wasps responded to less than 0.2 μW cm^{-2}; at 653 nm the threshold was at about 0.95 μW cm^{-2}. The differences in the spectral sensitivities of these species, particularly in whether they can respond to red light or not, may indicate a variety of photopigments.

Covering the compound eyes, ocelli, or larval stemmata with an opaque black paint, or destroying them by cautery, has demonstrated that the photoperiodic response can continue in the absence of the "organized photoreceptors" (Tanaka, 1951; de Wilde *et al.,* 1959; Lees, 1964; Geldiay, 1971). Illumination of different parts of the body, however, has indicated that the photoreceptors are in the head, and presumably in the brain. Lees (1964), for example, maintained virginoparae of *M. viciae* in a general body illumination of LD 14:10 and then attached the aphids to microilluminators for an additional 2 hr per day. When the supplementary illumination was applied to the middorsal line of the head, the aphids produced virginoparous daughters (the long-day response, equivalent to LD 16:8), but when the microilluminators were attached elsewhere, oviparae were produced (the short-day response, LD 14:10). Lees concluded that the photoreceptors were in the underlying protocerebrum. A more precise localization of the mechanism (photoreceptor plus clock), to the Group I neurosecretory cells and areas slightly lateral to these cells, has since been made by systematically destroying parts of the protocerebrum by radio frequency microcautery (Steel and Lees, 1977).

Unequivocal proof that the photoperiodic receptors are within the brain has been obtained in elegant surgical experiments with the silkmoth *Antheraea pernyi* (Williams and Adkisson, 1964). In these experiments diapausing pupae were plugged into holes in an opaque board in such a way that some of the pupae received long-day illumination (LD 16:8) at the front and short-day illumination at the rear, and others the opposite combination. In still further pupae, the brains were excised and replanted either back into the head or into the tip of the abdomen. The results clearly showed that photoperiodic sensitivity was controlled by the photoperiod "seen" by the brain, whether in the head or in the abdomen; that seen by the brainless head or the normal abdomen was inconsequential. Furthermore, since the response was evident in "loose-brain" preparations, the experiment also demonstrated that the humoral effector system and the clock were also brain-centered—although conclusive evidence of the latter strictly requires the reciprocal transfer of brains between insects possessing different clock characteristics (e.g., different critical day lengths) and the subsequent demonstration of those characteristics in the recipient animals. Later experiments involving the transplantation of progressively smaller pieces of brain tissue suggested that both receptor and clock were located in a "tiny mass" just lateral to the medial neurosecretory cells (Williams, 1969).

Almost nothing is known about the "concrete" physiology of time measurement in insect photoperiodism. Consequently, we are still restricted to the kind of analysis in which the organism is treated like a "black box," exposing populations of insects to different experimental light and temperature cycles, on the one hand, and observing the proportion entering diapause, on the other. Despite this restriction to a purely formal approach, much has been learned about the properties of the clock. However, this approach has also given rise to a plethora of models according to both species and, sometimes, apparently to the authors' interpretations. One of the intentions of this chapter is to rationalize some of these apparent differences.

It is axiomatic that realistic models must be based on sound experimental evidence or theory. Thus, they may become useful in describing presumed events in time measurement, in comparing different species, and in designing further lines of investigation. For models based on circadian rhythmicity, there is a conceptual difficulty in that the entry into diapause occurs only once in a particular insect and, moreover, is not an event (like eclosion, for example) that can be observed directly; all we can measure is the final result, whether the individual is in diapause or not. Therefore, experiments based on the "resonance" principle (see below), which may reveal circadian rhythmicity in the photoperiodic response, are very "indirect," and it is considered essential that a parallel study of an *overt* circadian rhythmicity should be carried out, preferably in the same species (Pittendrigh and Minis, 1964). It also becomes important to demonstrate that the chosen overt periodicity possesses the same properties as, or properties very similar to, the presumed circadian oscillation involved in photoperiodic time measurement.

ACCOUNT OF MODELS FOR PHOTOPERIODIC INDUCTION

Hourglasses. When explicitly formulated, hourglasses in insect photoperiodism are seen as mechanisms that are set in motion at the dawn—or more usually the *dusk*—transition of the photoperiod and run their time course in a temperature-compensated fashion. Short and long nights may then be distinguished by whether "dawn arrives early" to illuminate a particular light-sensitive portion of the night (i.e., the short night or summer, nondiapause pathway), or whether it "arrives late" and fails to illuminate this light-sensitive point (i.e., the long night or autumnal, diapause pathway). Such a model was implicit in the work of several early workers (Dickson, 1949; Way and Hopkins, 1950; Lees, 1953) and has more recently received extensive experimental support in work on the green vetch aphid, *Megoura viciae* (Lees, 1968, 1973). Night-length hourglasses, such as that in *M. viciae,* differ from the circadian mechanisms discussed below in that they execute a *single* act of time measurement, even in experimentally extended "nights": they do not reset themselves (as does an oscillation); they require a period of illumination (= "day") to "prime" the mechanism or to "turn the hourglass over."

Bünning's Hypothesis. A totally different kind of model was proposed by Erwin Bünning, initially to account for photoperiodism in plants (Bünning, 1936), but later introduced to explain the phenomenon in insects (Bünning and Joerrens, 1960). This entirely original proposition suggested that photoperiodic time measurement was a function of the organism's circadian system; it thus had the attraction of equating photoperiodism with the control of overt daily activity cycles and suggested that both had a common origin. In its original form, the model supposed that the endogenous daily cycle comprised a 12-hr "photophilic" (light-requiring) half-cycle and a 12-hr "scotophilic" (dark-requiring) half-cycle, terms that are equivalent to the "subjective day" and "subjective night" of later authors (Pittendrigh, 1960). When entrained to a natural or an artificial light cycle, the former coincided with the light portion of the cycle, and the latter with the dark. Bünning also envisaged that the onset of the photophil was phase-locked to dawn. Consequently, when the photoperiod was short, light was restricted to the photophil and long night effects were produced, but when the photoperiod increased, light extended into the scotophil and produced long-day (short-night) effects. The essential elements of this model, therefore, were (1) its basis in circadian rhythmicity and (2) a temporal interaction between environmental light and a particular light-sensitive phase of the oscillation.

External Coincidence. The external coincidence model of Pittendrigh and Minis (1964) and Pittendrigh (1966) is a more explicit version of Bünning's general hypothesis. It recognizes that model's dual requirement for light (entrainment and induction) but is based on a more complete understanding of the phenomenon of entrainment, derived from a study of pupal eclosion in *Drosophila pseudoobscura*. In particular, it recognizes that the light-sensitive phase of the oscillation (hereafter referred to as the photoinducible phase, ϕ_i) seems more restricted, in time, than Bünning's scotophil. It also recognizes that the photoperiodic oscillation is not "phase-locked" to dawn; rather, there is a determinate phase relationship between ϕ_i and the entraining light cycle. In its latest form (Pittendrigh, 1966), it was proposed that the photoperiodic oscillation, like that controlling pupal eclosion in *D. pseudoobscura,* is reset to a narrow range of phases by light pulses in excess of about 12 hr; after these longer pulses, therefore, the oscillation effectively commences its motion in darkness at the same phase (equivalent to ct 12) regardless of the length of the preceding light period. The photoinducible phase (ϕ_i) was thought to lie at about ct 21. Consequently, in long-night regimes (LD 12:12), ϕ_i falls in the dark, and the short-day response (diapause induction or maintenance) ensues, whereas in short-night regimes (LD 16:8), ϕ_i falls in the light (hence "external coincidence") and diapause is averted or terminated (Figure 3). Since the photoperiodic oscillation is reset by each photoperiod, it effectively measures night length as if it were an "hourglass." The evidence for such a model is presented in a later section.

Internal Coincidence. The internal coincidence model recognizes the important fact that the circadian system of higher organisms is almost certainly of a multioscillator construction, and the model suggests that at least some of these oscillators are coupled to dawn and others to dusk. Consequently, as the photoperiod either shortens or lengthens with the seasons, the *internal* phase relationships between these constituent subsystems change (Pittendrigh, 1960, 1972, 1974). In some photoperiods, for example, phases may coincide, whereas in others they may not; and it is easy to imagine short-lived metabolic reactants that need to be brought together for the next step in an inductive process. An explicit version of internal coincidence was independently proposed by Tyshchenko (1966). This model comprised two circadian oscillations, one phase-set by dawn, the other by dusk. At short day-length (LD 12:12), "active" phases were held in antiphase, whereas in long day-lengths (LD 16:8) or ultrashort day-lengths (LD 6:18), they coincided to avert or reduce the incidence of diapause. This type of model differs from external coincidence in that light has only a single role—that of entrainment.

The Resonance Model. Pittendrigh (1972, 1974), again basing his arguments on the multioscillator nature of the circadian system, suggested that circadian rhythmicity might be involved in photoperiodism, but not necessarily in time measurement *per se*. In other words, whatever the actual mechanism used for night-length measurement (i.e., hourglasses or oscillations), the *success* with which time measurement is effected is a function of the proximity of the multioscillator circadian system to resonance with its entraining cycle. This proposition has its basis in the various observations that organisms "do better," or at least "differently," when driven by light cycles whose periodicities are close to the natural circadian period (τ) or modulo τ, than when far from τ (i.e., modulo $\tau + \frac{1}{2}\tau$) (Went, 1959; Pittendrigh and Minis, 1972; Saunders, 1972). It is probable, for example, that the internal temporal disorder generated in the latter cycles affects the way in which physiological functions, including time measurement, are discharged.

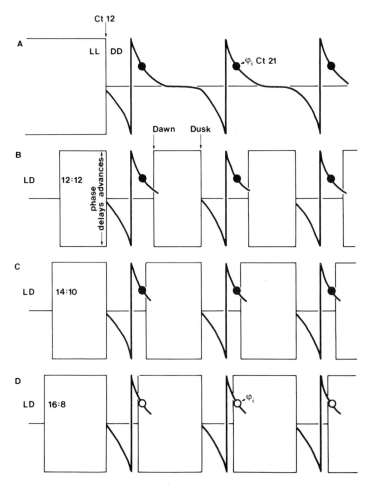

Fig. 3. The external coincidence model for the photoperiodic clock (after Pittendrigh, 1966). The photoperiodic oscillation (shown here as the phase-response curve for *Drosophila pseudoobscura*) always commences its dark freerun at the same phase (ct 12), so that in long-night regimes (B and C), the photoinducible phase, ϕ_i (at about ct 21) falls in the dark, but in a short-night regime (D), ϕ_i falls in the light.

Other Models. The last model worthy of mention is that proposed by Truman (1971) for the silkmoth *Antheraea pernyi.* Like Bünning's general hypothesis, it is based on a parallel study of a circadian rhythm in the same organism. Its essential features are an oscillation entrained by the light cycle and dictating "gates" through which brain hormone may be released, and a second component, timed from dawn and lasting about 11½ hr, which imposes an *inhibition* on hormone release. In short-day (diapause-maintaining) photoperiods, the hormone gates fall in the inhibitory zone; in long-day (diapause-terminating) regimes, they do not. The similarities of this model with internal coincidence are obvious. This model has also been elaborated to account for time measurement in the European corn borer, *Ostrinia nubilalis* (Beck, 1974a,b; 1975), despite the strong evidence that night-length measurement in that species is effected by an hourglass (Pittendrigh, 1974; Skopik and Bowen, 1976).

From the rather brief account set out here, it is evident that three controversial issues exist:

1. Is time measurement effected by an hourglass, or by some aspect of the entrained steady-state of the circadian system?
2. Where circadian rhythmicity *is* involved, is it a *direct* involvement (i.e., in time measurement itself), or an indirect modification of another mechanism (i.e., affecting internal temporal order)?
3. If circadian rhythmicity is causally involved in time measurement itself, does photoperiodic induction rely on "external" or "internal" coincidence?

In the following sections, experimental evidence for and against these various models is described.

HOURGLASSES IN INSECT PHOTOPERIODISM. The most persuasive evidence of an hourglass mechanism in insect photoperiodism comes from the extensive work of Lees (1966, 1968, 1973) on the green vetch aphid, *Megoura viciae.* This insect produces successive generations of wingless, parthenogenetic virginoparae during the summer months, but in the autumn when nights exceed a critical value (9.75 hr), oviparae are produced that subsequently lay diapausing winter eggs.

The most powerful experimental protocols for investigating the nature of time measurement in photoperiodism (i.e., whether hourglasses or oscillations are involved) are (1) the interruption of the dark period with a supplementary light pulse (= "night interruption" experiments), and (2) the use of abnormal light-cycle lengths, particularly when a short light component is coupled to a variety of extended "nights" to provide cycles of great length (= "resonance" experiments). In both, a periodic ($\sim$ 24 hr) occurrence of diapause incidence is evident in species with a circadian clock (see below), but not in those that rely exclusively on an hourglass.

In *M. viciae,* abnormal light cycles have demonstrated the overriding importance of night length. Furthermore, with resonance experiments using a light period of 8 hr coupled with dark periods up to 60 hr ($T68$), the long-night response (ovipara production) became evident as soon as the "night" exceeded the critical value; it then remained level, even up to $T68$, without any evidence of circadian resonance (Figure 4). In night-interruption experiments using a 1-hr pulse to systematically scan the extended "night" of an LD 8:64 ($T72$) regime, the short-night response (virginopara production) was obtained only when the pulse fell 8 hr after "dusk" (at zeitgeber time 16) and nowhere else in the extended "night" (Figure 5A). Once again, therefore, evidence for circadian rhythmicity was lacking. Experiments of the "bistability" type (see "Bünning's Hypothesis," above) have also failed to produce evidence of a circadian involvement in *Megoura* (Hillman, 1973).

In common with many other insect species, *M. viciae* shows two "peaks" of short-night effect in night-interruption experiments where $T = 24$ hr. In a cycle of LD 13.5:10.5 ($T24$), one of these occurred about 2 hr after "dusk"; the other was more pronounced and occurred when the light pulse fell during the last 6 hr of the night. Lees (1966) showed that this response—and in particular, the positions of these peaks—was unaltered when the light period accompanying the 10.5 hr of darkness was extended to 25.5 hr (LD 25.5:10.5, $T36$) or shortened to 8 hr (LD 8:10.5, $T18.5$). These results were interpreted as evidence that night length was of crucial importance and that time measurement began at "dusk" rather than at "dawn." It was also considered inconsistent with any circadian involvement (but see section below on circadian oscillations). "Early" and "late" light breaks in *M. viciae* were also shown to have quite different modes of action. The short-night effect generated by the first pulse falling 1½ hr after "dusk," for example, can be reversed by a subsequent dark period that exceeds the critical night length (9.75 hr) (Figure 5B). In another series of experiments, the hours following the interrupting pulse were kept at 12 hr (a long night), but the hours of darkness *preceding* the pulse were systematically

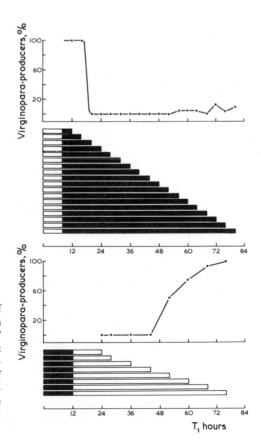

Fig. 4. The production of wingless virginoparae of *Megoura viciae* in photoperiodic regimes in which the length of the cycle was varied (i.e., "resonance" experiments), but the length of the light component held at 8 hr *(upper)* or the length of the dark component held at 12 hr *(lower)*. Note the absence of periodic maxima of short-day effect (low virginopara-production), which would be expected if the *Megoura* clock contained an obvious circadian component. (After Lees, 1965.)

increased. In this case, the terminal 12 hr of light functioned as a long night (ovipara production) until the light pulse fell between the seventh and tenth hours of the night, where it functioned as a "late" interruption, and virginoparae were produced. The effects of a late interruption were therefore clearly irreversible (Figure 5C).

The "clock" in *M. viciae* is thought to be a dark-period hourglass that measures night length without reference to the insect's circadian system. The function of the light component—which must be at least 4 hr in length to act as "day" (Lees, 1971)—is merely to "prime" or "turn the hourglass over." Time measurement is seen as a mechanism consisting of a complex sequence of biochemical reactions distinguished on the basis of their responses to light (Lees, 1968). During the first 3 hr of darkness, the timing mechanism can be reversed by low-intensity blue light (see the section on photoreception and spectral

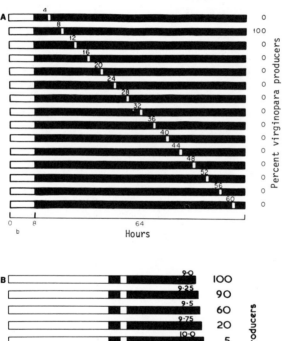

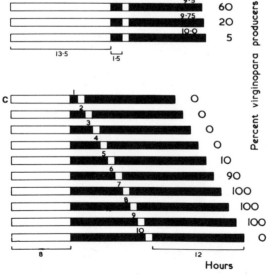

Fig. 5. Night-interruption experiments in *Megoura viciae*. (A) In a cycle of $T72$ with long-day effects (100% virginopara production) occurring only when the scanning pulse fell about 8 hr after dusk. (From Lees, 1970.) (B) The reversibility of an "early" night interruption when followed by more than the critical night length (9.75 hr). (C) A 1-hr pulse scans the night, but is followed in all cases by a dark period greater than the critical night length (12 hr). When the pulse falls early in the night, its long-day effect (virginopara production) is overridden by the following 12 hr of darkness; when it falls late in the night, it is not. (After Lees, 1970. Reprinted with permission of the author.)

sensitivity above). From the third to the fourth hour of the night the photoreceptor is insensitive. Between the fifth hour and 9.75 hr, the system is again photoreceptive, but the effects of light at this point are irreversible by subsequent dark exposure. Finally, the hours of darkness after 9.75 hr are "insensitive" to light because an uninterrupted "residue" of 9.75 hr or more darkness is always left. The hourglass reaction, as Lees sees it, is therefore a complex one, operated in nature by the "dawn" transition of the photoperiod extending "backwards" to coincide with Stage 3, as day length increases, whereupon virginoparae are produced.

Resonance or "T experiments" have also been applied to several other insect species, notably Lepidoptera, without revealing a circadian "involvement" in time measurement. In the pink boll worm moth, *Pectinophora gossypiella,* for example, an 8-hr photoperiod (Adkisson, 1966) or a 12-hr photoperiod (Adkisson, 1964; Pittendrigh and Minis, 1971) coupled with various extended nights, to give Ts of 24, 36, 48, 60, and 72 hr, showed a high incidence of diapause at T24 (LD 8:16 or LD 12:12) and then a decline at longer T values without any evidence of circadian resonance (Figure 6). In the codling moth, *Carpocapsa pomonella,* Peterson and Hamner (1968) found a similar lack of resonance in cycles from T12 (LD 8:4) to T72 (LD 8:64).

Bünning (1969) exposed larvae of the cabbage butterfly, *Pieris brassicae,* to regimes of LD 12:12 (T24), LD 12:24 (T36), and LD 12:36 (T48), with the night of each systematically interrupted by 30 min pulses of light. In each case, long-day effects (diapause prevention) were observed when the supplementary pulses fell about 15 hr after "dusk" or about 15 hr before "dawn" of the main light component (Figure 7). Once again, therefore, these results constituted evidence against the participation of the circadian system in photoperiodic induction.

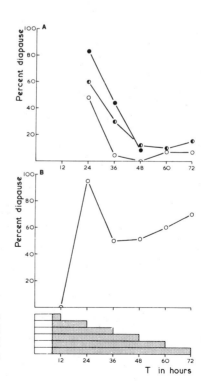

Fig. 6. Results of "resonance" experiments in (A) *Pectinophora gossypiella* (data from Adkisson, 1964, 1966; Pittendrigh and Minis, 1971), and (B) *Carpocapsa pomonella* (Peterson and Hamner, 1968). Note the absence of a "positive" resonance in both species.

More recently, the resonance technique has been applied to the European corn borer *Ostrinia nubilalis* (Bowen and Skopik, 1976; Skopik and Bowen, 1976). With diapause termination (the pupation of diapause larvae) used as the indication of "long-day" effects, a 16-hr light period was coupled to various extended "nights" to give cycles of $T24$ (LD 16:8), $T36$ (LD 16:20), $T48$ (LD 16:32), and $T60$ (LD 16:44). After 30 days, all of the larvae in the first regime had terminated diapause, but pupation in the others was negligible. Evidence of circadian rhythmicity was therefore absent, and the results indicated that it was not the 16 hr of light that were measured, but the length of the dark. In a converse experiment, 8 hr of darkness were coupled to extended "days"; all larvae terminated diapause (pupated) in all regimes ($T24$–$T60$). The results were interpreted as evidence that an 8-hr dark period was measured by an hourglass mechanism, regardless of T (and therefore of the circadian system). While this interpretation is undoubtedly correct, the insects in the second experiment (extended light) might have produced a "constant light" response. It is also a pity, perhaps, that a resonance experiment using a 12-hr photoperiod was not attempted. This experiment (like those described below in the section on circadian oscillations for *Nasonia vitripennis* and *Sarcophaga argyrostoma*) would have shown diapause maintenance at $T24$ (LD 12:12) and $T48$ (LD 12:36), but diapause termination at $T36$ (LD 12:24) and $T60$ (LD 12:48) if the circadian system were involved, but no termination in *any* regime if it was not, because in all cycles D was greater than 8 hr. Lastly, despite the conclusion that night length is measured by an hour-glass, we must still consider Pittendrigh's (1972, 1974) observation (from data obtained by Beck, 1962a) that diapause incidence in *O. nubilalis* is maximal when T is close to τ, thereby suggesting *some* circadian involvement. We must also consider the observation (Pittendrigh, 1966; Saunders, 1975b)

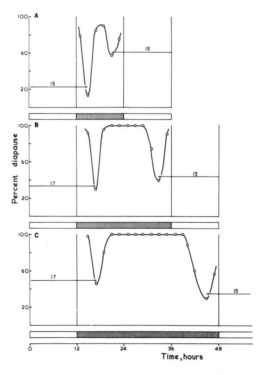

Fig. 7. The diapause-inhibiting effects of 30-min night interruptions in *Pieris brassicae:* (A) in LD 12:12 ($T24$); (B) in LD 12:24 ($T36$); (C) in LD 12:36 ($T48$). Note that two peaks of long-day response are observed in each regime, the first 15–17 hr after dawn (zt 15–17), the second about 15 hr before dusk. There is no evidence of a peak 24 hr after the first, which would be expected (in C) at zt 41 if the circadian system were involved in photoperiodism in this species. (After Bünning, 1969. Reprinted with permission of Pergamon Press, Ltd., Oxford.)

that the circadian system in *D. pseudoobscura* (and *S. argyrostoma*) is effectively "damped out" by extended light periods, to continue its "motion" at the start of the dark at near-constant phase, and is therefore in a position to measure the duration of darkness as if it *were* an hourglass, despite the fact that the system is oscillatory.

PECTINOPHORA GOSSYPIELLA AND THE EXTERNAL COINCIDENCE MODEL. At this point, we must make a digression to consider photoperiodic induction in the pink boll worm moth, *Pectinophora gossypiella*. The extensive work on this species carried out by Pittendrigh and Minis (1964), Minis (1965), and Pittendrigh (1966) gave rise to the external coincidence model and included a number of tests of that proposition (Pittendrigh and Minis, 1971) and, therefore, of the role of circadian rhythmicity in photoperiodic induction itself.

The origins of the external coincidence model lie in Bünning's hypothesis (see above) and in Adkisson's (1964) observations that systematic night interruptions in cycles of $T24$ (LD 6:18, LD 12:12, and LD 13:11) with a 1-hr supplementary light pulse produce *two* discrete points of long-day effect (diapause prevention), one (peak A) about 14 hr after "dawn," the other (peak B) about 14 hr before "dusk," in all cycles tested. Similar results have since been obtained in a wide range of insect species (Saunders, 1976b). Pittendrigh and Minis (1964) noted the striking parallels between this type of response and the entraining effects of asymmetrical "skeleton" photoperiods on the pupal eclosion rhythm of *Drosophila pseudoobscura* (Chapter 7), and they suggested that the bimodal response was powerful, if circumstantial, evidence of the involvement of the circadian system in the photoperiodic clock. The reader must be referred to the original papers (Pittendrigh and Minis, 1964; Pittendrigh, 1966) for details of the explicit formulation; the essential features of its most recent version (Pittendrigh, 1966), however, are sufficiently set out in the section on external coincidence above.

Pittendrigh and Minis (1971) compared photoperiodic induction in *P. gossypiella* with three overt circadian periodicities: oviposition, egg hatch, and pupal eclosion. The several tests of external coincidence that were carried out were based on the assumption that the photoinducible phase (ϕ_i) possessed a fixed phase relationship to the overt systems; in particular, it occurred about 5 hr before pupal eclosion, at a phase (ct 21) that corresponded to the position of peak B in night-interruption experiments, and also to the end of the critical night.

In the first test, the concurrent effects of a short-day light cycle (LD 8:16 or LD 10:14) and of a temperature cycle (20–29°C) upon diapause induction and pupal eclosion were investigated (Figure 8). In the short-day light cycle alone, the median of pupal eclosion (ϕ_r) occurred soon after "dawn." With the addition of the temperature cycle, however, ϕ_r occurred a few hours after the point of lowest temperature. Thus, as the temperature cycle was displaced later relative to the light cycle, the phase of the eclosion rhythm was displaced to the right. Since ϕ_i was assumed to lie about 5 hr before ϕ_r for eclosion, it too was assumed to be displaced to the right. Figure 8 shows that when the assumed position of ϕ_i was drawn into the light, diapause inhibition (long-day effects) occurred. The result was thus in accordance with prediction from the external coincidence model. Results of experiments using daily periods of chilling in *Nasonia vitripennis* (Saunders, 1967) can also be interpreted in this way.

A second test, again using the concurrent analysis of induction and a circadian "indicator" (oviposition or eclosion), was based on the knowledge that in entrainment of the *D.*

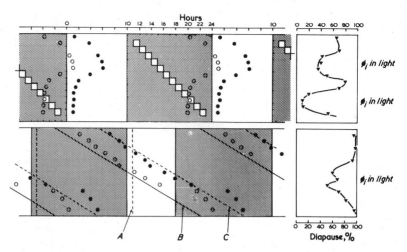

Fig. 8. Concurrent light and temperature cycles in *Pectinophora gossypiella* as a test of the external coincidence model. *(Upper)* The phase reference points for pupal eclosion (●) and the photoinducible phase, ϕ_i (O), in asymmetrical skeleton photoperiods, showing diapause inhibition when ϕ_i is illuminated. *(Lower)* The same but in a light cycle (LD 8:16) and a sinusoidal temperature cycle (20–29°C). A-normal phase of the rhythm in LD 8:16, B-low part of temperature cycle, C-normal phase of the rhythm to the temperature cycle. Note that diapause inhibition occurs when ϕ_i is drawn into the light. (After Pittendrigh and Minis, 1971. Reproduced from *Biochronometry*, Fig. 10, p. 226, with the permission of the National Academy of Sciences, Washington, D.C.)

pseudoobscura eclosion rhythm (period τ) to an environmental zeitgeber (period T), the entraining light pulse had to fall in the late subjective night (or early subjective day) to cause a phase advance when $T < \tau$, but the pulse must fall in the early subjective night to cause a phase delay when $T > \tau$ (see Chapter 7). Therefore, simply by changing the period (T) of the driving light cycle, the pulse could be brought to illuminate different phases of the oscillation. If ϕ_i is a "reality" and lies at ct 21 as suggested, illumination of this phase should bring about long-day responses.

The experiment was carried out twice with *P. gossypiella*, once (Pittendrigh and Minis, 1964; Minis, 1965) with 15-min pulses, entraining cycles of T20 hr 40 min to T25, and oviposition as the measure of phase, and again (Pittendrigh and Minis, 1971) with 8-hr pulses, T20–T27, and pupal eclosion. In both tests the overt rhythmicity adopted the expected phase relationships (Figure 9), but the diapause responses were *not* as predicted. In the shorter cycles (T20 and T21), for example, ϕ_i ought to have been illuminated by the 8-hr pulse to produce a low incidence of diapause, whereas in the longer cycles (T24–T27), ϕ_i should have fallen in the dark to give a high incidence of diapause. Figure 9 shows that all diapause incidences were high, with the highest being in the *shorter* cycles. Clearly, this result is in conflict with prediction from the model. It should be noted, however, that a similar experimental design with *Sarcophaga argyrostoma*, as part of a more extensive resonance experiment (Figure 11), *does* produce the predicted response: practically no diapause at T19.2, T21, and T23, but almost 100% diapause at T24, T26, and T30 (Saunders, 1973a).

A third test of external coincidence was based on a comparison of two strains of *P. gossypiella* selected for emergence time: the "early" strain emerging from the pupa about 5 hr before the "late" (see Chapter 7). Once again basing the test on the assumption that ϕ_i lies about 5 hr before ϕ_r (eclosion), it was predicted that the critical day length for the two strains should have altered by a predictable amount. The results showed that the critical day length for "late" was indeed shorter than "early" after 4–5 generations. However, after 6–8 generations of selection, the results for "late" also showed that the photoperiodic responses at strong, short day lengths (LD 11:13 and LD 12:12) were *lower in "amplitude."* This may mean that the apparent shift in critical day length merely reflects a lowered response in all day lengths. The results of this experiment, therefore, remained equivocal and provided no clear evidence in favor of external coincidence.

Although some experimental evidence, and the result of one test, were consistent with the external coincidence model in *P. gossypiella*, others were at best equivocal, while still others were in direct contradiction of it. The validity of the model (for *P. gossypiella*) was further called into question by the discovery that red light cycles (> 600 nm) failed to initiate or entrain the overt rhythmicities studied (although red light was not without effect on τ), but that the photoperiodic clock could differentiate between 12 hr of red light per day (98% diapause) and 14 hr of red light per day (17% diapause) (Pittendrigh *et al.*, 1970), even though the constituent oscillations within the circadian system must have been in an unsynchronized condition. The interpretation of this experiment could, of course, be that ϕ_i is part of a "separate" oscillation concerned with photoperiodic induction and coupled to the light cycle by quite a different pigment (absorbing in the red). However, the failure of all attempts to produce "positive" resonance with this species (Adkisson, 1964, 1966; Pittendrigh and Minis, 1971; Figure 6), even with the possibly more rewarding period of diapause reactivation (Pittendrigh and Minis, 1971), seems to suggest that photoperiodic induction is not carried out by any sort of oscillatory clock: perhaps *P. gossypiella*, like the other Lepidoptera examined above, must join the ranks of those insects that measure night length by a nonoscillatory hourglass or interval timer.

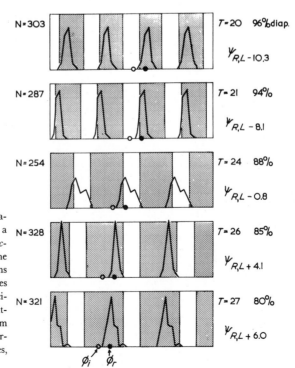

Fig. 9. Pupal eclosion and the induction of diapause when T is close to τ ($T20$–$T27$) as a test of the external coincidence model in *Pectinophora gossypiella*. The polygons and the closed circles show the distributions and means (ϕ_r) of eclosion in each regime; the open circles mark the supposed phases of the photoinducible phase (ϕ_i). See text for details. (After Pittendrigh and Minis, 1971. Reproduced from *Biochronometry*, Fig. 14, p. 236, with the permission of the National Academy of Sciences, Washington, D.C.)

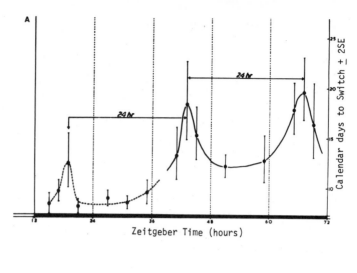

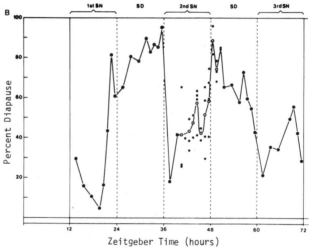

Fig. 10. Evidence of a circadian component in the insect photoperiodic clock from night interruption experiments. (A) Two-hr pulses of light scanning the dark of an LD 12:60 (*T*72) cycle in *Nasonia vitripennis*. (From "Circadian Clock in Insect Photoperiodism," by D. S. Saunders, *Science*, 1970, *168*, 601–603, Fig. 2. Copyright 1970 by the American Association for the Advancement of Science. Reprinted with permission.) (B) One-hr pulses in LD 12:60 (*T*72) in *Sarcophaga argyrostoma* (from Saunders, 1976. Reprinted with permission of Springer-Verlag, Heidelberg). In both species, pulses falling in successive subjective nights (zt 12–24, zt 36–48, zt 60–72) bring about long-day responses (low diapause, or a delayed switch to the production of diapause), whereas pulses falling in successive subjective days (zt 24–36, zt 48–60) do not.

CIRCADIAN OSCILLATIONS IN INSECT PHOTOPERIODISM

Evidence. Positive evidence of the involvement of the circadian system in photoperiodic time measurement has come from the study of four insect species: the parasitic wasp, *Nasonia vitripennis;* its flesh-fly host, *Sarcophaga argyrostoma;* the mosquito *Aëdes atropalpus* (Beach and Craig, 1977); and the carabid beetle *Pterostichus nigrita* (Thiele, 1977). In *N. vitripennis* and *S. argyrostoma*, night interruptions in extended cycles (*T*48 or *T*72) show "peaks" of long-day effect (uninterrupted development) at roughly 24-hr intervals (Figure 10) (Saunders, 1970, 1976b), and a periodic occurrence of high and low incidence of diapause is seen, in both species, in resonance experiments (Figure 11) (Saunders, 1973a, 1974). Additional evidence of the close association between the circadian system and photoperiodism is also available from symmetrical "skeleton" photoperiods in the "zone of bistability" (Pittendrigh, 1966; Saunders, 1975b, 1976b) (Figure 17). In *A. atropalpus,* night interruption experiments in a cycle of *T*48 showed two "peaks" of long-day effect, 24 hr apart; and in *P. nigrita,* resonance experiments have shown that maturation of both males and females occurs at *T*24, *T*48, and *T*72, but not, or to a lesser extent, at *T*36 or *T*60. Here we will note that although showing that the circadian system is somehow involved in photoperiodic time measurement, these results do not, with any certainty, tell us whether circadian rhythmicity is involved in time measurement *per se,* or merely as an indirect modification of another mechanism. We will, however, return to consider these alternatives later in the chapter.

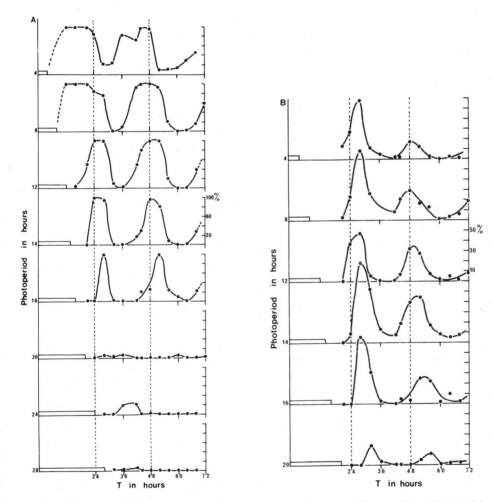

Fig. 11. Evidence of a circadian component in the insect photoperiodic clock from "resonance" experiments. (A) *Nasonia vitripennis* in cycle from *T*12 to *T*72, containing 4–28 hr of light (from Saunders, 1974. Reprinted with permission of Pergamon Press, Ltd., Oxford.) (B) *Sarcophaga argyrostoma* in cycles from *T*20 to *T*72 containing 4–20 hr of light (from Saunders, 1973a).

Sarcophaga argyrostoma and the External Coincidence Model. A comparison of the "photoperiodic oscillation" in *S. argyrostoma* with the circadian system controlling pupal eclosion in that species (Saunders, 1976a) reveals several close similarities: first, both rhythmic systems are sensitive to the phase-resetting effects of light during the *larval* but not the intrapuparial stages of development; second, both possess the same type of "weak" or Type 1 phase-response curve (Winfree, 1970) to short light pulses; and third, both appear to be reset by light pulses greater than 12 hr to a narrow range of phases (Figure 12), so that the oscillations "restart" their motion, at dusk, at *a near-constant phase* (Saunders, 1976a). Thus, not only are the two circadian oscillations (photoperiodism and eclosion) sufficiently similar to allow the latter, overt rhythm to be used as a "measure of phase" for the covert photoperiodic oscillation (as recommended by Pittendrigh and Minis, 1964), but their phase relationships to the entraining light cycles are comparable with those for *D. pseudoobscura* (Pittendrigh, 1966) and, moreover, consistent with the essential features of external coincidence. In this section, therefore, photoperiodic induction in *S. argyrostoma* is discussed in terms of that model.

In order to use the eclosion rhythm in *S. argyrostoma* in an analysis of photoperiodic induction, the free-running oscillation was perturbed at all circadian times (after a transition from LL to DD in the first 24 hr of larval life) by single light pulses of 1–20 hr duration, to obtain a "family" of phase-response curves. Particular attention was paid to the phase relationship (ψ) of the reset peaks of eclosion to the light, and to their degree of arrhythmicity (R), because these parameters were thought to be of most significance in an analysis of the photoperiodic clock.

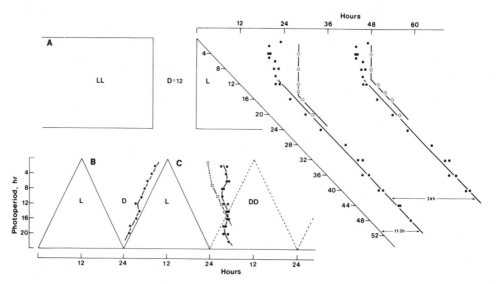

Fig. 12. Comparisons between the photoperiodic clock and the rhythm of pupal eclosion in *Sarcophaga argyrostoma*. (A) Medians of pupal eclosion (ϕ_r) following a final photoperiod of between 4 and 48 hr ($\bullet$) compared with peaks of resonance (from Figure 11) ($\bigcirc$), showing that both oscillatory systems obtain their principal time cue from "dusk," once the photoperiod exceeds about 12 hr. (B) Phase relationship between ϕ_r and the light cycle when the latter is continued up to eclosion. (C) Phase relationship between ϕ_r ($\bullet$) when photoperiod is discontinued at puparium-formation, compared with the calculated positions of ϕ_i ($\bigcirc$). Note how ϕ_i phase-leads ϕ_r by about 2 hr for cycles containing between 10 and 16 hr of light. (From Saunders, 1976a. Reprinted with permission of Springer-Verlag, Heidelberg.)

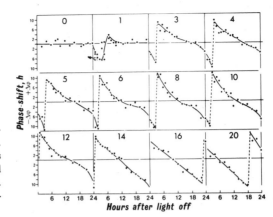

Fig. 13. *Sarcophaga argyrostoma:* Phase-response curves for the pupal eclosion rhythm. First instar larvae exposed to 1- to 20-hr pulses of white light (240 μW cm^{-2}), starting at all times after transfer from LL to DD (ct 12). (After Saunders, 1978a. Reprinted with permission of Springer-Verlag, Heidelberg.)

The phase-response curve for 1-hr pulses of white light (240 μW cm^{-2}) was of the "weak" Type 1 with small phase delays (< 6 hr) in the early subjective night (ct 12–18) and small phase advances (3–4 hr) in the late subjective night (ct 18–24). Pulses of 5 hr or more gave rise to larger phase shifts and to "strong" Type 0 response curves (see Winfree, 1970, and Chapter 7). Pulses of 3 and 4 hr, on the other hand, were ambiguous in the sense that the response curves could not be attributed to either Type 1 or Type 0 with any certainty (Figure 13). These data were then used to calculate theoretical entrained steady-states to a variety of complete and "skeleton" photoperiods; and these theoretical values were compared with those obtained experimentally, and with diapause-induction data obtained in the same or similar experimental light regimes (Saunders, 1978a).

Highly arrhythmic cultures were found after several different kinds of light treatment: (1) After resetting pulses 3–5 hr in duration, starting 3–5 hr after the LL/DD transition. In particular, a 4-hr pulse timed to begin 4 hr after this transition was identified as Winfree's (1970, 1972) "singular stimulus" (T*S*), since pulses shorter than this gave rise to Type 1 resetting curves, and pulses longer than this value to Type 0 curves; (2) When the hours of darkness between the LL/DD transition and the beginning of the resetting pulse (D hours), and the duration of the light pulse (L hours) added up to a value (D + L) of close to 12, 36, 60, 84, or 108 hr (modulo $\tau + \frac{1}{2}\tau$), whereas when D + L was close to 24, 48, 72, 96, or 120 hr (modulo τ), eclosion patterns were rhythmic (Figure 14). Much of this arrhythmia can be attributed to the fact that the light pulse falls on that part of the

Fig. 14. *Sarcophaga argyrostoma:* Arrhythmicity (R values) of the pupal eclosion rhythm in reset cultures as a function of D + L (the time between LL/DD and the beginning of the light pulse [D hours] + the length of the light pulse [L hours]). When D + L is close to 12, 36, 60, 84, or 108 hr (modulo $\tau + \frac{1}{2}\tau$), arrhythmicity is high; when D + L is close to 24, 48, 72, 96, or 120 hr (modulo τ), it is low. (O) L > D; (●) D > L. (After Saunders, 1978a. Reprinted with permission of Springer-Verlag, Heidelberg.)

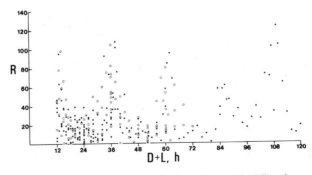

oscillation where maximum phase advances are generated, and this seems to indicate a failure to achieve proper entrainment; (3) In cultures subjected to very short or very long photoperiods ($T24$) for seven to nine cycles.

The entrained steady state of the eclosion rhythm in *S. argyrostoma* (both theoretical and experimental) was compared with diapause induction in the following light regimes: complete photoperiods (all $T24$); symmetrical "skeleton" photoperiods formed from two 1-hr pulses ($T24$); and asymmetrical "skeleton" photoperiods formed from a longer "main" pulse and a second 1-hr scanning pulse ($T24$ and $T72$). In nearly every case, theoretical steady states were in very close agreement with those determined experimentally. Even more striking was the close agreement with diapause induction data. In those instances where the agreement was not close, the differences were readily attributable to properties of the phase-response curve in larvae as they aged (Saunders, 1978a).

A comparison of eclosion and diapause induction in complete photoperiods is shown in Figure 15. Computed data for theoretical populations of larvae that were exposed to one and eight consecutive light cycles are shown as open circles. Both sets of computed data show a phase relationship in which the eclosion peaks (ϕ_r) occur in the latter half of the night for pulses of 1–12 hr but "cross over" the "dawn" threshold for pulses of 14, 16, and 20 hr. Experimentally derived eclosion data (closed circles and squares) show the same general phase relationship to the photoperiod, serious divergence being apparent only with very short pulses (< 3 hr) and with very long pulses (20 hr). Even more striking is the comparison between the phase of the eclosion rhythm and the diapause response, shown to the right (closed triangles). This comparison indicates that short-day–long-night effects (a high incidence of diapause) occur when ϕ_r lies in the dark, but diapause is averted when ϕ_r passes from the dark into the light. Since in an earlier paper it was established that the putative photoinducible phase (ϕ_i) (ct 21.5) lies close to ϕ_r (ct 23.5) (Saunders, 1976a), the remarkable similarity of these observations to presumed events in the external coincidence model is obvious.

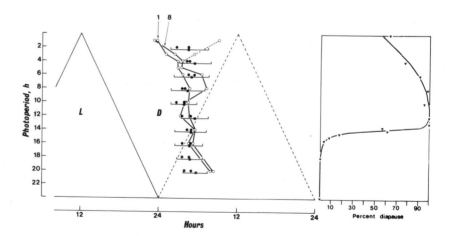

Fig. 15. *Sarcophaga argyrostoma:* Computed and experimentally determined phases of eclosion (ϕ_r) compared with diapause incidence in complete photoperiods ($T24$). (O) computed data for theoretical cultures exposed to 1 and 8 cycles respectively; (●) experimental phases; (▼) diapause incidence. (Data from Saunders, 1971, 1978a. Reprinted with permission of Springer-Verlag, Heidelberg.)

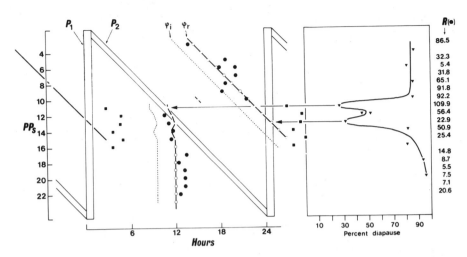

Fig. 16. *Sarcophaga argyrostoma:* Computed (O) and experimentally determined (● and ■) phases of eclosion compared with diapause incidence (▲) in symmetrical skeleton photoperiods (PP$_s$) formed from two 1-hr pulses of light. R: arrhythmicity values. Horizontal arrows indicate phases at which ϕ_r (or a phase close to it) coincide with P$_1$ or P$_2$. (●) experimental populations in which P$_1$ commenced at ct 16; (■) experimental populations in which P$_1$ commenced at ct 22. (Data from Saunders, 1975b, 1978a. Reprinted with permission of Springer-Verlag, Heidelberg.)

In Figure 16, computed steady states for the eclosion rhythm in *S. argyrostoma*, starting at all initial circadian phases, are shown in relation to skeleton photoperiods formed from two 1-hr pulses of light. As in *D. pseudoobscura* (Pittendrigh and Minis, 1964), the circadian system accepts P$_1$ as "dawn" and P$_2$ as "dusk" when the skeleton is short (< PP$_s$10) and achieves a phase relationship that reflects this. When P$_1$ and P$_2$ are initially far apart, however, the system undergoes a phase jump, takes the shorter "interpretation," and accepts P$_2$ as "dawn" and P$_1$ as "dusk." At intermediate skeletons (PP$_s$11 to PP$_s$15), there were *two* possible steady states determined by the phase of the oscillation that is first illuminated by P$_1$ and by which interval (the longer or the shorter) is seen first. This area is called the "zone of bistability" by Pittendrigh (1966).

Experimental populations of *S. argyrostoma* achieved a remarkably similar phase relationship to the skeleton regime. In addition, it is evident that diapause induction is high before *and* after the phase jump when the oscillation takes the two pulses to signify a short day length, but it dips to a low value when the accepted interval becomes "long," or when the computed values of ϕ_r coincide with either of the light pulses, an observation that is, of course, consistent with external coincidence.

An even more powerful test of the similarity between eclosion and diapause induction is that afforded by the behavior of the oscillatory system within the zone of bistability (Figure 17). Two skeleton regimes were selected within this zone: one (LD 1:9:1:13, or PP$_s$11), if taken as "day" by the photoperiodic oscillation, would be read as a short day and would give rise to a high incidence of diapause; its "mirror image" (LD 1:13:1:9, or PP$_s$15), however, if selected, would be read as a long day and would give rise to a low incidence of diapause. The results show that according to the skeleton offered and the phase at which P$_1$ is first seen, the computed eclosion peaks, the observed eclosion peaks, *and* the diapause data are all in remarkably close agreement.

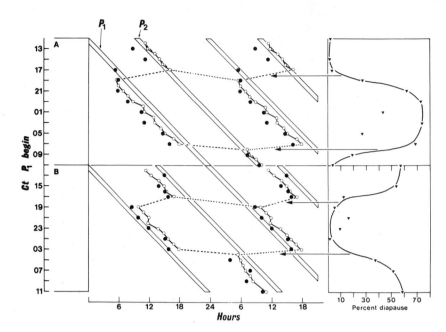

Fig. 17. *Sarcophaga argyrostoma:* Computed (O) and experimentally determined (●) phases of eclosion (ϕ_r) compared with diapause incidence (▲) in symmetrical skeleton photoperiods (PP$_s$) in the "zone of bistability." (A) PP$_s$11 (LD 1:9:1:13) with P$_1$ beginning at all circadian times. (B) PP$_s$15 (LD 1:13:1:9) with P$_1$ beginning at all circadian times. Horizontal arrows show where a phase jump occurs. (Data from Saunders, 1975b, 1978a. Reprinted with permission of Springer-Verlag, Heidelberg.)

The behavior of the circadian system in the zone of bistability was first described by Pittendrigh (1966) for *D. pseudoobscura,* and the close similarities between this behavior and the photoperiodic induction of flowering in *Lemna perpusilla* (Hillman, 1964) were considered among the most persuasive evidence in favor of circadian rhythmicity being causally involved in photoperiodic time measurement. It is therefore of interest that applications of this experimental protocol to *P. gossypiella* (Pittendrigh and Minis, 1971) and to *M. viciae* (Hillman, 1973) have both failed to indicate this association, results that are consistent with the presumed "hourglass" nature of night-length measurement in those species. *S. argyrostoma,* therefore, is only the second organism in which this test has been successfully applied and, of course, the first animal species. The complexity of the test and its outcome surely leave little doubt that photoperiodic induction of diapause in *S. argyrostoma* is a function of the circadian system and strongly suggest that eclosion and diapause induction are governed by a similar—or perhaps the same—circadian pacemaker.

In asymmetrical skeleton photoperiods (*T*24) formed from a 10-hr "main" light component (P$_1$) and a 1-hr scanning pulse (P$_2$), computed steady states for ϕ_r show, first, phase delays ($-\Delta\phi$) and then phase advances ($+\Delta\phi$) as P$_2$ scans the "night" (Figure 18). When all initial circadian phases are taken into account, there is a zone of bistability between LD 10:4:1:9 and LD 10:6:1:7. Before the phase jump, the scanning pulse is taken as the terminator of an asymmetrical skeleton; after the phase jump, it is taken as its initiator. The experimentally determined values of ϕ_r were in good agreement for those cultures that saw only one cycle of the skeleton regime (closed squares), but they were poorer, particularly for the first part of the night, for those that saw six cycles (closed circles). The explanation

of this poor simulation is outside the scope of this chapter but is discussed in detail by
Saunders (1978a).

Comparison of calculated values of ϕ_r with the diapause induction data (closed triangles) shows that diapause incidence was high when the skeleton formed from P_1 and P_2
was "short" (i.e., both before and after the phase jump) but dipped to low values when
ϕ_r—or some phase close to it—coincided either with the "dawn" transition of P_1 or with
P_2.

These experiments show that the entrained steady state of the circadian system, as
exemplified by the eclosion rhythm, can be used to account for photoperiodic induction in
S. argyrostoma, according to the principles of external coincidence. The circadian system,
however, is almost certainly of a multioscillator "construction" (Saunders, 1972), and it
becomes relevant to ask what role (if any) arrhythmicity plays in induction. If at least some
types of arrhythmicity reflect an incoherence between constituent oscillations in the individual as well as *between* individuals—and it is by no means clear that they do—arrhythmicity must have an effect on the success with which night-length measurement is achieved.

The most striking "type" of arrhythmicity is that shown in Figure 14, which suggests
that entrainment fails when T is close to $\tau + \frac{1}{2}\tau$. This effect further suggests that the
internal temporal disorder that results from such regimes might upset the effectiveness of
night-length measurement, whereas at $T =$ modulo τ, temporal order is maintained. In
cycles of $T24$, the decline in diapause incidence at ultrashort day lengths (< 5 hr) might
similarly be attributed to an internal disorder, this time due to the slow approach to steady
state in an initially scattered group of oscillations when exposed to trains of "weak" pulses
(Saunders, 1978a). Arrhythmicity at the "singularity" (T*S*), however, is not likely to
have much significance in photoperiodism.

Experimental results for *S. argyrostoma* in a wide range of light cycles therefore

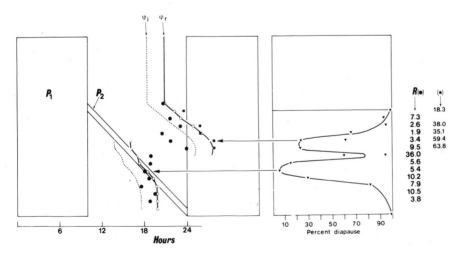

Fig. 18. *Sarcophaga argyrostoma:* Computed (○) and experimentally determined (● and ■) phases of eclosion
(ϕ_r) compared with diapause incidence (▲) in asymmetrical skeleton photoperiods ($T24$) formed from a longer
"main" light pulse (P_1) and a 1-hr "scanning" pulse (P_2). (●) experimentally determined data for cultures
exposed to six successive cycles; (■) data for one cycle. Horizontal arrows show phases where ϕ_r (or a phase
close to it) coincide with P_1 or P_2. (Data from Saunders, 1975b, 1978a. Reprinted with permission of Springer-
Verlag, Heidelberg.)

remain consistent with external coincidence, but with certain modifications. The most important of these is the recognition that the circadian system in *S. argyrostoma,* like that in other multicellular organisms, is of a multioscillator nature, and that the degree of internal organization or disorganization within this "population" plays its part in the accuracy with which time measurement is effected. The model proposed for *S. argyrostoma,* therefore, is external coincidence with elements from Pittendrigh's (1972) "resonance" model. At this point, however, it must again be stressed that this interpretation is by no means certain, particularly in the absence of detailed knowledge of the concrete physiological events involved in photoperiodic time measurement.

Nasonia vitripennis and the Internal Coincidence Model. In a second species showing "positive" resonance, *N. vitripennis,* the nature of time measurement is open to interpretation in terms of *internal* coincidence (Saunders, 1974). Particularly if the results shown in Figure 11 are redrawn as an extended circadian surface (Figure 19, top panel), it is

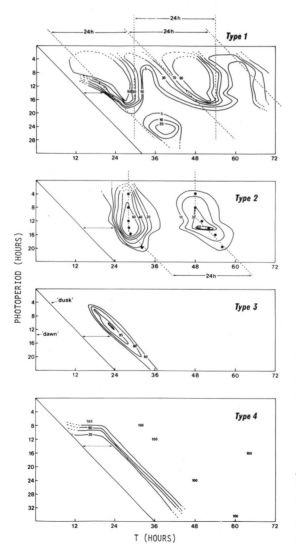

Fig. 19. "Extended circadian surfaces" for four insect species showing four apparently different types of photoperiodic clock. The surfaces (Pittendrigh, 1972) show "contours" connecting points of equal diapause incidence in abnormal light–dark cycles ("resonance" experiments) in which the hours of light (L), of darkness (D), and the period of the LD cycle (= *T*) are varied. The photoperiod (= L) is shown to the left of each panel as a light "wedge" with "dawn" and "dusk" indicated. The horizontal arrows between "dusk" and the ascending slopes of the first diapause "mountain" indicate the importance of night-length measurement. Type 1: *Nasonia vitripennis* (Saunders, 1974). Type 2: *Sarcophaga argyrostoma* (Saunders, 1973a). Type 3: *Ostrinia nubilalis* (Beck, 1962a). Type 4: *Panonychus ulmi* (Lees, 1953). Details of these surfaces and their possible significance may be found in the text. (Reprinted by permission of Springer-Verlag, Heidelberg.)

clear that the ascending slopes of the diapause maxima are parallel to "dusk" and the descending slopes are parallel to "dawn." With a 20-hr photoperiod, the two "components" appear to coalesce, and diapause is eliminated at all T values. With a 24-hr photoperiod, on the other hand, a discrete peak of diapause reappears at $T36-T42$. These results, particularly the wedge-shaped "mountains" of diapause in Figure 19 suggest the interaction of separate "dawn" and "dusk" oscillations, according to the internal coincidence model. The differences between the photoperiodic clocks in *S. argyrostoma* and *N. vitripennis* are further discussed in terms of external and internal coincidence in Saunders (1978b).

AN ATTEMPTED RATIONALIZATION OF THE VARIOUS PROPOSITIONS TO ACCOUNT FOR PHOTOPERIODIC INDUCTION IN INSECTS

Any attempt to reach general conclusions about the nature of the insect photoperiodic clock is hampered by the small number of species that have been adequately investigated. Nevertheless, comparisons are greatly facilitated by following Pittendrigh's (1972, 1974) suggestion that the available information is best displayed by "extended circadian surfaces" in which "iso-induction contours" joining all points of equal diapause incidence are shown in relation to the duration of darkness (D) and of light (L) (viz., Pittendrigh's [1972] treatment of Beck's [1962a] data for *O. nubilalis*). Modified circadian surfaces in which the photoperiod (L) is shown as a "light wedge" and the contours plotted as a function of L and T (Saunders, 1973a, 1974) are shown in Figure 19. Such plots enable one, at a glance, to appreciate the relative roles of L, D, and T; the shape of the diapause maxima; and whether they occur singly or in multiples along the T axis.

A survey of the available information on the relative importance of D and L, and of the more extensive "resonance" experiments, indicates the existence of four "types" of insect clock, which are exemplified in Figure 19 by *Nasonia vitripennis* (Type 1) (Saunders, 1974); *Sarcophaga argyrostoma* (Type 2) (Saunders, 1973a); *Ostrinia nubilalis* (Type 3) (Beck, 1962a); and the red spider mite *Panonychus ulmi* (Type 4) (Lees, 1953).

In Types 1 and 2, the circadian system is thought to be causally and probably directly involved in time measurement because the "mountains" of high diapause incidence repeat themselves with a circadian frequency in the extended "night." Type 1, of which *N. vitripennis* is the only example at present, is here identified as an example of internal coincidence, and Type 2 *(S. argyrostoma)* of external coincidence, for the various reasons outlined above. The mosquito *Aëdes atropalpus* may also be of Type 2 (Beach and Craig, 1977). In Type 2, the oscillatory system is reset by light pulses in excess of about 12 hr to a narrow range of phases in such a way that it "measures" night length as if it were an hourglass (Pittendrigh, 1966; Saunders, 1976a), and temporal organization within the population of oscillations probably plays its part in the effectiveness of this night-length measurement. The validation of this distinction between internal and external coincidence will almost certainly have to await more detailed knowledge of the physiological events in photoperiodic induction; meanwhile, however, the models and their designations to these two species are adopted as adequate working hypotheses.

In Type 3 *(O. nubilalis)*, comparable data from resonance experiments are not available, but evidence suggests that the *single* diapause "mountain" does not occur again in the extended night. This, in turn, suggests that the circadian system may not be directly involved in time measurement. Night length is clearly of "central" importance (Beck,

1962a), but the observation that induction is maximal when T is close to τ (Pittendrigh, 1972, 1974) indicates that whatever the mechanism used to measure night length (an hour-glass?), the success with which measurement is achieved is affected by the closeness of the multioscillator circadian system to resonance with the environmental driver. More limited data from *P. gossypiella, C. pomonella,* and *Grapholitha molesta* (Dickson, 1949) suggest that these species also fall into Type 3.

Type 4 clocks, exemplified by *P. ulmi* (Lees, 1953) and the aphid *M. viciae* (Lees, 1973), appear to measure night length without reference to the circadian system. Induction of diapause or the winter morph becomes maximal once the critical night length is passed, whatever the length of L, and then remains at a consistently high level over an extremely wide range of D. They may be regarded, therefore, as "pure" hourglasses.

The four "types" of clock, however, are probably not mutually exclusive. It is possible, for example, that merely reducing the temperature—and therefore increasing the length of the sensitive period—might convert Type 3 into either Type 2 or Type 4. Conversely, raising the temperature might convert Type 4 into Type 3 or 2. Evidence comes from the observation in *S. argyrostoma* that at low temperature, the resonance peaks become inapparent, leaving only the "hourglass" nature of night-length measurement (Saunders, 1973a), whereas a rise in temperature flattens out the second and third resonance peaks before the first. Skopik and Bowen's (1976) resonance data for *O. nubilalis,* using diapause *termination,* resemble Type 4, rather than Type 3, because all long Ts (36, 48, 60) were diapause-maintaining, whereas $T24$ (LD 16:8) was not. This finding raises the possibility that a Type 3 surface is indicated for diapause *induction* in this species—particularly at the high temperature ($30°C$) at which the experiments were performed—merely because the larval sensitive period is not long enough to accommodate a sufficient *number* of long nights.

There are almost certainly other types of mechanism to be found in the insects. For example, the cabbage butterfly, *Pieris brassicae,* may "measure" *day*length by a nonoscillatory timer (Bünning, 1969); and complex combinations of oscillators and hourglasses have been proposed to account for data obtained from species such as *Carpocapsa pomonella* (Hamner, 1969).

A comparison of the formal properties of the photoperiodic clocks in *M. viciae* and *S. argyrostoma,* however, reveals a number of close similarities. In the flesh fly, although the clock is clearly based on circadian rhythmicity, the "photoperiodic oscillation" measures night length as an hourglass. Its circadian nature is revealed only in long cycles ($T48$ or $T72$, for example). Discrimination between short and long night-lengths is brought about (if the external coincidence model is followed) by whether dawn illuminates or fails to illuminate ϕ_i. The fall in diapause incidence at ultrashort day lengths (< 5 hr), so characteristic of many insect photoperiodic response curves, is here attributed to the weaker resetting powers of short light pulses, to the relatively long time taken by the oscillatory system to reach steady state in these cycles, and to a consequent scatter of phases within the multioscillator circadian system. In *M. viciae,* a remarkably similar picture is presented by Lees (1968, 1973), but in different words. Thus, night length is also measured by an hourglass timer, and the function of the light component is to "prime" the dark-period hourglass. As in *S. argyrostoma,* photoperiodic induction is then dependent on coincidence between dawn and a light-sensitive region (phase) late in the night (Lees's Stage 3). Finally, as the photoperiod becomes less than about 6 hr, "the critical night-length is increased, and timing accuracy lost." In both species, therefore, the formal properties of the clock, as presented, are of the "external coincidence" type.

Perhaps, then, night-length measurement in *M. viciae* (Type 4) is accomplished by a *redundant* oscillation that achieves only a single time-measuring "cycle" before its extinction. This suggestion, which is derived from Bünning (1969), is particularly attractive if one seeks simplicity in biological theories. In this view, the important consideration in insect photoperiodism is the theoretical (and possibly "real") difference between internal and external coincidence.

REFERENCES

Adkisson, P. L. Action of the photoperiod in controlling insect diapause. *American Naturalist,* 1964, *98,* 357–374.

Adkisson, P. L. Internal clocks and insect diapause. *Science* (Washington), 1966, *154,* 234–241.

Atwal, A. S. Influence of temperature, photoperiod, and food on the speed of development, longevity, fecundity, and other qualities of the diamond-back moth *Plutella maculipennis* (Curtis) (Tineidae, Lepidoptera). *Australian Journal of Zoology,* 1955, *3,* 185–221.

Baker, F. C. The effect of photoperiodism on resting, treehole, mosquito larvae. *Canadian Entomologist,* 1935, *67,* 149–153.

Barry, B. D., and Adkisson, P. L. Certain aspects of the genetic factors involved in the control of larval diapause of the pink bollworm. *Annals of the Entomological Society of America,* 1966, *59,* 122–125.

Beach, R. F. The required day number and timely induction of diapause in geographic strains of the mosquito *Aëdes atropalpus. Journal of Insect Physiology,* 1978, *24,* 449–455.

Beach, R. F., and Craig, G. B., Jr. Night length measurements by the circadian clock controlling diapause induction in the mosquito *Aëdes atropalpus. Journal of Insect Physiology,* 1977, *23,* 865–870.

Beck, S. D. Photoperiodic induction of diapause in an insect. *Biological Bulletin of the Marine Biological Laboratory, Woods Hole,* 1962a, *122,* 1–12.

Beck, S. D. Temperature effects on insects: Relation to periodism. *Proceedings of the North Central Branch, Entomological Society of America,* 1962b, *17,* 18–19.

Beck, S. D. *Insect Photoperiodism.* New York: Academic Press, 1968.

Beck, S. D. Photoperiodic determination of insect development and diapause. *Journal of Comparative Physiology,* 1974, *90,* 275–295; 1974b, *90,* 297–310; 1975, *103,* 227–245.

Beck, S. D., and Hanec, W. Diapause in the European corn borer, *Pyrausta nubilalis* (Hubn). *Journal of Insect Physiology,* 1960, *4,* 304–318.

Beck, S. D., Cloutier, E. J., and McLeod, D. G. R. Photoperiod and insect development. *Proceedings of the 23rd Biological Colloquium, Oregon State University,* 1962, pp. 43–64.

Bell, R. A., and Adkisson, P. L. Photoperiodic reversal of diapause induction in an insect. *Science* (Washington), 1964, *144,* 1149–1151.

Blake, G. Control of diapause by an "internal clock" in *Anthrenus verbasci* (L.) (Col., Dermestidae). *Nature* (London), 1959, *183,* 126–127.

Bowen, M. F., and Skopik, S. D. Insect photoperiodism: The "T-experiment" as evidence for an hour-glass mechanism. *Science* (Washington), 1976, *192,* 59–60.

Bradshaw, W. E. Major environmental factors inducing the termination of larval diapause in *Chaoborus americanus* Johannsen (Diptera: Culicidae). *Biological Bulletin of the Marine Biological Laboratory, Woods Hole,* 1969, *136,* 2–8.

Bradshaw, W. E. Geography of photoperiodic response in diapausing mosquito. *Nature* (London), 1976, *262,* 384–386.

Bünning, E. Die endogene Tagesrhythmik als Grundlage der photoperiodischen Reaktion. *Bericht der Deutschen botanischen Gesellschaft,* 1936, *54,* 590–607.

Bünning, E. Common features of photoperiodism in plants and animals. *Photochemistry and Photobiology,* 1969, *9,* 219–228.

Bünning, E., and Joerrens, G. Tagesperiodische antagonistische Schwankungen der Blau-Violett und Gelbrot-Empfindlichkeit als Grundlage der photoperiodischen Diapause-Induktion bei *Pieris brassicae. Zeitschrift für Naturforschung,* 1960, *15,* 205–213.

Clay, M. E., and Venard, C. E. Larval diapause in the mosquito, *Aëdes triseriatus:* Effect of diet and temperature on photoperiodic induction. *Journal of Insect Physiology,* 1972, *18,* 1441–1446.

Danilevskii, A. S. *Photoperiodism and Seasonal Development of Insects* (1st ed.). Edinburgh & London: Oliver and Boyd, 1965.

Denlinger, D. L. Induction and termination of pupal diapause in *Sarcophaga* (Diptera; Sarcophagidae). *Biological Bulletin of the Marine Biological Laboratory, Woods Hole,* 1972, *142,* 11–24.

Dickson, R. C. Factors governing the induction of diapause in the oriental fruit moth. *Annals Entomological Society of America,* 1949, *42,* 511–537.

Dingle, H. The experimental analysis of migration and life-history strategies in insects. In L. Barton Browne (Ed.), *Experimental Analysis of Insect Behaviour.* Berlin: Springer-Verlag, 1974, pp. 329–342.

Dumortier, B., and Brunnarius, J. L'information thermopériodique et l'induction de la diapause chez *Pieris brassicae* L. *Compte Rendu Hebdomadaire des Séances de l'Académie des Sciences, Paris D.,* 1977, *284,* 957–960.

Fernandez, A. T., and Randolph, N. M. The susceptibility of houseflies reared under various photoperiods to insecticide residues. *Journal of Economic Entomology,* 1966, *59,* 37–39.

Fukuda, S. Déterminisme hormonale de la diapause chez le ver de soie. *Bulletin de la Société Zoologique de France,* 1963, *88,* 151–179.

Geispitz, K. F. The mechanisms of acceptance of light stimuli in the photoperiodic reaction of Lepidoptera larvae. *Zoologicheskii Zhurnal SSSR,* 1957, *36,* 548–560.

Geldiay, S. Control of adult reproductive diapause in *Anacridium aegyptium* L. by direct action of photoperiod on the cerebral neurosecretory cells. *Proceedings of the XIII International Congress Entomology, Moscow,* 1971, *1968,* 379–380.

Gibbs, D. Reversal of pupal diapause in *Sarcophaga argyrostoma* by temperature shifts after puparium formation. *Journal of Insect Physiology,* 1975, *21,* 1179–1186.

Goryshin, N. I. The relation between light and temperature factors in the photoperiodic reaction in insects. *Entomologicheskoe Obozrenie,* 1955, *34,* 9–14.

Goryshin, N. I. The influence of diurnal light and temperature rhythms on diapause in Lepidoptera. *Entomologicheskoe Obozrenie,* 1964, *43,* 43–46.

Goryshin, N. I., and Kozlova, R. N. Thermoperiodism as a factor in the development of insects. *Zhurnal Obshchei Biologii,* 1967, *28,* 278–288.

Goryshin, N. I., and Tyshchenko, V. P. Thermostability of the process of perception of photoperiodic information in the moth *Acronycta rumicis* (Lepidoptera, Noctuidae). *Doklady Akademii Nauk SSSR,* 1970, *193,* 458–461.

Hamner, W. M. Hour-glass dusk and rhythmic dawn timers control diapause in the codling moth. *Journal of Insect Physiology,* 1969, *15,* 1499–1504.

Hillman, W. S. Endogenous circadian rhythms and the response of *Lemna purpusilla* to skeleton photoperiods. *American Naturalist,* 1964, *98,* 323–328.

Hillman, W. S. Non-circadian photoperiodic timing in the aphid *Megoura. Nature* (London), 1973, *242,* 128–129.

Hoelscher, C. E., and Vinson, S. B. The sex ratio of a hymenopterous parasitoid, *Campoletis perdistinctus,* as affected by photoperiod, mating, and temperature. *Annals of the Entomological Society of America,* 1971, *64,* 1373–1376.

Kogure, M. The influence of light and temperature on certain characters of the silkworm, *Bombyx mori. Journal of the Department of Agriculture, Kyushu University,* 1933, *4,* 1–93.

Lees, A. D. The significance of the light and dark phases in the photoperiodic control of diapause in *Metatetranychus ulmi* Koch. *Annals of Applied Biology,* 1953, *40,* 487–497.

Lees, A. D. The role of photoperiod and temperature in the determination of parthenogenetic and sexual forms in the aphid *Megoura viciae* Buckton. I. The influence of these factors on *apterous virginoparae* and their progeny. *Journal of Insect Physiology,* 1959, *3,* 92–117.

Lees, A. D. The role of photoperiod and temperature in the determination of parthenogenetic and sexual forms in the aphid *Megoura viciae.* III. Further properties of the maternal switching mechanism in apterous aphids. *Journal of Insect Physiology,* 1963, *9,* 153–164.

Lees, A. D. The location of the photoperiodic receptors in the aphid *Megoura viciae. Journal of Experimental Biology,* 1964, *41,* 119–133.

Lees, A. D. Is there a circadian component in the *Megoura* photoperiodic clock? In J. Aschoff (Ed.), *Circadian Clocks.* Amsterdam: North-Holland, 1965, pp. 351–356.

Lees, A. D. Photoperiodic timing mechanisms in insects. *Nature* (London), 1966, *210,* 986–989.

Lees, A. D. Photoperiodism in insects. In A. C. Giese (Ed.), *Photophysiology.* Vol. 4. New York: Academic Press, 1968, pp. 47–137.

Lees, A. D. Insect clocks and timers. Inaugural lecture, Imperial College of Science and Technology, 1 December 1970.

Lees, A. D. The relevance of action spectra in the study of insect photoperiodism. In M. Menaker (Ed.), *Biochronometry*. Washington, D.C.: National Academy of Sciences, 1971, pp. 372–380.

Lees, A. D. Photoperiodic time measurement in the aphid *Megoura viciae*. *Journal of Insect Physiology*, 1973, *19*, 2279–2316.

MacLeod, E. G. Experimental induction and elimination of adult diapause and autumnal coloration in *Chrysopa carnea* (Neuroptera). *Journal of Insect Physiology*, 1967, *13*, 1343–1349.

Marcovitch, S. Plant lice and light exposure. *Science* (Washington), 1923, *58*, 537–538.

Masaki, S. The response of a "short-day" insect to certain external factors: The induction of diapause in *Abraxas miranda* Butl. *Japanese Journal of Applied Entomology and Zoology*, 1958, *2*, 285–294.

Menaker, M., and Gross, G. Effects of fluctuating temperature on diapause induction in the pink bollworm. *Journal of Insect Physiology*, 1965, *11*, 911–914.

Minis, D. H. Parallel peculiarities in the entrainment of a circadian rhythm and photoperiodic induction in the pink bollworm *(Pectinophora gossypiella)*. In J. Aschoff (Ed.), *Circadian Clocks*. Amsterdam: North-Holland, 1965, pp. 333–343.

Müller, H. J. Uber den Einfluss der Photoperiode auf Diapause und Körpergrösse der Delphacide *Stenocranus minutus* Fabr. *Zoologischer Anzeiger*, 1958, *160*, 294–311.

Müller, H. J. Formen der Dormanz bei Insekten. *Nova Acta Leopold*, 1970, *35*, 7–27.

Norris, K. H., Howell, F., Hayes, D. K., Adler, V. E., Sullivan, W. N., and Schechter, M. S. The action spectrum for breaking diapause in the codling moth, *Laspeyresia pomonella* (L.) and the oak silkworm, *Antheraea pernyi* Guer. *Proceedings of the National Academy of Sciences, USA*, 1969, *63*, 1120–1127.

Norris, M. J. The influence of daylength on imaginal diapause in the red locust, *Nomadacris septemfasciata*. *Entomologia experimentalis et applicata*, 1959, *2*, 154–168.

Novak, V. J. A. *Insect Hormones* (3rd ed.). London: Methuen, 1966.

Paris, O. H., and Jenner, C. E. Photoperiodic control of diapause in the pitcher plant midge, *Metriocnemus knabi*. In R. B. Withrow (Ed.), *Photoperiodism and Related Phenomena in Plants and Animals*. Washington, D.C.: American Association for the Advancement of Science, 1959, pp. 601–624.

Perez, Y., Verdier, M., and Pener, M. P. The effect of photoperiod on male sexual behaviour in a north adriatic strain of the migratory locust. *Entomologia Experimentalis et Applicata*, 1971, *14*, 245–250.

Peterson, B. M., and Hamner, W. M. Photoperiodic control of diapause in the codling moth. *Journal of Insect Physiology*, 1968, *14*, 519–528.

Pittendrigh, C. S. Circadian rhythms and the circadian organization of living systems. *Cold Spring Harbor Symposia Quantitative Biology*, 1960, *25*, 159–184.

Pittendrigh, C. S. On temporal organization in living systems. *Harvey Lectures Series*, 1961, *56*, 93–125.

Pittendrigh, C. S. The circadian oscillation in *Drosophila pseudoobscura* pupae: A model for the photoperiodic clock. *Zeitschrift für Pflanzenphysiologie*, 1966, *54*, 275–307.

Pittendrigh, C. S. Circadian surfaces and the diversity of possible roles of circadian organization in photoperiodic induction. *Proceedings of the National Academy of Sciences, U.S.A.*, 1972, *69*, 2734–2737.

Pittendrigh, C. S. Circadian oscillations in cells and the circadian organization of multicellular systems. In F. O. Schmitt and F. G. Worden (Eds.), *The Neurosciences Third Study Program*. Cambridge, Mass.: MIT Press, 1974, pp. 437–458.

Pittendrigh, C. S., and Minis, D. H. The entrainment of circadian oscillations by light and their role as photoperiodic clocks. *American Naturalist*, 1964, *98*, 261–294.

Pittendrigh, C. S., and Minis, D. H. The photoperiodic time measurement in *Pectinophora gossypiella* and its relation to the circadian system in that species. In M. Menaker (Ed.), *Biochronometry*. Washington, D.C.: National Academy of Sciences, 1971, pp. 212–250.

Pittendrigh, C. S., and Minis, D. H. Circadian systems: Longevity as a function of circadian resonance in *Drosophila melanogaster*. *Proceedings of the National Academy of Sciences, USA*, 1972, *69*, 1537–1539.

Pittendrigh, C. S., Eichhorn, J. H., Minis, D. H., and Bruce, V. G. Circadian systems. VI. Photoperiodic time measurement in *Pectinophora gossypiella*. *Proceedings of the National Academy of Sciences, USA*, 1970, *66*, 758–764.

Ring, R. A. Maternal induction of diapause in the larvae of *Lucilia caesar* L. (Diptera, Calliphoridae). *Journal of Experimental Biology*, 1967, *46*, 123–136.

Ryan, R. B. Maternal influence on diapause in a parasitic insect, *Coeloides brunneri* Vier. (Hymenoptera: Braconidae). *Journal of Insect Physiology*, 1965, *11*, 1331–1336.

Saunders, D. S. Larval diapause induced by a maternally-operating photoperiod. *Nature* (London), 1965, *206*, 739–740.

Saunders, D. S. Larval diapause of maternal origin. II. The effect of photoperiod and temperature on *Nasonia vitripennis*. *Journal of Insect Physiology*, 1966a, *12*, 569–581.

Saunders, D. S. Larval diapause of maternal origin. III. The effect of host shortage on *Nasonia vitripennis*. *Journal of Insect Physiology*, 1966b, *12*, 899–908.

Saunders, D. S. Time measurement in insect photoperiodism: Reversal of a photoperiodic effect by chilling. *Science* (Washington), 1967, *156*, 1126–1127.

Saunders, D. S. Photoperiodism and time measurement in the parasitic wasp, *Nasonia vitripennis*. *Journal of Insect Physiology*, 1968, *14*, 433–450.

Saunders, D. S. Circadian clock in insect photoperiodism. *Science* (Washington), 1970, *168*, 601–603.

Saunders, D. S. The temperature-compensated photoperiodic clock "programming" development and pupal diapause in the flesh-fly, *Sarcophaga argyrostoma*. *Journal of Insect Physiology*, 1971, *17*, 801–812.

Saunders, D. S. Circadian control of larval growth rate in *Sarcophaga argyrostoma*. *Proceedings of the National Academy of Sciences, USA*, 1972, *69*, 2738–2740.

Saunders, D. S. The photoperiodic clock in the flesh-fly, *Sarcophaga argyrostoma*. *Journal of Insect Physiology*, 1973a, *19*, 1941–1954.

Saunders, D. S. Thermoperiodic control of diapause in an insect: Theory of internal coincidence. *Science* (Washington), 1973b, *181*, 358–360.

Saunders, D. S. Evidence for "dawn" and "dusk" oscillators in the *Nasonia* photoperiodic clock. *Journal of Insect Physiology*, 1974, *20*, 77–88.

Saunders, D. S. Manipulation of the length of the sensitive period, and the induction of pupal diapause in the flesh-fly, *Sarcophaga argyrostoma*. *Journal of Entomology, Series A*, 1975a, *50*, 107–118.

Saunders, D. S. "Skeleton" photoperiods and the control of diapause and development in the flesh-fly, *Sarcophaga argyrostoma*. *Journal of Comparative Physiology*, 1975b, *97*, 97–112.

Saunders, D. S. Spectral sensitivity and intensity thresholds in *Nasonia* photoperiodic clock. *Nature* (London), 1975c, *253*, 732–734.

Saunders, D. S. The circadian eclosion rhythm in *Sarcophaga argyrostoma:* Some comparisons with the photoperiodic "clock." *Journal of Comparative Physiology*, 1976a, *110*, 111–133.

Saunders, D. S. *Insect Clocks*. New York: Pergamon Press, 1976b.

Saunders, D. S. An experimental and theoretical analysis of photoperiodic induction in the flesh-fly, *Sarcophaga argyrostoma*. *Journal of Comparative Physiology*, 1978a, *124*, 75–95.

Saunders, D. S. Internal and external coincidence and the apparent diversity of photoperiodic clocks in the insects. *Journal of Comparative Physiology*, 1978b, *127*, 197–207.

Skopik, S. D., and Bowen, M. F. Insect photoperiodism: An hour-glass measures photoperiodic time in *Ostrinia nubilalis*. *Journal of Comparative Physiology*, 1976, *111*, 249–259.

Steel, C. G. H., and Lees, A. D. The role of neurosecretion in the photoperiodic control of polymorphism in the aphid *Megoura viciae*. *Journal of Experimental Biology*, 1977, *67*, 117–135.

Tanaka, Y. Studies on hibernation with special reference to photoperiodicity and the breeding of the Chinese Tussar silkworm. V. *Journal of Sericultural Science* (Tokyo), 1951, *20*, 132–138.

Tauber, M. J., and Tauber, C. A. Quantitative response to daylength during diapause in insects. *Nature* (London), 1973, *224*, 296–297.

Thiele, H. U. Measurement of day-length as a basis for photoperiodism and annual periodicity in the carabid beetle *Pterostichus nigrita* F. *Oecologia* (Berlin), 1977, *30*, 331–348.

Truman, J. W. The role of the brain in the ecdysis rhythm of silkmoths: Comparison with the photoperiodic termination of diapause. In M. Menaker (Ed.), *Biochronometry*. Washington, D.C.: National Academy of Sciences, 1971, pp. 483–504.

Tyshchenko, V. P. Two-oscillatory model of the physiological mechanism of insect photoperiodic reaction. *Zhurnal Obshchei Biologii*, 1966, *27*, 209–222.

Tyshchenko, V. P., Goryshin, N. I., and Azaryan, A. G. The role of circadian processes in insect photoperiodism. *Zhurnal Obshchei Biologii*, 1972, *33*, 21–31.

Vinogradova, E. B., and Zinovjeva, K. B. Maternal induction of larval diapause in the blowfly, *Calliphora vicina*. *Journal of Insect Physiology*, 1972, *18*, 2401–2409.

Way, M. J., and Hopkins, B. A. The influence of photoperiod and temperature on the induction of diapause in *Diataraxia oleracea* L. *Journal of Experimental Biology*, 1950, *27*, 365–376.

Went, F. W. The periodic aspect of photoperiodism and thermoperiodicity. In R. B. Withrow (Ed.), *Photoperiodism and Related Phenomena in Plants and Animals*. Washington, D.C.: American Association for the Advancement of Science, 1959, pp. 551–564.

Wilde, J. de. Perception of the photoperiod by the Colorado potato beetle, (*Leptinotarsa decemlineata* Say.). *Proceedings of the Xth International Congress of Entomology, Montreal, 1956*, 1958, *2*, 213–218.

Wilde, J. de. Photoperiodism in insects and mites. *Annual Reviews of Entomology*, 1962, *7*, 1–26.

Wilde, J. de, and Bonga, H. Observations on threshold intensity and sensitivity of different wavelengths of photoperiodic response in the Colorado beetle (*Leptinotarsa decemlineata* Say.). *Entomologia Experimentalis et Applicata*, 1958, *1*, 301–307.

Wilde, J. de, Duintjer, C. S., and Mook, L. Physiology of diapause in the adult Colorado beetle *(Leptinotarsa decemlineata)*: The photoperiod as a controlling factor. *Journal of Insect Physiology*, 1959, *3*, 75–85.

Williams, C. M. Physiology of insect diapause. IV. The brain and prothoracic glands as an endocrine system in the cecropia silkworm. *Biological Bulletin of the Marine Biological Laboratory, Woods Hole,* 1952, *103,* 120–138.

Williams, C. M. Photoperiodism and the endocrine aspects of insect diapause. *Symposia of the Society for Experimental Biology, Cambridge,* 1969, *23,* 285–300.

Williams, C. M., and Adkisson, P. L. Physiology of insect diapause. XIV. An endocrine mechanism for the photoperiodic control of pupal diapause in the oak silkworm, *Antheraea pernyi. Biological Bulletin of the Marine Biological Laboratory, Woods Hole,* 1964, *127,* 511–525.

Williams, C. M., Adkisson, P. L., and Walcott, C. Physiology of insect diapause. XV. The transmission of photoperiodic signals to the brain of the oak silkworm, *Antheraea pernyi. Biological Bulletin of the Marine Biological Laboratory, Woods Hole,* 1965, *128,* 497–507.

Winfree, A. T. Integrated view of resetting a circadian clock. *Journal of Theoretical Biology,* 1970, *28,* 327–374.

Winfree, A. T. Slow dark-adaptation in Drosophila's circadian clock. *Journal of Comparative Physiology,* 1972, *77,* 418–434.

23

Photoperiodism in Vertebrates

KLAUS HOFFMANN

INTRODUCTION

Annual cycles in many functions have been demonstrated in practically all groups of vertebrates. Starting with the work of Rowan (1925) in birds and of Baker and Ranson (1932) and of Bissonette (1932) in mammals, it has been shown that the photoperiod (i.e., the light fraction of the 24-hr day and its seasonal changes) influences the annual cycle, especially in those species living in medium or higher latitudes. In recent years, much progress has been made in analyzing the time-measuring mechanisms involved, as well as in unveiling the physiological mechanisms that participate in the seasonal changes and their regulation by photoperiod. Most of this work has been concerned with the cycle in reproduction, and thus, this function is discussed here in greatest detail. Since there seem to be definite differences in the physiological mechanisms in different vertebrate groups, the discussion deals with these groups separately. Because of the author's bias, emphasis is placed on the situation in mammals.

MAMMALS

Annual cycles in mammalian species are well known. The antler cycle in deer, the rutting seasons in carnivores, and the changes of pelage color in the stoat serve as a few well-known examples. To achieve a high survival rate of the young, the external conditions prevailing during birth, lactation, and early development are of prime importance. In accordance with the gestation time, mating takes place in spring or summer, as in ferrets, voles, and hamsters, or in fall or winter, as in sheep, goats, and deer. In both situations, it has been shown that photoperiod can regulate the time of mating. However, the photope-

KLAUS HOFFMANN   Max-Planck-Institut für Verhaltensphysiologie, D-8131 Andechs, West Germany.

riodic effects may be opposite, depending on when sexual activity takes place. Thus, in animals that mate in spring, such as the ferret or the hamster, short photoperiods induce gonadal regression, and long photoperiods hasten recrudescence or development; the opposite effect appears in animals mating in fall or winter, like sheep or deer. These differences are not surprising since photoperiod is not the "ultimate factor" directly determining the most advantageous time for reproduction but is a "proximate factor" that gives the most reliable and noise-free information on the season and allows the organism to prepare in advance for the times to come (Baker, 1938, see also Chapter 20).

In some species, the proper timing of birth is achieved by delayed implantation, which may also be influenced by photoperiod, for example, in the mink and the badger (Allais and Martinet, 1978; Canivec and Bonnin, 1979). Besides reproduction, other functions that change with the season may be governed by photoperiod, as has been shown for the antler cycle in deer (Goss, 1976) or the molt of several species. In the Djungarian hamster, not only gonadal activity but also body weight and pelage color display a prominent annual cycle subject to photoperiodic regulation (Figala, Hoffmann, and Goldau, 1973; Hoffmann, 1979a). However, most studies have been concerned with reproduction. Since the majority of work on the physiological mechanism of the photoperiodic reaction has been focused— among long-day breeders on hamsters and the ferret, and among short-day breeders on sheep—discussion of this work is emphasized.

THE PHOTOPERIODIC SIGNAL

In two species of hamsters, it has been shown that there is a rather marked "critical photoperiod" dividing light times that induce regression from those that maintain gonadal activities or further recrudescence (Elliott, 1976; Hoffmann, 1979a). In the golden hamster, this photoperiod is at 12½ hr of light per day; in the Djungarian hamster, a more northern species, it is at about 13 hr. Such sharp borderlines suggest that the animals are able to measure those photoperiods rather precisely. Formerly, theories prevailed that assumed that this time measurement is achieved by a kind of hourglass or interval timer, determining either the length of the light time or of the dark time of the daily cycle. An alternative hypothesis was advanced by Bünning as early as 1936, suggesting that an endogenous daily rhythm of light sensitivity might underlie photoperiodic time measurement. As has been pointed out by Pittendrigh (1972), in the "Bünning hypothesis" light has a dual function: it entrains the presumed endogenous cycle of sensitivity, and it induces either stimulation or no stimulation, depending whether light coincides with a particular phase of the rhythm of sensitivity (for a fuller review, see Follett, 1973).

Evidence of the existence of such a coincidence model of photoperiodic time measurement has recently been presented for two mammalian species, the golden hamster (Elliott, 1976) and a vole (Grocock and Clarke, 1974). The most elegant demonstration of circadian involvement in the photoperiodic mechanism is found in the work of Elliott (1976). He was able to show that 1 hr of light per circadian cycle may induce either a short-day or a long-day response, depending on the circadian phase into which the light pulse falls. In his experiments, he made use of the fact that circadian cycles can be entrained to light–dark cycles differing from 24 hr, and that the phase angle between zeitgeber cycle and biological cycle depends on the difference in frequency between the two cycles (see Chapter 7).

It has been known for some time that a short light time in which the following dark time is interrupted by a light pulse (skeleton photoperiod) can give the same results as full long photoperiods. In order to be effective, such light interruptions may be quite brief. For stimulation of testicular recrudescence in the Djungarian hamster, 8 hr of light plus 1 min of light in the middle of the dark time daily were as effective as full 16-hr photoperiods (Hoffmann, 1979b). Such findings are of interest in context with the possible function of the pineal and of melatonin in transducing the photoperiodic effects (see p. 456).

All these experiments indicate that in mammals, *light* falling into a certain phase of the circadian cycle of photosensitivity causes the stimulatory photoperiodic response. However, these experiments have been performed only on some species of spring and summer breeders, in which short photoperiods induce regression while long photoperiods instigate recrudescence. Of fall breeders, experiments on the effects of skeleton photoperiods have been performed only on rams (Garnier, Ortavant, Mansard, and Terqui, 1977; Ravault and Ortavant, 1977; Lincoln, 1978). While the results demonstrate that there are zones in the daily cycle that are sensitive to the lighting conditions, it is not yet clear whether light or darkness during the sensitive phase is responsible for the photoperiodic response.

PHOTOPERIODIC EFFECTS ON PUBERTY

In many mammals with distinct but extended breeding periods, the age at which puberty is reached depends on the season of birth (see Sadleir, 1969; Lincoln and Mac-Kinnon, 1976; Hoffmann, 1978a). In general, puberty is reached only during the adult mating season. In species with rapid development, as in some rodents and hares, animals born early in the year may mature rapidly and reproduce within the same season, while in animals born at the end of the breeding season, puberty may be delayed until the beginning of the next season.

In several species, it has been shown that photoperiod may also regulate gonadal development in juveniles. Djungarian hamsters maintained from birth in long photoperiods have large and fully functional testes at the age of 40 days, while in short photoperiods, testicular development is delayed up to about 180 days of age. Similar effects were observed on pelage color and on body weight in this species (Hoffmann, 1978a). It should be noted, however, that marked species differences may occur. Thus, in golden hamsters, which as adults show strong photoperiodic reactions, gonadal development in juveniles is not influenced by the lighting conditions (Gaston and Menaker, 1967; Reiter, Sorrentino, and Hoffman, 1970). The physiological basis for the different behavior in the two hamster species is unknown. Similarly, in young lemmings, no effect of photoperiod on testicular development was observed, while pelage color was markedly influenced in the same animals (Hasler, Buhl, and Banks, 1976). Such findings should warn against broad generalizations.

SPONTANEOUS PROCESSES AND PHOTOPERIODIC REFRACTORINESS

In several mammalian species that show strong reactions to photoperiodic manipulations, an endogenous circannual cycle of gonadal size and/or activity may persist in the absence of changes in photoperiod (see Chapter 21). This is true in particular of species whose sexual competence is retained for several years. Here, the changing photoperiod apparently only synchronizes the annual cycle and is not its immediate cause. In experiments without proper control groups, it may be difficult to judge whether changes in gonadal state are due to the influence of photoperiod or to the endogenous process (Lincoln, 1978).

Even in species with a short life span, like the golden and the Djungarian hamsters, spontaneous changes in gonadal state and activity may occur. After short photoperiods have induced regression, this state is not maintained indefinitely. After some time, spontaneous recrudescence sets in (Reiter, 1972a, 1975; Turek, Elliott, Alvis, and Menaker, 1975b; Hoffmann, 1973). In these cases, gonads remained large and active for the rest of the observation (80 weeks in golden hamsters—Reiter, 1972a; 2 years in young Djungarian hamsters—Hoffmann, unpublished), although the short photoperiods that normally lead to regression were maintained throughout.

Such observations indicate that after some time, the neuroendocrine–gonadal axis becomes insensitive or "refractory" to the inhibitory effect of short photoperiods. This photorefractoriness has been the object of intensive study in the golden hamster. It has been shown that a prolonged exposure to long photoperiods is necessary to break refractoriness and render the system again sensitive to the inhibitory effect of short photoperiods. The time necessary is somewhat variable in different animals, but in general 11 weeks of long photoperiods sufficed to break refractoriness in practically all animals (Reiter, 1972a; Stetson, Matt, Watson-Whitmyre, 1976, 1977; Bittman, 1978). It has also been shown that exposure to short photoperiods *per se* is not sufficient to induce refractoriness. Although complete gonadal regression is not required, some inhibition of the neuroendocrine–gonadal axis is apparently necessary for the initiation of refractoriness to short photoperiods (Zucker and Morin, 1977; Turek and Losee, 1979).

While refractoriness to short photoperiods in hamsters has been amply demonstrated, there is no indication of a refractoriness to long photoperiods in this group. Regression brought about by short days can be stopped and reversed by long photoperiods at any time (Stetson, Watson-Whitmyre, and Matt, 1977; Hoffmann, 1978b). However, in ferrets, it has been found that estrus may end spontaneously in long photoperiods, and that treatment with short photoperiods renders the animals again sensitive to the stimulatory effect of long photoperiods, while during continuous exposure to long photoperiods, estrus occurs again spontaneously in only some animals (Thorpe and Herbert, 1976a).

ORGANS AND PHYSIOLOGICAL PROCESSES INVOLVED

Experimental work to analyze the physiological mechanism underlying photoperiodic action has started from two directions. On the one side, research has centered on following the pathway of light effecting photoperiodic responses and on determining the structures and processes involved. On the other side, the endocrine events that are responsible for development and regression of the gonads and accessory structures have been investigated. In both fields, considerable progress has been made in recent years. Much less effort has been invested in studying the underlying physiology of nonreproductive functions that are governed by photoperiod.

THE PATHWAY OF LIGHT. All available evidence indicates that in mammals, the photoperiodically effective light cycle is perceived by the retina. After bilateral orbital enucleation, or sectioning of the optic nerves, the same effect as after exposure to short photoperiods or to constant dark was observed (golden hamster—Hoffman and Reiter, 1965; Reiter, 1974a; Rusak and Morin, 1976; ferret—Thomson, 1954; Herbert, Stacey, and Thorpe,

1978; gerbil—Dixit, Sharma, and Agrawal, 1977). This effect corresponds to the general finding that, at least in adult mammals, circadian rhythms freerun after blinding and are no longer influenced by the schedule of illumination (Rusak and Zucker, 1975, 1979).

In mammals, four projections from the retina are known: the primary optic tract (POT), the superior (SAOT) and the inferior (IAOT) accessory optic tract, and the retinohypothalamic tract (RHT), which directly connects the retina with the suprachiasmatic nuclei (Moore, 1974, 1978). Rusak and Morin (1976) observed undisturbed photoperiodic reactions in golden hamsters with a partially or completely lesioned POT and SAOT. They suggested that the RHT is the most probable pathway involved in conveying photoperiodic information. At that time, no IAOT had been detected in hamsters (Eichler and Moore, 1974), but more recently, such a tract has been described (Lin, Alexander, and Giolli, 1976). In ferrets, lesions of the primary or accessory optic tract also did not interfere with the accelerating effect of long photoperiods (Thorpe and Herbert, 1976b). In young Djungarian hamsters, sensitivity to photoperiod starts at an age of about 13 days (Frieling, 1979). The age at which direct retinohypothalamic projections to the suprachiasmatic nuclei appear is not known in this species; in the rat, it is at about 17 days (Campbell and Ramaley, 1974). In general, the evidence suggests that the RHT is the pathway of light in the photoperiodic mechanism. This has also been suggested for entrainment of circadian rhythms by light (Rusak and Zucker, 1979). A direct proof of this assumption by selectively interrupting the RHT has not yet been possible without partial or complete destruction of the nuclei suprachiasmatici because of their close proximity to the optic chiasm. These nuclei also play an essential role in the photoperiodic mechanism.

THE SUPRACHIASMATIC NUCLEI. Studies in the golden hamster show the suprachiasmatic nuclei to be an essential component of the photoperiodic mechanism. Their bilateral destruction prevents the inhibitory effect of short photoperiods or of blinding on the neuroendocrine axis (Rusak and Morin, 1976; Stetson and Watson-Whitmyre, 1976). This finding cannot be explained by the simultaneous interruption of the RHT and its photic information, since this should mimic rather than abolish the effect of constant dark or short photoperiods.

The suprachiasmatic nuclei are involved in the regulation and the entrainment of circadian rhythms; many rhythms disappear or are at least greatly disturbed after their destruction (Moore, 1977, 1978; Rusak and Zucker, 1979). Since a circadian rhythm of photosensitivity underlies the photoperiodic mechanism, lesions of these nuclei may abolish the rhythm. It is not clear why this impairment mimics the results of long rather than short photoperiods (Turek and Campbell, 1979). However, bilateral destruction of this nucleus also abolishes circadian rhythms in the pineal gland (Klein, 1973; Axelrod, 1974), and the latter effect may be of importance (see p. 457).

THE PINEAL GLAND. Starting with the pioneering work of Czyba, Girod, and Durand (1964) and of Hoffman and Reiter (1965) in the golden hamster, it has been shown again and again—in this species (Reiter, 1978a) as well as in the Djungarian hamster (Hoffmann, 1974), the vole (Farrar and Clarke, 1976), and the ferret (Thorpe and Herbert, 1976b)—that pinealectomy prohibits the effects of short photoperiods or of blinding, which normally instigate gonadal regression in long-day breeders. This effect is not restricted to the gonadal system. In the Djungarian hamster, pinealectomy also prevents the change into the whitish winter pelage (Hoffmann, 1977).

From these and other findings, it has been concluded by many authors that the pineal organ has exclusively inhibitory effects on the hypophyseal–gonadal axis, and that these effects are enhanced by short photoperiods or darkness but are abolished by long photoperiods. Especially Reiter (1973, 1978a) has promoted this view and has suggested that in long photoperiods, the animals are "physiologically pinealectomized," and that hence under such conditions, removal of the pineal gland has no noticeable effect on reproductive status. It is assumed that the pineal has to be "challenged" by short photoperiods in order to demonstrate its antigonadotrophic function.

While such conclusions can be drawn from experiments performed so far in the golden hamster—and also in rats—work in other species suggests that the pineal may also be involved in the transduction of the effects of long photoperiods. In the Djungarian hamster, pinealectomy significantly delayed testicular development, or recrudescence under long photoperiods, in each of five independent experiments (Hoffmann and Küderling, 1975, 1977; Brackmann and Hoffmann, 1977; Hoffmann, 1978b). In ferrets, removal of the pineal gland prevented the acceleration of estrus onset caused by long photoperiods (Herbert, 1971). Such findings are certainly not in agreement with the above-mentioned hypothesis, which postulates that pinealectomy has the same effect as long photoperiods, regardless of the schedule of illumination. In this context, further observations by Herbert (1972; Herbert et al., 1978) are of particular interest. In ferrets kept under natural light conditions, pinealectomy prevented neither onset nor end of estrus; both occurred initially at regular and later at irregular intervals. However, synchronization with the seasons was lost in spite of the large natural fluctuation of photoperiod to which the animals were exposed. These observations, together with those mentioned before, suggest that the pineal is neither progonadotrophic nor antigonadotrophic *per se*, but that it is an essential organ for the transduction of photoperiodic effects, and thus for the synchronization of the annual gonadal cycle.

Not only pinealectomy but also interference with its sympathetic innervation can suppress photoperiodic effects. Surgical interruption of the nervi conarii, which innervate the pineal, or extirpation of the superior cervical ganglia from which the postganglionic fibers derive, or chemical sympathectomy has been shown to prevent the effects of short photoperiods in hamsters and voles (Reiter, 1972b; Charlton, Grocock, and Ostberg, 1976; Farrar and Clarke, 1976). Decentralization of these ganglia, or transecting the descending pathways destined for the pineal gland, had the same effect (Reiter, 1972b). In ferrets, superior cervical ganglionectomy, like pinealectomy, prevented the acceleration of estrus onset by long photoperiods (Herbert, 1969). In general, it can be stated that any procedure that interrupts the pathway from the suprachiasmatic nuclei to the pineal has essentially the same effect as pinealectomy. These findings suggest that this pathway is essential for the transduction of photoperiodic effects.

MELATONIN. The pineal is considered a neurochemical transducer in which neuronal information, modified by the conditions of illumination, is converted into chemical messages (Axelrod, 1974; Moore and Klein, 1974; Binkley, 1976). So far, it has not been established with certainty which substance or substances produced in the pineal are responsible for conveying the photoperiodic effects. Two groups of compounds have been mainly discussed; polypeptides and indolamines. Of the latter, especially the effect of melatonin (N-acetyl-5-methoxytryptamine) has been intensively investigated in photoperiodic mammals. Since its half-life in the organism is short, and since early experiments with injection of melatonin revealed no measurable effects (Reiter, 1969), melatonin has been implanted in many investigations, either in beeswax or in Silastic tubing, thus assuring a sustained release.

In many photoperiodic species, drastic effects were observed after melatonin implantation. Rust and Meyer (1969) found that in male weasels, melatonin implantation prevented induction of testicular recrudescence and of molt into summer pelage by long photoperiods in winter, while in summer, it induced testicular involution and molt into the winter fur. Similarly, in Djungarian hamsters in winter state, implanted melatonin delayed the growth of testes and the molt into summer pelage after exposure to long photoperiods (Hoffmann, 1972, 1973). In the golden hamster, melatonin could induce regression of testes in long photoperiods or prevent premature recrudescence in long days (Turek et al., 1975a; Turek, Desjardins, and Menaker, 1976b); similar effects were reported for the white-footed mouse (Lynch and Epstein, 1976). In ferrets, injection of melatonin induced premature anestrus in long photoperiods and thus also simulated the action of short days (Thorpe and Herbert, 1976).

From such findings, it might be concluded that melatonin is an antigonadotrophic hormone, and that high levels of circulating melatonin induce gonadal involution or prevent recrudescence. However, when melatonin was implanted in sexually active Djungarian or golden hamsters, and the animals were at the same time exposed to short photoperiods, this treatment abolished the effect of short photoperiods; that is, it had just the opposite effect of that observed in long photoperiods, preventing rather than causing regression (Hoffmann, 1974; Reiter, Vaughan, Blask, and Johnson, 1974; Turek et al., 1976b). Thus, the results were similar to those obtained by pinealectomy.

So far, it is difficult to interpret these rather diverging results. Nevertheless, several generalizations seem possible. Although there is some variation due to dose and method of application, at least in hamsters the data indicate that sustained availability of exogenous melatonin counteracts the stimulatory effects of long photoperiods as well as the inhibitory effects of short photoperiods. Furthermore, while often drastic effects of melatonin application were observed in photoperiodic mammals, the same dose and way of application caused no detectable effect in nonphotoperiodic species (Turek et al., 1976b). Moreover, even in photoperiodic species, melatonin had effects only at times when the photoperiod could influence gonadal state. Thus, before puberty, no effect of melatonin was observed in golden hamsters (Turek, 1979a); in this species, sexual development until puberty is independent of photoperiod. In the Djungarian hamster, in which gonadal development depends on photoperiod (Hoffmann, 1978a), implantation of melatonin caused a delay of sexual maturation in long photoperiods (Brackmann, 1977). Spontaneous recrudescence in short photoperiods could not be prevented by melatonin in either species of hamster (Hoffmann, 1973; Turek and Losee, 1978). In ferrets, photorefractoriness to long photoperiods could be broken either by exposure to short photoperiods or by injection of melatonin (Thorpe and Herbert, 1976b).

In general, the findings related so far suggest that exogenous melatonin, and especially its implantation and thus sustained availability, interferes with and sometimes mimics photoperiodic effects, but that it is neither antigonadotrophic nor progonadotrophic per se. In view of such findings, it has been concluded by some authors that melatonin is not involved in transmitting the photoperiodic effects on the neuroendocrine axis, or that the site of action is the pineal itself, where it might regulate the synthesis and/or release of the true antigonadotrophic substance (e.g., Reiter *et al.*, 1974; Reiter, Blask, Johnson, and Rudeen, 1976). The latter hypothesis has not been supported in experiments with pinealectomized hamsters, in which application of melatonin had effects similar to those observed in controls (Hoffmann and Küderling, 1977; Turek, 1977a; Tamarkin, Hollister, Lefebvre, and Goldman, 1977a; Goldman, Hall, Hollister, Roychoudhury, Tamarkin, and Westrom, 1979). While all these findings show only that exogenous melatonin can have drastic effects in photoperiodic mammals (at times when photoperiodic manipulation can be effective), several other lines of evidence strongly suggest that melatonin is involved in conveying the photoperiodic information.

In every vertebrate species studied so far, pineal as well as plasma melatonin shows a marked daily cycle, with high values at night and low values during the day; the same is true of the activity of serotonin *N*-acetyltransferase (NAT), which is generally considered the rate-limiting enzyme in the conversion of serotonin to melatonin (Axelrod, 1974; Binkley, 1976; Stephens and Binkley, 1978). Hence, implantation and thereby continuous availability of melatonin can be considered unphysiological. It seems possible that it is not only the amount of melatonin but also its temporal pattern of release that is important for conveying the photoperiodic message.

Recent experiments support such an assumption. Tamarkin, Westrom, Hamill, and Goldman (1976b; Tamarkin, Lefebvre, Hollister, and Goldman 1977b) reported that one injection of melatonin daily can induce gonadal involution in hamsters kept in long photoperiods; but the result depended not only on dosage but also on the time of injection. A repetition of these experiments by Reiter *et al.* (1976) confirmed the results but also demonstrated that pinealectomy or procedures that interrupt the sympathetic pathway to the pineal can render the same injections ineffective. While these findings seemed to contradict the assumption that the pattern of available melatonin acts directly on the neuroendocrine axis, further experiments with pinealectomized or ganglionectomized hamsters have shown that here, melatonin injections are effective if they are repeated thrice daily in 3-hr intervals; thus, an intact and functional pineal is not necessary (Tamarkin *et al.*, 1977a; Goldman *et al.*, 1979). Though there are still considerable variations and inconsistencies in the reports on the effect of exogenous melatonin in photoperiodic species, in general the evidence supports the hypotheses that melatonin is involved in the transduction of the photoperiodic signal, and that the amount as well as the temporal pattern of availability is important.

This hypothesis is further supported by the fact that the production and release of melatonin are highly light-sensitive. Continuous light suppressed the nocturnal peak of NAT activity and of pineal and plasma melatonin in practically every case studied. While darkness during the normal light time had no effect, light during the dark time led to a rapid decrease of pineal NAT activity and of pineal and plasma melatonin (Axelrod, 1974; Rollag and Niswender, 1976; Klein, 1978; Tamarkin, Reppert, and Klein, 1979). In the rat, Illnerova *et al.* (Illnerova, Backström, Sääf, Wetterberg, and Vangbo, 1978; Illnerova, Vanacek, Krecek, Wetterberg, and Sääf, 1979) have shown that exposure to only 1 min of light in the dark time induced a precipitous decline of pineal NAT activity and of pineal and plasma melatonin; if applied at midnight or later, the values remained low for the rest of the night. This finding means that a very brief exposure to light during the dark time can drastically alter the pattern of melatonin production and release. The same effect has recently been found in Djungarian hamsters (Hoffmann, Illnerova, and Vanecek, 1980), in which an identical night-interruption schedule induced testicular recrudescence and thus had the same effect as full long photoperiods (Hoffmann, 1979b). In sheep, the temporal pattern of peripheral melatonin concentration accurately reflected the duration of darkness in artificial light regimes (Rollag and Niswender, 1976); under natural conditions, the pattern varied with the season and thus with the length of the light period (Arendt, 1979). In the golden hamster the phase relationship of the cycle of pineal melatonin content to the cycle of illumination differed in long and short photoperiods (Tamarkin *et al.,* 1979). In general, it can be stated that all light exposures that have been shown to influence gonadal state also change the pattern of melatonin production in the pineal and melatonin levels in the circulation.

Further support for the assumption that the temporal pattern of melatonin release is involved in transducing the photoperiodic signal is rendered by the fact that all surgical manipulations that suppress the effect of short photoperiods or of blinding on gonadal state in hamsters (Reiter, 1978a) also suppress the nocturnal peak in melatonin. Thus, destruction of the suprachiasmatic nuclei, or denervation of the pineal gland by extirpation or decentralization of the superior cervical ganglion, abolishes the pineal rhythms (Axelrod, 1974; Klein, 1978). These observations were made in the rat; however, the suppression of the nocturnal peak of pineal melatonin content after ganglionectomy has also been found in the hamster (Panke, Rollag, and Reiter, 1979).

While all the results mentioned so far support, or at least are in agreement with, the hypothesis that melatonin is involved in the transmission of photoperiodic effects to the hypothalamus–pituitary–gonadal axis, there are some publications that are at variance with this assumption. Knigge and Sheridan (1976) found that immunization against melatonin led to regression of testes in blinded as well as in sighted hamsters. However, the specificity of the antibody was not tested, and the fact that in blinded controls hypothalamic LHRH was increased as compared with sighted controls, whereas in the immunized animals it was decreased, suggests that blinding and immunization affected the testes by different mechanisms. A similar study was conducted by Brown, Basinska, Bubenik, Sibony, Grota, and Stancer (1976) with male hamsters that were immunized against melatonin and N-acetyl-serotonin and were kept in short photoperiods. The effect of short photoperiods was not abolished by the immunization. Again, specificity was not fully tested, and it is also noteworthy that in the controls, pinealectomy did not prevent but only attenuated gonadal regression. In general, though these studies do not support the hypothesis of melatonin involvement in the photoperiodic process, they also do not prove the contrary. A detailed discussion of the impact of these results has been given by Reiter (1978b).

One further point needs to be mentioned. While most investigations have concerned themselves with the effect of melatonin, it has also been described that melatonin-free pineal extracts may have inhibitory effects on the hypothalamic–hypophysial–gonadal axis. Polypeptides are under discussion (Ebels and Benson, 1978). Particularly the effect of arginine vasotocin (AVT), which was thought to be produced in the mammalian pineal gland, has been studied recently (Vaughan and Blask, 1978). Most of these studies were performed in species in which no or only very slight photoperiodic effects can be observed. It should also be noted that in recent investigations, AVT could not be found in mammalian pineals (Dogterom, Snijdewint, Pevet, and Swaab, 1980). In general, while more information is certainly necessary, the hypothesis that melatonin is an essential factor in the transduction of the photoperiodic message, and that not only its amount but also the temporal pattern of its synthesis and release are important, seems to me the best-supported and the most promising assumption. The site of physiological action of melatonin is so far elusive.

ENDOCRINE ASPECTS

In most examples mentioned so far, changes in gonads or accessory organs were presented as criteria for the effects of photoperiodic manipulation, since these are easily measured. In a considerable number of cases, plasma and pituitary hormones were also determined, and drastic changes were found. Especially the changes in levels of gonadal steroids and gonadotrophins, and the mechanisms underlying these changes, are discussed here. So far, there is evidence that three types of mechanism contribute to the photoperiodic regulation of gonadotrophin release and thus of gonadal state.

GONADAL STEROIDS. The physiological testicular atrophy in photoperiodic mammals is accompanied by a reduction—and in many cases, complete cessation—of spermatogenesis and a drastic decline in androgen levels, as is also indicated by the involution of the androgen-dependent accessory glands. Data on changes in androgen levels, induced by natural or experimental changes in length of photoperiod, have been presented in male hamsters (Berndtson and Desjardins, 1974), in rams (Lincoln, Peet, and Cunningham, 1977), in male minks (Nieschlag and Bienek, 1975), in male badgers (Maurel, 1978), and in stags (Lincoln, Youngson, and Short, 1970), to quote only a few examples. It should be noted that in some species, marked circadian variations in androgen levels may occur. In Djungarian hamsters, the values for plasma testosterone at dusk were about 12 times higher than those at dawn (Hoffmann and Nieschlag, 1977). If such variations are not taken into consideration, they might mar the photoperiod-dependent differences. In females, noninductive photoperiods led to cessation of estrus cycles and ovulation, to marked histological changes in the ovary, to uterine involution, and to changes in the levels of ovarian steroids (Reiter, 1968, 1974a; Seegal and Goldman, 1975; Legan, Karsch, and Foster, 1977; Van Horn and Resko, 1977; Plotka, Seal, Schmoller, Karns, and Keenlyne, 1977).

Inhibitory photoperiods not only cause gonadal involution but also lead to a marked diminution or even a complete cessation of sexual behavior, an effect that is similar to that observed after gonadectomy, although the changes brought about by noninductive photoperiods are more gradual. While this decline is partially due to the decrease in steroid levels, several findings indicate that other factors depending on photoperiod also contribute. Exogenous testosterone was more effective in restoring copulatory behavior in castrated male hamsters that were maintained in long photoperiods than in those exposed to short days (Morin and Zucker, 1978; Campbell, Finkelstein, and Turek, 1978). In castrated red deer stags, restoration of full-scale sexual behavior by testosterone was possible only during the normal rutting season, but not in the normal sexually quiescent season (Lincoln, Guinnes, and Short, 1972). Such findings might reflect photoperiodically altered sensitivity of the appropriate brain areas to androgens, or a contribution of gonadotrophins to sexual behavior.

GONADOTROPHINS. Gonadal activity is regulated by gonadotrophins, and changes in gonadal size and activity, induced by photoperiodic manipulation, should reflect changes in gonadotrophin production and release. Accordingly, in many mammals, drastic decreases in plasma and pituitary luteinizing hormone (LH) and follicle-stimulating hormone (FSH) have been observed in nonstimulatory photoperiods, especially in males. Lowered LH and

FSH levels were found in the golden hamster (Berndtson and Desjardins, 1974; Turek *et al.*, 1975b), the vole (Worth, Charlton, and MacKinnon, 1973), the ram (Pelletier and Ortavant, 1975a; Lincoln *et al.*, 1977), and the stag (Mirarchi, Howland, Scanlon, Kirkpatrick, and Sanford, 1978), to mention only a few examples. In females, the situation is more complex. In sexually active animals, there are marked variations in gonadotrophin levels during the estrus cycle, and these may be drastically changed under the influence of nonstimulatory photoperiods. Thus, in the golden hamster, in long photoperiods females are cyclic and show a prominent surge of LH and FSH at proestrus, while in short photoperiods the animals cease to show estrus cycles but exhibit a comparable peak of LH and FSH every day (Seegal and Goldman, 1975; Bridges, Tamarkin, and Goldman, 1976). A similar daily cycle of gonadotrophins occurs in female hamsters that are acyclic during lactation (Bridges and Goldman, 1975). The daily surge of LH persists after ovariectomy, which demonstrates that it does not depend on ovarian steroids. To me, these findings are difficult to reconcile with the generally accepted model of the estrus cycle in rodents, which postulates that the gonadotrophin surge at proestrus is the result of a positive feedback action of estrogen (J. Hoffmann, 1973). The existence of a daily gonadotrophin surge in acyclic hamsters rather poses the question of which factors suppress this surge in three out of four days in normal cyclic animals. Relatively few careful determinations of gonadotrophin values in different photoperiodic conditions have been made in females of other photoperiodic species; in ewes and mares, the data suggest that tonic gonadotrophin secretion is not very different in the breeding and in the nonbreeding season, except for the preovulatory surge at estrus (Yuthasastrokosol, Palmer, and Howland, 1975; Walton, McNeilly, McNeilly, and Cunningham, 1977; Oxender, Noden, and Hafs, 1977).

At least two factors contribute to the decrease of gonadotrophins in nonstimulatory photoperiods observed in many mammals. In two species, there is clear evidence that an altered sensitivity of the gonadotrophin control centers to negative steroid feedback is involved, a mechanism that was suggested by J. Hoffmann in 1973. Recent experiments in male hamsters show that the rise in plasma gonadotrophins after castration can be prevented or attenuated by exogenous testosterone in both long and short photoperiods; however, much smaller doses are effective after prolonged exposure to short photoperiods (Tamarkin, Hutchison, and Goldman, 1976a; Turek, 1977b). Stimulation of short-day hamsters by long photoperiods again reduces feedback sensitivity (Ellis and Turek, 1979). After prolonged exposure to short photoperiods, a spontaneous decrease in feedback sensitivity is observed, corresponding to the spontaneous testicular recrudescence in intact animals under these conditions (Ellis, Losee, and Turek, 1979). Pinealectomy, which prevents the gonadal reaction to short photoperiods, also prevents, at least partially, an increase in sensitivity to the negative feedback of gonadal steroids (Turek, 1979b). Similarly, in castrated rams, exogenous testosterone induces a more pronounced reduction in plasma LH values in nonstimulatory than in stimulatory photoperiods (Pelletier and Ortavant, 1975b). In ovariectomized ewes kept under natural conditions, plasma LH levels were high at all seasons, but in animals in which estradiol was implanted, thus providing a constant level, marked annual changes with high levels of LH only in the normal breeding season were observed; similar results were obtained by photoperiodic manipulation (Legan *et al.*, 1977; Legan and Karsch, 1979). These examples show that changes in the sensitivity of the hypothalamus–pituitary axis to negative feedback of gonadal steroids are a component of the photoperiodic mechanism regulating gonadal involution and recrudescence.

Several observations suggest that photoperiod can also alter gonadotrophin release independently of gonadal steroid hormones. In male hamsters that had been maintained in short photoperiods for several weeks and were then castrated, LH and FSH levels increased only slightly above the low values measured before castration, while in long photoperiods, a marked increase was found (Turek, Elliott, Alvis, and Menaker, 1975c). In male snowshoe hares that were trapped at different seasons and castrated, pituitary LH and FSH values 45 days later were only higher than in intact controls during the breeding season, while outside the breeding season, the same low values were measured in both castrated and intact hares (Davis and Meyer, 1973). In castrated rams, plasma LH levels were markedly higher in stimulatory than in nonstimulatory photoperiods (Pelletier and Ortavant, 1975a); in ovariectomized mares, plasma LH was higher in the breeding season than in the nonbreeding season (Garcia and Ginther, 1976).

Taken together, all these observations suggest that photoperiod-induced changes in gonadotrophin levels are due to at least two mechanisms, one depending on feedback effects from gonadal steroids, the other independent of gonadal factors. The relative contribution of these two mechanisms may differ from species to species, or even between sexes of the same species. Thus, in ovariectomized ewes, no seasonal change in plasma LH was detected (Legan *et al.*, 1977), while in castrated rams, marked changes were observed (Pelletier and Ortavant, 1975a).

PROLACTIN. In most photoperiodic mammals examined, differences in pituitary and plasma prolactin values were observed between long and short photoperiods. In golden hamsters of both sexes, Reiter and his colleagues (Reiter *et al.*, 1974; Reiter and Johnson, 1974a,b; Reiter, 1976) always found that gonadal regression, brought about by short photoperiods or by blinding, was accompanied by a marked diminution in pituitary prolactin content. Any procedure that interfered with the effect of short photoperiods on gonads, like pinealectomy or melatonin implantation, completely or at least partially prevented the decline in prolactin values. Although these workers did not observe significant changes in plasma prolactin caused by photoperiodic treatment, other authors have reported markedly lower values after exposure to short photoperiods in this species (Bex, Bartke, Goldman, and Dalterio, 1978; Matthews, Benson, and Richardson, 1978; Bartke, Goldman, Bex, Kelch, Smith, Dalterio, and Doherty, 1980).

In male golden hamsters, there is increasing evidence that prolactin participates in mediating the effect of short photoperiods on the gonads. Repeated injections of ovine prolactin, or ectopic pituitary homografts, delayed and attenuated regression of testes and accessory glands caused by short days or by blinding, or induced premature recrudescence (Bartke, Croft, and Dalterio, 1975; Bartke *et al.*, 1978; Bartke *et al.*, 1980; Bex *et al.*, 1978; Matthews *et al.*, 1978; Reiter and Ferguson, 1979). Since LH binding was markedly higher in animals injected with ovine prolactin or bearing pituitary homografts, and since injection of LH and FSH alone did not increase testicular size or plasma testosterone values, it is assumed that the main effect of prolactin is to increase the binding capacity of the Leydig cells for LH, although the finding that exogenous prolactin also increases FSH release might suggest that the effect is at least partially pituitary-mediated (Bex and Bartke, 1977; Bex *et al.*, 1978; Bartke *et al.*, 1980).

In general, the action of prolactin alone cannot account for the marked changes in testicular activity brought about by photoperiod in the hamster, as evidenced by the work on gonadotrophin regulation reported above. Moreover, it seems doubtful whether the results obtained in the golden hamster can be generalized to other species. While in the hamster photoperiodic treatment causes parallel changes in LH, FSH, and prolactin, in other species an inverse relationship between prolactin and the gonadotrophins has been observed. In the ram, high plasma prolactin values were measured in the sexually quiescent phase, and these values decreased toward the sexually active phase, while the initially low LH and FSH values increased, and changes in photoperiod had the opposite effects on prolactin and on gonadotrophins (Pelletier, 1973; Ravault, 1976; Lincoln, McNeilly, and Cameron, 1978; Schanbacher and Ford, 1979). In stags, prolactin and gonadotrophins also showed a reverse relationship (Mirarchi *et al.,* 1978). Both ram and stag are short-day breeders. It thus seems possible that the action of prolactin in this group differs from that in the hamster, and that the mechanism described in the golden hamster is limited to long-day breeders, to rodents, or even only to the golden hamster. Comparative studies are urgently needed.

BIRDS

Birds were the first vertebrates in which photoperiodic reactions were described (Rowan, 1925), and there is now a vast and ever-increasing literature on photoperiodism in this group. Photoperiodic effects were found in more than 50 species (Farner, Lewis, and Darden, 1973; Farner, 1975; Farner and Follett, 1980; Murton and Westwood, 1977). While the function measured to indicate photoperiodic effects is usually reproduction, molt, fat deposition, and migratory restlessness have also been demonstrated to be influenced by day length. Even the preferred direction during migration depends on the phase of the annual cycle and can be changed by photoperiodic treatment, as has been shown in the indigo bunting (Emlen, 1969). Seasonal dimorphism of plumage, as found in ptarmigans, can also be controlled by photoperiod (Høst, 1947; Stokkan, 1979). It should be pointed out that in birds, as in long-lived mammals, there are many demonstrations of a circannual cycle—in gonadal size and activity, in molt, and in other functions—that can, under suitable conditions, persist in spite of the fact that the photoperiod remains unchanged (Chapter 21). Here the photoperiod apparently synchronizes the annual cycle rather than causing it.

In the bulk of photoperiodic work in birds, gonadal size and activity—and more recently, changes in gonadotrophins—have been measured to assay photoperiodic effects. Since in females in most cases only partial ovarian development is induced by photoperiod, while final development depends on other sources of information (e.g., weather conditions and the presence and behavior of a partner), in the majority of studies males have been used. It should be stressed, however, that the basic principle holds for both sexes. There are many excellent recent reviews that cover many aspects of bird photoperiodism (e.g., Farner and Follett, 1980; Farner, 1975; Murton and Westwood, 1977; Turek, 1978; Follett and Davies, 1975; Follett and Robinson, 1980); here, only some general features will be mentioned, and similarities and especially differences to the situation in mammals are discussed. As far as I am aware, in all bird species studied in sufficient detail, long photoperiods stimulate gonadal development and recrudescence. Hence, findings in birds are compared here with findings in long-day mammals, and in particular in hamsters, since this mammalian group has been most thoroughly studied.

KLAUS HOFFMANN

In practically all avian species that react to photoperiod, long light times—applied in late fall, winter, or early spring—can prematurely induce gonadal development. There is a minimum threshold for the length of the light period to be stimulatory. As has been shown in males of several species, above this threshold the rate of development depends on the length of the photoperiod, at least within a certain range, longer light times resulting in faster development (Farner and Wilson, 1957; Farner, 1975; Farner and Follett, 1980; Follett and Robinson, 1980). Such findings have so far not been reported in mammals, and the rather precisely defined critical photoperiods in hamsters suggest that here, photoperiodic stimulation is an all-or-nothing phenomenon once it has surpassed the threshold and is independent of the absolute length of the stimulatory photoperiod. However, systematic quantitative examinations of this question are not available in mammals. One further point should be mentioned: in some bird species, paradoxical effects of ultrashort photoperiods have been reported that have not yet been explained; they may be the result of the artificial experimental situation (Farner, Donham, Lewis, Mattocks, Dardon, and Smith, 1977).

Reactions to long photoperiods are remarkably fast in birds, as evidenced by rapid testicular development. A significant rise of gonadotrophin levels has been found even before the end of the first long photoperiod to which birds were exposed, as was demonstrated in Japanese quail and in two species of passerines (Follett, Mattocks, and Farner, 1974; Follett and Robinson, 1980). In this respect, the avian photoperiodic response seems to differ from that found in mammals.

Birds were the first vertebrates in which evidence for a circadian oscillator of photosensitivity underlying photoperiodic time measurement was obtained (Hamner, 1963). Since then, a considerable amount of evidence in different bird species has been amassed to support this contention (Follett, 1973; Follett et al., 1974; Farner, 1975; Turek, 1978). In this respect, data on both birds and mammals point to the same formal mechanism of photoperiodic time measurement. Because in both groups only a few species have been studied so far, it seems premature to claim that this finding holds for all photoperiodic avian and mammalian species. Photoperiodic reactions have probably been developed several times, and the fact that in lizards an hourglass mechanism of photoperiodic time measurement has been demonstrated (see p. 465) should warn against premature generalizations. The data so far available on birds and mammals, however, all support the assumption of a circadian mechanism underlying photoperiodic time measurement.

While in the majority of avian species long photoperiods hasten development, it is more difficult to make generalizations about the effect of short photoperiods. Wide species differences exist in the timing and duration of the breeding season. Apparently, in some pigeons and waterfowl, breeding may be ended by the influence of short photoperiods (Murton and Westwood, 1977). A species in which this was experimentally shown is the Japanese quail, which has been widely used for the investigation of photoperiodic effects on gonadal and gonadotrophin activity. Here, gonadal growth is initiated by long photoperiods, and as long as these conditions are maintained, the gonads remain large and active. Exposure to short photoperiods induces gonadal regression and a decline in plasma gonadotrophin levels. However, whether a photoperiod is considered long or short depends on the previous photoperiodic conditions. Thus, photoperiods that are stimulatory in the regressed condition can induce regression if they follow longer photoperiods (Follett and

Robinson, 1980). To my knowledge, this is the first demonstration in vertebrates that the critical photoperiod may depend on previous conditions. This phenomenon may be more widespread. In the Japanese quail, the effect of short photoperiods can be immediately reversed by again exposing the birds to long photoperiods (Follett and Robinson, 1980). In some other species, there is also evidence that short photoperiods can end prematurely and inverse testicular development, if this has been initiated by long light times (see Gwinner, 1977, and Figure 2 in Turek, 1978).

Photoperiodic Refractoriness

In the majority of avian species, there is a marked photoperiodic refractoriness; in fact, this phenomenon was first described in birds and has been discussed intensively (Farner and Follett, 1980; Farner, 1975; Murton and Westwood, 1977; Follett and Robinson, 1980). In birds moved into long photoperiods in winter or spring, testes develop and reach full size and activity. After some time, however, testes regress in many species without any change in the photoperiodic regime, and they may remain regressed and apparently refractory to the effects of long photoperiods. Similarly, under natural conditions, gonads often regress when the photoperiods are still much longer than those that caused development or are even still lengthening. In order to break refractoriness and render the birds again sensitive to the stimulatory effect of long photoperiods, a prolonged exposure to short photoperiods is required. It is evident that here, the situation is just the opposite of that in hamsters, in which *short* photoperiods induce regression while recrudescence is spontaneous, and an exposure to *long* photoperiods is necessary to break refractoriness and render the animals again sensitive to the influence of short photoperiods.

Organs and Physiological Processes Involved

Light Perception. While in mammals photoperiodic control depends exclusively on the retina, in birds it has been definitely established that extraretinal photoreceptors are predominantly or even exclusively responsible for conveying the photoperiodic message. This effect was first shown in the domestic mallard (Benoit, 1935) and has since been demonstrated also in a variety of passerine species and in the quail (for reviews, see Benoit, 1970; Menaker, 1971; McMillan, Underwood, Elliott, Stetson, and Menaker, 1975; Menaker and Underwood, 1976). While for the mallard, Benoit (1970) suggested that both the retina and the extraretinal photoreceptors participate in gonadal stimulation, more recent experimentation, and a critical evaluation of old and new experiments, suggests that the retina is not involved in photostimulation in birds, at least not in the sparrow (McMillan *et al.*, 1975).

The site and nature of the extraretinal photoreceptors is not yet clear. Experiments with direct encephalic illumination suggest that most of the photoreceptors lie either within the ventromedial hypothalamus or in sites ventral thereto (Yokoyama, Oksche, Darden, and Farner, 1978). The spectral characteristics of the light penetrating into the brain, as well as the possible nature of the extraretinal photoreceptors, have recently been discussed by Hartwig and van Veen (1979).

Pineal Gland. The assumption that the extraretinal photoreceptors involved in the photoperiodic reaction in birds are localized within the pineal has not been supported in experimental studies. Although the pineal, at least of the chicken, is clearly light-sensitive (Binkley, Riebman, and Reilly, 1978; Deguchi, 1979), experiments on the photoperiodic reaction in pinealectomized and blinded birds have shown that neither the eyes nor the pineal are essential for the photoperiodic reaction (Menaker, 1971; Oishi and Lauber, 1973; Menaker and Oksche, 1974; Menaker and Underwood, 1976). In general, the experiments performed so far suggest that the eyes and the pineal may, at best, serve auxiliary roles in the reception of photoperiod but are not the main photoreceptors involved.

Besides the question of whether the pineal is involved as a photoreceptor in the photoperiodic reaction, it must also be asked whether it has *any* role in avian photoperiodism, a question that is suggested by the observations in mammals. As already mentioned, most of the available evidence indicates that it has not. However, there are several isolated findings that suggest that the pineal gland might play some role in regulating the annual cycle, at least in some species, though the evidence is not consistent (for review and discussion, see Ralph, 1970; Menaker and Oksche, 1974; Turek, 1978; Gwinner and Dittami, 1980). In general, it seems obvious that the contribution of the avian pineal to the photoperiodic mechanism, if it does exist, is different from that found in mammals.

Endocrine Aspects

As has already been mentioned, stimulatory photoperiods in winter or spring cause a very rapid increase in plasma LH and FSH levels, followed by an increase in gonadal size and somewhat later in testosterone in males. Experiments with gonadectomized birds clearly show that the photoperiod can alter gonadotrophin secretion directly, and changes in feedback sensitivity need not be involved, though they might contribute to some extent (see Follett and Robinson, 1980, for review and discussion). It is assumed that the elevated gonadotrophin values in long days represent an increase of GnRH output from the hypothalamus. Experiments with hypothalamic lesions, or with implantation of sexual steroids or inhibitors, suggest that the basal infundibular nucleus of the hypothalamus is essentially involved in photoperiodically regulated gonadotrophin release, and that the anterior hypothalamus also plays an essential role (Davies and Follett, 1975; Yokoyama *et al.,* 1978). Gonadal regression, spontaneous or induced, is anticipated by a rapid decrease of gonadotrophin levels.

The physiological basis of spontaneous regression and photorefractoriness is unknown; several hypotheses for its mechanism have been proposed (Follett and Robinson, 1980). One of these assumes that antigonadal effects of thyroidal hormones may be involved. Especially in ducks, but also in other groups, it has been found that levels of thyroxin and of androgens show a nearly inverse relationship in the annual cycle, with highest values of T_4 at the time of gonadal regression (Murton and Westwood, 1977; Assenmacher and Jallageas, 1978). Thyroidectomy and application of exogenous thyroxin have been shown to interfere with the annual cycle in several bird species (Wieselthier and van Tienhoven, 1972; Chandola and Thapliyal, 1978).

From observations on the circadian pattern of plasma corticosterone and of prolactin in different seasons, and from injections of these hormones at different phase angles, Meier and colleagues have concluded that the phase relationship of these two hormones is causally involved in governing the annual cycle of reproduction, as well as of fat metabolism and of migratory activity, in the white-throated sparrow (Meier, 1976). These findings would lend support to the internal coincidence model of photoperiodic action (Pittendrigh, 1972). It must be stressed, however, that the changes observed in testicular size were usually minor, that is, about 3- or 4-fold as compared to about 50- to 100-fold after photostimulation. Moreover, these results have so far been observed in one species only. Studies in other species and other laboratories are urgently needed.

LOWER VERTEBRATES

Annual cycles of a host of functions are widespread in poikilothermic vertebrates. Though these have been studied much less intensively than birds or mammals, photoperiodic effects, especially on gonadal state and activity, have been reported in a number of species of fish and Reptilia and in some Amphibia (for reviews, see Harrington, 1959; van Tienhoven, 1968; Schwassmann, 1971; Licht, 1971a; de Vlaming, 1974; Fischer, 1974). It is very difficult to make any generalizations on the photoperiodic mechanism in these poikilotherms, since temperature has a major influence on the annual cycle, replacing or often superseding the effect of photoperiod. The same photoperiodic treatment may have drastically different effects, depending not only on the phase of the annual cycle but also on ambient temperature (e.g., Licht, 1971b; Fischer, 1974). Moreover, strong interspecific differences exist, and different findings have been reported even in different populations of the same species (Fischer, 1974). Together with the paucity of data in these groups, a comparison with the situation in birds and mammals seems premature.

Several points deserve mentioning, however. To my knowledge, there is as yet no conclusive proof of circadian involvement in the photoperiodic time measurement of any lower vertebrate. Baggerman (1972) has shown in the stickleback that short photoperiods, in which the dark time was interrupted by a 2-hr light pulse, could induce development similar to that caused by full photoperiods. Effects of light pulses, depending on the time of day of application, have also been reported in catfish (Vasal and Sundararaj, 1975). While such findings are not conclusive evidence of circadian involvement, they are at least suggestive. In the lizard *Anolis,* Underwood (1978) has recently provided convincing evidence that in this species, photoperiodic time measurement is based not on a circadian rhythm of photoperiodic sensitivity but on an hourglass mechanism that measures the absolute length of the light period. Further studies are necessary to determine whether such findings can be generalized, and in view of the different mechanisms of photoperiodic time measurement described in different insect species (Chapter 22), caution is necessary.

Little seems to be known about the photoreceptors involved in the perception of photoperiodic signals in lower vertebrates, though extraretinal photoreception has been described in all groups. In the lizard *Anolis,* Underwood (1975) has shown that neither the lateral eyes nor the parietal eye is essential for conveying the photoperiodic message. From these experiments, it cannot be excluded that the extraretinal photoreceptors involved are located within the pineal body. However, experiments on the entrainment of circadian rhythms by light in lizards have conclusively demonstrated that extraretinal photoreceptors must also reside within the brain (Underwood and Menaker, 1976); hence, the situation here may be similar to that found in birds.

Finally, it must be mentioned that there is evidence of pineal involvement in the photoperiodic process in some reptiles and fishes (e.g., Hoffman, 1970; Levey, 1973; de Vlaming and Vodicnic, 1978), though generalizations seem premature at present. While most workers on photoperiodic influences in lower vertebrates have used morphological criteria, endocrine changes have also been measured (e.g., Whitehead, Bromage, Breton, and Matty, 1979). There is an excellent recent review on testicular regulation in lower vertebrates (Callard, Callard, Lance, Bolaffi, and Rosset, 1978); in general, the hypothalamus–pituitary–gonad system and its regulation seem to be similar to that in birds and mammals.

Concluding Remarks

An attempt has been made here to present a condensed review of the photoperiodic regulation of annual cycles in vertebrates. Emphasis has been placed on recent developments, and especially on the analysis of the underlying physiological mechanisms. This is a rapidly developing field, and some of the generalizations and oversimplifications made in this chapter will soon be obsolete. An admittedly subjective view of the present state of this field has been attempted, in order to point out some of the present ideas and concepts, and to stimulate further work. Because of the rigid limitations in space set by the editor, the fields covered and the work and publications quoted had to be limited. Especially the lower vertebrates have been unduly neglected.

It should be stressed that while photoperiodic regulation of the annual cycle is widespread in the animal kingdom, photoperiod is only one of the many factors that may influence and synchronize the annual cycle. Hardly any mention of the important work on these other factors has been made here. For the many possibilities, Chapter 20 should be consulted.

References

Allais, C., and Martinet, L. Relation between daylight ratio, plasma progesterone levels and timing of nidation in mink *(Mustela vison)*. *Journal of Reproduction and Fertility,* 1978, *54,* 133–136.

Arendt, J. Radioimmunoassayable melatonin: Circulating patterns in man and sheep. *Progress in Brain Research,* 1979, *52,* 249–258.

Assenmacher, I., and Jallageas, M. Annual endocrine cycles and environment in birds with special reference to male ducks. In I. Assenmacher and D. S. Farner (Eds.), *Environmental Endocrinology.* Berlin, Heidelberg, New York: Springer, 1978.

Axelrod, J. The pineal gland: A neurochemical transducer. *Science,* 1974, *184,* 1341–1348.

Baggerman, B. Photoperiodic responses in the stickleback and their control by a daily rhythm of photosensitivity. *General and Comparative Endocrinology,* 1972, *Suppl. 3,* 1972, 466–476.

Baker, J. R. Evolution of breeding seasons. In G. R. de Beer (Ed.), *Evolution* (Essays presented to T. S. Goodrich). Oxford: Clarendon Press, 1938.

Baker, J. R., and Ranson, R. M. Factors affecting the breeding of the field mouse *(Microtus agrestis)*. I. Light. *Proceedings of the Royal Society of London,* Series B, 1932, *110,* 313–322.

Bartke, A., Croft, B. T., and Dalterio, S. Prolactin restores plasma testosterone levels and stimulates testicular growth in hamsters exposed to short day-length. *Endocrinology,* 1975, *97,* 1601–1604.

Bartke, A., Goldman, B. D., Bex, F. J., and Dalterio, S. Mechanism of reversible loss of reproductive capacity in a seasonally-breeding mammal. *International Journal of Andrology,* 1978, *Suppl. 2,* 345–353.

Bartke, A., Goldman, B. D., Bex, F. J., Kelch, R. P., Smith, M. S., Dalterio, S., and Doherty, P. C. Effects of prolactin on testicular regression and recrudescence in the golden hamster. *Endocrinology,* 1980, *106,* 167–172.

Benoit, J. Rôle des yeux dans l'action stimulante de la lumière sur le développement testiculaire chez le Canard. *Comptes Rendus de la Société de Biologie* (Paris), 1935, *118*, 669–671.

Benoit, J. Etude de l'action des radiations visibles sur la gonadostimulation et de leur pénétration intra-cranienne chez les oiseaux et les mammifères. In J. Benoit and I. Assenmacher (Eds.), *La Photorégulation de la Reproduction chez les Oiseaux et les Mammifères*. Paris: CNRS, 1970.

Berndtson, W. E., and Desjardins, C. Circulating LH and FSH levels and testicular function in hamsters during light deprivation and subsequent photoperiodic stimulation. *Endocrinology*, 1974, *95*, 195–205.

Bex, F. J., and Bartke, A. Testicular LH binding in the hamster: Modification by photoperiod and prolactin. *Endocrinology*, 1977, *100*, 1223–1226.

Bex, F., Bartke, A., Goldman, B. D., and Dalterio, S. Prolactin, growth hormone, luteinizing hormone receptors, and seasonal changes in testicular activity in the golden hamster. *Endocrinology*, 1978, *103*, 2069–2080.

Binkley, S. Comparative biochemistry of the pineal gland of birds and mammals. *American Zoologist*, 1976, *16*, 57–65.

Binkley, S. A., Riebman, J. B., and Reilly, K. B. The pineal gland: A biological clock in vitro. *Science*, 1978, *202*, 1198–1201.

Bissonette, T. H. Modification of mammalian sexual cycles. I. Reactions of ferrets *(Putorius vulgaris)* of both sexes to electric light added after dark in November and December. *Proceedings of the Royal Society of London*, Series B, 1932, *110*, 322–336.

Bittman, E. L. Photoperiodic influences on testicular regression in the golden hamster: Termination of scotorefractoriness. *Biology of Reproduction*, 1978, *17*, 871–877.

Brackmann, M. Melatonin delays puberty in the Djungarian hamster. *Naturwissenschaften*, 1977, *64*, 642–643.

Brackmann, M., and Hoffmann, K. Pinealectomy and photoperiod influence testicular development in the Djungarian hamster. *Naturwissenschaften*, 1977, *64*, 341–342.

Bridges, R. S., and Goldman, B. D. Diurnal rhythms in gonadotropins and progesterone in lactating and photoperiod induced acyclic hamsters. *Biology of Reproduction*, 1975, *13*, 617–622.

Bridges, R., Tamarkin, L., and Goldman, B. Effects of photoperiod and melatonin on reproduction in the Syrian hamster. *Annales de Biologie animale, Biochimie, Biophysique*, 1976, *16*, 399–408.

Brown, G. M., Basinska, J., Bubenik, G., Sibony, D., Grota, L. J., and Stancer, H. C. Gonadal effects of pinealectomy and immunization against *N*-acetilindolalkylamines in the hamster. *Neuroendocrinology*, 1976, *22*, 289–297.

Bünning, E. Die endogene Tagesrhythmik als Grundlage der photoperiodischen Reaktion. *Berichte der Deutschen Botanischen Gesellschaft*, 1936, *54*, 590–607.

Callard, I. P., Callard, G. V., Lance, V., Bolaffi, J. L., and Rosset, J. S. Testicular regulation in nonmammalian vertebrates. *Biology of Reproduction*, 1978, *18*, 16–43.

Campbell, C. B. G., and Ramaley, J. A. Retinohypothalamic projections: Correlation with onset of the adrenal rhythm in infant rats. *Endocrinology*, 1974, *94*, 1201–1211.

Campbell, C. S., Finkelstein, J. S., and Turek, F. W. The interaction of photoperiod and testosterone on the development of copulatory behaviour in castrated male hamsters. *Physiology and Behavior*, 1978, *21*, 409–415.

Canivec, R., and Bonnin, M. Delayed implantation is under environmental control in the badger (*Meles meles* L.). *Nature*, 1979, *278*, 849–850.

Chandola, A., and Thapliyal, J. P. Regulation of reproductive cycles of tropical spotted munia and weaverbird. In I. Assenmacher and D. S. Farner (Eds.), *Environmental Endocrinology*. Berlin, Heidelberg, New York: Springer, 1978.

Charlton, H. M., Grocock, C. A., and Ostberg, A. The effects of pinealectomy and superior cervical ganglionectomy on the testis of the vole, *Microtus agrestis. Journal of Reproduction and Fertility*, 1976, *48*, 377–379.

Czyba, J. C., Girod, C., and Durand, N. Sur l'antagonisme épiphysohypophysaire et les variations saisonnières de la spermatogénèse chez le hamster doré *(Mesocricetus auratus)*. *Comptes Rendus des Séances de la Société de Biologie*, 1964, *158*, 742–745.

Davies, D. T., and Follett, B. K. The neuroendocrine control of gonadotropin release in the Japanese quail. *Proceedings of the Royal Society of London*, Series B, 1975, *191*, 285–315.

Davis, G. J., and Meyer, R. K. Seasonal variation in LH and FSH of bilaterally castrated snowshoe hares. *General and Comparative Endocrinology*, 1973, *20*, 61–68.

Deguchi, T. A circadian oscillator in cultured cells of chicken pineal gland. *Nature*, 1979, *282*, 94–96.

de Vlaming, V. L. Environmental and endocrine control of teleost reproduction. In C. Schreck (Ed.), *Control of Sex in Fishes*. Blacksburg, Virginia: Sea Grant and V.P.I. & S.U. Press, 1974.

de Vlaming, V. L., and Vodicnik, M. J. Seasonal effects of pinealectomy on gonadal activity in the goldfish, *Carassius auratus*. *Biology of Reproduction*, 1978, *19*, 57–63.

Dixit, V. P., Sharma, O. P., and Agrawal, M. The effects of light deprivation/blindness on testicular function of gerbil (*Meiones hurrianae* Jerdon). *Endocrinologie*, 1977, *70*, 13–18.

Dogterom, J., Snijdewint, F. G. M., Pevet, P., and Swaab, D. F. Studies on the presence of vasopression, oxytocin and vasotocin in the pineal gland, subcommissural organ and fetal pituitary gland: Failure to demonstrate vasotocine in mammals. *Journal of Endocrinology*, 1980, *84*, 115–123.

Ebels, I., and Benson, B. A survey of the evidence that unidentified pineal substances affect the reproductive system in mammals. In R. J. Reiter (Ed.), *The Pineal Gland and Reproduction*. Basel: Karger, 1978.

Eichler, V. B., and Moore, R. Y. The primary and accessory optic system in the golden hamster. *Acta Anatomica*, 1974, *89*, 359–371.

Elliott, J. A. Circadian rhythms and photoperiodic time measurement in mammals. *Federation Proceedings*, 1976, *35*, 2339–2346.

Ellis, G. B., and Turek, F. W. Time course of the photoperiod-induced change in sensitivity of the hypothalamic–pituitary axis to testosterone feedback in castrated male hamsters. *Endocrinology*, 1979, *104*, 625–630.

Ellis, G. B., Losee, S. H., and Turek, F. W. Prolonged exposure of castrated male hamsters to a nonstimulatory photoperiod: Spontaneous change in sensitivity of the hypothalamic–pituitary axis to testosterone feedback. *Endocrinology*, 1979, *104*, 631–635.

Emlen, S. T. Bird migration: Influence of physiological state upon celestial orientation. *Science*, 1969, *165*, 716–718.

Farner, D. S. Photoperiodic controls in the secretion of gonadotropins in birds. *American Zoologist*, 1975, *15* (Suppl. 1), 117–135.

Farner, D. S., and Follett, B. K. Reproductive periodicity in birds. In E. J. W. Barrington (Ed.), *Hormones and Evolution*. London: Academic Press, 1980.

Farner, D. S., and Wilson, A. C. A quantitative examination of testicular growth in the white-crowned sparrow. *Biological Bulletin*, 1957, *113*, 254–267.

Farner, D. S., Lewis, R. A., and Darden, T. R. Photoperiodic control mechanisms. In P. L. Altman and D. S. Dittmer (Eds.), *Biology Data Book* (2nd ed.). Vol. 2. Bethesda, Md.: Federation of American Societies of Experimental Biology, 1973.

Farner, D. S., Donham, R. S., Lewis, R. A., Mattocks, P. W., Dardon, R. R., and Smith, J. P. The circadian component in the photoperiodic mechanism of the house sparrow, *Passer domesticus*. *Physiological Zoology*, 1977, *50*, 247–268.

Farrar, G. M., and Clarke, J. R. Effect of chemical sympathectomy and pinealectomy upon gonads of voles (*Microtus agrestis*) exposed to short photoperiod. *Neuroendocrinology*, 1976, *22*, 134–143.

Figala, J., Hoffmann, K., and Goldau, G. Zur Jahresperiodik beim Dsungarischen Zwerghamster *Phodopus sungorus* Pallas. *Oecologia*, 1973, *12*, 89–118.

Fischer, K. Die Steuerung der Fortpflanzungszyklen bei männlichen Reptilien. *Fortschritte der Zoologie*, 1974, *22*, 362–390.

Follett, B. K. Circadian rhythms and photoperiodic time measurement in birds. *Journal of Reproduction and Fertility*, 1973, *Suppl. 19*, 5–18.

Follett, B. K., and Davies, D. T. Photoperiodicity and the neuroendocrine control of reproduction in birds. *Symposia of the Zoological Society* (London), 1975, *35*, 199–224.

Follett, B. K., and Robinson, J. E. Photoperiod and gonadotrophin secretion in birds. In R. J. Reiter and B. K. Follett (Eds.), *Progress in Reproductive Biology*. Vol. 5. Basel: Karger, 1980.

Follett, B. K., Mattocks, P. W., and Farner, D. S. Circadian function in the photoperiodic induction of gonadotropin secretion in the white-crowned sparrow, *Zonotrichia leucophrys* gambelli. *Proceedings of the National Academy of Sciences of the USA*, 1974, *71*, 1666–1669.

Frieling, R. Untersuchungen zur Spermatogenese und zum Einfluss der Photoperiode auf die Hodenentwicklung beim Dsungarischen Hamster (*Phodopus sungorus* Pallas). Doctoral thesis, Universität München, 1979.

Garcia, M. C., and Ginther, O. J. Effects of ovariectomy and season on plasma luteinizing hormones in mares. *Endocrinology*, 1976, *98*, 958–962.

Garnier, D. H., Ortavant, R., Mansard, P. X., and Terqui, M. Influence de la lumière sur le variations de la testostéronémie chez le bélier: Mise en évidence d'une phase photosensible au cours du rythme diurne. *Comptes Rendus Hebdomadaires de Séances de l'Académie de Sciences, Paris*, Serie D, 1977, *284*, 61–64.

Gaston, S., and Menaker, M. Photoperiodic control of hamster testis. *Science*, 1967, *158*, 925–928.

Goldman, B., Hall, V., Hollister, C., Roychoudhury, P., Tamarkin, L., and Westrom, W. Effects of melatonin on the reproductive system in intact and pinealectomized male hamsters maintained under various photoperiods. *Endocrinology*, 1979, *104*, 82–88.

Goss, R. J. Photoperiodic control of antler cycles in deer. III. Decreasing versus increasing day lengths. *Journal of Experimental Zoology*, 1976, *197*, 307–312.

Grocock, C. A., and Clarke, J. R. Photoperiodic control of testis activity in the vole, *Microtus agrestis*. *Journal of Reproduction and Fertility*, 1974, *39*, 336–347.

Gwinner, E. Photoperiodic synchronization of circannual rhythms in the European starling *(Sturnus vulgaris)*. *Naturwissenschaften*, 1977, *64*, 44.

Gwinner, E., and Dittami, J. Pinealectomy affects the circannual testicular rhythm in European starlings. *Journal of Comparative Physiology*, 1980, *136*, 345–348.

Hamner, W. M. Diurnal rhythm and photoperiodism in testicular recrudescence of the house finch. *Science*, 1963, *142*, 1294–1295.

Harrington, R. W. Photoperiodism in fishes in relation to the annual sexual cycle. In R. B. Withrow (Ed.), *Photoperiodism and Related Phenomena in Plants and Animals*. Washington, D.C.: AAAS, 1959.

Hartwig, H. G., and van Veen, T. Spectral characteristics of visible radiation penetrating into the brain and stimulating extraretinal photoreceptors. *Journal of Comparative Physiology*, 1979, *130*, 277–282.

Hasler, J. F., Buhl, A. E., and Banks, E. M. The influence of photoperiod on growth and sexual function in male and female collared lemmings *(Dicrostonyx groenlandicus)*. *Journal of Reproduction and Fertility*, 1976, *46*, 323–329.

Herbert, J. The pineal gland and light-induced oestrus in ferrets. *Journal of Endocrinology*, 1969, *43*, 625–636.

Herbert, J. The role of the pineal gland in the control by light of the reproductive cycle of the ferret. In G. E. W. Wolstenholme and J. Knight (Eds.), *The Pineal Gland* (A Ciba Foundation Symposium). Edinburgh: Churchill Livingstone, 1971.

Herbert, J. Initial observations on pinealectomized ferrets kept for long periods in either daylight or artificial illumination. *Journal of Endocrinology*, 1972, *55*, 591–597.

Herbert, J., Stacey, P. M., and Thorpe, D. H. Recurrent breeding seasons in pinealectomized or optic-nerve-sectioned ferrets. *Journal of Endocrinology*, 1978, *78*, 389–397.

Hoffman, R. A. The epiphysial complex in fish and reptiles. *American Zoologist*, 1970, *10*, 191–199.

Hoffman, R. A., and Reiter, R. J. Pineal gland: Influence on the gonads of male hamsters. *Science*, 1965, *148*, 1609–1611.

Hoffmann, J. C. The influence of photoperiods on reproductive function in female mammals. In R. O. Greep (Ed.), *Handbook of Physiology*. Section 7, Vol. 2, Part 1. Washington, D.C.: American Physiological Society, 1973.

Hoffmann, K. Melatonin inhibits photoperiodically induced testis development in a dwarf hamster. *Naturwissenschaften*, 1972, *59*, 218–219.

Hoffmann, K. The influence of photoperiod and melatonin on testis size, body weight, and pelage colour in the Djungarian hamster *(Phodopus sungorus)*. *Journal of Comparative Physiology*, 1973, *95*, 267–282.

Hoffmann, K. Testicular involution in short photoperiods inhibited by melatonin. *Naturwissenschaften*, 1974, *61*, 364–365.

Hoffmann, K. Die Funktion des Pineals bei der Jahresperiodik der Säuger. *Nova Acta Leopoldina*, 1977, *46*, 217–229.

Hoffmann, K. Effects of short photoperiods on puberty, growth and moult in the Djungarian hamster *(Phodopus sungorus)*. *Journal of Reproduction and Fertility*, 1978a, *54*, 29–35.

Hoffmann, K. Photoperiodic mechanism in hamsters: The participation of the pineal gland. In I. Assenmacher and D. S. Farner (Eds.), *Environmental Endocrinology*. Berlin, Heidelberg, New York: Springer, 1978b.

Hoffmann, K. Photoperiod, pineal, melatonin and reproduction in hamsters. *Progress in Brain Research*, 1979a, *52*, 397–415.

Hoffmann, K. Photoperiodic effects in the Djungarian hamster: One minute of light during darktime mimics influence of long photoperiods on testicular recrudescence, body weight and pelage colour. *Experientia*, 1979b, *35*, 1529–1530.

Hoffmann, K., and Küderling, I. Pinealectomy inhibits stimulation of testicular development by long photoperiods in a hamster *(Phodopus sungorus)*. *Experientia*, 1975, *31*, 122–123.

Hoffmann, K., and Küderling, I. Antigonadal effects of melatonin in pinealectomized Djungarian hamsters. *Naturwissenschaften*, 1977, *64*, 339–340.

Hoffmann, K., and Nieschlag, E. Circadian rhythm of plasma testosterone in the male Djungarian hamster *(Phodopus sungorus)*. *Acta Endocrinologica*, 1977, *86*, 193–199.

Hoffmann, K., Illnerova, H., and Vanecek, J. Pineal *N*-acetyl-transferase activity in the Djungarian hamster. *Naturwissenschaften*, 1980, *67*, 408–409.

Høst, P. Effects of light on the moults and sequences of plumage in the willow ptarmigan. *Auk*, 1942, *59*, 388–403.

Illnerova, H., Backström, M., Sääf, J., Wetterberg, L., and Vangbo, B. Melatonin in rat pineal gland and plasma; Rapid parallel decline after light exposure at night. *Neuroscience Letters,* 1978, *9,* 189–193.

Illnerova, H., Vanecek, J., Krecek, J., Wetterberg, L., and Sääf, J. Effect of one minute exposure to light at night on rat pineal serotonin *N*-acetyltransferase and melatonin. *Journal of Neurochemistry,* 1979, *32,* 673–675.

Klein, D. C. The role of serotonin *N*-acetyltransferase in the adrenergic regulation of indole metabolism in the pineal gland. In J. Barchas and E. Usdin (Eds.), *Serotonin and Behavior.* New York: Academic Press, 1973.

Klein, D. C. Pineal gland as a model of neuroendocrine control systems. In S. M. Reichlin, R. J. Baldessarini, and J. B. Martin (Eds.), *The Hypothalamus.* New York: Raven Press, 1978.

Klein, D. C., and Moore, R. Y. Pineal *N*-actyltransferase and hydroxy-indole-O-methyltransferase: Control by the retinohypothalamic tract and the suprachiasmatic nucleus. *Brain Research,* 1979, *174,* 245–262.

Knigge, K. M., and Sheridan, M. N. Pineal function in hamsters bearing melatonin antibodies. *Life Sciences,* 1976, *19,* 1235–1238.

Legan, S. J., and Karsch, F. J. Neuroendocrine regulation of the estrous cycle and seasonal breeding in the ewe. *Biology of Reproduction,* 1979, *20,* 74–85.

Legan, S. J., Karsch, F. J., and Foster, D. L. The endocrine control of seasonal reproductive function in the ewe: A marked change in response to the negative feedback action of estradiol on luteinizing hormone secretion. *Endocrinology,* 1977, *101,* 818–824.

Le Gros Clark, W. E., McKeown, T., and Zuckerman, S. Visual pathways concerned in gonadal stimulation in ferrets. *Proceedings of the Royal Society of London,* Series B, 1939, *126,* 449–468.

Levey, I. L. Effects of pinealectomy and melatonin injections at different seasons on ovarian activity in the lizard *Anolis carolinensis. Journal of Experimental Zoology,* 1973, *185,* 169–174.

Licht, P. Regulation of the annual testis cycle by photoperiod and temperature in the lizard *Anolis carolinensis. Ecology,* 1971a, *52,* 240–252.

Licht, P. Response of the male reproductive system to interrupted-night photoperiods in the lizard *Anolis carolinensis. Zeitschrift für vergleichende Physiologie,* 1971b, *73,* 274–284.

Lin, H., Alexander, M., and Giolli, R. A. The accessory optic fiber system of the golden hamster with special reference to the retino-hypothalamic projection. *Anatomical Record,* 1976, *186,* 451–460.

Lincoln, G. A. Induction of testicular growth and sexual activity in rams by a "skeleton" short-day photoperiod. *Journal of Reproduction and Fertility,* 1978, *52,* 179–181.

Lincoln, G. A., and MacKinnon, P. C. B. A study of seasonally delayed puberty in the male hare, *Lepus europaeus. Journal of Reproduction and Fertility,* 1976, *46,* 123–128.

Lincoln, G. A., Youngson, R. W., and Short, R. V. The social and sexual behaviour of the red deer stag. *Journal of Reproduction and Fertility,* 1970, *Suppl. 11,* 71–103.

Lincoln, G. A., Guiness, F., and Short, R. V. The way in which testosterone controls the social and sexual behavior of the red deer stag *(Cervus elaphus). Hormones and Behavior,* 1972, *3,* 375–396.

Lincoln, G. A., Peet, M. J., and Cunningham, R. A. Seasonal and circadian changes in the episodic release of follicle-stimulating hormone, luteinizing hormone and testosterone in rams exposed to artifical photoperiods. *Journal of Endocrinology,* 1977, *72,* 337–349.

Lincoln, G. A., McNeilly, A. S., and Cameron, C. L. The effects of a sudden decrease or increase in daylength on prolactin secretion in the ram. *Journal of Reproduction and Fertility,* 1978, *52,* 305–311.

Lynch, G. R., and Epstein, A. L. Melatonin induced changes in gonads, pelage and thermogenic characters in the white-footed mouse, *Peromyscus leucopus. Comparative Biochemistry and Physiology,* 1976, *53C,* 67–68.

Matthews, M. J., Benson, B., and Richardson, D. L. Partial maintenance of testes and accessory organs in blinded hamsters by homoplastic anterior pituitary grafts or exogenous prolactin. *Life Sciences,* 1978, *23,* 1131–1138.

Maurel, D. Seasonal changes of the testicular and thyroid functions in the badger, *Meles meles* L. In I. Assenmacher and D. S. Farner (Eds.), *Environmental Endocrinology.* Berlin, Heidelberg, New York: Springer, 1978.

McMillan, J. P., Underwood, H. A., Elliott, J. A., Stetson, M. H., and Menaker, M. Extraretinal light perception in the sparrow. IV. Further evidence that the eyes do not participate in photoperiodic photoreception. *Journal of Comparative Physiology,* 1975, *97,* 205–213.

Meier, A. H. Chronoendocrinology of the white-throated sparrow. *Proceedings of the 16th International Ornithological Congress,* Canberra, 1976, pp. 355–368.

Menaker, M. Rhythms, reproduction, and photoperception. *Biology of Reproduction,* 1971, *4,* 295–308.

Menaker, M., and Oksche, A. The avian pineal organ. In D. S. Farner and J. R. King (Eds.), *Avian Biology.* Vol. 4. New York: Academic Press, 1974.

Menaker, M., and Underwood, H. Extraretinal photoreception in birds. *Photochemistry and Photobiology,* 1976, *23,* 299–306.

Mirarchi, R. E., Howland, B. E., Scanlon, P. F., Kirkpatrick, R. L., and Sanford, L. M. Seasonal variation in plasma LH, FSH, prolactin, and testosterone concentrations in adult male white-tailed deer. *Canadian Journal of Zoology,* 1978, *56,* 121–127.

Moore, R. Y. Visual pathways and the central neural control of diurnal rhythms. In F. O. Schmitt and F. G. Worden (Eds.), *The Neurosciences Third Study Program.* Cambridge, Mass.: MIT Press, 1974.

Moore, R. Y. Central neural control of circadian rhythms. In W. F. Ganong and L. Martini (Eds.), *Frontiers in Neuroendocrinology.* Vol. 5. New York: Raven Press, 1977.

Moore, R. Y. The innervation of the mammalian pineal gland. In R. J. Reiter (Ed.), *The Pineal Gland and Reproduction.* Basel: Karger, 1978.

Moore, R. Y., and Klein, D. C. Visual pathways and the central neural control of a circadian rhythm in pineal serotonin *N*-acetyltransferase activity. *Brain Research,* 1974, *71,* 17–33.

Morin, L. P., and Zucker, I. Photoperiodic regulation of copulatory behaviour in the male hamster. *Journal of Endocrinology,* 1978, *77,* 249–258.

Murton, R. K., and Westwood, N. J. *Avian Breeding Cycles.* Oxford: Clarendon Press, 1977.

Nieschlag, E., and Bienek, H. Endocrine testicular function in mink during the first year of life. *Acta Endocrinologica,* 1975, *79,* 375–379.

Oishi, T., and Lauber, J. K. Photoreception in the photosexual response of quail. I. Site of photoreceptor. *American Journal of Physiology,* 1973, *225,* 155–158.

Oxender, W. D., Noden, P. A., and Hafs, H. D. Estrus, ovulation and serum progesterone, estradiol, and LH concentrations in mares after an increased photoperiod during winter. *American Journal of Veterinary Research,* 1977, *38,* 203–207.

Panke, E. S., Rollag, M. D., and Reiter, R. J. Pineal melatonin concentrations in the Syrian hamster. *Endocrinology,* 1979, *104,* 194–197.

Pelletier, J. Evidence for photoperiodic control of prolactin release in rams. *Journal of Reproduction and Fertility,* 1973, *35,* 143–147.

Pelletier, J., and Ortavant, R. Photoperiodic control of LH release in the ram. I. Influence of increasing and decreasing light photoperiods. *Acta Endocrinologica,* 1975a, *78,* 435–441.

Pelletier, J., and Ortavant, R. Photoperiodic control of LH release in the ram. II. Light-androgens interaction. *Acta Endocrinologica,* 1975b, *78,* 442–450.

Pittendrigh, C. S. Circadian surfaces and the diversity of possible roles of circadian organization in the photoperiodic induction. *Proceedings of the National Academy of Sciences of the USA,* 1972, *69,* 2734–2737.

Plotka, E. D., Seal, U. S., Schmoller, G. C., Karns, P. D., and Keenlyne, K. D. Reproductive steroids in the white-tailed deer *(Odocoileus virginianus borealis).* I. Seasonal changes in the female. *Biology of Reproduction,* 1977, *16,* 340–343.

Ralph, C. L. Structure and alleged function of avian pineals. *American Zoologist,* 1970, *10,* 217–235.

Ravault, J. P. Prolactin in the ram: Seasonal variation in the concentration of blood plasma from birth to three years. *Acta Endocrinologica,* 1976, *78,* 435–441.

Ravault, J. P., and Ortavant, R. Light control of prolactin secretion in sheep. Evidence for a photoinducible phase during a diurnal rhythm. *Annales de Biologie Animale, Biochimie, Biophysique,* 1977, *17,* 459–473.

Reiter, R. J. Changes in the reproductive organs of cold-exposed and light deprived female hamsters *(Mesocricetus auratus). Journal of Reproduction and Fertility,* 1968, *16,* 217–222.

Reiter, R. J. Pineal-gonadal relationship in male rodents. In C. Gual (Ed.), *Progress in Endocrinology.* Amsterdam: Excerpta Medica Foundation, 1969.

Reiter, R. J. Evidence for refractoriness of the pituitary-gonadal axis to the pineal gland and its possible implication in annual reproductive cycles. *Anatomical Record,* 1972a, *173,* 365–371.

Reiter, R. J. Surgical procedures involving the pineal gland which prevent gonadal degeneration in adult male hamsters. *Annales d'Endocrinologie,* 1972b, *33,* 571–581.

Reiter, R. J. Comparative physiology: Pineal gland. *Annual Review of Physiology,* 1973, *35,* 305–328.

Reiter, R. J. Circannual reproductive rhythms in mammals related to photoperiod and pineal function: A review. *Chronobiologia,* 1974a, *1,* 365–395.

Reiter, R. J. Pineal regulation of hypothalamicopituitary axis: Gonadotrophins. In E. Knobil and W. H. Sawyer (Eds.), *Handbook of Physiology.* Section 7, Vol. 4., Part 2. Washington, D.C.: American Physiological Society, 1974b.

Reiter, R. J. Exogenous and endogenous control of the annual reproductive cycle in the male golden hamster: Participation of the pineal gland. *Journal of Experimental Zoology,* 1975, *191,* 111–119.

Reiter, R. J. Regulation of pituitary gonadotrophins by the mammalian pineal gland. In Anand Kumar (Ed.), *Neuroendocrine Regulation of Fertility.* Basel: Karger, 1976.

Reiter, R. J. Interaction of photoperiod, pineal and seasonal reproduction as exemplified by findings in the hamster. In R. J. Reiter (Ed.), *The Pineal Gland and Reproduction.* Basel: Karger, 1978a.

Reiter, R. J. *The Pineal.* Vol. 3. Montreal: Eden Press, 1978b.

Reiter, R. J. and Ferguson, B. N. Delayed reproductive regression in male hamsters bearing intrarenal pituitary homografts and kept under natural winter photoperiods. *Journal of Experimental Zoology,* 1979, *209,* 175–180.

Reiter, R. J., and Johnson, L. Y. Depressant action of the pineal gland on pituitary luteinizing hormone and prolactin in male hamsters. *Hormone Research,* 1974a, *5,* 311–320.

Reiter, R. J., and Johnson, L. Y. Pineal regulation of immunoreactive luteinizing hormone and prolactin in light-deprived female hamsters. *Fertility and Sterility,* 1974b, *25,* 958–964.

Reiter, R. J., Sorrentino, S., Jr., and Hoffman, R. A. Early photoperiodic conditions and pineal antigonadal function. *International Journal of Fertility,* 1970, *15,* 163–170.

Reiter, R. J., Vaughan, H. K., Blask, D. E., and Johnson, L. Y. Melatonin: Its inhibition of pineal antigonadotrophic activity in male hamsters. *Science,* 1974, *185,* 1169–1171.

Reiter, R. J., Blask, D. E., Johnson, L. Y., Rudeen, P. K., Vaughan, M. K., and Waring, P. J. Melatonin inhibition of reproduction in the male hamster: Its dependency on time of day of administration and on an intact and sympathetically innervated pineal gland. *Neuroendocrinology,* 1976, *22,* 107–116.

Rollag, M. D., and Niswender, G. D. Radioimmunoassay of serum concentrations of melatonin in sheep exposed to different lighting regimes. *Endocrinology,* 1976, *98,* 482–489.

Rowan, W. Relation of light to bird migration and development changes. *Nature,* 1925, *115,* 494–495.

Rusak, B., and Morin, L. P. Testicular responses to photoperiod are blocked by lesions of the suprachiasmatic nuclei in golden hamsters. *Biology of Reproduction,* 1976, *15,* 366–374.

Rusak, B., and Zucker, I. Biological rhythms and animal behavior. *Annual Review of Psychology,* 1975, *26,* 137–171.

Rusak, B., and Zucker, I. Neural regulation of circadian rhythms. *Physiological Reviews,* 1979, *59,* 449–526.

Rust, C. C., and Meyer, R. K. Hair Color, molt and testis size in male short-tailed weasels treated with melatonin. *Science,* 1969, *165,* 921–922.

Sadleir, R. M. F. S. *The Ecology of Reproduction in Wild and Domestic Mammals.* London: Methuen, 1969.

Schanbacher, B. D., and Ford, J. J. Photoperiodic regulation of ovine spermatogenesis: Relationship to serum hormones. *Biology of Reproduction,* 1979, *20,* 719–726.

Schwassmann, H. O. Biological rhythms. In W. S. Hoar and D. J. Randall (Eds.), *Fish Physiology.* Vol. 6. New York: Academic Press, 1971.

Seegal, R. F., and Goldman, B. D. Effects of photoperiod on cyclicity and serum gonadotropins in the Syrian hamster. *Biology of Reproduction,* 1975, *12,* 223–231.

Stephens, J. L., and Binkley, S. Daily change in pineal *N*-acetyltransferase activity in a diurnal mammal, the ground squirrel. *Experientia,* 1978, *34,* 1523–1524.

Stetson, M. H., and Watson-Whitmyre, M. Nucleus suprachiasmaticus: The biological clock in the hamster? *Science,* 1976, *191,* 197–199.

Stetson, M. H., Matt, K. S., and Watson-Whitmyre, M. Photoperiodism and reproduction in golden hamsters: Circadian organisation and the termination of photorefractoriness. *Biology of Reproduction,* 1976, *14,* 531–537.

Stetson, M. H, Watson-Whitmyre, M., and Matt, K. S. Termination of photorefractoriness in golden hamsters—photoperiodic requirements. *Journal of Experimental Zoology,* 1977, *202,* 81–88.

Stokkan, K. A. Testosterone and daylength-dependent development of comb size and breeding plumage of male willow ptarmigan *(Lagopus lagopus lagopus)*. *Auk,* 1979, *96,* 106–115.

Tamarkin, L., Hutchison, J. S., and Goldman, B. D. Regulation of serum gonadotropins by photoperiod and testicular hormone in the Syrian hamster. *Endocrinology,* 1976a, *99,* 1528–1533.

Tamarkin, L., Westrom, W. K., Hamill, A. I., and Goldman, B. D. Effect of melatonin on the reproductive system of male and female Syrian hamsters: A diurnal rhythm in sensitivity to melatonin. *Endocrinology,* 1976b, *99,* 1534–1541.

Tamarkin, L., Hollister, C. W., Lefebvre, N. G., and Goldman, B. D. Melatonin induction of gonadal quiescence in pinealectomized Syrian hamsters. *Science,* 1977a, *198,* 935–955.

Tamarkin, L., Lefebvre, N. G., Hollister, C. W., and Goldman, B. D. Effect of melatonin administered during the night on reproductive function in the Syrian hamster. *Endocrinology,* 1977b, *101,* 631–634.

Tamarkin, L., Reppert, S. M., and Klein, D. C. Regulation of pineal melatonin in the Syrian hamster. *Endocrinology,* 1979, *104,* 385–389.

Thomson, A. P. D. The onset of oestrus in normal and blinded ferrets. *Proceedings of the Royal Society of London,* Series B, 1954, *142,* 116–135.

Thorpe, P. A., and Herbert, J. The effects of lesions of the accessory optic tract terminal nuclei on the gonadal response to light in ferrets. *Neuroendocrinology,* 1976a, *22,* 250–258.

Thorpe, P., and Herbert, J. Studies on the duration of the breeding season and photorefractoriness in female ferrets pinealectomized or treated with melatonin. *Journal of Endocrinology,* 1976b, *70,* 255–262.

Turek, F. W. Antigonadal effects of melatonin in pinealectomized and intact male hamsters. *Proceedings of the Society for Experimental Biology and Medicine,* 1977a, *155,* 31–34.

Turek, F. W. The interaction of the photoperiod and testosterone in regulating serum gonadotropin levels in castrated male hamsters. *Endocrinology,* 1977b, *101,* 1210–1215.

Turek, F. W. Diurnal rhythms and the seasonal reproductive cycle in birds. In I. Assenmacher and D. S. Farner (Eds.), *Environmental Endocrinology.* Berlin, Heidelberg, New York: Springer, 1978.

Turek, F. W. Effect of melatonin on photic-independent and photic-dependent testicular growth in juvenile and adult male golden hamsters. *Biology of Reproduction,* 1979a, *20,* 1119–1122.

Turek, F. W. Role of the pineal gland in photoperiod-induced changes in hypothalamic–pituitary sensitivity to testosterone feedback in castrated male hamsters. *Endocrinology,* 1979b, *104,* 636–640.

Turek, F. W., and Campbell, C. S. Photoperiodic regulation of neuroendocrine–gonadal activity. *Biology of Reproduction,* 1979, *20,* 32–50.

Turek, F. W., and Losee, S. H. Melatonin-induced testicular growth in golden hamsters maintained on short days. *Biology of Reproduction,* 1978, *18,* 299–305.

Turek, F. W., and Losee, S. H. Photoperiodic inhibition of the reproductive system: A prerequisite for the induction of the refractory period in hamsters. *Biology of Reproduction,* 1979, *20,* 611–616.

Turek, F. W., Desjardins, C., and Menaker, M. Melatonin: Antigonadal and progonadal effects in male golden hamsters. *Science,* 1975a, *190,* 280–282.

Turek, F. W., Elliott, J. A., Alvis, J. D., and Menaker, M. Effect of prolonged exposure to nonstimulatory photoperiods on the activity of the neuroendocrine–testicular axis of golden hamsters. *Biology of Reproduction,* 1975b, *13,* 475–481.

Turek, F. W., Elliott, J. A., Alvis, J. D., and Menaker, M. The interaction of castration and photoperiod in the regulation of hypophysial and serum gonadotropin levels in male golden hamsters. *Endocrinology,* 1975c, *96,* 854–860.

Turek, F. W., Desjardins, C., and Menaker, M. Differential effects of melatonin on the testes of photoperiodic and nonphotoperiodic rodents. *Biology of Reproduction,* 1976a, *15,* 94–97.

Turek, F. W., Desjardins, C., and Menaker, M. Melatonin-induced inhibition of testicular function in adult golden hamsters. *Proceedings of the Society for Experimental Biology and Medicine,* 1976b, *151,* 502–506.

Underwood, H. Extraretinal light receptors can mediate photoperiodic photoreception in the male lizard *Anolis carolinensis. Journal of Comparative Physiology,* 1975, *99,* 71–78.

Underwood, H. Photoperiodic time measurement in the male lizard *Anolis carolinensis. Journal of Comparative Physiology,* 1978, *125,* 143–150.

Underwood, H., and Menaker, M. Extraretinal photoreception in lizards. *Photochemistry and Photobiology,* 1976, *23,* 227–243.

Van Horn, R. N., and Resko, J. A. The reproductive cycle of the ring-tailed lemur *(Lemur catta):* Sex steroid levels and sexual receptivity under controlled photoperiods. *Endocrinology,* 1977, *101,* 1579–1586.

van Tienhoven, A. *Reproductive Physiology of Vertebrates.* Philadelphia, London, Toronto: W. B. Saunders, 1968.

Vasal, S., and Sundararaj, B. I. Responses of the regressed ovary of the catfish, *Heteropneustes fossilis* (Bloch), to interrupted-night photoperiods. *Chronobiologia,* 1975, *2,* 224–239.

Vaughan, M. K., and Blask, D. E. Arginine vasotocin—A search for its function in mammals. In R. J. Reiter (Ed.), *The Pineal Gland and Reproduction.* Basel: Karger, 1978.

Walton, J. S., McNeilly, J. R., McNeilly, A. S., and Cunningham, F. J. Changes in concentrations of follicle-stimulating hormone, luteinizing hormone, prolactin and progesterone in the plasma of ewes during the transition from anoestrous to breeding activity. *Journal of Endocrinology,* 1977, *75,* 127–136.

Whitehead, C., Bromage, N. R., Breton, B., and Matty, A. J. Effect of altered photoperiod on serum gonadotrophin and testosterone levels in male rainbow trout. *Journal of Endocrinology,* 1979, *81,* 139P–140P.

Wieselthier, A. S., and van Tienhoven, A. The effect of thyroidectomy on testicular size and the photorefractory period in the starling (*Sturnus* vulgaris L.). *Journal of Experimental Zoology,* 1972, *179,* 331–338.

Worth, R. W., Charlton, H. M., and MacKinnon, P. C. P. Field and laboratory studies on the control of luteinizing hormone secretion and gonadal activity in the vole, *Microtus agrestis. Journal of Reproduction and Fertility,* 1973, *Suppl. 19,* 89–99.

Yokoyama, K., Oksche, A., Darden, T. R., and Farner, D. S. The sites of encephalic photoreception in photoperiodic induction of the growth of the testes in the white-crowned sparrow, *Zonotrichia leucophrys gambelii. Cell and Tissue Research,* 1978, *189,* 441–467.

Yuthasastrokosol, P., Palmer, W. M., and Howland, B. E. Luteinizing hormone, oestrogen and progesterone levels in peripheral serum of unoestrous and cyclic ewes as determined by radioimmunoassay. *Journal of Reproduction and Fertility,* 1975, *43,* 57–65.

Zucker, I., and Morin, L. P. Photoperiodic influences on testicular regression, recrudescence and the induction of scotorefractoriness in male golden hamsters. *Biology of Reproduction,* 1977, *17,* 493–498.

24

Annual Rhythms in Man

Jürgen Aschoff

> We are told by a grave Author, an eminent French Physician, that Fish being a prolifick Dyet, there are more children born in Roman Catholic Countries about Nine Months after Lent, than at any other Season.
> —Jonathan Swift, 1729.

Preface

The main part of this chapter had to be written in the middle of an ongoing study, in which I attempt to analyze vital statistics on conception rates, mortality, and suicides from all over the world. The data sources were in part easily accessible in specific publications, such as those of the World Health Organization, but often they were available only from serials not easy to find. In presenting a general view at the present stage of my investigation, I am confronted with the difficulty that information from several geographical areas is still missing, and that the data collected so far are not satisfactorily homogeneous with regard to the time spans they cover. Hence, more data and more analytical procedures are needed until reliable answers can be given to some of the questions developed so far. However, even the preliminary findings seem to me to be of sufficient interest to risk publication (and the criticism of jumping to conclusions).

In an introductory section, I briefly touch on seasonal rhythms in physiological functions, while I have disregarded the seasonality of diseases as being out of the scope of this handbook. The interested reader is referred to the still highly valuable monograph of Rudder (1952). A more recent, condensed but quite comprehensive survey on human seasonal rhythms in physiology and pathology has been published by Hildebrandt (1962) (cf. also Smolensky, Halberg, and Sargent, 1972).

Jürgen Aschoff Max-Planck-Institut für Verhaltensphysiologie, D-8131 Andechs, West Germany.

JÜRGEN ASCHOFF

The investigation of seasonal rhythms in the physiology of man began at the turn of the century, initiated, among others, by Malling-Hansen (1886), who first described periodic changes in the growth rate of children, and Lindhard (1917), who measured his own respiration and alveolar CO_2 content throughout one year at $76°46'$ northern latitude. Lindhard concluded that the periodicity that he found in the sensitivity of the respiratory center to CO_2 was "due first and foremost to the variation in the intensity of sunlight." Impulses then came from Dorno's (1919) recordings of seasonal variations in ultraviolet radiation, and from the concurrent discoveries on health effects of UV-irradiation, extensively discussed by Rudder (1952) with regard to skeleton growth and the metabolic processes related to it. Ten years later, Hildebrandt (1962) was able to list more than 30 physiological variables for which seasonal rhythms had been described. Although there is not, as far as I know, a more recent review that summarizes our knowledge in this field, I have resisted the temptation to write a new one. Rather, it seems to me useful to demonstrate seasonal rhythms in a few representative examples and to refer to some of the factors that have been considered as causes for seasonality.

According to Figure 1, Swedish, Scottish, and German children more or less agree in the variations of their growth rate, which shows a major peak in spring or early summer for the increase in height, and predominantly two peaks for the gain in body mass. Curves with similar patterns have been found in weight gains of patients with tuberculosis: the phases were opposite in the northern and southern hemispheres (Strandgaard, 1923), and there was a peculiar dependence of amplitude on northern latitude (Nylin, 1929). In most of the more than 15 papers published on the subject, light and ambient temperature have been considered as the main factors influencing growth rate. However, Sanders (1934) concluded:

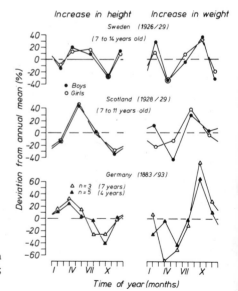

Fig. 1. Seasonal rhythms in growth rate of children. Data sources: *(top)* Nylin, 1929; *(middle)* Orr and Clark, 1930; *(bottom)* Camerer, 1893.

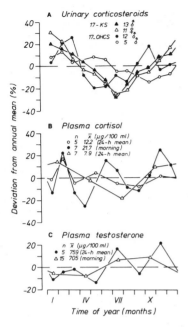

Fig. 2. Seasonal rhythms in urinary corticosteroid excretion and in plasma hormone levels. Data sources: (A) (▲△) Watanabe and Yoshida, 1956; (●) Hale *et al.*, 1966; (O) Reinberg, Lagoguey, Cesselin, Touitou, Legrand, Delassalle, Antreassian, and Lagoguey, 1978. (B) (△) Weitzman *et al.*, 1975; (●) Philip and Hanson, 1974; (O) Reinberg *et al.*, 1978. (C) (△) Smals, Kloppenborg, and Benraad, 1976; (●) Reinberg *et al.*, 1978.

the causal agents proposed by different investigators cannot be considered definite. It does seem probable that temperature, radiation, nutrition, habits of life, as well as diseases, are all contributing elements.

The increase in blood hemoglobin levels in spring has also been attributed to sunshine, but Coulthard (1958), summarizing data from 11 studies, objects:

> in all the surveys known of to me the haemoglobin level commences to rise between December and January. Whatever the factor which promotes this ... it clearly cannot be sunshine or warmth.

From variations in urinary corticosteroid excretion (Figure 2), it has been concluded that low ambient temperatures are stimulatory for the adrenals (Watanabe and Yoshida, 1956) and high temperatures depressive (Hale, Ellis, and Williams, 1966); but in view of the bimodal patterns in some of the data on plasma cortisol, it has also been suggested that both low and high temperatures could be stimulatory (Watanabe, 1964). Although the curves for plasma cortisol agree less than those for urinary excretion, a seasonal (possibly bimodal) rhythm seems to exist, as also in the level of plasma testosterone.

To illustrate the diversity of other phenomena that have been studied for seasonal variations, the incidence of menarch (reviewed by Bojlen and Bentzon, 1974), the threshold for tooth pain (Pöllmann and Harris, 1978), and the alertness of locomotive drivers (Hildebrandt, Rohmert, and Rutenfranz, 1973) might be mentioned. It is thus difficult to doubt that there is a seasonal temporal order within the human organism. This order most likely interacts with the circadian order (see Chapters 12 and 17), resulting in systematic changes of circadian phase, amplitude, or mean level over the year. Such variations in circadian parameters have been documented for the excretion of urinary electrolytes (Lobban, 1974, 1977; Mills and Waterhouse, 1973), oral temperature (Palmai, 1962; Horne and Coyne,

1975), plasma cortisol and growth hormone (Weitzman, Graaf, de Sassin, Hansen, Godtlibsen, Perlow, and Hellman, 1975), and birthrate (Erkinaro, 1972). One must still be aware of the possibility that without any variation in the mean (circadian) level of a variable, a rhythm in seasonal level might erroneously be inferred from mere changes in circadian phase. Seasonal changes in circadian parameters, on the other hand, may well reflect changes in habit, as suggested by Lobban (1974, 1977) for Eskimos.

In search of causes, I see little use in discussing to what extent seasonal variations found in the physiology of man are based on endogenous, rhythmic processes. If there is a circannual system, similar to that of animals (see Chapter 21), the question still remains what the external factors (zeitgebers) are by which it is controlled. Answers might partly be provided by the statistical data discussed in the following section.

Mortality, Suicides, and Conception Rates

Treatment of Data

Vital statistics on general mortality, suicides, and birthrates (converted into conception rates) were collected from as many countries as possible. The monthly raw data were normalized to an equivalent 30-day month length and then expressed as percentage deviations from the annual mean. Examples of curves obtained by this procedure are shown in Figure 3. Seasonal rhythms are apparent in all three events, but the curves differ with regard to amplitude and to the seasons at which maxima and minima occur. For further analyses, a sine function was fitted to each curve, and two parameters were then derived from it: the acrophase (in months), that is, the phase of the maximal value; and the relative amplitude, that is, the percentage variation of the maximum from the yearly mean. Curves with two or more maxima (cf. the suicides in Sweden in 1956–1959 and the conceptions in Italy in 1968–1972) were not included in this computation; if only a single minor maximum appeared (usually in December or January; cf. the conception rates in Sweden), the data were treated like unimodal curves.

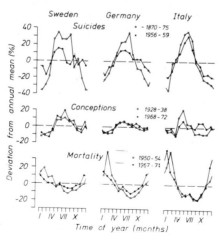

Fig. 3. Seasonal rhythms in suicides, conception rates, and mortality according to vital statistics from Sweden, Germany, and Italy.

As can be seen in Figure 4, the amplitude of the rhythms in suicides was above 25% in several European countries and in Japan during the second half of the last century, after which it has steadily declined in most of these countries. As opposed to the amplitude, there was nearly no change in the acrophases: over a time span of 100 years, maximal suicides always occurred in May or June. It should be noted that the stability in phase and the uniform and drastic decrease in amplitude were not related to the absolute numbers of suicides, as indicated in the uppermost diagram of Figure 4.

The data on conception rates have been split arbitrarily into three groups. Some European countries had small amplitudes already before the turn of the century, but the acrophases slowly drifted from May to July (Figure 5, left). In other countries, the rhythms decreased in amplitude (especially drastic in Japan), but kept their acrophase constant at April–May (Figure 5, middle). In Scandinavian countries (Figure 5, right), the amplitude remained constant at an intermediate level, while the acrophases were quite late already in 1920.

In the data from mortality statistics, decreases in amplitude over the last 50 years prevail (Figure 6, left and right diagram), concurrently with slow but steady advances of the acrophases. In only a few countries, neither phase nor amplitude seems to have changed (Figure 6, middle). (Recall that total mortality represents death by all kinds of diseases. Various diseases are known to result in maximal death rates at *different* times of the year.

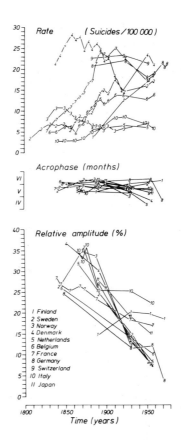

Fig. 4. Seasonal rhythms in suicides in 10 European countries and in Japan; long-term trends in suicide rates, in acrophase, and in relative amplitude.

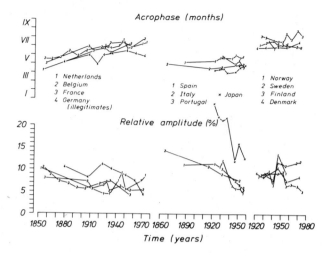

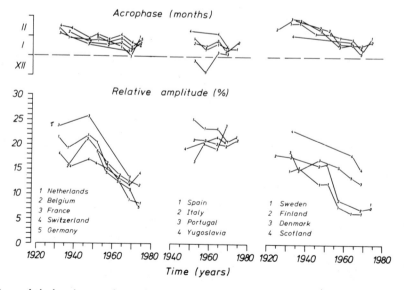

Fig. 5. Seasonal rhythms in conception rates in 11 European countries and Japan; long-term trends in acrophase and in relative amplitude.

Hence, a change in acrophase for total mortality could result from merely a change in the combination of causes for death.)

Several statements can now be made:

1. There are definite seasonal rhythms in suicides, conception rates, and mortality.
2. Although sociocultural influences interfere (see below), it is hard to deny a biological basis for all three rhythms, especially in view of the stable and uniform acrophases in some rhythms (cf. the suicides).
3. There must be factors in the environment that either produce these rhythms or synchronize endogenous (circannual) rhythms. These correlations are especially evident in rhythms that have the same acrophase over the whole hemisphere and in which this phase has remained unchanged over decades (cf. suicides, Figure 4).

Fig. 6. Seasonal rhythms in general mortality in 12 European countries; long-term trends in acrophase and relative amplitude.

4. The steady decreases in amplitude suggest a decrease in the "effectiveness" of the environmental factors or a decrease in the responsiveness of the human organism. Most likely, these changes are related to industrialization and the increase in standard of living over the last 100 years. Cowgill (1966a) stated in one of her studies on the season of birth that the amplitude is increased by "lack of industrialization, poverty, and rural living." Momiyama and Katayama (1972), who have described the "deseasonalization" of mortality in the world, consider central heating a major causative factor.

The plausible reasons for the worldwide deseasonalization do not give clues to the natural environmental factors that cause seasonality or contribute to its timing. A comparison of data from different latitudes might be useful for the analysis of this problem.

Dependence on Latitude

As can be seen in Figure 7, the relative amplitude of the rhythm in mortality is minimal in areas close to the equator and reaches maximal values in the northern hemisphere at about 40° latitude. The acrophases are predominantly fixed to January in the northern hemisphere and to July in the southern hemisphere. However, this six-month shift in phase occurs not at the equator but about 10° north of it. This phenomenon agrees with the range in which amplitudes are minimal. Together, these findings suggest the existence of a "biological equator" located somewhat north of the geographical equator and possibly related to the meteorological equator (at about 6°N), which is characterized by "maximal ground temperatures, converging winds, as well as maximal cloudiness and rainfall" (Flohn, 1950).

There are at least two seasonal rhythms in the environment whose amplitude reaches

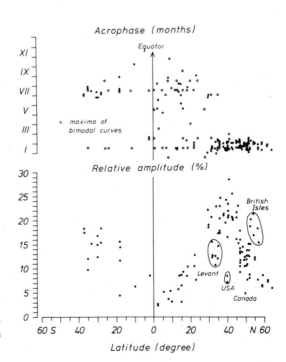

Fig. 7. Seasonal rhythms in mortality; dependence of acrophase and relative amplitude on latitude.

maximal value at about 40°N: the monthly ambient temperature and the monthly duration of sunshine (Figure 8). Duration of sunshine takes into account the mean monthly cloudiness (Landsberg, 1965). Ambient temperature could be considered a causal factor, as close correlations have been found between temperature and mortality by various authors (e.g., Katayama and Momiyama-Sakamoto, 1972), and the months of minimal temperature coincide with the mortality acrophases (compare Figures 7 and 8). However, the relative amplitude in mortality is more strongly correlated with the amplitude in duration of sunshine (Figure 9, left) than with the amplitude of ambient temperature (Figure 9, right). I fully agree with the statement of Campbell and Beets (1979) that "correlation studies exploring simple one-to-one correspondences between climatological variables and health statistics must be considered inadequate." Hence, further analyses ought to include other factors, for instance, the seasonal rhythm of total heat exchange, which reaches a maximal amplitude just below 40°N (Albrecht, 1961). Nevertheless, it is useful to indicate that duration of sunshine—a variable so far neglected in studies of this kind—might be a contributing factor.

The data of conception rates (Figure 10) differ from those of mortality in two major ways: the acrophases show a strong dependence on latitude, and the amplitudes reach maximal values not at 40°N but at about 20°–25°N (if the exceptionally high values from three Levant countries are disregarded). The steady advances of acrophases with decreasing northern latitude, first described by Batschelet and co-workers (1973), become delays south

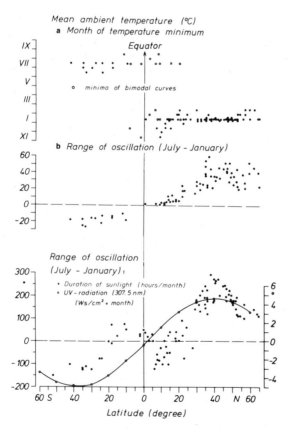

Fig. 8. *(Top)* Seasonal rhythms of mean monthly ambient temperature; month of minimum and range of oscillation drawn as a function of latitude. *(Bottom)* Seasonal rhythms of duration of sunshine (from local records, cloudiness included; left ordinate) and of UV radiation (theoretical curve; right ordinate); dependence of range of oscillation on latitude. Data sources: sunshine—Landsberg, 1965; UV radiation—Schulze, 1970.

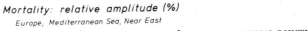

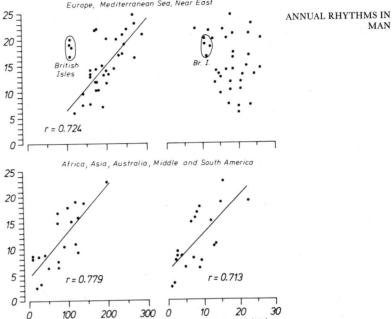

Fig. 9. Seasonal rhythms in mortality; relative amplitude drawn as a function of the seasonal range of oscillation (July–January) in duration of sunshine *(left)* and in ambient temperature *(right)*. British Isles not included in correlation coefficient *(r)*.

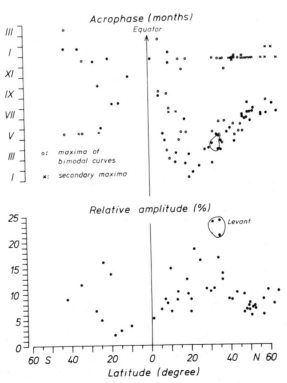

Fig. 10. Seasonal rhythms in conception rates; dependence of acrophase and relative amplitude on latitude.

of about 20°–25°N, that is, at the latitude of maximal amplitudes. These peculiar patterns of phase and amplitude have no relationship with the changes in range of oscillation as displayed by ambient temperature or monthly sunshine (cf. Figure 8). There is, however, another parameter in the seasonal rhythm of sunshine that is of interest. If the *mean annual duration of sunshine* (taken again from a map in Landsberg, 1965) is drawn as a function of latitude, a distinct maximum appears between 20° and 30°N, and a second one between 20° and 30°S. (Note that this differs from the latitude at which the *amplitude* of *monthly* duration of sunshine reaches its maximum; cf. Figure 8). Hence, it is not surprising that a positive correlation is indicated between mean annual sunshine and conception amplitude, and a negative correlation between sunshine and conception acrophase (Figure 11); caution in interpreting these correlations is warranted, however, in view of the sub-Poissonian distribution of data! Unfortunately, the scarcity of data from equatorial and more southern regions does not allow one to draw strong conclusions.

In view of the still incomplete data base, I refrain from speculating on how the mean annual duration of sunshine might affect the phase and amplitude of the seasonal rhythm in conception rate. Moreover, it is not yet clear whether sunshine is a controlling factor at all, because the correlations shown in Figure 11 are inconsistent, and one has to acknowledge arguments that have led several authors to emphasize the important role played by ambient temperature (Mills and Senior, 1930; Huntington, 1938; MacFarlane and Spalding, 1960). It is, in fact, somewhat puzzling that at all latitudes between 30° and 50°N, acrophases of conception rate occur when the ambient temperature reaches approximately 18.5°C—a value considered "optimal" for conception by Mills and Senior (1930). Finally, it has to be mentioned that contrary to the seasonal rhythms in mortality and suicides, conception rates are under strong social–cultural influences. This is indicated in Figure 10

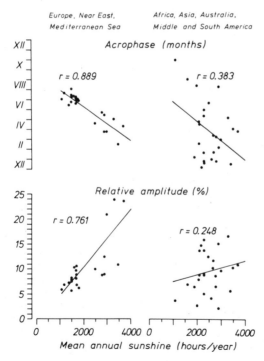

Fig. 11. Seasonal rhythms in conception rates; acrophase (above) and relative amplitude (below) drawn as a function of the mean annual duration of sunshine.

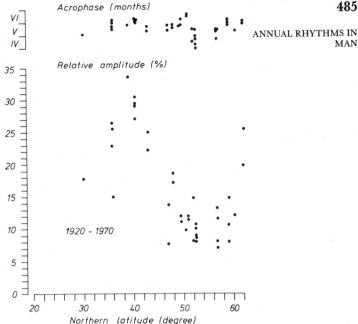

Fig. 12. Seasonal rhythms in suicides; dependence
of acrophase and relative amplitude on latitude.

by the consistency of secondary maxima in December, which can occur at all northern
latitudes and are most likely an expression of cultural habits. The same probably applies
to some of the trends in acrophases shown in Figure 5. Cowgill (1966a,b) has discussed
these phenomena in detail; she concluded that in the northern new world, "the season of
births pattern is largely culturally controlled—in contrast to that of Europe where it is
largely meteorologically determined" (1966b). (It is for this reason that data from the USA
and from Canada were not included in Figure 11, and also not in Figure 9).

Most interesting are the data on suicides, which unfortunately are available for only
parts of the northern hemisphere (Figure 12). The pattern of phases in the suicide rhythm
is not, as I had expected, similar to that of the conception rate, nor is it the reverse of it, as
an earlier pilot analysis had suggested (Aschoff, 1967). Instead, the suicide rhythm follows
the mortality pattern: the acrophases are independent of latitude, and the amplitudes reach
maximal values at about 40°N. The two sets of data differ only insofar as the suicide
amplitudes are somewhat larger than those of the mortality rhythms and insofar as the
acrophases of suicides occur in May instead of in January. These preliminary findings
strongly suggest the incorporation of data from violence and rapes, which are known to
have seasonal rhythms with acrophases in early summer; at the present stage of the investigation, it is hard to predict whether their acrophase pattern follows that of conception
rates or of suicides.

Concluding Remarks

Seasonal rhythms in the physiology of man are now well documented, and many more
rhythms will be described in coming years. There is also evidence that psychological func-

tions and emotional states vary with the time of year in a systematic manner (Hellpach, 1965; Myers and Davies, 1978). Hence, temporal order in synchrony with the seasons may eventually turn out to be as profound as the circadian temporal order. It seems hard to object to the hypothesis that these rhythms play an important role in the seasonal rhythms of general mortality, suicides, and conception rates, and that, on the other hand, there must be environmental (natural) factors that control these rhythms and that are responsible for the remarkable phenomenon of a "biological equator." Such a statement does not deny possible influences from sociocultural factors. They may increasingly override the influence of the natural factors, as especially indicated by the long-term trends in conception acrophases, and they most likely have caused the decrease in amplitudes over past decades. The deseasonalization is a "denaturalization," brought about by industrialization and urbanization, that is, by increased standards of living. This view is supported by the observation that the amplitude in conception rates is inversely correlated with socioeconomic status (Pasamanick, Dinitz, and Knobloch, 1960). The natural factors, however, against which we have become increasingly shielded, remain to be determined.

REFERENCES

Albrecht, F. Der jährliche Gang der Komponenten des Wärme- und Wasserhaushaltes der Ozeane. *Berichte des deutschen Wetterdienstes,* 1961, *79,* 3–24.

Aschoff, J. Adaptive cycles: Their significance for defining environmental hazards. *International Journal of Biometeorology,* 1967, *11,* 255–278.

Batchelet, E., Hillman, D., Smolensky, M. and Halberg, F. Angular–linear correlation coefficient for rhythmometry and circannually changing human birth rates at different geographic latitudes. *International Journal of Chronobiology,* 1973, *1,* 183–202.

Bojlen, K. and Bentzon, M. W. Seasonal variation in the occurrence of menarche. *Danish Medical Bulletin,* 1974, *21,* 161–168.

Camerer, W. Untersuchungen über Massenwachsthum und Längenwachsthum der Kinder. *Jahrbuch für Kinderheilkunde und psychische Erziehung,* 1893, *36,* 249–293.

Campbell, D. E., and Beets, J. L. The relationship of climatological variables to selected vital statistics. *International Journal of Biometeorology,* 1979, *23,* 107–114.

Coulthard, A. J. The annual cycle of blood haemoglobin levels. *Clinica Chimica Acta,* 1958, *3,* 226–233.

Cowgill, U. M. Season of birth in man. Contemporary situation with special reference to Europe and the southern hemisphere. *Ecology,* 1966a, *47,* 614–623.

Cowgill, U. M. The season of birth in man: The northern new world. *The Kroeber Anthropological Society Papers,* 1966b, *35,* 1–21.

Dorno, C. *Physik der Sonnen- und Himmelsstrahlung.* Braunschweig: Fr. Vieweg & Sohn, 1919.

Erkinaro, E. Seasonal changes of circadian rhythms of human birth in northern Finland. *Experientia,* 1972, *28,* 910.

Flohn, H. Neuere Anschauungen über die allgemeine Zirkulation der Atmosphäre und ihre klimatische Bedeutung. *Erdkunde,* 1950, *4,* 141–162.

Hale, H. B., Ellis, J. P., and Williams, E. W. Seasonal changes among endocrine–metabolic indices of men residing in a subtropical climate. *USAF School of Aerospace Medicine,* 1966, SAM-TR-66-114, 1–14.

Hellpach, W. *Geopsyche.* Stuttgart: Ferdinand Enke Verlag, 1965.

Hildebrandt, G. Biologische Rhythmen und ihre Bedeutung für die Bäder- und Klimaheilkunde. In A. Amelung and A. Evers (Eds.), *Handbuch der Bäder- und Klimaheilkunde.* Stuttgart: F. K. Schattauer Verlag, 1962, pp. 730–785.

Hildebrandt, G., Rohmert, W., and Rutenfranz, J. Über jahresrhythmische Häufigkeitsschwankungen der Inanspruchnahme von Sicherheitseinrichtungen durch die Triebfahrzeugführer der Deutschen Bundesbahn. *Internationales Archiv für Arbeitsmedizin,* 1973, *31,* 73–80.

Horne, J. A., and Coyne, I. Seasonal changes in the circadian variation of oral temperature during wakefulness. *Experientia,* 1975, *31,* 1296–1298.

Huntington, E. *Season of Birth.* London: Wiley, 1938.

Katayama, K., and Momiyama-Sakamoto, M. The seasonal variation of stroke mortality and its relationship to its temperature in Japan. *Papers in Meteorology and Geophysics*, 1972, *23*, 329–345.

Landsberg, H. E. Global distribution of solar and sky radiation. In E. Rodenwaldt and H. J. Jusatz (Eds.), *World Maps of Climatology*. Berlin-Heidelberg-New York: Springer-Verlag, 1965.

Lindhard, J. Contribution to the physiology of respiration under arctic climate. *Meddelelser om Grønland*, 1917, *44*, 77–175.

Lobban, M. C. Seasonal variations in daily patterns of renal excretion in modern Eskimo children. *Journal of Interdisciplinary Cycle Research*, 1974, *5*, 295–301.

Lobban, M. C. Seasonal changes in daily rhythms of renal excretion and activity patterns in an arctic Eskimo community. *Journal of Interdisciplinary Cycle Research*, 1977, *8*, 259–263.

MacFarlane, W. V., and Spalding, D. Seasonal conception rates in Australia. *Medical Journal of Australia*, 1960, *1*, 121–124.

Malling-Hansen, R. *Perioden in Gewichte der Kinder und in der Sonnenwärme*. Kopenhagen, 1886.

Mills, C. A., and Senior, F. A. Does climate affect the human conception rate? *Archives of Internal Medicine*, 1930, *46*, 921–929.

Mills, J. N., and Waterhouse, M. Circadian rhythms over the course of a year in a man living alone. *International Journal of Chronobiology*, 1973, *1*, 73–79.

Momiyama, M., and Katayama, K. Deseasonalization of mortality in the world. *International Journal of Biometeorology*, 1972, *16*, 329–342.

Myers, D. H., and Davies, P. The seasonal incidence of mania and its relationship to climatic variables. *Psychological Medicine*, 1978, *8*, 433–440.

Nylin, G. Periodical variations in growth, standard metabolism and oxygen capacity of the blood in children. *Acta Medica Scandinavica*, 1929, *31*, 1–207.

Orr, J. B., and Clark, M. L. Seasonal variation in the growth of school-children. *Lancet*, 1930, *2*, 365–367.

Palmai, G. Diurnal and seasonal variations in deep body temperature. *Medical Journal of Australia*, 1962, *2*, 989–991.

Pasamanick, B., Dinitz, S., and Knobloch, H. Socio-economic and seasonal variations in birth rates. *The Milbank Memorial Fund Quarterly*, 1960, *38*, 248–254.

Philip, B. A., and Hanson, K. H. Circannual cycles in morning plasma cortisol levels in man in Fairbanks, Alaska. In L. E. Scheving, F. Halberg, and J. E. Pauly (Eds.), *Chronobiology*. Stuttgart: Georg Thieme Verlag, 1974, pp. 256–261.

Pöllman, L., and Harris, P. H. P. Rhythmic changes in pain sensitivity in teeth. *International Journal of Chronobiology*, 1978, *5*, 459–464.

Reinberg, A., Lagoguey, M., Cesselin, F., Touitou, Y., Legrand, J. C., Delassalle, A., Antreassian, J., and Lagoguey, A. Circadian and circannual rhythms in plasma hormones and other variables of five healthy young human males. *Acta Endocrinologica*, 1978, *88*, 417–427.

Rudder, B. de. *Grundriss einer Meteorobiologie des Menschen*. Berlin-Göttingen-Heidelberg: Springer-Verlag, 1952.

Sanders, B. S. *Environment and Growth*. Baltimore: Warwick & York, 1934.

Schulze, R. *Strahlenklima der Erde*. Darmstadt: Dr. Dietrich Steinkopff Verlag, 1970.

Smals, A. G. H., Kloppenborg, P. W. C., and Benraad, T. J. Circannual cycle in plasma testosterone levels in man. *Journal of Clinical Endocrinology and Metabolism*, 1976, *42*, 979–982.

Smolenksy, M., Halberg, F., and Sargent, F., II. Chronobiology of the life sequence. In S. Ito, K. Ogata, and H. Yoshimura (Eds.), *Advances in Climatic Physiology*. Tokyo: Igaku Shoin Ltd., 1972, pp. 281–318.

Strandgaard, N. J. Seasonal variation of the weight of tuberculous patients. *Acta Medica Scandinavica*, 1923, *57*, 275–299.

Swift, J. A modest proposal. In *A Tale of a Tub and Other Satires*. London: J. M. Dent, 1975, p. 255.

Watanabe, G. I. Seasonal variation of adrenal cortex activity. *Archives of Environmental Health*, 1964, *9*, 192–200.

Watanabe, G. I., and Yoshida, S. Climatic effect on urinary output of neutral 17-ketosteroids. *Journal of Applied Physiology*, 1956, *9*, 456–460.

Weitzman, E. D., Graaf, A. S. de, Sassin, J. F., Hansen, T., Godtlibsen, O. B., Perlow, M., and Hellman, L. Seasonal pattern of sleep stages and secretion of cortisol and growth hormone during 24 hour periods in northern Norway. *Acta Endocrinologica*, 1975, *78*, 65–76.

PART IV

Rhythms not Directly Related to Environmental Cycles

25

Short-Term Rhythms in Activity

Serge Daan and Jürgen Aschoff

In the behavior patterns of some animals, bouts of activity and rest alternate with a higher frequency than once per day. Such patterns (Figure 1) have been termed *polyphasic* (Szymanski, 1920) as opposed to *monophasic* activity patterns. This distinction represents the artificial dichotomy of a continuum with a single solid daily block of activity at one extreme, through bimodal distributions to high-frequency patterns in which circadian components can no longer be discerned. These short-term rhythms differ from the circarhythms in that they do not correspond with any known environmental periodicity. However, they sometimes display strikingly precise oscillatory features and cannot be overlooked as an important ingredient in the temporal organization of behavior.

In this chapter we consider in the class of short-term rhythms the periodic recurrence of a behavior in any part of the daily cycle with frequencies in the range of 10^{-3} to 5.10^{-5} Hz, that is, with periods in the range of 20 min to 6 hr. This category excludes both the circarhythms and high-frequency rhythms in the nervous system and in muscular dynamics as associated with the integration of movements. Ultradian rhythms within this range that are not obviously related to behavior, such as phases of rapid eye movements (REM), are treated in Chapter 26.

Short-term rhythms in activity are known in laboratory rats and mice (Szymanski, 1920) but occur more conspicuously in other small mammals, such as shrews (Crowcroft, 1954) and voles (Davis, 1933). They characterize the alternation of grazing and rumination in cattle (Hughes and Reid, 1951) and other ruminants, such as roedeer (Bubenik, 1960). Ultradian rhythms in locomotion have also been described in free-ranging howler monkeys (Altman, 1959) and in caged rhesus monkeys (Delgado-Garcia, Grau, DeFeudis, DelPozo, Jimenez, and Delgado, 1976). Polyphasic patterns of sleep–wakefulness are further characteristic of the early ontogenetic stages of monophasic species, as in human infants (Kleit-

SERGE DAAN   Zoology Department, Groningen State University, Haren, 9750 AA, The Netherlands.
JÜRGEN ASCHOFF   Max-Planck-Institut für Verhaltensphysiologie, D-8131 Andechs, West Germany.

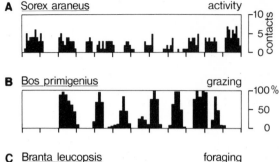

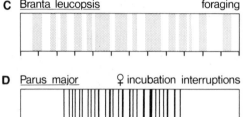

time of day in hours

Fig. 1. Examples of short-term rhythms in activity. (A) Locomotor activity in a common shrew (after Crowcroft, 1954, Figure 4). (B) Grazing activity (% of time) in eight bullocks (after Hughes and Reid, 1951, Figure 1). (C) Foraging bouts in a family of barnacle geese (two parents and six juveniles) on Spitsbergen (unpublished observations by M. van Eerden and S. Daan, July 30, 1978). (D) Absence from the nest in an incubating female great tit (after Kluyver, 1950, Figure 4).

man and Engelmann, 1953; and see Chapter 14). Kleitman (1963) actually proposed that a basic rest–activity cycle (BRAC) continues also in adult humans throughout the day, expressing itself at night in the alternation between REM and non-REM sleep. Since Kleitman's proposal, 90- to 110-min oscillations have been reported in humans for a variety of behavioral measures, such as oral behavior and vigilance and performance in verbal and spatial matching tasks (Klein and Armitage, 1979). Among passerine birds, males and females often take alternating shifts in attentiveness at the nest, resulting in more-or-less regular short-term incubation rhythms (e.g., Kluyver, 1950; Drent, 1975). Barnacle geese, on their breeding grounds in the Arctic, feed and rest in a 1- to 2-hr periodicity around the clock (Figure 1C). Other examples are found in Aschoff's (1962) review.

In most instances, short-term activity patterns are related to foraging and food intake. Bouts of activity commonly are times of concentrated feeding, alternating with other behaviors, for example, incubation, sleep, or rest. Both causal and functional analysis of short-term rhythms have scarcely begun. It is known only in some instances that the rhythm reflects the natural behavior of the species in the field and is not a pattern induced by a constant laboratory environment. The following discussion concentrates on the short-term rhythms in voles of the genus *Microtus*, for which most of the empirical evidence is available.

CAUSAL CONSIDERATIONS

The short-term activity rhythm in voles is basically a rhythm of food intake alternating with digestive pauses. The rhythms often appear as a stable pattern phase-locked to the daily cycle (Figure 2). It appears in measures of wheel-running activity (Davis, 1933; Erkinaro, 1969), feeding and drinking (Lehmann, 1976a) and oxygen consumption (Wie-

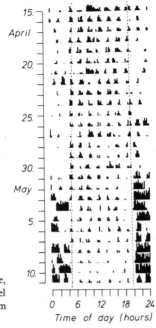

Fig. 2. The daily distribution of wheel-running activity in a field vole, *Microtus agrestis*. Vertical bars are proportional to the number of wheel revolutions per 15 min. Dashed lines represent sunrise and sunset. (From Erkinaro, 1969.)

gert, 1961). The properties of the rhythm are related to a species's metabolic demands. This effect is detected, for instance, when the feeding rhythms of voles of different sizes are compared (Figure 3). The period of the rhythm increases with body weight with a log–log regression coefficient of 0.30 (Daan and Slopsema, 1978). Since metabolic rates in mammals increase with the 0.73d power of body weight (W), this implies that the energy used in metabolism per meal cycle increases with $W^{1.03}$, or virtually linearly. The relationship strongly suggests that meal frequency is adapted to metabolic rate in these voles as much as the rhythms of lung ventilation and heart rate in mammals in general (Stahl, 1962). The short-term rhythm of feeding can be further adjusted to the balance of deficit and incentive,

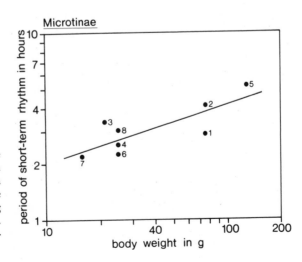

Fig. 3. Relation between the period (t) of the short-term activity rhythm and body weight in the lemmings and voles (Microtinae). Data points represent eight different species. The regression is log t (hours) = 0.002 + 0.30 log W (grams). (From Daan and Slopsema, 1978. Reprinted with permission of Springer-Verlag, Heidelberg.)

just as pulse and ventilation frequency are adjusted to metabolic needs and oxygen pressure. The high rate of food intake in lactating voles *(Microtus arvalis)* is partially achieved by an increase in the frequency of the feeding rhythm. The same response is observed when the nutritious value of the food is reduced (Figure 4). In rats and mice, the frequency of the rhythm is slightly larger in young than in old animals, as expected on the basis of size and metabolic differences (review in Aschoff, 1962).

While the short-term rhythm in voles seems to be related to metabolism, this does not imply that it is generated by a metabolic process. Several authors (e.g., Davis, 1933) have suggested that the process of stomach filling alternating with digestive pauses is responsible. However, the rhythm of energy intake may, of course, be timed by a nervous pacemaker just as well as heart and lung rhythms are. The evidence in support of one or the other of these alternatives is restricted. Unfortunately, stochastic properties of the rhythmic phenomenon observed tell us little about the generating mechanisms, as Lehmann (1976b) has pointed out. A negative serial correlation between successive periods (or between, e.g., bouts of activity and rest) indicates that the generating system is more precise than our detection of the critical phase in the overt rhythm. Such negative correlations, as calculated for short-term rhythms in voles and lemmings (Erkinaro, 1973; Lehmann, 1976a), are therefore not indicative of an endogenous oscillator comparable to circadian pacemakers. Little direct experimental evidence bears on the problem. It is known that stomach deafferentation does not influence the polyphasic activity pattern in rats (Bash, 1939). The persistence of a periodicity of feeding attempts in a field vole when no food was available (Daan and Slopsema, 1978) also suggests that stimuli arising from the state of depletion of the gastrointestinal tract can not be solely responsible for the short-term rhythm. Yet such stimuli, as certainly are involved in meal patterns of the rat (Magnen, 1967), of course, may modify the rhythm.

The alternative hypothesis of central timing could hold either a 2-hr endogenous oscillator or the circadian system responsible. The behavioral evidence available today does not distinguish between these possibilities. The solutions may well be different for different

Microtus arvalis

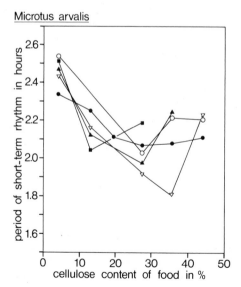

Fig. 4. Effect of food quality on the period of the short-term feeding rhythm in the common vole. The cellulose content of food was manipulated by mixing standard rat chow ("Muracon") with alfalfa. Each symbol represents one individual.

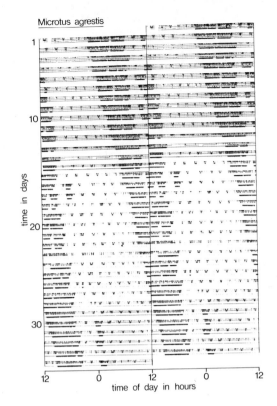

Microtus agrestis

Fig. 5. Circadian rhythm of various behaviors in the field vole, *Microtus agrestis,* in constant conditions (LL 0.01 lux). Channels from upper to lower: (1) presence in nestbox; (2) feeding; (3) drinking; (4) wheel running. (From Lehmann, 1976a. Reprinted with permission of Springer-Verlag, Heidelberg.)

species. In Crowcroft's (1954) data on activity of the shrew *Sorex araneus* (Figure 1A), the pronounced activity rhythm with a period of 2.0–2.4 hr bears no relationship to the circadian or external day. The rhythm continued throughout night and day without any fixed phasing relative to lights and darkness. On the other hand, the data available for voles invariably show a fixed-phase relationship with the daily light–dark cycle (e.g., Erkinaro, 1969; Mossing, 1975). Quite commonly, the rhythm is expressed differently during the light and dark portions of the 24 hr, usually more clearly in the light. In both *Microtus agrestis* and *M. arvalis,* when kept in constant conditions (LL or DD), the 2-hr rhythm of feeding appears only in the subjective day of the freerunning circadian cycle (Lehmann, 1976a; Daan and Slopsema, 1978). The subjective night is characterized by more diffuse feeding patterns, together with wheel running, which is absent during the subjective day (Figure 5). There is good correspondence from day to day in the phases of meals relative to the circadian cycle as it is identified by wheel running. Such data suggest that the circadian system in voles does play a role in the timing of meals at short intervals. Whether or not a 2-hr oscillator is involved in addition is a matter of speculation.

Functional Considerations

The diversity of phenomena belonging to the class of short-term rhythms lends futility to any search for a general function served. Yet some basic considerations may be advanced. A functional approach may emphasize the temporal organization either with respect to the

SERGE DAAN AND
JÜRGEN ASCHOFF

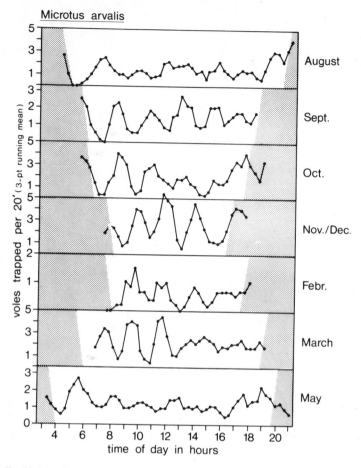

Fig. 6. Daily distributions of trappings of the common vole, *Microtus arvalis;* 196 traps were checked every 20 min, and the numbers caught averaged and smoothed in threes. (From Daan and Slopsema, 1978.)

external world or with respect to the internal milieu of the organism. Alternatively, one may view short-term rhythms as the by-product of physiological feedback loops. Yet, they are certainly stable elements in the temporal organization of behavior, which as a whole is functionally adjusted to the evolutionary needs of the animal's genes.

While the supply of oxygen is a virtually continuous process in most organisms (except for submersed air breathers, such as whales and water beetles), the intake of food occurs in more-or-less periodic fashion. The availability of oxygen is as good as constant, but food may be scarce or abundant, patchy or uniformly distributed. Discontinuous feeding may provide the spare time needed either for other vital activities or merely as a buffer, allowing the animal to extend its feeding time when intake rate slows down. The patterns of interrupted feeding are adaptive to the type of food and to the animal's requirements. For each combination, there should be some optimal arrangement of meals and digestive pauses. This arrangement may be especially critical with food that is relatively hard to process in the gastrointestinal tract and is probably true for the efficient breakdown of celluloses in vegetable matter with the help of microbial enzymes. It is likely that grazers, especially, benefit from a regular rhythmic pattern of stomach filling. Many of the pronounced short-term activity rhythms do indeed stem from animals like voles, cattle, and geese that rely on intestinal fermentation of bulky food (Daan and Slopsema, 1978). Apart from slow energy input, fast energy expenditure may also promote the rhythmic regularity of meal timing; the small shrews with their high metabolic rates (Gebzcynski, 1965) would fall in this category.

In the voles, activity bouts above ground in daytime as needed for regular feeding are associated with a risk of being killed, for example, by aerial raptors. Such risk may vary in the course of the day. In the face of varying risk, it is probably a good strategy to adhere to fixed temporal schedules day after day (see Chapter 15). The common vole *(Microtus arvalis)* does this, indeed, in cage as well as in field conditions. Moreover, the feeding trips are made more-or-less synchronously, so that the 2-hr rhythm can be detected also at the population level (Figure 6). At least under some circumstances, this pattern may lead to the additional benefit of reduction of predatory risk by safety in numbers: a vole taking his meal at the same time of day as his conspecifics may have a slightly smaller chance of predation than if he chooses a different time (Daan and Slopsema, 1978). This may be one explanation of the circadian regulation of meals in voles, since this is a way to guarantee synchronous phases within the population.

Optimal timing with respect to predatory risk is a hypothesis for the function of vole 2-hr rhythms and is unlikely to be generally valid. Less specific hypotheses will be more difficult to investigate. Some general considerations may include the role of short-term rhythms in preparing the animal's physiological readiness for a recurrent behavior pattern. The rhythm may be the organism's way of guaranteeing that several variables of physiological and motivational state will reach appropriate levels in synchrony, which may contribute to an optimal coordination of behavior and at the same time allow for energy savings that accrue from, for example, reduced alertness between meals. These, in turn, are more specific elaborations on a general theme of functional order in the daily patterning of behavior. In the same vein, oscillatory patterns may be thought of as generally contributing to the stability of behavioral organization (Aschoff and Wever, 1961; Wilke, 1977). It is not quite clear to which testable hypotheses such considerations on the meaning of short-term rhythms for the internal milieu may lead. In the absence of environmental cycles matched by short-term rhythms, research into their role in the coordination of behavior is thoroughly needed.

References

Altman, S. A. Field observations on a howling monkey society. *Journal of Mammalogy*, 1959, *40*, 317–330.

Aschoff, J. Spontane lokomotorische Aktivität. *Handbuch der Zoologie*, 1962, 8(11); 1–76.

Aschoff, J., and Wever, R. Biologische Rhythmen und Regelung. *Bad Oeynhausener Gespräche*, 1961, *5*, 1–15.

Bash, K. W. An investigation into a possible organic basis for the hunger drive. *Journal of Comparative and Physiological Psychology*, 1939, *28*, 109–133.

Bubenik, A. N. Le rhythme nycthéméral et le régime journalier des ongulés sauvages. Problèmes theoriques. Rhythme d'activité du chevreuil. *Mammalia*, 1960, *24*, 1–58.

Crowcroft, P. The daily cycle of activity in British shrews. *Proceedings of the Zoological Society* (London), 1954, *123*, 715–729.

Daan, S., and Slopsema, S. Short term rhythms in foraging behavior of the common vole, *Microtus arvalis*. *Journal of Comparative Physiology*, 1978, *127*, 215–227.

Davis, D. H. S. Rhythmic activity in the short-tailed vole, *Microtus*. *Journal of Animal Ecology*, 1933, *2*, 232–238.

Delgado-Garcia, J. M., Grau, C., DeFeudis, P., DelPozo, F., Jimenez, J. M., and Delgado, J. M. R. Ultradian rhythms in the mobility and behavior of rhesus monkeys. *Experimental Brain Research,* 1976, *25,* 79–91.

Drent, R. H. Incubation. In D. S. Farner and J. R. King (Eds.), *Avian Biology.* Vol. 5. New York: Academic Press, 1975, pp. 333–420.

Erkinaro, E. Der Phasenwechsel der lokomotorischen Aktivität bei *Microtus agrestis* (L.), *M. arvalis* (Pall.) and *M. oeconomous* (pall.). *Aquilo, Series Zoologica,* 1969, *8,* 1–31.

Erkinaro, E. Short-term rhythm of locomotor activity within the 24 hr. period in the Norwegian lemming, *Lemmus lemmus* and watervole *Arvicola terrestris. Aquilo, Series Zoologica,* 1973, *14,* 46–58.

Gebzcynski, M. Seasonal and age changes in the metabolism and activity of *Sorex arameus* Linnaeus, 1758. *Acta Theriologica,* 1965, *10,* 303–331.

Hughes, G. P., and Reid, D. Studies on the behaviour of cattle and sheep in relation to the utilization of grass. *Journal of Agricultural Science,* 1951, *41,* 360–366.

Klein, R., and Armitage, R. Rhythms in human performance: 1½-hour oscillations in cognitive style. *Science,* 1979, *204,* 1326–1328.

Kleitman, N. *Sleep and Wakefulness.* Chicago: University of Chicago Press, 1963.

Kleitman, N., and Engelman, T. G. Sleep characteristics of infants. *Journal of Applied Physiology,* 1953, *6,* 269–282.

Kluyver, H. N. Daily routines of the great tit, *Parus* m. *major* L. *Ardea,* 1950, *38,* 99–135.

Lehmann, U. Short-term and circadian rhythms in the behaviour of the vole, *Microtus agrestis* (L.). *Oecologia,* 1976a, *23,* 185–199.

Lehmann, U. Stochastic principles in the temporal control of activity behaviour. *International Journal of Chronobiology,* 1976b, *4,* 233–266.

Magnen, J. le. Habits and food intake. In C. F. Code and W. Heidel (Eds.), *Handbook of Physiology, Section 6. Alimentary Canal.* Vol. 1. Baltimore: Williams & Wilkins, 1967, pp. 11–30.

Mossing, T. Measuring small mammal locomotory activity with passage counters. *Oikos,* 1975, *26,* 237–239.

Stahl, W. R. Similarity and dimensional methods in biology. *Science,* 1962, *137,* 205–212.

Szymanski, J. S. Aktivität und Ruhe bei Tieren und Menschen. *Zeitschrift für Allgemeine Physiologie,* 1920, *18,* 105–162.

Wiegert, R. G. Respiratory energy loss and activity patterns in the meadow vole, *Microtus pennsylvanicus pennsylvanicus. Ecology,* 1961, *42,* 245–252.

Wilke, J. T. Ultradian biological periodicities in the integration of behavior. *International Journal of Neuroscience,* 1977, *7,* 125–143.

26

Temporal Characteristics of Sleep

Wilse B. Webb and Michael G. Dube

Introduction

The mode of viewing sleep as a biological rhythm has not been clearly articulated, although there has been an increasing rapprochement between sleep research and the concepts and methods of biological rhythm research. This chapter first reviews a background of that interrelationship. The prominent phenomena of sleep are then reviewed in terms of the core property of biological rhythms—the temporal characteristics of sleep. These include both the time properties of the patterns of sleep as it appears in the circadian cycle and the timing of within-sleep events of the sleep structure. A discussion of the major changes in these time characteristics associated with ontogeny, phylogeny, and time schedules follows. The next section considers the possible extension of ultradian events, seen clearly in sleep, into wakefulness. An exploration of the role of the central nervous system in sleep rhythmicity concludes the chapter.

A Background of Sleep and Other Biological Rhythms

Sleep has a long history as a modifier variable of other physiological variables. Kleitman began *Sleep and Wakefulness* (1963) with seven chapters on the "Functional Differences between Sleep and Wakefulness." In these chapters, he reviewed the data on the differences in sleep and waking of the musculature, nervous system, blood circulation, digestion, metabolism, body temperature, and excretion. The intimacy of the relationship between sleep and other systems is seen in his historical citations and the relative extensiveness of the references.

Wilse B. Webb and Michael G. Dube   Department of Psychology, University of Florida, Gainesville, Florida 32601.

WILSE B. WEBB AND
MICHAEL G. DUBE

In his discussion of temperature, Kleitman noted that

> the effect of sleep on body temperature has long been a topic for debate. It is not that anyone
> doubts that the body temperature falls during the night, but the fall can conceivably be due to
> rest in the horizontal position and muscular relaxation. In addition, the fact that one's temper-
> ature begins to decrease long before bedtime, and follows its usual 24-hour course even if one
> stays awake the whole night, has been interpreted as showing that sleep is not directly responsible
> for the low night temperature. (p. 58)

The concerns of Kleitman were by no means new, or his alone. The issue of sleep and
biological rhythms, in fact, emerged as early as 1875. Fraisse (1963) noted that

> It has been known for a long time that the pulse, blood pressure, and especially temperature of
> the body present day–night variations in humans as well as in many animals. There is about
> 1.8°F. difference in the human temperature between the minimum at night and the maximum
> in the afternoon. In 1875, physiologists already attributed this rhythm to the alternation of light
> and darkness which brought with it the alternation of activity and rest; they therefore thought it
> possible to reverse this by substituting nocturnal for diurnal activity. The results of their exper-
> iments remained very controversial, however, until Toulouse and Pieron found in 1907 that the
> temperature change was reversed in the case of nurses changing from day to night duty. This
> reversal was gradual and was not completed until after 30 or 40 days. During the first few weeks
> the rise in temperature, which usually takes place in the mornings and the early part of the
> afternoon, grew gradually less marked, until it finally changed to an increasingly rapid drop.
> (p. 25)

This background formulates the problem. Are time characteristics of biological events
within sleep dependent on sleep *per se,* or are they endogenously determined changes
independent of sleep? This question could be answered only by experimentally separating
the systems. Sleep variations in human subjects were used in five experimental models:

1. Measurements of biological systems while subjects rested but did not sleep during
   regular sleep periods
2. Measurements of biological systems while subjects remained awake and active during the regular sleep period
3. Displacement of the regular sleep periods to other times within the 24 hr
4. Imposition of non-24-hr schedules
5. Removal of time cues

In the first three of these designs, sleep was typically the control variable similar to
the use of light–dark schedules in lower animals. In the later designs, while sleep regimes
were typically modified, such changes were generally of secondary consideration. In all
designs, primary attention was given to the retention or variations of temporal patterns of
other systems. For example, Lewis and Lobban (1957) reported extensively on excretory
rhythms in days of varied length (Model 4), but the report on sleep was as follows: "The
quality of sleep for these subjects was at least as good as the sleep which they normally
enjoyed in Great Britain, in a comfortable bed, during the hours of darkness." The extensive studies by Aschoff and his colleagues using the Model 5 design focused on "activity
units," temperature, and urinary measures but, until recently, gave no data on sleep itself
(Aschoff, 1965).

We shall not review these interactions of sleep with other systems but refer to three
chapters of Kleitman (1963): Chapter 15, "The 24-Hour Sleep-Wakefulness and Body-
Temperature Rhythms"; Chapter 16, "24-Hour Variation in Activity and Performance";
and Chapter 17, "24-Hour Variation in Visceral Activity." We also refer to the recent

books of Conroy and Mills (1970) and Mills (1973) and to other chapters of this book (see
Chapters 12, 17, and 18).

501

TEMPORAL
CHARACTERISTICS OF
SLEEP

Sleep as a Biological Rhythm

In the late 1960s sleep research began to consider sleep and sleep subcharacteristics
within the context of biological rhythms. Specifically, the timing of sleep onset and termination or the timing of within-sleep events such as REM sleep became of focal interest.

Clearly, there is growth of interest in sleep as a biological rhythm. Since 1968, the
Brain Information Service of the UCLA Center for Health Sciences has published an
annual bibliography of worldwide sleep literature (1972). In 1969, in recognition of the
growing literature in the area, the category of *biorhythms* was introduced. The number of
articles about biorhythms rose from 16 in 1969 to 91 in 1977; the percentages increased
from 2.5% to 4.9%.

Dimensions of Sleep

There are two major objective components of sleep: the patterns of sleep and the structure of sleep.

The term *patterns of sleep* refers to the interrelation between sleep and waking. The
basic unit of sleep patterns is defined by sleep onset and termination. These units are typically measured in a 24-hr or circadian context, and a number of interacting components
result: total sleep time, number of sleep episodes, episode lengths, and placement descriptors
(e.g., diurnal ratios or onset and termination time averages).

Sleep structure refers to within-sleep characteristics, and these are conventionally
indexed by the electroencephalogram (EEG). In the adult human, there are five reliably
recognizable subunits or "stages" of sleep (Webb, 1971). Four stages (1–4) are generally
related to the "depth" of sleep. A fifth stage is identified by a Stage 1 EEG pattern and a
number of concomitant physiological states, for example, changes in the electromyogram
(EMG), penile erections, and rapid eye movements (REM). This stage is typically designated State 1–REM. In human subjects, this stage is closely associated with dreaming.
Brief episodes of awakening are identifiable within a sleep period and are designated Stage
0.

Temporal Characteristics of Human Sleep

Because of the wide variations resulting from species and age variables (see below),
the description of temporal components of sleep must be restricted to a limited age range
within species. We shall describe the young human adult characteristics.

Sleep patterns are generally measured by questionnaires or self-reports over time
periods (sleep diaries). Sleep diary data of 102 college students (18–22 years old) have been
carefully examined for their time components and will serve as the primary base of the
description of sleep patterns (White, 1974).

Sleep diaries reveal surprising complexities in describing total sleep time. Within a 2-

week sample, the population figure for sleep per night is 7.5 hr (SD = 0.85); total sleep on week nights is 7.4 hr (SD = 0.92) and on weekends 7.9 hr (SD = 1.07); and total sleep per 24 hr is 7.9 hr (SD = 0.82). The latter figure reflects the presence of naps. In spite of the variations in methods of data collection (questionnaires and diaries), estimates of average sleep length in young adults yield highly similar results (McGhie and Russell, 1962; O'Connor, 1964; Terman and Hocking, 1913; Tune, 1968, 1969; White, 1974). Essentially, the average total sleep of young adults for each 24 hr is 7½ hr, with a standard deviation of about 1 hr and with variation on weekends and weekdays.

The standard deviations reflect substantial between-subject differences. There are also substantial within-subject variations, as was seen in several statistics: the *average* of the *within*-subject standard deviations of sleep length across 2 weeks was 1.53 hr; the correlation of sleep time between one week and the next was 0.68; and 20% of the subjects had sleep lengths that varied by 1 hr or more during a 2-week period (White, 1974).

Naps are a significant component of sleep patterns in college populations (White, 1974). There was an average of 1.6 naps per week (SD = 1.3), with 2.6 hr per week (SD = 2.8) of sleep. Only 16% reported no naps during a 2-week interval, and 42% reported five or more naps during that interval. O'Connor (1964), in a questionnaire study of college students, found 7% reporting napping as "almost always" and 28% as "fairly often." Clearly, circumstances sharply affect these variations from a uniphasic nocturnal pattern. Using a presumably noncollege young adult population (20–29 years), Tune reported on two studies using 8-week sleep logs. In one study, 60% showed no naps (1969), and in a second study, there was an average of only one nap in 8 weeks (1968).

Again, referring to the college population, all subjects took their major sleep period at night (White, 1974). However, there was large between-subject and within-subject variability relative to sleep onset times. The population's within-week onset time was 12 midnight, but the standard deviation was 0.99 hr, while the weekend onset time was 1:30 A.M, with a standard deviation of 1.27. The within-subject *average* standard deviation of sleep onset time across a 2-week period was 1.58 hr. Only 30% uniformly went to bed within a half hour of the same time each night.

Figure 1 presents a typical night of sleep graphed by stages. Summary figures of the overall distribution of sleep stages have been taken from a normative group of young adult (16–19 years) males measured five nights in the laboratory under controlled conditions (Williams, Karacan, and Hursch, 1974). The percentage means and associated standard deviations were as follows: Stage 0, 1.87 (1.59); Stage 1, 4.02 (1.35); Stage 2, 49.05 (7.48); Stage 3, 5.76 (1.87); Stage 4, 17.28 (5.47); and Stage 1–REM: 22.02 (3.26). These figures clearly indicate that the various sleep stages occupy different temporal segments of the total sleep period.

An additional temporal characteristic is the differential distribution of the stages across the sleep period. Figure 2 displays the hourly distribution for a group of 30 young adults across the sleep period.

We shall further detail the ultradian cycling within sleep in a later section.

COMPARATIVE ASPECTS

The significant effects of phylogeny on sleep can be seen in a comparison of the sleep of the rat and the human. The structural component of the sleep of the rat has two "stages":

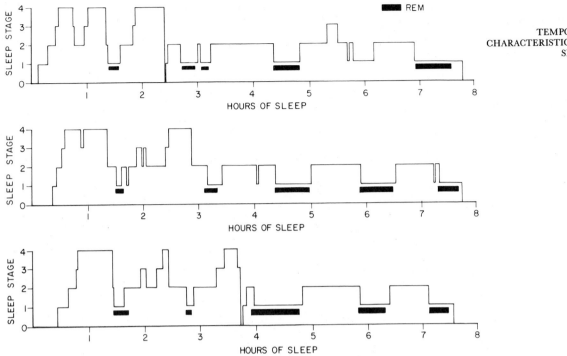

Fig. 1. Three nights of sleep for a single subject. Hours across the baseline and stages on the vertical. Bars are REM periods.

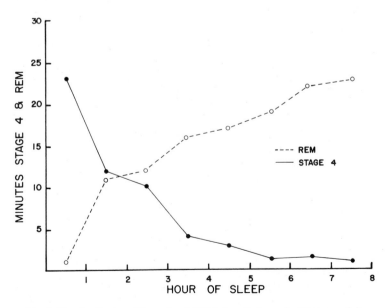

Fig. 2. The distribution of Stage 4 and REM sleep by hours for 30 young adults.

a slow-wave sleep stage (SWS) and an "activated" sleep stage, in which the cortical EEG is essentially identical to the waking EEG. Because some animals do not have conjugate eye movements (REMs), the "activated" sleep period is more often measured by loss of muscle tonus or by theta waves in hippocampal electrodes. As a consequence, this stage is most commonly referred to as *paradoxical sleep* (PS). This stage of sleep differs in other significant ways from human REM sleep. The interval from onset to onset of episodes is about 8 min, and episodes average about 2.5 min in length (Webb and Friedmann, 1970). The episodes do not become longer across a sleep period. The episodes are, however, significantly longer in interval and length during the light phase than in the dark phase. They constitute 20% of sleep during the light phase and 16% during the dark phase. Figure 3 displays the pattern of PS in rats.

The patterns of the sleep of the rat and the human also show marked phylogenetic differences. The sleep of the rat is highly polyphasic. The number of episodes in 24 hr range from about 45 to 90, with episode length extending from 1 min to 105 min (Webb and Friedmann, 1969). While there is a tendency toward nocturnal wakefulness, about 40% of the episodes occur during the dark phase. The ratio of total day–night sleep is 1.47, and the total amount is about 13 hr per 24 hr (Van Twyver, 1969).

Wide differences in both structure and pattern are seen across species. In structure, primates have a five-stage pattern of sleep, with the stages essentially identical in EEG criteria to those of man, although the proportional distribution differs (Bert, Ayats, Martino, and Collomb, 1967). The sleep structure of cats shows two distinct stages of slow-wave sleep (Ursin, 1971). Ruminant animals, in particular, as well as other species, have a significant segment of "drowsiness" (Ruckebusch, 1972). The measurement and characterization of amphibian and reptilian sleep is in considerable dispute (Tauber, 1974). Birds show distinct episodes of slow-wave sleep and paradoxical sleep, although episode lengths tend to be shorter than in mammals and paradoxical sleep does not exceed 10% of total sleep time in any species studied (Tauber, 1974).

The range of variations in sleep and the extent of phylogenetic data available on animal sleep can be seen in two reviews of cross-species data (Zepelin and Rechtschaffen, 1974; Allison and Cicchetti, 1976). The Zepelin–Rechtschaffen review reports three measures: total sleep time, "paradoxical sleep" percentage, and "sleep cycle length" (the average length of an SWS episode and the succeeding PS episode). The data include 53 species

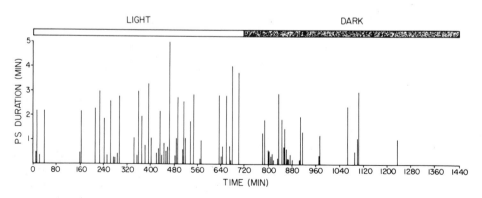

Fig. 3. Paradoxical or activated sleep of the rat across 24 hr.

representing 12 orders and 33 families. Total sleep time is reported on 49 species, PS on 40 species, and the sleep cycles on 24 species.

Allison and Cicchetti confined their analyses to PS amounts and SWS amounts. They listed 39 species and 13 orders for these variables. They stated that there were only 24 species for which sleep cycle data were available and that there were "few data available" on the variable of "the placement of sleep within the 24 hours."

The data of the Zepelin–Rechtschaffen paper display a wide range in the reported variables. Examples of very long total sleep time are water opossum (19.4 hr), little brown bat (19.9 hr), armadillo (18.1 hr), and owl monkey (17 hr). Short total sleep times reported were roe deer (2.6 hr), goat and sheep (3.8 hr), and African elephant (3.3 hr). Percentages of PS ranged from 33.7% in the water opossum to 5.6% in the mouse. Cycle length extended from 124 min in the Asian elephant to 6.5 min in the chinchilla.

Zepelin and Rechtschaffen found total sleep time to be substantially negatively correlated with brain weight (−0.71), which was itself highly correlated with metabolism estimates (0.96), life span (0.85), and gestation period (0.85). Allison and Cicchetti reported a 0.68 correlation between metabolic rate estimates and SWS (which, in turn, is highly correlated with total sleep time and brain weight). Zepelin and Rechtschaffen found PS time negatively correlated with brain weight (−0.54), which undoubtedly reflects PS time correlation with total sleep time (0.76). When percentage of PS is used, the correlation with brain weight and the associated measures drops to 0.10, which is not significant. Cycle length is highly correlated with brain weight (0.92). Allison and Cicchetti, in addition, found significant negative correlation of SWS amounts with ratings of the "exposure" of the sleep habitat (protected versus unprotected) (−0.58) and ratings of the predatory danger to the species (−0.54).

These reviews reflect the limitations and measurement problems inherent in the data on cross-species sleep characteristics. As noted elsewhere (Webb, 1975), each measure poses formidable problems. Desirable data on any given species would be those collected in the natural environment across 24-hr periods with valid measurements of patterns and sleep structure. Measurement problems generally preclude the simultaneous fulfillment of these requirements. Sleep habitats (e.g., burrowing) or wide-ranging territories pose difficulties in accurate measurement. If electrophysiological measures are imposed for accuracy, the natural behavior repertoire is sharply restricted. Because of typical circadian variations, measures of less than 24 hr are essentially useless if not downright misleading.

Particularly critical for biological rhythm interest is the almost total lack of data on such variables as number and placement of sleep episodes.

What biological-rhythm-oriented sleep research exists in the animal literature is limited to the effects of food as a competing zeitgeber and to the manipulation of light–dark cycles. Mouret and Bobillier (1971) have reported that the limitation of food to the light phase of an LD 12 : 12 cycle caused albino rats to lose their diurnal sleep rhythm and to distribute their sleep equally between the light and dark phases. This pattern was accompanied by an increase in their total PS amount. Dube (1978) has replicated this study and extended the analysis to show that the sleep distribution actually assumes an 8-hr periodicity under these conditions, although his pigmented animals showed no PS increase. A redistribution of rat sleep has also been shown to result from 1-hr food access during the light period, with a dip in the light-period sleep peak anticipating feeding by 2 or 3 hr (Dube, 1976).

When these freerunning conditions were instituted following a light–dark cycle, during 7 days of continuous recording, the sleep rhythm continued in the same form with only a slight period change in accord with its nature as an endogenous circadian rhythm. Mitler, Lund, Sokolove, Pittendrigh, and Dement (1977) have shown in mice, however, that after a long period in constant illumination, the sleep rhythm can desynchronize and become "damped and/or polyphasic." This finding is similar to results obtained on activity rhythms under certain conditions of illumination (Hoffmann, 1971; Pittendrigh, 1974). Particularly noteworthy in this case, however, is the fact that simultaneously recorded wheel-running rhythms remained intact, suggesting either that constant illumination caused the sleep rhythm to become uncoupled from some common oscillator or that sleep and wheel-running rhythms have independent driving mechanisms. Female baboons exposed to constant light for 3 years have been shown to retain intact their slow-wave sleep and paradoxical sleep rhythms (Yamaoka and Hagino, 1972).

Short light–dark cycles have been found to exert a considerable effect on the distribution of rat sleep. On schedules such as LD 6 : 6, LD 2 : 2, LD 1 : 1, LD 10 min : 10 min, LD 5 min : 5 min, LD 2.5 min : 2.5 min, paradoxical sleep has been found to occur predominantly during the dark phase rather than during the light phase as it does under normal conditions (Borbély, Huston, and Waser, 1975; Borbély, 1976; Johnson, Adler, and Sawyer, 1970). These effects are always superimposed on a freerunning circadian rhythm of sleep, which modulates their magnitude. The significance of these light cycle effects is obscured by a recent result in another rodent species. In hamsters subjected to short light-dark cycles, paradoxical sleep predominated during the light periods, and slow-wave sleep was unaffected (Tobler and Borbély, 1977).

Related to the above is the finding that the lights-off transition can reliably trigger a PS episode in a slow-wave-sleeping rat (Lisk and Sawyer, 1966; Johnson *et al.,* 1970). Lights-on is an ineffective stimulus, however, and pairing lights-off with a tone fails to produce a conditioned response. The eyes appear necessary for this triggering to occur, but the pineal gland does not.

ONTOGENETIC ASPECTS

Dramatic changes occur in temporal characteristics of both the structural and the pattern components of sleep in association with aging. We first consider the changes in sleep structure.

In human sleep, there are significant changes in the REM stages in both amount and interval timing as a function of age. Since the initial report of Roffwarg, Muzio, and Dement (1966), it has been clear that "active" sleep comprises a proportionately large segment of human neonatal sleep. Roffwarg reported 50% compared to the 20%–25% of Stage 1–REM in adults. However, it is clear that the exact amount and the developmental course of "active" sleep are highly dependent on the measurement criteria. There are six associated states used as indices: (1) rapid eye movements; (2) irregular respiration; (3) small body movements; (4) irregular heart rate; (5) absence of a chin EMG; and (6) a continuous low-amplitude EEG pattern. Using the presence of four or more of these criteria, Parmelee *et al.* (1967) reported 84% active sleep in 29-week prematures, 58% in 39-week conceptional-aged infants, and 40% in full-term neonates. However, using criteria 1, 2, and 3 (above) applied simultaneously during 20-sec epochs, they found only 15% "active" sleep in 29-week-old infants, with an increase in "active" sleep to full term.

Ellingson (1975) reported the development rate in a group of infants of the "mature" EEG and REM pattern (the adult pattern) at three conceptional ages to be 41–45 weeks = 10%; 46–50 weeks = 62%; 50 weeks plus = 100%. With the use of this stabilized criterion the amount of REM is about 30% at the end of the first year. Williams *et al.* (1974) reported the decline in amounts from the age of 3–5 years of about 30% to a stabilized level between 22% and 28% at about age 10. In the 70s, men show a slight decrease in REM.

In the sleep of other species, the course of REM (or PS) amounts follows a "maturity law." Altricial animals show a high percentage of PS at birth compared with maturity; precocial animals tend to show little differences in proportion of PS from birth through maturity (Verley and Garma, 1975).

The REM cycle, defined as the time between REM period onsets, shows age changes. The neonate has an interval of 50–60 min (Roffwarg *et al.,* 1966). The interval

> increases from about 90 minutes in the 3-5 year old group to between 105 and 120 minutes at age 8 and remains there through 29 for both sexes. Average REM cycle length is between 92 and 108 minutes for age 30 through 80 for women and age 30 through 69 for men. REM cycle length for 70–80 year old men was higher than any other age group; it averaged 130 min. (Williams *et al.,* 1974)

The occurrence of "spindles" (rhythmic 12–14 Hz waves) associated with adult Stage 2 sleep appears from about the second month and is fully developed typically by the fourth month. The amount and character of Stage 2 sleep show minimal changes from this point (Keane, Smith, and Webb, 1977).

Slow-wave sleep, Stage 0, and Stage 1 sleep show dramatic changes in amounts with continued aging. Slow-wave sleep begins a significant decline in the 30s. The decline is sharper in males than in females (Williams *et al.,* 1974). However, a recent computer analysis suggests that this sharp decline may be primarily a decline in the amplitude of slow-wave sleep, while the frequency measure (1–2 Hz) may continue intact (Smith, Karacan, and Yang, 1977).

Stage 1 sleep amounts increase steadily with age, from 2%–3% in 10-year-olds to 8%–10% in 60-year-olds. Females generally have less Stage 1 across age groups. Time awake after sleep onset changes very little from early childhood through age 50 in women and age 40 in men. After that time there is a sharp rise in awake time and number of awakenings (Williams *et al.,* 1974).

Impressive changes are associated with the patterns of sleep and aging. Again, availability of data focuses on human sleep. These data are primarily observations of younger subjects and self-reports of older subjects.

Figure 4 shows the changes in total sleep per 24 hr. It is a composite of a number of studies (Kleitman and Engelmann, 1953; O'Connor, 1964; Parmelee, Schultz, and Disbrow, 1961; Reynolds and Mallay, 1933; Terman and Hocking, 1913), and the time scale differences shold be noted. The general picture portrayed is essentially a linear decline over the first 6 months and a reduction of some 2½ hr in the first year. This is followed by another linear decline from the first year to the late teens of about 6 hr, and then a general stabilizing of sleep amounts into the 70s.

There are two aspects of periodicity of sleep patterns for which data are available:

WILSE B. WEBB AND
MICHAEL G. DUBE

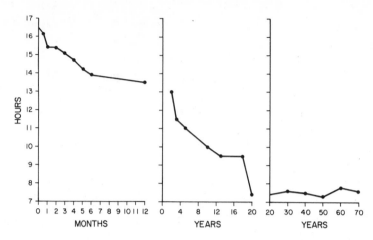

Fig. 4. Total sleep per 24 hr. Note the three different time units used for aging.

diurnal placement and number of episodes. These are interactive, since nonnocturnal sleep periods appear as naps. The diurnal shift of sleep into the night period has been assessed by Parmelee *et al.* (1961) on 46 infants, using a night period of 7 P.M. to 7 A.M., and by Kleitman and Engelmann (1953) on 18 infants, using a night period of 8 P.M. to 8 A.M. These data are shown in Figure 5.

The course of the nocturnal placement of sleep from the sixth month can be only crudely plotted since nonnocturnal sleep follows the course of changes in the extent of napping. Two early studies carefully assessed the amount of day sleep in children from the ages of 2 to 6 years (Reynolds and Mallay, 1933; Shinn, 1932). When the results of the two studies are averaged, the amount of day sleep in the populations declined as follows: 2 years = 81 min; 3 years = 70 min; 4 years = 50 min; 5 years = 15 min. This decline was a joint function of the decreased length of the sleep period and the dropping out of the sleep period entirely. Shinn (1932) reported that a day sleep period was present in 96% of the 2-year-old observations but in only 50% of the 5-year-old observations. Reynolds and Mallay noted that only 50% of the 2-year-olds slept every day, only 8% of the 3-year-olds slept every day, and none of the 4-year-olds slept every day. Evidence from a number of studies indicates that naps increase in older subjects (Webb and Swinburne, 1971). The extent to which this is a release from work routines or a distinct change in the rhythmic structure of sleep is difficult to assess since college students, who are less time-locked to routine work schedules, show a substantial number of nap periods (White, 1974).

The animal aging studies are surprisingly limited. One study reported no changes with age in total sleep time of rats when 19-day-old and 19-month-old rats were compared (Smielkova and Svorad, 1968). A more extensive study found only "indications" of reduced sleep time and shorter sleep episodes in aged rats and no diminution of SWS amplitude or PS sleep ratio (Zepelin, Whitehead, and Rechtschaffen, 1972).

TIME SCHEDULES OF SLEEP AND WAKEFULNESS

A binary system such as sleep and waking placed in a circadian time unit of 24 hr yields three primary change variables relative to sleep: the time of wakefulness preceding sleep periods, the length of sleep periods, and the onset and termination timing. These three variations are interactive and can yield a remarkable range of patterns. As a result of these interactions, experimental designs present difficult problems.

Again, focusing on the larger body of data available on human subjects, a number of systematic relationships have emerged.

Prior wakefulness and onset latency show an essentially negative log linear relationship (Agnew and Webb, 1971). With increased prior wakefulness, there is a systematic increase in Stage 4 sleep and a decrease in awake time after sleep onset (Webb and Agnew, 1977).

In human sleep, because of the differential time distribution within sleep, curtailment of sleep length or its extension necessarily disproportionately effects REM sleep and has a limited affect on the amount of Stage 4 sleep down to about 4 hr (see Figure 2). Since Stage 2 is generally linearly distributed across the sleep period, it is reduced or extended proportionately to the variation in sleep amount.

Studies have experimentally restricted the length of sleep and demonstrated performance decrements (Webb and Agnew, 1965; Wilkinson, 1969). Limited restrictions have been imposed for 8 weeks (Webb and Agnew, 1974a), and gradual reductions have been introduced (Friedmann, Globus, Huntley, Mullaney, Naitoh, and Johnson, 1977). The later studies indicated a limit of about 4.5 hr as a minimal requirement. Restricted sleep has been shown to systematically lengthen the subsequent free sleep period (Webb and Agnew, 1975a).

A variant of the sleep-period-length studies has focused on short and long sleep defined by the subject's status relative to group norms or individual differences in natural sleep length. A very short (about 1 hr) subject has been recorded (Meddis, Pearson, and Langford, 1973), as well as less extreme short periods (4–5.5 hr) (Jones and Oswald, 1968). In the less extreme studies, the short sleepers show evidence of more "compact" sleep, with a slight increase in Stage 4 and little reduction in REM sleep, and long sleepers show enhanced amounts of REM sleep (and Stage 2) (Webb and Agnew, 1970; Hartmann, Baekeland, Zwilling, and Hoy, 1971).

It is clear that REM sleep is responsive to circadian time. If one assumes a "standard" sleep period from 11 P.M. to 7 A.M., there is an increased REM "tendency" across the sleep period and into the early morning period (about 7 A.M.–10 A.M.), with a decreasing ten-

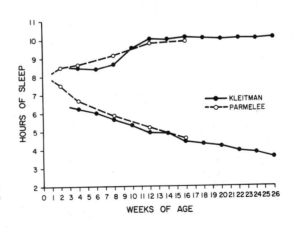

Fig. 5. Number of infants' hours of sleep in 24 hr. Upper line is the sleep from 7 P.M. to 7 A.M.; the lower line from 7 A.M. to 7 P.M.

dency to a low point at sleep onset time (11 P.M.)(Webb and Agnew, 1967). This systematic tendency is demonstrated by the latency of REM sleep relative to sleep onset time at the time points across a circadian day (Webb and Agnew, 1977). The other stages of sleep show only a limited response to onset time of sleep (Webb and Agnew, 1977). With controlled prior wakefulness, sleep latencies are shortest during the "normal" sleep period (11 P.M.–7 A.M.) and continuously rise to a maximum across time to a peak just prior to the normal sleep period (Webb and Agnew, 1975b).

Other circadian effects are discussed in the ultradian rhythm section.

A detailed study of sleep in a freerunning environment (Webb and Agnew, 1974b) shows sleep onsets and terminations approximating the patterns well established by the extensive work of Aschoff and his associates. Total amount of sleep is increased, naps are frequent occurrences, and while sleep stages display the dynamics associated with schedule variations (above), the total proportions of sleep stages approximate entrained environment proportions. A claim is made for a double-rhythm effect (circadian influences and freerunning influences). A recent paper has reported freerunning sleep patterns in a nonisolated blind subject (Miles, Raynal, and Wilson, 1977). A bicircadian sleep–wake regime (48 hr) has been reported in time-isolated environments (Aschoff, Gerecke, and Wever, 1967; Chouvet, Mouret, Coindet, Siffre, and Jouvet, 1974).

A number of studies have assessed sleep in non-24-hr schedules. These have used schedules of 90 min (60 min W–30 min S) (Carskadon and Dement, 1975), 3 hr (2 hr W–1 hr S) (Weitzman, Nogeire, Perlow, Fukushima, Sassin, MacGregor, Gallagher, and Hellman, 1974), 3.5 hr (2.5 hr W–1 hr S) (Moses, Hord, Lubin, Johnson, and Naitoh, 1975), and 9 hr, 12 hr, 18 hr, 30 hr, 36 hr (Webb and Agnew, 1977), and 48 hr (Webb, 1978). In general, again the sleep stages reflect the dynamics of time schedules (above). The data further indicate that the greater the degree of difference from a circadian schedule, the less the total sleep obtained during the scheduled sleep periods (Webb and Agnew, 1975b).

ULTRADIAN RHYTHMS AND SLEEP

Ultradian rhythms are those with time sequences shorter than circadian rhythms. When considered in relationship to sleep, these may be arbitrarily divided into events that have been primarily viewed as sleep-defined phenomena and events, continuous throughout the 24 hr, that may be extensions of or related to sleep-defined rhythms. Examples of the first group would be such variables as REM episodes or spindles. The second group would show time characteristics similar to those occurring in sleep but present in the waking state.

ULTRADIAN RHYTHMS WITHIN SLEEP

A landmark article entitled "Regularly Occurring Periods of Eye Motility and Concomitant Phenomena during Sleep" (Aserinsky and Kleitman, 1953) initiated a research focus that was to dominate sleep research through the 1960s and 1970s. These "regularly occurring" periods were the Stage 1–REM periods of sleep, and their presence in other animals was quickly established (Dement, 1958). The presence and general parameters and associated changes with phylogeny, ontogeny, and time schedules have been noted in earlier sections. Our focus here is on the interval characteristics of this ultradian event within sleep.

It must be noted that this is not a precisely timed event. Table I presents REM time data from the normative studies of Williams *et al.* (1974) on 10 females and 11 males between the ages of 20 and 29. These were highly standardized recordings from 11 P.M. to 7 A.M. and are from the second, third, and fourth nights of laboratory recording. Clearly, the substantial standard deviations both for the first REM latency and for the REM cycle length (onset to onset of REM episodes) indicate a highly variable timing. This variability reflects both between- and within-subject variability. However, the hope that this is a precise system within subjects but variant between subjects is not supported by available data. Hartmann, in an early study (1968), defined *cycle length* as the end of a REM episode to the end of the next episode. While this definition adds some variability due to changing REM episode length across the night, the range of variability within subjects was substantial. For 15 young adults measured eight or nine nights, the average range of cycle length was 63 min. The smallest range was 38 min (66–104 min) and the largest was 102 min (68–170 min).

Globus (1970) defined cycle length by an autocorrelation procedure. Ten subjects slept from 6 to 10 nights in the laboratory. Autocorrelations were obtained for each night, and the time period of highest agreement was used to define a cycle length. While the mean cycle length for the population was 101.5 min, the mean period of the subjects ranged from 85.5 min to 112.4 min, and within subjects the standard deviation of the cycles ranged from 6.2 min to 24.7 min. The average standard deviation was 12.7 min, which yields an average range within subjects similar to Hartmann's: 72 min versus 63 min.

A particular avenue of search for the source of these variabilities has been to posit a time lock between REM and real clock time or to consider REM sleep-dependent. Thus, if REM timing is real-time-"locked," variability may be attributable to variations in between-subject "clock settings," or if sleep-dependent, the variations may be a function of different sleep onset times. Globus explored this question by varying onset times for two subjects in the afternoon (1966). In one subject, sleep-onset-time dependency was clearly apparent; the other showed some evidence of "real"-time responding. A different approach was used by Moses *et al.* (1977). In a study in which sleep was broken into naps, the naps were "compressed" into a continuous sleep period and REM intervals determined. No difference was obtained in the compressed period intervals when compared with within sleep intervals, and as a result, sleep dependency was hypothesized. In a recent elaborate analysis, Schulz, Dirlich, and Zulley (1975) concluded that the onset of the first REM period was tied to sleep onset but that within-sleep REM showed a phase shift of 5–10 min per day. These data suggest that REM intervals may be neither sleep-dependent

TABLE I. THREE-NIGHT MEANS OF 11 MALE AND 10 FEMALE YOUNG ADULTS' REM MEASURES

		Female	Male
Latency of first REM	M	100.2	88.3
	SD	44.2	21.3
REM cycle length	M	115.6	106.5
	SD	48.1	17.5

(except for the first episode) nor real-time-locked but operating on an endogenous freerunning rhythm. As we note in the following section, the issue of sleep dependent–independent phasing of REM enters into the problem of REM as a part of the waking period.

Other aspects of the timing of ultradian rhythms of sleep variables have been explored. Lubin, Nute, Naitoh, and Martin (1973) fit a damped sinusoid to delta (slow-wave) activity with a period of approximately 100 min. Silverstein and Levy (1976) intensively explored "spindle" activity by a computer detection system based on the sigma frequency range (12.25–15.5 Hz/sec). They found large subject-to-subject variations in total amounts and a concentration of spindles in Stage 2 (essentially none in Stage 1 and Stage 1–REM, and intermediate amounts in Stages 3 and 4). The amounts were generally stable across the night.

The most extensive temporal analysis of intrasleep periods is that reported by Keane *et al.* (1977). This paper used computer analysis of sleep activity. Cycle lengths of beta, delta, and sigma frequencies and REM density showed periods ranging from 85 min to 106 min with standard deviations between 12 min and 21 min. No age effect was noted in cycle lengths. However, an age change was present relative to the first half versus the last half of the sleep period. The amount of beta occurring in the first half increased with age, while the opposite was true of delta frequencies. Finally, an intensive analysis of rapid eye movements and REM within sleep and eye movement measures during waking has been reported (De La Pena, Zarcone, and Dement, 1973). Total REM amount was found to be independent of a number of submeasures (e.g., intensity measures). Eye movement measures within sleep were correlated with waking eye-movement measures taken from, for example, viewing pictures.

Ultradian Sleep Rhythms and Wakefulness

The relationship between sleep and ultradian rhythms is framed by two questions. Are the rhythms of systems that are ultradian different when the organism is asleep from when it is awake? Are ultradian rhythms that are noted in sleep continuous across the waking period? The effect of sleep on the frequency and amplitude of other rhythms is reviewed elsewhere and not considered in this chapter. As an example, hormonal secretions are typically ultradian; their relationship to sleep is reviewed by Aschoff (1979). However, the second question has been a provocative one in sleep research.

Certainly, a part of the interest in the extension of an ultradian rhythm across the 24 hr stems from the concept of the basic rest–activity cycle (BRAC) suggested by Nathaniel Kleitman. Extending his earlier thoughts (1939) about an alternating sleep–wakefulness "evolution," Kleitman incorporated the established presence of the approximately 90-min REM cycle in sleep into a call for a recognition of this as a marker of a continuously present BRAC (1963, 1967, 1969). Clearly, the implication was that it is a basic cycle that is present across time but merely obvious in the measurement properties during sleep. Kleitman cited, as basic supportive data, the continuous gastric motility cycles of about 90 min reported by Wada (1922).

As noted above, the time dimensions of REM sleep have continued to be examined and remain problematic. An added dimension has been the search for cycling of non-REM measures across the 24 hr. Friedmann and Fisher (1967) reported an average cycle duration of 96 min of "orality" in waking human subjects in confinement. Orality was measured by time of "eating, drinking, smoking, etc." This finding was replicated by Oswald, Merrington, and Lewis (1970). Friedmann also reported on orality cycles in schizophrenics (1968) and obese patients (1972). Kripke reported 10–20 cycle–day rhythms in delta amplitude and operant lever presses for water (1970). Globus, Drury, Phoebus, and Boyd (1971) found 100-min cycles in a visual signal-detection task. Lavie, Levy, and Coolidge (1975) reported cycles of about 90 min in perceptual illusions and urine flow (Lavie and Kripke, 1977), and Hiatt, Kripke, and Lavie (1975) reported on a waking cycle of fantasies. In addition, Kripke, Halberg, Crowley, and Pegram (1970) have reported on ultradian cycling in rhesus monkeys, and Sterman (1972) and Sterman, Lucas, and MacDonald (1972) have reported an ultradian-rhythm REM cycle of about 20 min in the sleep of the cat and behavioral and EEG responses in the waking cat of about 20 min.

A general review of ultradian rhythms in sleep and wakefulness and analytical problem solving was published by Kripke (1974). Orr, Hoffman, and Hegge (1974) and Orr and Naitoh (1976) have discussed analytical techniques associated with ultradian rhythms and have argued for an application of a demodulation procedure. They have subsequently applied this procedure to heart rate and behavioral measures (Orr and Hoffman, 1974; Orr, Hoffman, and Hegge, 1976).

What, then, is the status of the concept of a BRAC of about 90 min? In human subjects, it is clear that within sleep, the average interval between REM periods is about 100 min. However, both within subjects and between subjects, this timing is not precise. The interval shows developmental changes from birth to maturity, and the onset is sensitive to circadian effects relative to sleep onset. An analogue of REM cycles is clearly present in most vertebrates, but the cycle length shows a wide range.

Is this periodic REM event in humans an apparent index of a 90-min (circa) cycle that extends across the 24 hr? It has been argued (above) that this is a sleep-dependent rhythm, that it is time-dependent, that onset is sleep-dependent, and that the interval is a freerunning endogenous rhythm. A more complex argument has contended that it is an endogenous rhythm whose phase, frequency, and amplitude may be influenced by the sleep–wake conditions (Kripke, 1974). An intriguing and overlooked theory was stated by Shapiro (1970). He noted that 85.5 min is the value of Schuler's constant for the gyrocompass and is equal to

$$\frac{1}{2\pi} \sqrt{\frac{R}{G}}$$

where R = the radius of the earth and G is acceleration due to gravity at the earth's surface. He suggested that the "90-min" cycle was of geophysical origin.

SLEEP AND HORMONAL RHYTHMS

With the development of sensitive micromeasurement techniques, the relationship between anterior pituitary hormones and sleep states has been subjected to extensive investigation and these studies have recently been well reviewed (Aschoff, Ceresa, and Halber, 1974; Daly and Evans, 1974; Hedlund, Franz, and Kenny, 1975; Krieger and Aschoff, 1978; Rubin, Poland, Rubin, and Govin, 1974; Takahashi, 1974; Weitzman, 1974). Particular attention is called to a discussion by Aschoff (1979), which integrates the consideration of sleep and waking, endocrine rhythms, and circadian rhythms. In the following summary, references have been omitted, as all are included in one or more of the cited reviews.

It has become clear that ACTH–cortisol, growth hormone, prolactin, and gonadotropin cycles all have important temporal relations with the sleep–waking rhythm. The ACTH–cortisol rhythm, for example, shows a trough during the initial hours of nocturnal sleep and a peak in the latter hours when REM sleep is maximal. This underlying pattern has superimposed numerous peaks reflecting the episodic nature of ACTH release. Despite these temporal relations, however, there does not appear to be a close neurophysiological link between ACTH and the sleep–waking rhythm. Subjects deprived of sleep for 1 or 2 nights still show the nocturnal episodes of increased ACTH–cortisol secretion evident in normal subjects. Further, acute inversion of the sleep–waking rhythm can dissociate REM episodes from the ACTH rhythm for periods of 1–2 weeks, and shortening or lengthening of the sleep–waking rhythm requires several days for the ACTH–cortisol rhythm to correspondingly shorten or lengthen. Ten days on 3-hr (ultradian) sleep–waking schedules also fails to disrupt the plasma cortisol rhythm.

Studies in blind subjects have shown that perception of the light–dark cycle is not necessary to maintain the ACTH–cortisol rhythm. These subjects show a circadian rhythm of episodic ACTH release, with the transition from sleep to waking correlated with the early morning rise in plasma cortisol. The consistent synchronization of the circadian ACTH–cortisol rhythm with the sleep–waking rhythm indicates that while the ACTH rhythm does not require the sleep–waking rhythm in order to persist, sleep cues are an important determinant of its circadian phase relationships.

Growth hormone (GH), on the other hand, has been shown to require sleep in the normal subject in order for significant secretion to occur. GH is secreted during the first few hours of nocturnal sleep when the EEG pattern of slow-wave sleep, Stages 3 and 4, predominates. A peak is usually reached between 1 and 2 hr after sleep onset, with a return to presleep levels by the 4th hour. During the rest of the day, plasma GH levels usually remain very low.

GH secretion is elevated during naps taken in the afternoon, when Stages 3 and 4 tend to occur, but not during naps taken in the morning, when REM sleep tends to occur. If sleep onset is delayed or prevented for 12 hr, a corresponding immediate delay of GH secretion takes place, with the sleep-related release occurring when the subject has a sustained sleep period. Infants younger than 3 months and very old subjects fail to show a sleep-related GH release, apparently because of the small amount or absence of Stages 3 and 4 in these groups.

Despite this close relationship, dissociation of slow-wave sleep and GH secretion is possible. Deprivation of slow-wave sleep by stimuli that lighten sleep but do not awake the subject results in blunting of the GH response. However, flurazepam, which reduces slow-wave sleep after several days' administration, does not affect GH release. Conversely, imipramine, medroxyprogesterone acetate, and free fatty acid infusion all attenuate or abolish the GH peak without affecting slow-wave sleep.

Prolactin secretion is also episodic and displays a circadian rhythm that increases throughout the night, reaching a peak in the last hour or two of the normal sleep period. Following awakening, a rapid fall in concentration takes place, with low values reached 3–

5 hr later. Sleep onset delay and early awakening produce immediate corresponding shifts in the prolactin peak, and daytime naps result in increased prolactin secretion. Partial or complete inversion of the sleep–waking rhythm causes an immediate shift of the episodes of prolactin secretion to the new sleep schedule. Thus, as in the case of GH, the nocturnal rise in prolactin secretion appears to be dependent on sleep.

The 24-hr pattern of secretion of the two gonadotropins LH and FSH has a complex form because of maturational and sex differences. In prepubertal children, no difference in mean serum LH levels between sleeping and waking exists; however, in pubertal boys and girls, there is a major augmentation of episodic LH release during sleep periods. These episodes appear to have a 70- to 90-min period, with secretion beginning during non-REM (NREM) sleep and terminating in close temporal proximity to REM sleep. Acute sleep-cycle reversal in pubertal boys produces an increase in LH concentrations during the day sleep period; however, nocturnal waking LH concentrations are higher than daytime waking concentrations.

Both LH and FSH are released episodically during the day and night in adult men and women. Adult males show random episodic secretion of both LH and FSH during the entire 24-hr period, with no differences occurring in relation to either the sleep–waking rhythm or to specific sleep stages.

In adult women, the pattern of LH release depends on the phase of the menstrual cycle. Early in the menstrual cycle, LH secretion decreases during the first few hours of nocturnal sleep, followed by a rise in the latter half of the sleep period. Acute inversion of the 24-hr sleep–waking rhythm during this phase produces the same decrease of LH concentration during the first part of the daytime sleep period as occurred during the first few hours of nocturnal sleep. During the periovulatory phase, LH release during sleep is similar to that of adult men, but with a greater rhythmicity of secretory episodes. During the LH surge, episodic secretion continues, with a large increment occurring in the latter hours of the sleep period or at the time of awakening. These results demonstrate a time-locked relationship between the ovulatory cycle and the sleep–waking rhythm in the control of gonadotropin secretion.

The Central Nervous System and Sleep Rhythms

Historically, neurophysiological and biochemical studies of sleep have been concerned with the mechanisms of the sleep process itself and not with its temporal placement. This work, which has been extensively reviewed elsewhere (Gillin, Mendelson, Sitaram, and Wyatt, 1978; Holman, Elliott, and Barchas, 1975; Jouvet, 1972, 1973, 1974; Karnovsky and Reich, 1977; Moruzzi, 1972, 1974), has revealed sleep to be an active neural process. The firing of individual neurons, for example, does not come to a halt during sleep and may actually exceed waking rates in different brain regions during various sleep stages. The main anatomical regions involved in sleep–waking processes appear to be the raphe nuclear complex, the locus ceruleus, the reticular activating system–diffuse thalamic system, the preoptic region, and the area postrema-nucleus of the tractus solitarius.

During the past 10 years, considerable work has been performed investigating the role of various neurotransmitters in the regulation of the sleep process. Particular attention has been paid to the biogenic amines. However, their role in sleep is far from clear. Serotonin has been proposed as an important neurotransmitter in the operation of the sleep system, primarily on the basis of studies using cats (Jouvet, 1972, 1973, 1974). Research on rats, employing means that more specifically intervene in the serotonergic system, has produced negative results and has raised serious questions about the serotonergic theory of sleep (Bouhuys and Van Den Hoofdakker, 1977; Ross, Trulson, and Jacobs, 1976). The catecholamines, in particular norepinephrine, have been regarded as playing a role in the production of REM sleep.

Acetylcholine has also been implicated in sleep processes. Its application to many areas of the central nervous system has been known for some time to induce sleep (Hernández Peón, 1965). This lack of anatomical specificity, however, makes assessing its role in normal animals difficult. More recent studies implicate it in REM sleep processes (Gillin *et al.,* 1978; Holman *et al.,* 1975). The role of polypeptides and other neurotransmitters has also been considered (Gillin *et al.,* 1978; Karnovsky and Reich, 1977), but in every case, the thrust of these investigations has been toward the mechanisms of the components of the sleep response and not their temporal placement. At the present time, therefore, the role of neurochemistry in the temporal placement of sleep is unknown.

Lesion studies, however, have shed some light on the mechanisms controlling the placement of sleep. The processes that control the circadian distribution of sleep do not appear to depend on the integrity of brain-stem sleep mechanisms. Destruction of the anterior and intermediary raphe nuclei, reducing total sleep time to only 3.5% of normal, does not prevent the normal circadian distribution of the sleep time that remains (Jouvet, 1974).

The hypothalamus appears to be an important center in the timing of a number of rhythms. Stephan and Zucker (1972) have reported that lesions of the suprachiasmatic nucleus (SCN) eliminate activity and drinking rhythms in the rat, and other studies have implicated this nucleus as a possible timing center for the circadian rhythms of pineal serotonin N-acetyltransferase activity (Moore and Klein, 1974); hypothalamopituitary regulation of adrenal function (Moore and Eichler, 1972); luteinizing-hormone secretion (Butler and Donovan, 1971); food intake (Nagui, Nishio, Nakagawa, Nakamura, and Fukuda, 1978); brain temperature (Stephan and Nunez, 1977); heart rate (Saleh and Winget, 1977); estrous cyclicity (Stetson and Watson-Whitmyre, 1976); and several other rhythms. These results suggest that the SCN plays a key role in the mammalian circadian system.

Ibuka and Kawamura (1975) have shown that SCN lesions also abolish the sleep rhythm in rats, and this finding has been confirmed by a number of other studies (Coindet, Chouvet, and Mouret, 1975; Dube, 1978; Ibuka, Inouye, and Kawamura, 1977; Stephan and Nunez, 1977). These studies all find the SWS and PS rhythms of SCN-lesioned animals to be flat, even in the presence of light–dark cycles. Whether the SCN is functioning as a central oscillator or a coupling mechanism or in some more complex way is at present unknown. Also the anatomical and physiological connections involved between most of these rhythms (including sleep) and the SCN are unknown. It has been established, however, that the light–dark entrainment of these rhythms depends on a direct retinohypothalamic projection (Moore and Eichler, 1976; Ibuka *et al.,* 1977).

In addition to the SCN role in sleep rhythm production, it has been reported by Mouret, Coindet, and Chouvet (1974) that in rats, pinealectomy leads to an increase of PS during the dark period and a decrease during the light period, while leaving SWS unaffected. Thus, the pineal may be involved in the circadian variation of PS and its phase relationships with SWS.

Another question, as yet unanswered, concerns the neural processes producing the cyclical alternation of NREM and REM sleep. Batsel (1960) has shown in the dog that spontaneous cyclic fluctuations of activity are inherent in the physiology of the upper reticular formation. Recently, Hobson, McCarley, and Wyinski (1975) (also McCarley and Hobson, 1975) have suggested that a reciprocal interaction existing between neurons of the locus ceruleus and subceruleus and those of the gigantocellular tegmental field (FTG) may serve as a physiological basis of the sleep cycle oscillation. Hobson (1977) has recently stated this "reciprocal interaction hypothesis" in more specific physiological terms. He proposed that

> ... the giant cells are cholinergic and cholinoceptive and excitatory to post-synaptic elements including one another. Self-excitation is then possible within the FTG generatory pool. FTG neurons are reciprocally interconnected with two groups of aminergic cells: The raphe and locus coeruleus which use norepinephrine as their transmitter. Both aminergic groups are inhibitory to self and other. At any given time, the excitability of FTG population is thus an inverse function of the level of activity in the aminergic populations (and vice versa). (p. 173)

This model is supported by the behavior of these cell populations during waking, NREM, and REM episodes.

REFERENCES

Agnew, H. W., Jr., and Webb, W. B. Sleep latencies in human subjects: Age prior wakefulness and reliability. *Psychonomic Science,* 1971, *24*(6), 253–254.

Allison, T., and Cicchetti, D. V. Sleep in mammals: Ecological and constitutional correlates. *Science,* 1976, *194,* 732–734.

Aschoff, J. Circadian rhythms in man. *Science,* 1965, *148,* 1427–1432.

Aschoff, J. Circadian rhythms: General features and endocrinological aspects. In D. T. Krieger (Ed.), *Endocrine Rhythms.* New York: Raven Press, 1979.

Aschoff, J., Gerecke, U., and Wever, P. Desynchronization of human circadian rhythms. *Japanese Journal of Physiology,* 1967, *17,* 450–457.

Aschoff, J., Ceresa, F., and Halber, F. (Eds.). Chronobiological aspects of endocrinology. In *Chronobiologia,* 1974, *1*(Suppl. 1).

Aserinsky, E., and Kleitman, N. Regularly occurring periods of eve motility and concomitant phenomena during sleep. *Science,* 1953, *118,* 273–274.

Batsel, H. L. Electroencephalographic synchronization and desynchronization in the chronic "cerveau isole" of the dog. *Electroencephalography and Clinical Neurophysiology,* 1960, *12,* 421–430.

Bert, J., Ayats, H., Martino, A., and Collomb, H. Le sommeil nocturne chez le babouin *Papio papio. Folia Primatologica,* 1967, *6,* 28–43.

Borbély, A. A. Sleep and motor activity of the rat during ultra-short light–dark cycles. *Brain Research,* 1976, *114,* 305–317.

Borbély, A. A. Huston, J. P., and Waser, P. G. Control of sleep states in the rat by short light–dark cycles. *Brain Research,* 1975, *95,* 89–101.

Bouhuys, A. L., and Van Den Hoofdakker, R. H. Effects of midbrain raphe destruction on sleep and locomotor activity in rats. *Physiology and Behavior,* 1977, *19,* 535–541.

Butler, J. E. M., and Donovan, B. T. The effect of surgical isolation of the hypothalamus upon reproductive function in the guinea pig. *Journal of Endocrinology,* 1971, *50,* 507–514.

Carskadon, M. A., and Dement, W. C. Sleep studies on a 90 minute day. *Electroencephalography and Clinical Neurophysiology,* 1975, *39,* 145–155.

Chouvet, G., Mouret, J., Coindet, J., Siffre, M., and Jouvet, M. Periodicité bicircadienne du cycle veille—Sommeil dans des condition hors du temps. Etude polygraphique. *Electroencephalography and Clinical Neurophysiology,* 1974, *37,* 367–380.

Coindet, J., Chouvet, G. and Mouret, J. Effects of lesions of the suprachiasmatic nuclei on paradoxical sleep and slow wave sleep circadian rhythms in the rat. *Neuroscience Letters,* 1975, *1,* 243–247.

Conroy, R. T., and Mills, J. N. *Human Circadian Rhythms.* Baltimore: Williams & Wilkins, 1970.

Daly, J. R., and Evans, J. I. Daily rhythms of steroid and associated pituitary hormones in man and their relationship to sleep. *Advances in Steroid and Biochemical Pharmacology,* 1974, *4,* 61–110.

De La Pena, A., Zarcone, V., and Dement, W. C. Correlation between measures of eye movements of wakefulness and sleep. *Psychophysiology,* 1973, *10*(5), 488–500.

Dement, W. C. The occurrence of low voltage, fast electroencephalogram patterns during behavioral sleep in the cat. *Electroencephalography and Clinical Neurophysiology,* 1958, *10,* 291–296.

Dube, M. G. Food as a zeitgeber: Effect of one hour light phase food access on sleep in the rat. *Sleep Research,* 1976, *5,* 214.

Dube, M. G. Aspects of the physiology of bio-behavioral chronometry. *JSAS Catologue of Selected Documents in Psychology,* 1978, *8.*

Ellingson, R. J. Ontogenesis of sleep in the human. In G. C. Lairy and P. Salzarulo (Eds.), *The Experimental Study of Human Sleep.* New York: Elsevier, 1975.

Fraisse, P. *The Psychology of Time.* New York: Harper & Row, 1963.

Friedmann, J., Globus, G., Huntley, A., Mullaney, D., Naitoh, P., and Johnson, L. Performance and mood during and after gradual sleep reduction. *Psychophysiology,* 1977, *14,* 245–250.

Friedmann, S. Oral activity cycles in mild chronic schizophrenia. *American Journal of Psychiatry,* 1968, *125,* 743–751.

Friedmann, S. On the presence of a variant form of instinctual regression: Oral drive cycles in obesity-bulimia. *Psychoanalytic Quarterly,* 1972, *41,* 364–383.

Friedmann, S., and Fisher, C. On the presence of a rhythmic diurnal, oral and instinctual drive cycle in man. *Journal of American Psychoanalytical Association,* 1967, *15,* 317–343.

Gillin, J. C., Mendelson, W. B., Sitaram, N., and Wyatt, R. J. The neuropharmacology of sleep and wakefulness. *Annual Review of Pharmacology and Toxicology,* 1978, *18,* 563–579.

Globus, G. G. Rapid eye movement cycle in real time. *Archives of General Psychology,* 1966, *15,* 654–659.

Globus, G. G. Quantification of the sleep cycle as a rhythm. *Psychophysiology,* 1970, *7,* 244–253.

Globus, G., Drury, R., Phoebus, E., and Boyd, R. Ultradian rhythms in human performance. *Perceptual and Motor Skills,* 1971, *33,* 1171–1174.

Hartmann, E. The ninety-minute sleep dream cycle. *Archives of General Psychiatry,* 1968, *18,* 280–286.

Hartmann, E., Baekeland, F., Zwilling, G., and Hoy, P. Sleep need: How much sleep and what kind. *American Journal of Psychiatry,* 1971, *127,* 1001–1008.

Hedlund, L. W., Franz, J. M., and Kenny, A. D. *Biological Rhythms and Endocrine Function.* New York: Plenum Press, 1975.

Hernández Péon, R. Central neurohumoral transmission in sleep and wakefulness. In K. Akert, C. Bally, and J. P. Schade (Eds.), *Progress in Brain Research, Vol. 18: Sleep Mechanisms.* Amsterdam: Elsevier, 1965.

Hiatt, J. F., Kripke, D. F., and Lavie, P. Relationships among psychophysiologic ultradian rhythms. *Chronobiologia Supplement,* 1975, *1,* 30.

Hobson, J. A. The reciprocal interaction model of sleep cycle control: Implications for PGO wave generation and dream amnesia. In R. R. Drucker-Colin and J. L. McGaugh (Eds.), *Neurobiology of Sleep and Memory.* New York: Academic Press, 1977.

Hobson, J. A., McCarley, R. W., and Wyinski, P. W. Sleep cycle oscillation: Reciprocal discharge by two brainstem neuronal groups. *Science,* 1975, *189,* 55–58.

Hoffmann, K. Splitting of the circadian rhythm as a function of light intensity. In M. Menaker (Ed.), *Biochronometry.* Washington, D.C.: National Academy of Sciences, 1971.

Holman, R. B., Elliott, G. R., and Barchas, J. D. Neuroregulators and sleep mechanisms. *Annual Review of Medicine,* 1975, *26,* 499–520.

Ibuka, N., and Kawamura, H. Loss of circadian rhythm in sleep–wakefulness cycle in the rat by suprachiasmatic nuclear lesions. *Brain Research,* 1975, *96,* 76–81.

Ibuka, N., Inouye, S. I. T., and Kawamura, H. Analysis of sleep–wakefulness rhythms in male rats after suprachiasmatic nucleus lesions and ocular enucleation. *Brain Research,* 1977, *122,* 33–47.

Johnson, J. H., Adler, N. T., and Sawyer, C. H. Effects of various photoperiods on the temporal distribution of paradoxical sleep in rats. *Experimental Neurology,* 1970, *27,* 162–171.

Jones, H. S., and Oswald, I. Two cases of healthy insomnia. *Electroencephalography and Clinical Neurophysiology*, 1968, *24*, 378–380.

Jouvet, M. The role of monoamines and acetylcholine-containing neurons in the regulation of the sleep–waking cycle. *Ergebnisse der Physiologie*, 1972, *64*, 166–307.

Jouvet, M. Serotonin and sleep in the cat. In J. Barchas and E. Usdin (Eds.), *Serotonin and Behavior*. New York: Academic Press, 1973.

Jouvet, M. The role of monoaminergic neurons in the regulation and function of sleep. In O. Petre-Quadens and J. D. Schlag (Eds.), *Basic Sleep Mechanisms*. New York: Academic Press, 1974.

Karnovsky, M. L., and Reich, P. Biochemistry of sleep. *Advances in Nurochemistry*, 1977, *2*, 213–275.

Keane, B., Smith, J., and Webb, W. B. Temporal distribution and ontogenetic development of EEG activity during sleep. *Psychophysiology*, 1977, *14*(3), 315–321.

Kleitman, N. *Sleep and Wakefulness* (1st ed.). Chicago: University of Chicago Press, 1939.

Kleitman, N. *Sleep and Wakefulness* (2nd ed.). Chicago: University of Chicago Press, 1963.

Kleitman, N. Phylogenetic, ontogenetic and environmental determinants in the evolution of sleep–wakefulness cycles. In S. S. Kety, E. V. Evarts, and H. L. Williams (Eds.), *Sleep and Altered States of Consciousness* (Research Publications of the Association for Research in Nervous and Mental Disease, Vol. 45). Baltimore: Williams & Wilkins, 1967.

Kleitman, N. Basic rest activity cycle in relation to sleep and wakefulness. In A. Kales (Ed.), *Sleep: Physiology and Pathology*. Philadelphia: Lippincott, 1969.

Kleitman, N., and Engelmann, T. Sleep characteristics of infants. *Journal of Applied Physiology*, 1953, *6*, 269–282.

Krieger, D., and Aschoff, J. Endocrine and other biological rhythms. In L. DeGroot, L. Martini, J. Potts, D. Nelson, A. Winegra, W. Odell, E. Steinberg, and G. Cahill (Eds.), *Metabolic Basis of Endocrinology*. New York: Grune & Stratton, 1978.

Kripke, D. F. An ultradian biological rhythm associated with perceptual deprivation and REM sleep. *Psychosomatic Medicine*, 1970, *34*, 221–234.

Kripke, D. F. Ultradian rhythms in sleep and wakefulness. In E. D. Weitzman (Ed.), *Advances in Sleep Research*. Vol 1. New York: Spectrum, 1974.

Kripke, D. F., Halberg, F., Crowley, T. J., and Pegram, G. V. Ultradian rhythms in rhesus monkeys. *Psychophysiology*, 1970, *7*, 307–308.

Lavie, P., and Kripke, D. F. Ultradian rhythms in urine flow in waking humans. *Nature*, 1977, *269*, 142–143.

Lavie, P., Levy, M., and Coolidge, F. Ultradian rhythms in the perception of the spiral aftereffect. *Physiological Psychology*, 1975, *3*(2), 144–146.

Lewis, P. R., and Lobban, M. C. Disassociation of diurnal rhythms in human subjects living on abnormal time routines. *Quarterly Journal of Experimental Physiology*, 1957, *42*, 371–386.

Lisk, R. D., and Sawyer, C. H. Induction of paradoxical sleep by lights-off stimulation. *Proceedings of the Society of Experimental Biology and Medicine*, 1966, *123*, 664–667.

Lubin, A., Nute, C., Naitoh, P., and Martin, W. EEG data activity during human sleep as a damped ultradian rhythm. *Psychophysiology*, 1973, *10*(1) 27–35.

McCarley, R. W., and Hobson, J. A. Neuronal excitability modulation over the sleep cycle: A structural and mathematical model. *Science*, 1975, *189*, 58–60.

McGhie, A., and Russell, S. M. The subjective assessment of normal sleep patterns. *Journal of Mental Science*, 1962, *107*, 188–202.

Meddis, R., Pearson, A. J. D., and Langford, G. An extreme case of healthy insomnia. *Electroencephalography and Clinical Neurophysiology*, 1973, *35*, 213–214.

Miles, L., Raynal, D. M., and Wilson, M. A. Blind man living in normal society has circadian rhythm of 24.9 hours. *Science*, 1977, *198*, 421–423.

Mills, J. N. (d.). *Biological Aspects of Circadian Rhythms*. London: Plenum Press, 1973.

Mitler, M. M., Lund, R., Sokolove, P. G., Pittendrigh, C. S., and Dement, W. C. Sleep and activity rhythms in mice: A description of circadian patterns and unexpected disruptions in sleep. *Brain Research*, 1977, *131*, 129–145.

Moore, R. Y., and Eichler, V. B. Loss of a circadian adrenal corticosterone rhythm following suprachiasmatic lesions in the rat. *Brain Research*, 1972, *42*, 201–206.

Moore, R. Y., and Eichler, V. B. Central neural mechanisms in diurnal rhythm regulation and neuroendocrine responses to light. *Psychoneuroendocrinology*, 1976, *1*, 265–279.

Moore, R. Y., and Klein, D. C. Visual pathways and the central neural control of a circadian rhythm in pineal serotonin N-acetyltransferase activity. *Brain Research*, 1974, *71*, 17–33.

Moruzzi, G. The sleep-waking cycle. *Ergebnisse der Physiologie*, 1972, *64*, 1–165.

Moruzzi, G. Neural mechanisms of the sleep–waking cycle. In O. Petre-Quadens and J. D. Schlag (Eds.), *Basic Sleep Mechanisms*. New York: Academic Press, 1974.

Moses, J. M., Hord, D. J., Lubin, A., Johnson, L. C., and Naitoh, P. Dynamics of nap sleep during a 40-hour period. *Electroencephalography and Clinical Neurophysiology*, 1975, *39*, 627–633.

Moses, J., Lubin, A., Johnson, L. C., and Naitoh, P. Rapid eye movement cycle is a sleep dependent rhythm. *Nature*, 1977, *265*, 360–361.

Mouret, J. R., and Bobillier, P. Diurnal rhythms of sleep in the rat: Augmentation of paradoxical sleep following alteration of paradoxical sleep following alterations of the feeding schedule. *International Journal of Neuroscience*, 1971, *2*, 265–270.

Mouret, J., Coindet, J., and Chouvet, G. Effet de la pinéalectomie sur les états et rhythmes de sommeil du rat mâle. *Brain Research*, 1974, *81*, 97–105.

Nagui, K., Nishio, T., Nakagawa, H., Nakamura, S., and Fukuda, Y. Effect of bilateral lesions of the suprachiasmatic nuclei on the circadian rhythm of food intake. *Brain Research*, 1978, *142*, 384–389.

O'Connor, A. L. Questionnaire responses about sleep. M.A. thesis, University of Florida, 1964.

Orr, W. C., and Hoffman, H. J. A 90-minute cardiac biorhythm: Methodology and data analysis using modified periodograms and complex demodulation. *IEEE Transactions in Biomedical Engineering*, 1974, *21*, 130–143.

Orr, W. C., and Naitoh, P. The coherence spectrum: An extension of correlation analysis with applications to chronobiology. *International Journal of Chronobiology*, 1976, *3*, 171–192.

Orr, W. C., Hoffman, H. J., and Hegge, F. W. Ultradian rhythms in extended performance. *Aerospace Medicine*, 1974, *45*, 995–1000.

Orr, W. C., Hoffman, H. J., and Hegge, F. W. The chronobiology of performance: The assessment of time dependent changes in human behavior. *Chronobiologia*, 1976, *3*, 293–305.

Oswald, I., Merrington, J., and Lewis, H. Cyclical "on demand" oral intake by adults. *Nature*, 1970, *225*, 959–960.

Parmelee, A. H., Schultz, H. R., and Disbrow, M. A. Sleep patterns of the newborn. *Journal of Pediatrics*, 1961, *58*, 241–250.

Parmelee, A. H., Wenner, W., Akima, Y., Schultz, M., and Stern, E. Sleep states in premature infants. *Developmental Medicine and Child Neurology*, 1967, *9*, 70–77.

Pittendrigh, C. S. Circadian oscillations in cells and the circadian organization of multicellular systems. In F. O. Schmitt and F. G. Worden (Eds.), *The Neurosciences: Third Study Program*. Cambridge, Mass.: M.I.T. Press, 1974.

Reynolds, M. M., and Mallay, H. The sleep of children in a 24 hour nursery school. *Journal of Genetic Psychology*, 1933, *43*, 322–351.

Roffwarg, H., Muzio, J., and Dement, W. C. Ontogenetic development of the human sleep-dream cycle. *Science*, 1966, *152*, 604–619.

Ross, C. A., Trulson, M. E., and Jacobs, B. L. Depletion of brain serotonin following intraventribular 5,7-dihydroxytryptamine fails to disrupt sleep in the rat. *Brain Research*, 1976, *114*, 517–523.

Rubin, R. J., Poland, R. E., Rubin, L. E., and Gouin, P. R. The neuroendocrinology of human sleep. *Life Sciences*, 1974, *14*, 1041–1052.

Ruckebusch, Y. The relevance of drowsiness in the circadian cycle of farm animals. *Animal Behaviour*, 1972, *20*, 637–643.

Saleh, M. A., and Winget, C. M. Effect of suprachiasmatic lesions on diurnal heart rate rhythm in the rat. *Physiology and Behavior*, 1977, *19*, 561–564.

Schulz, H., Dirlich, G., and Zulley, J. Phase shift in the REM sleep rhythm. *Pflügers Archiv*, 1975, *212*, 203.

Shapiro, A. Comments on the 90-minute sleep-dream cycle. In E. Hartmann (Ed.), *Sleep and Dreaming*. Boston: Little, Brown, 1970.

Shinn, A. F. A study of sleep habits of two groups of pre-school children, one in Hawaii and one in the mainland. *Child Development*, 1932, *3*, 159–166.

Silverstein, L. D., and Levy, M. The stability of the sigma sleep spindle. *Electroencephalography and Clinical Neurophysiology*, 1976, *40*, 666–670.

Smielkova, A., and Svorad, D. The sleep cycle of the rat in early and late stages of ontogenesis. *Ceskoslovenska Fysiologie*, 1968, *17*, 63.

Smith, J., Karacan, I., and Yang, M. Ontogeny of delta activity during human sleep. *Electroencephalography and Clinical Neurophysiology*, 1977, *43*, 229–237.

Stephan, F. K., and Nunez, A. A. Elimination of circadian rhythms in drinking, activity, sleep and temperature by isolation of the suprachiasmatic nuclei. *Behavioral Biology*, 1977, *20*, 1–16.

Stephan, F. K., and Zucker, I. Circadian rhythms in drinking behavior and locomotor activity of rat are eliminated by hypothalamic lesions. *Proceedings of the National Academy of Sciences, USA,* 1972, *69,* 1583–1586.

Sterman, M. B. The basic rest activity cycle and sleep. Developmental considerations in man and cats. In C. D. Clemente, D. P. Purpura, and F. E. Mayer (Eds.), *Sleep and the Maturing Nervous System.* New York: Academic Press, 1972.

Sterman, M. B., Lucas, E. A., and MacDonald, L. R. Periodicity within sleep and operant performance in the cat. *Brain Research,* 1972, *38,* 327–341.

Stetson, M. H., and Watson-Whitmyre, M. Nucleus suprachiasmaticus: The biological clock in the hamster. *Science,* 1976, *191,* 197–199.

Takahashi, Y. Growth hormone secretion during sleep: A review. In M. Kawakami (Ed.), *Biological Rhythms in Neuroendocrine Activity.* Tokyo: Igaku Shoin, 1974.

Tauber, E. S. Phylogeny of sleep. In E. D. Weitzman (Ed.), *Advances in Sleep Research.* Vol. 1. New York: Spectrum, 1974, pp. 132–172.

Terman, L., and Hocking, A. The sleep of school children: Its distribution according to age and its relation to physical and mental efficiency. *Journal of Educational Psychology,* 1913, *4,* 138–147.

Tobler, I., and Borbély, A. A. Enhancement of paradoxical sleep by short light periods in the golden hamster. *Neuroscience Letters,* 1977, *6,* 275–277.

Tune, G. S. Sleep and wakefulness in normal human adults. *British Medical Journal,* 1968, *2,* 269–271.

Tune, G. S. Sleep and wakefulness in 509 normal human adults. *British Journal of Medical Psychology,* 1969, *42,* 75–80.

(UCLA) Chase, M. H., Stern, W. C., and Walter, P. L. (Eds.). *Sleep Research.* Los Angeles: Brain Information Service/Brain Research Institute, 1972–present.

Ursin, R. Differential effect of sleep deprivation on the two slow wave sleep stages in the cat. *Acta Physiologica Scandinavica,* 1971, *83,* 352–361.

Van Twyver, H. Sleep patterns of five rodent species. *Physiology and Behavior,* 1969, *4,* 901–908.

Verley, R., and Garma, L. The criteria of sleep stages during ontogeny in different animal species. In G. Lairy and P. Salzarulo (Eds.), *The Experimental Study of Human Sleep: Methodological Problems.* Amsterdam: Elsevier, 1975.

Wada, T. An experimental study of hunger in its relation to activity. *Archives of Psychological Monography,* 1922, *57,* 1.

Webb, W. B. Sleep as a biorhythm. In W. P. Colquhoun (Ed.), *Biological Rhythms and Human Performance.* London: Academic Press, 1971.

Webb, W. B. The adaptive functions of sleep patterns. In P. Levin and W. P. Koella (Eds.), *Sleep 1974.* Basel: Karger, 1975.

Webb, W. B. The forty-eight hour day. *Sleep,* 1978, *1,* 191–197.

Webb, W. B., and Agnew, H. W., Jr. Sleep: Effects of a restricted regime. *Science,* 1965, *150,* 1745–1747.

Webb, W. B., and Agnew, H. W., Jr. Sleep cycling within twenty-four hour periods. *Journal of Experimental Psychology,* 1967, *74,* 158–160.

Webb, W. B., and Agnew, H. W., Jr. Sleep stage characteristics of long and short sleepers. *Science,* 1970, *168,* 146–147.

Webb, W. B., and Agnew, H. W., Jr. The effects of a chronic limitation of sleep length. *Psychophysiology,* 1974a, *11,* 265–274.

Webb, W. B., and Agnew, H. W., Jr. Sleep and waking in a time-free environment. *Aerospace Medicine,* 1974b, *45,* 701–704.

Webb, W. B., and Agnew, H. W., Jr. The effects on subsequent sleep of an acute restriction of sleep length. *Psychophysiology,* 1975a, *12,* 367–370.

Webb, W. B., and Agnew, H. W., Jr. Sleep efficiency for sleep wake cycles of varied length. *Psychophysiology,* 1975b, *12,* 637–641.

Webb, W. B., and Agnew, H. W., Jr. Analysis of the sleep stages in sleep–wakefulness regimens of varied length. *Psychophysiology,* 1977, *14*(5), 445–450.

Webb, W. B., and Friedman, J. K. Length of sleep and length of waking interrelations in the rat. *Psychonomic Science,* 1969, *17*(1), 14–15.

Webb, W. B., and Friedman, J. K. Some temporal characteristics of paradoxical (LVF) sleep occurrence in the rat. *Electroencephalography and Clinical Neurophysiology,* 1970, *30,* 453–456.

Webb, W. B., and Swinburne, H. An observational study of sleep of the aged. *Perceptual and Motor Skills,* 1971, *32,* 895–898.

Weitzman, E. D. Temporal patterns of neuro-endocrine secretion in man: Relationship to the 24-hour sleep waking cycle. In J. Aschoff, F. Ceresa, and F. Halberg (Eds.), *Chronobiological Aspects of Endocrinology.* Stuttgart: F. K. Schattauer Verlag, 1974.

Weitzman, E., Nogeire, C., Perlow, M., Fukushima, D., Sassin, J., MacGregor, P., Gallagher, T., and Hellman, L. Effects of a prolonged 3-hour sleep wake cycle on sleep stages, plasma cortisol, growth hormone and body temperature in man. *Journal of Clinical Endocrinology and Metabolism,* 1974, *38,* 1018–1030.

White, R. *Sleep Parameters in College Students.* Dissertation, University of Florida, 1974.

Wilkinson, R. T. Sleep deprivation: Performance tests for partial and selective sleep deprivation. In L. A. Abt and B. F. Reiss (Eds.), *Progress in Clinical Psychology.* Vol. 8. New York: Grune & Stratton, 1969.

Williams, W., Karacan, I., and Hursch, C. *EEG and Human Sleep.* New York: Wiley, 1974.

Yamaoka, S., and Hagino, N. Influence of constant illumination on the circadian rhythm of sleep, paradoxical sleep and wakefulness in female baboons and rats. *Federation Proceedings,* 1972, *31,* 327.

Zepelin, H., and Rechtschaffen, A. Mammalian sleep, longevity and energy metabolism. *Brain Behavior Evolution,* 1974, *10,* 425–470.

Zepelin, H., Whitehead, W. E., and Rechtschaffen, A. Aging and sleep in the albino rat. *Behavioral Biology,* 1972, *7,* 65–74.

27

Cyclic Function of the Mammalian Ovary

Constance S. Campbell and Fred W. Turek

The maturation and release of eggs from the mammalian ovary occur at regular and predictable intervals that are species-specific. This cyclicity of the ovary has been the subject of intensive interdisciplinary investigation in the past several decades. At base, the ovarian cycle is a product of the interaction of a number of components of the neuroendocrine system. Tonic secretion of luteinizing hormone (LH) and follicle-stimulating hormone (FSH) from the pituitary is stimulated by the tonic release of luteinizing-hormone-releasing hormone (LH-RH) from the ventromedial arcuate region of the hypothalamus (Figure 1). In addition to this tonic component, there is a complex of trophic hormones (LH, FSH, and prolactin) released in large quantities from the pituitary on a regular, periodic basis in most mammals; this rhythmic component is dependent on the integrity of the preoptic–suprachiasmatic area of the hypothalamus. The tonic release of gonadotropins stimulates maturation of ovarian follicles and secretion of ovarian steroid hormones, notably estradiol. The cyclic release of gonadotropins results in ovulation and the secretion of more ovarian steroid hormones, notably progesterone. These ovarian steroids act both alone and in synergy in complex positive and negative feedback relationships to ensure the periodic release of gonadotropins.

This cyclic complex, in a vast number of species, has an important interaction with a variety of environmental periodicities. Diurnal light–dark cues play a critical role in the synchrony of ovarian rhythms in some species; stimuli arising from environmental light cycles are presumed to act on the cyclic center, the preoptic–suprachiasmatic region (Figure 1). Seasonal environmental variables, such as day length, temperature, food availability, and social interactions, can also exert a tremendous impact on ovarian rhythms.

Constance S. Campbell and Fred W. Turek   Department of Biological Sciences, Northwestern University, Evanston, Illinois 60201. The preparation of this review and the previously unpublished studies was supported by NIH grants HD–09885 and HD–10050 and NSF grant PCM–09955.

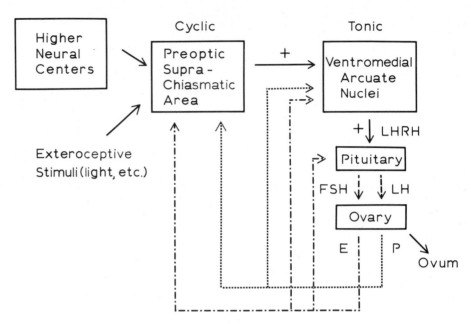

Fig. 1. Schematic representation of the events of the hypothalamic–pituitary axis and the hormonal relationships involved. Dotted lines represent feedback relationships of estradiol (E) and progesterone (P) on the hypothalamic–pituitary axis.

The purpose of this review is to integrate our current state of knowledge about the ovarian cycle, from morphological changes to neuroendocrine control, to the behavioral outputs and inputs of the system, and external factors that alter the characteristics of the cycle. In the interest of brevity, the development of cyclicity, aging, and changes in accessory reproductive tissues will not be covered in this chapter. To prevent the accumulation of an overwhelming bibliography, recent review articles have received considerable citation.

RHYTHMIC VARIABLES ASSOCIATED WITH THE OVARIAN CYCLE

THE CYCLE OF THE OVARY

The production of gametes and hormones in female mammals fluctuates rhythmically during the life span of the individual. Generally, ovarian cycles consist of three major phases: the follicular, the periovulatory, and the luteal phases. There are considerable species differences in the length of these phases, in the hormonal changes that accompany them, and in the role that exteroceptive stimuli play in their regulation. An exhaustive treatment of this topic is found in Zuckerman and Weir (1977).

FOLLICULAR PHASE. In the mature ovary, primary follicles consist of oocytes surrounded by a single layer of granulosa cells. With stimulation from pituitary hormones, the granulosa cells proliferate to form multiple layers, while the stroma cells surrounding the follicle form the theca interna and externa layers outside the basement membrane (Harrison and Weir, 1977). With further hormonal stimulation, this secondary follicle becomes fluid-filled inside a uniform wall, with the oocyte attached to one point and surrounded by granulosa cells destined to become the corona radiata (Figure 2) (Harrison and Weir, 1977). Only a certain number of follicles respond to gonadotropins by showing these maturational changes within a given cycle; the remaining follicles become atretic, showing degenerative changes beginning with the ovum and spreading to the rest of the follicle. Little is known about the basis of follicular recruitment and atresia (Schwartz and Hoffmann, 1972).

PERIOVULATORY PHASE. Ovulation occurs with a slow rupture of the follicle wall and steady exudation of follicular fluid, oocyte, and corona radiata, due to a release of proteolytic enzymes that break down thecal cells (Lipner, 1973). The number of ova ovulated is species-specific, and sometimes even strain- and breed-specific.

LUTEAL PHASE. When the ovum is extruded, the emptied follicle becomes a corpus luteum (Figure 2). In most species, both granulosa and theca cells form the corpora and undergo hypertrophy and hyperplasia to cause a progressive increase in size (Harrison and Weir, 1977). Only the function and hormonal control of the corpora lutea of the nonpregnant female are discussed here. In rabbits, voles, and cats, which are coitus-induced ovulators, there is no luteal phase, and the follicular phase is terminated simply by degeneration of the follicles (Rowlands and Weir, 1977). In rats, mice, and hamsters, the corpora are formed but apparently have little functional significance unless mating takes place (Yoshinaga, 1973). In a third group of species—guinea pigs, sheep, and primates—spontaneous ovulation is followed by the development of fully functional corpora lutea, which persist for as long as 6–15 days (Schwartz, 1973). If fertilization does not take place in the last two types of cyclers, degeneration of the corpora occurs, and corpora albicantia are

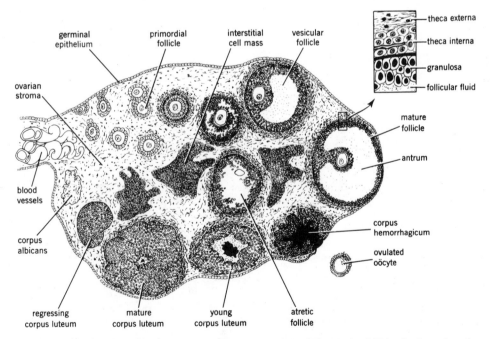

Fig. 2. Diagram of mammalian ovary, showing the sequential development of a follicle, the formation of a corpus luteum, and in the center, follicular atresia. A section of the wall of a mature follicle is enlarged at the upper right. (After Patten and Eskin. Reproduced with permission from Gorbman and Bern: *A Textbook of Comparative Endocrinology.* Copyright 1962, John Wiley, New York, N.Y.)

formed, which are composed primarily of scar tissue. Following the degeneration of the corpora, hormonal events are initiated that begin the ovarian cycle again.

The Cycle of Hormones

Follicular Phase. Morphological changes in the ovary occur in response to a cyclic discharge of pituitary hormones in conjunction with the release of ovarian hormones. The secondary surge of FSH released around the time of ovulation may be responsible for the recruitment of the cohort of follicles destined to ovulate in the next estrous cycle (Schwartz, Krone, Talley, and Ely, 1973). Antiserum to FSH (Welschen and Dullaart, 1976) and "folliculostatin," a nonsteroidal substance found in follicular fluid (Schwartz and Channing, 1977) both block this secondary rise of FSH and interfere with normal follicular maturation (Hoak and Schwartz, unpublished observations).

The growth and maturation of recruited follicles are maintained by continuous "tonic" secretion of pituitary gonadotropins. There is a rough dose–response relationship between the amount of LH and FSH secreted and the number of follicles that mature; the ratio of LH to FSH may be critical in this process as well (Schwartz and Hoffmann, 1972).

With follicular growth, there is an increase in estrogen secretion (Figure 3); this steroid probably derives primarily from thecal cells (Yoshinaga, 1973). However, recent evidence indicates that the theca interna synthesizes testosterone, which acts as a precursor for estradiol secretion by the adjacent granulosa cells (Dorrington, 1977). The total rate of estrogen secretion is dependent on the rate of secretion of each follicle and the number of follicles secreting (Schwartz and Hoffmann, 1972). Estrogen probably inhibits LH and keeps it at tonic levels in primates (Schwartz, 1973), while progesterone is primarily responsible for its regulation in breeding sheep (Legan and Karsch, 1979), and estradiol and progesterone synergize to regulate tonic LH in rats (Goodman, 1978a). This regulation appears to occur at the level of the ventromedial hypothalamus–arcuate region (Barraclough, 1973) (Figure 1). It is not known at this time what regulates the secretion of FSH during the follicular phase; estradiol alone in a wide range of doses cannot suppress FSH

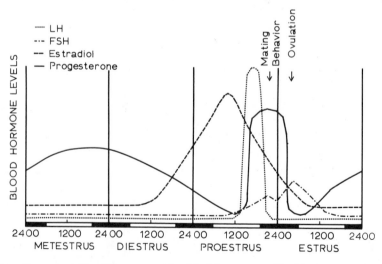

Fig. 3. Schematic representation of the estrous cycle of the laboratory rat. Blood hormone levels of LH, FSH, estradiol, and progesterone are represented in relation to behavioral estrus and ovulation.

to baseline (Campbell and Schwartz, 1977). Folliculostatin may be involved in some species (Schwartz and Channing, 1977).

PERIOVULATORY PHASE. The events surrounding ovulation differ considerably, depending on whether the female is a spontaneous or an induced ovulator. Spontaneously ovulating females shed ova in response to spontaneous changes in hormone levels; induced ovulators require a mating stimulus for ovulation.

Spontaneous Ovulation. Rising levels of estradiol are essential for triggering the release of ovulatory levels of LH in spontaneous cycling animals (Figure 3) (Schwartz, 1973). The site of action of estradiol appears to be the preoptic area of the brain in rats (Goodman, 1978b) (Figure 1). Coincidentally with the LH release, there is a surge of FSH and prolactin (Butcher, Collins, and Fugo, 1974). Whether the preovulatory surge of progesterone occurs before or after the LH surge in the rat has been debated (Goldman, Kamberi, Suteri, and Porter, 1969; Swerdloff, Jacobs, and Odell, 1972). Some have suggested that progesterone interacts with estradiol to trigger the surge (Swerdloff *et al.*, 1972); others have argued against this (Ferin, Tempone, Zimmering, and Vande Wiele, 1969).

With the release of ovulatory levels of gonadotropin, there occurs a sharp decrease in ovarian estrogen secretion. The cause of this decline is not well understood, but it is assumed that the morphological changes in the cells of the Graafian follicle are incompatible with estrogen secretion (Yoshinaga, 1973). On the other hand, progesterone may directly inhibit estradiol secretion (Greenwald, 1977).

Since spontaneous ovulators release a surge of LH without the stimulus of mating, a major question has been concerned with what signal is acting to trigger this surge. Arimura and Schally (1971) and others have shown an increased pituitary responsiveness on proestrus to hypothalamic LH-RH, which is estrogen-dependent. There is probably an additional neural signal associated with the circadian system that interacts with an ovarian signal to trigger LH, since the surge occurs at a particular time of day in most mammals (Everett, 1961) (see the section below on ovarian cycles and the circadian system). The surge mechanism is dependent on the integrity of the preoptic area (Barraclough, 1973) and the suprachiasmatic nuclei (Smalstig and Clemens, 1975).

Induced Ovulation. Estrogen secretion reaches high levels in induced ovulators, with a fairly constant number of follicles kept at ovulable size by a continuous process of maturation and regression. Release of gonadotropins requires a mating stimulus on this estrogen background (Everett, 1961). With the surge of LH, there occurs a sharp decrease in ovarian estrogen secretion. Presumably, the mechanisms by which estradiol secretion is decreased are similar in spontaneous and induced ovulators.

LUTEAL PHASE. With ovulation, the process of luteinization begins, but it differs greatly among species in terms of both morphology and function (Rothchild, 1966; Nalbandov, 1973). Unless mating occurs in rats, hamsters, and mice, and in induced ovulators, the corpora are not fully functional and do not secrete sufficient progestin to support the uterine changes associated with progestational proliferation. Following sterile mating, such species experience pseudopregnancy, a condition that resembles a spontaneous luteal phase of larger animals (Rowlands and Weir, 1977).

In animals with an active luteal phase, such as humans, cows, sheep, dogs, and guinea pigs, the corpora lutea remain functional for long periods of time, and progesterone secretion is prolonged even in the absence of a mating stimulus (Yoshinaga, 1973). In these species, tonic levels of LH appear to be adequate to maintain the corpora.

At the end of the luteal phase, there is regression of the corpora lutea; it is not known at present what causes this regression. There is also a concomitant decrease in progesterone secretion. With this decline, there is a loss of the negative feedback of ovarian hormones on pituitary function (Goodman, 1978a), tonic levels of gonadotropins once again stimulate follicular maturation, and the cycle begins again.

BEHAVIORAL ASPECTS OF THE OVARIAN CYCLE

ACTIVITY. It has long been known that there is an increase in activity associated with the period of behavioral heat in many species, including cats (Michael, 1973); rats (Wang, 1923–1925); mice (Guttman, Lieblich, and Gross, 1975); and hamsters (Finkelstein, Baum, and Campbell, 1978). The site of action of estrogen on locomotor activity appears to be localized in the basal anterior diencephalon (Wade, 1976).

More fine-grained analysis of the hamster activity rhythm has also shown a "scalloping" or earlier onset of activity on proestrus (Morin, Fitzgerald, and Zucker, 1977) (Figure 4). The functional importance of this earlier onset of activity during proestrus is not clear, although it may either increase the chances of an encounter with a male in solitary-living species such as the hamster, or it may be a component of proceptive behavior (Beach, 1976). In any case, activity is useful as a marker of hormonal events of the cycle; the time of ovulation in rats can be predicted from the onset of spontaneous wheel-running activity on proestrus (Sridaran and McCormack, 1977). Similarly, Fitzgerald and Zucker (1976) have shown a stable phase-angle difference between activity onset and behavioral heat onset in hamsters that are either entrained or freerunning in constant conditions.

SEXUAL BEHAVIOR. Female sexual behavior has been extensively studied and reviewed (Beach, 1976; Eayrs, Glass, and Swanson, 1977; Adler, 1978); only the temporal aspects of mating rhythms are discussed here.

In spontaneous ovulators, behavioral heat occurs in response to the secretion of progesterone on a background of estrogen, thus closely preceding ovulation (Feder and Marrone, 1977). This system ensures synchrony between copulation and the time most favorable for fertilization of the ova. Even in the higher primates, there is an increased incidence of mating around the time of ovulation; in the human female, the data are less clear (Eayrs *et al.*, 1977). The site of action of estrogen varies somewhat among species, from the preoptic–anterior hypothalamic area in the rat and the hamster to the ventromedial area in the rabbit (Lisk, 1973). Lesions of the suprachiasmatic nuclei render the female rat and hamster continuously receptive (Smalstig and Clemens, 1975; Stetson and Watson-Whitmyre, 1976). Increased gonadotropins in these animals may be inducing continuous high levels of estrogen (Smalstig and Clemens, 1975). The site of action of progesterone is species-dependent and generally diffuse (Feder and Marrone, 1977). In addition to estrogen and progesterone, LH-RH has been suggested as playing a role in the potentiation of estrous

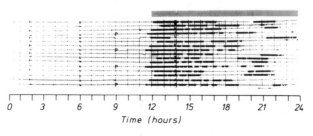

Time (hours)

Fig. 4. Portion of the activity record of a female hamster housed in LD 12 : 12 showing the estrous rhythm of wheel running. The time scale runs from left to right, with successive days' activity shown beneath each other. The day of proestrus is indicated by the symbol "P." The crosshatched bar at the top indicates the hours of darkness.

behavior and may exert its behavioral effects via stimulation of the medial preoptic area and the arcuate nucleus of the hypothalamus (Foreman and Moss, 1977).

Estrogen alone is sufficient for induction of behavioral heat in induced ovulators, although progesterone can facilitate it in the rabbit (Lisk, 1973). During the breeding season, there is no cycle of behavioral receptivity in induced ovulators; instead, females are continuously receptive.

The duration of the period of behavioral estrus is species-specific and is regulated by a number of factors. Copulatory stimulation eventually reduces receptivity in a wide variety of mammals (Adler, 1978). It seems unlikely that this effect is mediated hormonally (Carter, 1972); it may be due to a neural mechanism (Goldfoot and Goy, 1970). In addition, progesterone has been repeatedly shown to have biphasic effects on behavior—it terminates mating behavior as well as facilitating its onset in rats, mice, rabbits, ferrets, and guinea pigs (Morin, 1977). With termination of mating behavior, the animals undergo a behavioral refractoriness to the facilitatory effects of steroid administration. In those species in which progesterone is biphasic, the site of action of behavioral inhibition appears to be the midbrain (Feder and Marrone, 1977).

Those systems involved in the stimulus control of mating behavior also show predictable fluctuations with the ovarian cycle. Adler, Davis, and Komisaruk (1977) have found that the sensory field of the pudendal nerve (including the pelvic abdomen and thigh) increases in size and sensitivity on days of behavioral heat. In addition, releaser pheromone production shows a fluctuation over the ovarian cycle in a wide variety of female mammals, including New World primates (Epple, 1976), rodents (Johnston, 1977), and canids (Anisko, 1976). The data are controversial with respect to Old World monkeys (Michael, 1973; Goldfoot, Kravetz, Goy, and Freeman, 1976). These pheromones are found usually either in urine or in vaginal secretions or both and appear to be estrogen-dependent. Acoustic signals also appear to show cycle-related changes in some animals. Ultrasounds in female hamsters (Floody, Pfaff, and Lewis, 1977) and lemmings (Brooks and Banks, 1973) appear to be a form of sexual advertisement.

INGESTIVE BEHAVIOR. Feeding behavior shows dramatc fluctuations during the estrous cycle of many species. In the rat (Ter Haar, 1972) (Figure 5), guinea pig (Czaja and Goy, 1975), hamster (Morin and Fleming, 1978), rhesus monkey (Czaja and Goy, 1975), and ewe (Tartellin, 1968), there is an estrus-related decrease in feeding behavior. This depression is due to estrogen secretion, since estradiol administered to ovariectomized females has similar suppressive effects. The site of action of the steroid appears to be the ventromedial hypothalamus, although other areas may be involved as well (Wade, 1976). This decline in food intake in the late follicular phase, in combination with the previously discussed increase in activity levels, results in a decline in body weight (Wade, 1976). Food intake and activity level changes are not sufficient in every instance, however, to account for the entire change in body weight; metabolic changes caused by the hormones are clearly involved as well (Roy and Wade, 1977).

AGGRESSION AND EMOTIONALITY. It has been shown in a number of species that aggressiveness shows estrous-cycle-related fluctuations. Guinea pigs (Young, Dempsey, and Myers, 1935), hamsters (Wise, 1977), mice (Hyde and Sawyer, 1977), and primates (Rowell, 1972) all show a decrease in aggression coincident with sexual receptivity. Decreased aggression in the periovulatory phase of the cycle has been attributed to a rise in estrogen levels, and the increased aggression in the luteal phase has been linked to high progesterone levels (Eayrs *et al.,* 1977).

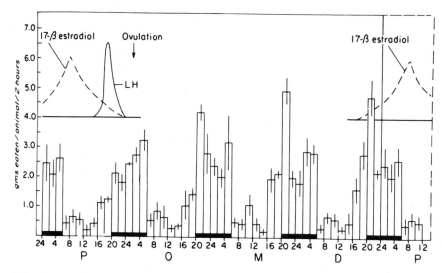

Fig. 5. Food intake (± SEM) by adult female rats through a 4-day estrous cycle as measured at 2-hr intervals. The hours of darkness are indicated, as are the timings of the preovulatory surge of 17 β-estradiol and luteinizing hormone (LH) and the time of ovulation in the colony. P = proestrus; 0 = oestrus; M = metestrus; D = diestrus. (From Ter Haar, 1972. Reprinted with permission of Academic Press.)

Changes in "emotionality" have been reported in rodents, with a decrease in this and other fear-related behaviors during behavioral estrus (Gray and Levine, 1964). The concept of "emotionality" in nonhumans has understandably been criticized, particularly since behaviors considered indices of "emotionality," such as ambulation and defecation, are themselves closely tied to the estrus-related cycles in activity and food intake described above (Birke and Archer, 1975). There has been controversy for centuries about menstrual-cycle-dependent changes in emotionality in women; considerable disagreement has continued as to whether the origins of such changes (if, indeed, they exist) are hormonal, psychological, a result of social factors, or a combination of these (Steiner and Carroll, 1977). Unfortunately, most of the work done on this problem to date has lacked appropriate controls and rigorous testing procedures, as well as careful definitions of concepts (Smith, 1975).

FACTORS THAT ALTER CHARACTERISTICS OF THE OVARIAN CYCLE WITHIN A GIVEN SPECIES

As described in the preceding sections, different species have estrous cycle types with sets of predictable characteristics. There is, however, a wide variety of environmental factors that act to dramatically alter these species-specific cycles. More comprehensive treatments of some of these factors have appeared elsewhere (Leatham, 1961; Sadleir, 1969; Whitten and Champlin, 1973; Herbert, 1977); only a brief review is included here.

LIGHT

In many species, the events of the ovarian cycle are strongly correlated with particular phases of the light–dark cycle. Since these events also occur in the absence of changes in environmental lighting, it appears that events of the estrous cycle are tied in with an endogenous circadian clock. Further discussion of the role of the daily light–dark cycle and the biological clock in control of the ovarian cycle will be reserved for the final section.

Exposure to constant light has species-specific effects on the estrous cycle. In female mice, the ovarian cycle appears to be largely unaffected by constant light, although some of the cycle events show temporal alterations (Campbell, Ryan, and Schwartz, 1976). In the hamster, only prolonged exposure (6–14 months) leads to a disruption of the estrous cycle (Kent, Ridgway, and Strobel, 1968). In the rat, constant bright light leads eventually to persistent vaginal cornification, constant behavioral estrus, cystic follicles, and anovulation (Lawton and Schwartz, 1967). The effects of bright LL on the rat cycle occur very rapidly, leading to major changes even in the first two cycles of this lighting regimen. During these early cycles, there is a complete suppression of gonadotropin surges and ovulation in some rats (McCormack and Sridaran, 1978; Campbell and Schwartz, 1978). In other rats in bright LL, however, all the hormonal events of the cycle and ovulation occur, but they freerun as a unit for a period of time prior to the eventual disruption. Interestingly, regardless of whether or not the estrous cycle is immediately disrupted, locomotor activity onsets show a reliable freerunning rhythm and thus dissociate from the ovarian cycle. Onsets of behavioral heat in these animals dissociate both from locomotor activity onsets and from the hormonal events of the estrous cycle (Campbell and Schwartz, 1978). The mechanism by which bright LL disrupts the rat estrous cycle is not known, but it does not appear to involve damage to retinal photoreceptors, since when animals in LL-induced persistent estrus are returned to normal light–dark cycles, they cycle normally (Brown-Grant, 1974). In contrast to bright constant light, dim constant light results only in a freerunning rhythm of the estrous cycle. Ovulation, the ovulatory surge of LH, and activity all show freerunning rhythms in dim LL and appear to maintain their usual phase relationships (Sridaran and McCormack, 1977); in addition, these animals do not develop the persistent estrous syndrome (McCormack and Sridaran, 1978). Constant darkness leads to anestrus in only a small proportion of animals, while the rest appear to cycle normally (Hoffman, 1973).

Aschoff and his co-workers (1975) have pioneered the use of phase-shifted light cycles to examine the interrelationships of individual circadian rhythms. This has been accomplished by studying relative rates of phase-shifting and the speed with which they reentrain to the new light cycle. Use of this paradigm has shown that the events of the hamster estrous cycle, both behavioral and hormonal, are very tightly coupled (Alleva, Waleski, Alleva, and Umberger, 1968) and respond as a unit to such manipulations. Under some conditions, however, the circadian activity rhythm dissociates from the other circadian-based estrous cycle rhythms and reentrains at a slower rate to photoperiod reversal (Finkelstein et al., 1978), demonstrating that under certain environmental conditions, a separation of these two may occur.

TEMPERATURE

Elevated temperatures are known to suppress ovarian activity, but at least some of these effects are indirect because of metabolic disturbances (Miller and Alliston, 1974). Rodents show a decrease in fertility in high temperatures but often eventually acclimatize. Reduced temperatures have similar effects on rodents that elevated temperatures do, with an initial ovarian anestrus followed by restoration of function due to adaptation (Herbert, 1977).

NUTRITION

The role of nutrition on reproduction has been extensively reviewed by several authors (Leatham, 1961; Sadleir, 1969). Underfeeding leads to anestrus in most domestic animals (Sadleir, 1969), as well as in rodents (Leatham, 1961) and humans (Frisch, 1978). When the female rat is placed on a restricted (50% of normal) diet, there is a cessation of vaginal cyclicity within two weeks, at the point at which the animals have lost 15% of their body weight. Tonic secretion of LH, FSH, progesterone, and estradiol in these animals is suppressed after three weeks of food restriction. These changes are accompanied by a dramatic increase in the rate of follicular atresia (Leikin and Campbell, 1978). Ovarian responsiveness to gonadotropin stimulation appears to be normal in underfed rats (Leatham, 1961), as does pituitary responsiveness to LH-RH and hypothalamic responsiveness to the negative and positive feedback effects of gonadal steroids (Howland, 1976). Since the above events of the cycle appear normal in these anestrous rats, LH surges may not occur because of a decrease in tonic gonadotropin secretion, which results in the absence of an estradiol positive feedback signal.

Overfeeding or "flushing" has been attempted in the past to accelerate the onset of breeding in domestic animals but has been generally ineffective (Sadleir, 1969). In fact, obesity has a deleterious effect on ovarian cyclicity. The cause is not understood, but it may be related to an impairment of steroid metabolism by fatty infiltration of the liver (Leatham, 1961).

SOCIAL FACTORS

In nonseasonal as well as seasonal species, the presence of a male can synchronize ovarian cycles within a population. This phenomenon has been demonstrated in sheep (Watson and Radford, 1960) and rodents (Whitten and Champlin, 1973). The data are clear in demonstrating that for many species, this synchronizing effect is mediated by urinary pheromones. The endocrine mechanism at the base of this *Whitten effect* has resisted efforts at clarification (Bronson, 1976). Ryan (1976) has observed a drop in progesterone with male exposure that could release the hypothalamic–pituitary axis from inhibition and lead to an increase in tonic gonadotropin secretion. What causes this progesterone drop is not known at this time.

Cyclicity can be reinduced in pregnant rodents by the introduction of a strange male, a phenomenon known as the *Bruce effect* (Whitten and Champlin, 1973). This effect also appears to be mediated by an olfactory stimulus that leads to an LH surge and may also alter secretion of prolactin and ACTH (Bronson, 1971). How these latter two hormones interact to induce ovulation and cyclicity is not understood.

The presence of conspecific females can inhibit cyclicity in mice; this has been called the *Lee–Boot effect*. This phenomenon also appears to be pheromone-induced, and it has been suggested that grouping leads to an increase in FSH and prolactin, which can stimulate corpora to secrete high levels of progesterone and induce a pseudopregnancy (Ryan and Schwartz, 1977).

Increasing population density itself can also lead to a decrease in ovarian cyclicity. Studies on field and penned populations of rodents and rabbits that undergo either natural or experimentally induced fluctuations in density show a reduction in fecundity with an increase in density (Sadleir, 1969; Christian, 1975). This is an exceedingly complex phenomenon, which probably involves a number of mechanisms. The Lee–Boot effect might play a part by suppressing cycles, but it is equally likely that the stressful effects of inter-male or interfemale aggression could alter breeding. Acyclicity could then be induced through an increased adrenocortical secretion, which could suppress gonadotropin secretion (Christian, 1975). Furthermore, stresses of this nature could alter implantation, pregnancy maintenance, fetal development, and the postnatal viability of offspring.

Interspecific Differences in the Temporal Occurrence of Ovarian Cycles

Seasonal versus Nonseasonal Breeders

FUNCTIONAL SIGNIFICANCE OF SEASONALITY. There is a variety of temporal patterns of ovarian cyclicity among mammals; these patterns are presumed to combine with lengths of gestation and lactation to maximize reproductive fitness. The vast majority of species are seasonal in that there is an increased incidence of cyclicity at specific times of the year. Although temperate-zone seasonal breeders show onsets of breeding that are species-specific to time of year, the birth of the young typically occurs in spring or summer, when survival of the young is optimal. Thus, if the gestation period is short (as in beavers, raccoons, and most rodents), females can have both conception and parturition within one optimal season. If, on the other hand, the time from conception to parturition is long, parturition occurs during the optimal season, but mating is pushed back to occur either in a suboptimal season (as in sheep, white-tailed deer, and wolves) or in the previous optimal season (as in horses, asses, and llamas) (Asdell, 1964). In other species (e.g., badgers, mink, and otters), the interval between conception and parturition is prolonged by delayed implantation to ensure that parturition will occur at the optimal time. Such a delay is commonly associated with the failure of the corpus luteum to develop fully.

Nonseasonal females generally include those for whom the environment is continually optimal (e.g., human beings, hippopotamuses, and guinea pigs); many of these are domesticated (e.g., laboratory rat, pig, and laboratory mouse) (Schwartz, 1973; Asdell, 1964; Sadleir, 1969).

CIRCANNUAL RHYTHMS. One question that has not been answered is the extent to which seasonal breeding in female mammals is an endogenous circannual rhythm. The only female mammal examined so far that shows an annual periodicity in reproduction without exogenous synchronizers is the ewe (Ducker, Bowman, and Temple, 1973). The female hamster shows a spontaneous restoration of cyclicity after being blinded for extended periods of time, but this effect is not part of an endogenous annual rhythm, since there is no subsequent loss of cyclicity (Reiter, 1974). Thus, in some species, environmental factors such as photoperiod may be solely responsible for the induction of annual reproductive cycles, whereas in other species, they serve simply to synchronize the reproductive cycle with the season of the year (see Chapter 20).

CONSTANCE S.
CAMPBELL AND FRED
W. TUREK

Light–Dark Cycles. In many seasonal animals, light–dark rhythms have a dual function. First, they appear to time the events of the estrous cycle, as has been demonstrated in the hamster (Alleva and Umberger, 1966), and in addition, they affect the timing and duration of the breeding season (Reiter, 1974). Little is understood, however, about how the two systems interact. For example, the classic "resonance light cycle" experiments and "T" experiments, which test if the circadian system is involved in photoperiodic time measurement, have never been performed in female mammals. In addition, the critical day length required for ovarian maintenance has not been precisely determined in any female mammal.

Temperature Cycles. In ewes, temperature cycles can act to synchronize breeding seasons in the absence of light–dark cues (Godley, Wilson, and Horst, 1966). Even in the presence of normal day-length changes, ewes are reproductively stimulated by lower temperatures and show an earlier onset of breeding (Duff and Bush, 1955). The physiological mechanisms involved are not known at present. Controlled experiments have not been done in other female mammals, however, and in light of the close relationship among temperature, day length, and nutrition, it is difficult to interpret most of the data on the effects of temperature. This problem is further complicated by the fact that many rodents respond to temperature changes by hibernating. It is not at all clear to what extent seasonal anestrus and hibernation in rodents are tied either in terms of physiological processes or in terms of the controlling factors.

Nutritional Cycles. Under natural conditions, the effects of the quality of available food are exceedingly difficult to separate from other environmental factors such as day length, temperature, rainfall, and population density.

Recently, it has been observed that seasonal cyclicity in the vole is directly controlled by the seasonal appearance of substances in their food. Winter-anestrous voles show an onset of breeding when given spring wheatgrass (Negus and Berger, 1977) and an inhibition of breeding when fed winter wheat (Berger, Sanders, Gardner, and Negus, 1977). This herbivore inhabits an unpredictable environment, and since photoperiod is not a very reliable signal for the onset of optimal breeding, the vole may rely upon chemical signals from plants to provide more dependable information on temperature and food availability, which are the most critical factors for the survival of offspring.

Social Factors. It has been observed in birds and reptiles that the presence of a male accelerates the onset of breeding in seasonal females. Similar observations have been made in domestic seasonal breeders, such as the sheep (Radford and Watson, 1957) and the goat (Signoret, 1976), and in wild ungulates (Grau, 1976). In mammals, these effects appear to be generally mediated by olfactory cues.

Neuroendocrine Correlates of Seasonality

Seasonal Changes in Hormones and Behavior. Few studies have been done on the nature of the reproductive system during seasonal anestrus, and little is known about how ovarian recrudescence is achieved following anestrus (Sadleir, 1969; Turek and Campbell, 1979). In anestrous females, there are follicular quiescence, reduced ovarian function, small and inactive sex accessory tissue, and regressed secondary sex characteristics. In mares, anestrus is characterized by episodic peaks of LH and estradiol, but low levels of progesterone when measurements were taken weekly (Oxender, Noden, and Hafs, 1977). In ewes, periodic spikes of LH and estradiol have also been observed from daily samples taken during anestrus (Yuthasastrakosol, Palmer, and Holland, 1975); progesterone levels were baseline. The female hamster has large daily peaks of LH, FSH, and progesterone during anestrus (Bridges and Goldman, 1975), as is shown in Figure 6; estradiol has not been measured. It has been presumed that these peaks are due to the absence of negative feedback from the quiescent ovary, but this has yet to be established. Prolactin measurements, taken infrequently, have shown levels to be low (Reiter, 1975); this hormone may be involved in gonadal regression in male hamsters (Bartke, Croft, and Dalterio, 1975), but its role in the female has not been studied.

The period of transition from anestrus to breeding has been studied in only a few species. Investigators have reported "silent ovulation," ovulation unaccompanied by behavioral estrus, just prior to the onset of seasonal breeding cycles (Legan, Karsch, and Foster, 1977). Presumably, without luteal progesterone, behavioral heat does not occur, and postovulatory progesterone from this "silent ovulation" is necessary for the expression of heat in the next cycle.

Legan *et al.* (1977) have reported an increase in tonic LH at the onset of the breeding season in the presence of unchanging high levels of estradiol in ovariectomized ewes with estrogen implants, and they suggested that the onset of cyclicity may occur through a reduction in the negative feedback effects of estradiol (Figure 7). Other parts of the system, such as positive feedback of estrogen on the proestrous surge of LH, and ovarian secretion of

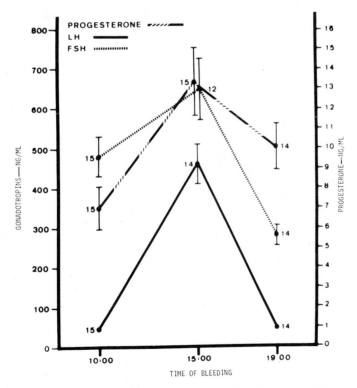

Fig. 6. Serum LH, FSH, and progesterone in photoperiod-induced-acyclic hamsters. Values are expressed as means ± SEM. The number adjacent to each mean is the *n* for that group. Animals were housed in LD 10 : 14 (lights on 0500–1500). (From Bridges and Goldman, 1975. Reprinted with permission.)

CONSTANCE S.
CAMPBELL AND FRED
W. TUREK

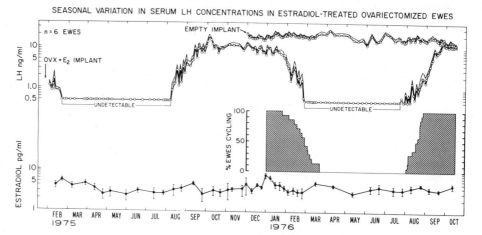

Fig. 7. Seasonal variation in serum LH concentrations in estradiol-treated ovariectomized ewes. The upper portion of the figure depicts mean ($\pm$ SEM) serum LH levels in two groups of 6 ewes each. One group was treated sc with Silastic capsules containing estradiol-17β immediately after ovariectomy (OVX + E$_2$ IMPLANT). The other group consisted of long-term ovariectomized ewes treated with empty Silastic implants beginning in December 1975 (EMPTY IMPLANT). The lower portion of the figure depicts mean ($\pm$ SEM) serum estradiol concentrations (closed circles) in the ewes receiving estradiol implants. The histogram illustrates the time courses of the onset and end of the anestrous season in 1976 as determined from observations of estrus in a group of 14 intact ewes. (From Legan *et al.*, 1977. Reprinted with permission.)

estradiol in response to LH stimulation, are intact in the anestrous ewe (Legan and Karsch, 1979), and only the negative feedback system appears to be altered. These data support the hypothesis of Hoffmann (1973) that the major mechanism for photoperiod-induced changes in reproductive function is an alteration of the negative feedback effects of ovarian hormones on pituitary gonadotropin release. During anestrus, sexual receptivity is absent, presumably because of a decrease in gonadal steroids; but in additon to the change in feedback sensitivity to gonadotropin secretion, there may also be a change in behavioral responsiveness to steroids during anestrus. In sheep (Lamond, 1964), there is a decreased incidence of estrogen-induced behavioral heat in anestrous as opposed to breeding ewes.

Sexual behavior is not the only type of behavior that is altered with season. Female Syrian hamsters show a decrease in locomotor activity levels when they are anestrous. This decline is not simply due to the presumed absence of estradiol, since restoration of this steroid to ovariectomized short-day females does not increase activity to the levels seen in ovariectomized long-day females given the same amount of estradiol (Figure 8a). Thus, this aspect of activity is less responsive to the stimulatory effects of estradiol in short-day animals than it is in long-day females. Another aspect of activity, its temporal distribution, is also altered during anestrus. Acyclic hamsters show their major peak of activity during the second half of the dark period, while cycling females have their most active time just at the offset of lights. Restoration of estradiol to anestrous females leads to an advance in this peak of activity so that the temporal pattern closely resembles the pattern seen in cycling females (Figure 8b).

The Role of the Pineal. When female hamsters are blinded or placed in LH 1 : 23 or LD 2 : 22, they become acyclic within 6 weeks (Reiter, 1974). This response can be blocked by pinealectomy, and also by chronic administration of the pineal product, melatonin (Reiter, Rudeen, and Vaughan, 1976). In addition to this progonadal effect of melatonin, when female hamsters on long days are injected daily with melatonin, they become anestrous within 7 weeks, regardless of the presence or absence of the pineal itself (Tamarkin, Hollister, Lefebvre, and Goldman, 1977). These latter antigonadal effects depend on the time of day, and the effects of melatonin generally vary with the mode of administration and the photoperiodic conditions, as well as with the timing of administration. Pinealectomy has also been shown to alter the onset of successive estrous periods in ferrets maintained in

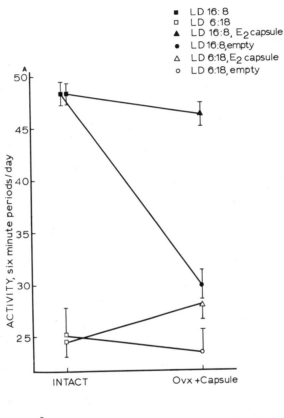

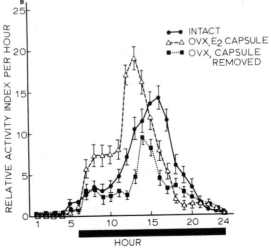

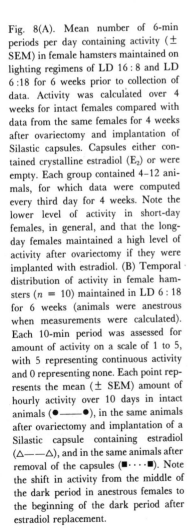

Fig. 8(A). Mean number of 6-min periods per day containing activity (± SEM) in female hamsters maintained on lighting regimens of LD 16 : 8 and LD 6 :18 for 6 weeks prior to collection of data. Activity was calculated over 4 weeks for intact females compared with data from the same females for 4 weeks after ovariectomy and implantation of Silastic capsules. Capsules either contained crystalline estradiol (E₂) or were empty. Each group contained 4–12 animals, for which data were computed every third day for 4 weeks. Note the lower level of activity in short-day females, in general, and that the long-day females maintained a high level of activity after ovariectomy if they were implanted with estradiol. (B) Temporal distribution of activity in female hamsters (*n* = 10) maintained in LD 6 : 18 for 6 weeks (animals were anestrous when measurements were calculated). Each 10-min period was assessed for amount of activity on a scale of 1 to 5, with 5 representing continuous activity and 0 representing none. Each point represents the mean (± SEM) amount of hourly activity over 10 days in intact animals (●——●), in the same animals after ovariectomy and implantation of a Silastic capsule containing estradiol (△——△), and in the same animals after removal of the capsules (■····■). Note the shift in activity from the middle of the dark period in anestrous females to the beginning of the dark period after estradiol replacement.

natural lighting conditions (Herbert, 1972). Herbert has suggested that anestrus is induced in nocturnal rodents by a short photoperiod, which acts via the pineal, while in the ferret, a diurnal carnivore, estrus is induced by long days via the pineal.

CONTINUOUS ESTROUS, POLYESTROUS, AND MONESTROUS CYCLERS

Female mammals that are seasonal may still show a variety of cycling patterns. Continuously estrous females, such as ferrets, have a pattern of continuous receptivity in the absence of the male for the duration of the breeding season, because of continuous follicular availability. Other seasonal breeders, such as the hamster, the mink, and the mare, have waves of recurring follicular cycles and thus more than one period of heat during the season, and they are considered polyestrous. A third type of seasonal breeder has only one period of heat per season (fox, dog) and one wave of follicular growth; these are monestrous (Asdell, 1964). It is assumed that these different reproductive strategies lead to maximal reproductive fitness and are determined by the interaction of environmental pressures with gestation length and duration of lactation. The latter factors are presumed to be less responsive to evolutionary pressures than are the temporal aspects of cyclicity (Sadleir, 1969).

THE RELATIONSHIP OF OVARIAN CYCLES TO THE CIRCADIAN SYSTEM

Although the events within the ovarian cycle occur at intervals that are much greater than 24 hr, there is a great deal of evidence to suggest that when an event does occur, it takes place at a specific time of day. The release of LH on proestrus, for example, occurs within a very limited time period (i.e., between 9 and 12 hr after the onset of light in animals exposed to LH 14 : 10) in rats maintained on a fixed light–dark cycle (Everett, 1961). Following a shift in the light regime, the LH surge assumes the same phase relationship to the new regime, suggesting that the events of the ovarian cycle are strongly correlated with particular phases of the light cycle (Hoffmann, 1973). Furthermore, if the LH surge is blocked by an injection of pentobarbital administered just prior to the surge, the LH surge occurs the next day at precisely the same time of day (Everett, 1961).

Additional support for the hypothesis that a daily signal triggers the LH surge on proestrus is found in studies of estrogen-primed ovariectomized rats, which show a daily release in LH at a time of day similar to that observed in intact animals on proestrus (Legan and Karsch, 1975). On the basis of data like these, it has been postulated that every 24 hr in the rat, there is an estrogen-sensitive phase during which estradiol, if it is elevated, induces the discharge of LH (Hoffmann, 1973). A daily signal is also responsible for the LH surge in the hamster (Norman, Blake, and Sawyer, 1973).

An examination of the events of the estrous cycle in hamsters exposed to constant light indicates that the daily signal involved in the estrous cycle is circadian in nature. Alleva, Waleski, and Alleva (1970) demonstrated that the onset of behavioral receptivity freeruns with a period greater than 96 hr in hamsters exposed to constant light, and that pituitary gonadotropin release and ovulation maintain their normal phase relationship to the onset of estrus. Furthermore, the 4-day estrous rhythm freeruns with a period that is four times that of the circadian activity rhythm (Figure 9) in dim constant light (Fitzgerald and Zucker, 1976). Administration of heavy water (D_2O) markedly lengthened the periods of both of these rhythms, with the maintenance of a stable phase angle between receptivity onset and activity onset before and after treatment (Fitzgerald and Zucker, 1976). These authors have suggested that a common circadian mechanism generates periodicities in estrus and activity. The correlation between these systems is further shown by exposing hamsters to constant light for a prolonged period; they show asynchronous ovulation and irregular cycles (Alleva *et al.*, 1968), together with a deterioration of the circadian activity rhythm (Stetson, Watson-Whitmyre, and Matt, 1977). The coupling between the activity rhythm and the estrous cycle is not absolute, however, since the circadian activity rhythm dissociates from the other circadian-based estrous cycle rhythms and reentrains at a slower rate following reversal of the photoperiod (Finkelstein *et al.*, 1978).

The signal controlling gonadotropin release could be either a direct neural signal or a neuroendocrine signal mediated by hormones that are themselves altered by light–dark signals. There is evidence to suggest that the adrenal gland is involved in the process (Mann, Korowitz, MacFarland, and Cost, 1976) since (1) the daily increase in adrenal secretion occurs earlier than the gonadotropin release on proestrus (Raps, Barthe, and Desaulles, 1971); (2) adrenal steroids can trigger the LH surge on a background of estrogen (Campbell and Schwartz, 1977); and (3) adrenalectomy can attenuate the LH surge (Campbell, Schwartz, and Firlit, 1977).

In addition to its role in regulating the precise timing of various events in the estrous cycle, the circadian system may also be involved in the timing of the breeding season in female mammals whose reproductive condition is regulated by the length of the day (see the section above on seasonal and nonseasonal breeders). Since this has been demonstrated

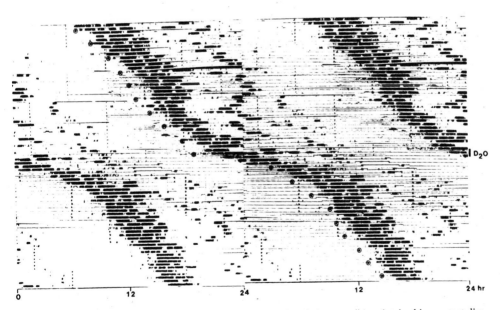

Fig. 9. Freerunning heat onset and wheel-running behavior of female hamster #4 maintained in constant dim illumination. The record has been doubled to permit visualization of the continuity of the freerunning rhythms. The days during which the animals were drinking 50% D_2O are indicated by a vertical bar to the right of the activity record. Heat onsets are designated by the circled stars. (From Fitzgerald and Zucker, 1976. Reprinted with permission.)

only in male mammals (Elliott, 1976), it is only an assumption at this time that the circadian system is also involved in photoperiodic time measurement in females of these species.

The search for the anatomical location of the circadian system involved in ovarian cyclicity has centered on the suprachiasmatic nuclei (SCN) of the hypothalamus. Numerous studies have demonstrated that the SCN are involved in the generation of a variety of different circadian rhythms (e.g., locomotor activity, adrenal corticosterone secretion, and pineal enzyme activity), since destruction of the SCN abolishes these rhythms (Moore and Klein, 1974; Moore and Eichler, 1976; Rusak, 1977). SCN lesions in female hamsters not only disrupt the circadian rhythm of locomotor acitivity but also induce persistent estrus regardless of the photoperiodic conditions (Stetson and Watson-Whitmyre, 1976). These results have been interpreted as indicating that the SCN are part of the circadian system involved in photoperiodic time measurement. Support for this hypothesis is found in the observation that male hamsters with lesions of the SCN remain reproductively competent irrespective of the photoperiod (Stetson and Watson-Whitmyre, 1976). However, it should be noted that destruction of the SCN also induces persistent estrus in the laboratory rat, a species whose reproductive condition is not regulated by the length of the day (Smalstig and Clemens, 1975). Thus, it is not known if a disruption of the circadian system in the hamster by lesions of the SCN interferes with the circadian clock involved in photoperiodic time measurement and/or with the clock involved in the timing of the temporal pattern of events within the estrous cycle. Further studies are clearly necessary to elucidate the precise role of the SCN and circadian organization in the control of the mammalian estrous cycle.

Acknowledgments

The authors wish to thank Dr. Kathleen D. Ryan and Dr. Charles E. McCormack for helpful criticism of the manuscript and Linda J. Swanson for preparation of a number of the figures. We wish to thank Drs. Sandra Legan, Bruce Goldman, Irving Zucker, and M. B. Ter Haar and their colleagues for permission to reproduce previously published data for this review, and Dr. Aubrey Gorbman for permission to reproduce the diagram of the mammalian ovary.

REFERENCES

Adler, N. T. On the mechanisms of sexual behavior and their evolutionary constraints. In J. S. Hutchison (Ed.), *Biological Determinants of Sexual Behavior*. New York: Wiley, 1978.

Adler, N. T., Davis, P. G., and Komisaruk, B. R. Variation in size and sensitivity of a genital sensory field in relation to the estrous cycle in rats. *Hormones and Behavior*, 1977, *9*, 334–344.

Alleva, J. J., and Umberger, E. J. Evidence for neural control of the release of pituitary ovulatory hormone in the golden Syrian hamster. *Endocrinology*, 1966, *78*, 1125–1129.

Alleva, J. J., Waleski, M. V., Alleva, F. R., and Umberger, E. J. Synchronizing effects of photoperiodicity on ovulation in hamsters. *Endocrinology*, 1968, *82*, 1227–1235.

Alleva, J. J., Waleski, M. V., and Alleva, F. R. A biological clock controlling the estrous cycle of the hamster. *Endocrinology*, 1970, *88*, 1368–1379.

Anisko, J. J. Communication by chemical signals in canidae. In R. L. Doty (Ed.), *Mammalian Olfaction, Reproductive Processes and Behavior*. New York: Academic Press, 1976.

Arimura, A., and Schally, A. V. Augmentation of pituitary responsiveness to LH-releasing hormone (LH–RH) by estrogen. *Proceedings of the Society for Experimental Biology and Medicine*, 1971, *136*, 290–293.

Aschoff, J., Hoffmann, K., Pohl, H., and Wever, R. Reentrainment of circadian rhythms after phase-shifts of the zeitgeber. *Chronobiologica,* 1975, *2,* 23–78.

Asdell, S. A. *Patterns of Mammalian Reproduction.* Ithaca, N.Y.: Cornell University Press, 1964.

Barraclough, C. A. Sex steroid regulation of reproductive neuroendocrine processes. In R. O. Greep and E. B. Astwood (Eds.), *Handbook of Physiology, Section 7, Endocrinology.* Vol. 2, Part 1. Washington, D.C.: American Physiological Society, 1973.

Bartke, A., Croft, B. T., and Dalterio, S. Prolactin restores plasma testosterone levels and stimulates testicular growth in hamsters exposed to short day-length. *Endocrinology,* 1975, *97,* 1601–1604.

Beach, F. A. Sexual attractivity, proceptivity and receptivity in female mammals. *Hormones and Behavior,* 1976, *7,* 105–138.

Berger, P. J., Sanders, E. H., Gardner, P. D., and Negus, N. C. Phenolic plant compounds functioning as reproductive inhibitors in *Microtus montanus. Science,* 1977, *195,* 575–577.

Birke, L. I. A., and Archer, J. Open-field behavior of oestrous and diestrous rats: Evidence against an "emotionality" interpretation. *Animal Behaviour,* 1975, *23,* 509–512.

Bridges, R. S., and Goldman, B. D. Diurnal rhythms in gonadotropins and progesterone in lactating and photoperiod-induced acyclic hamsters. *Biology of Reproduction,* 1975, *13,* 617–622.

Bronson, F. H. Rodent pheromones. *Biology of Reproduction,* 1971, *4,* 344–357.

Bronson, F. H. Urine marking in mice: Causes and effects. In R. L. Doty (Ed.), *Mammalian Olfaction, Reproductive Processes and Behavior.* New York: Academic Press, 1976.

Brooks, R. J., and Banks, E. M. Behavioral biology of the collared lemming (*Dicrostonyx groenlandicus* (traill)): An analysis of acoustic communication. *Animal Behaviour Supplement,* 1973, *6*(1), 1–83.

Brown-Grant, K. The role of the retina in the failure of ovulation in female rats exposed to constant light. *Neuroendocrinology,* 1974, *16,* 243–254.

Butcher, R. L., Collins, W. E., and Fugo, N. W. Plasma concentrations of LH, FSH, prolactin, progesterone and estradiol 17-B throughout the 4-day estrous cycle of the rat. *Endocrinology,* 1974, *94,* 1704–1708.

Campbell, C. S., and Schwartz, N. B. Steroid feedback regulation of luteinizing hormone and follicle-stimulating hormone secretion rates in male and female rats. *Journal of Toxicology and Environmental Health,* 1977, *3,* 61–95.

Campbell, C. S., and Schwartz, N. B. The impact of constant light on the estrous cycle of the rat. *The Physiologist,* 1978, *21,* 16.

Campbell, C. S., Ryan, K. D., and Schwartz, N. B. Estrous cycle in the mouse: Relative influences of continuous light and the presence of a male. *Biology of Reproduction,* 1976, *14,* 292–299.

Campbell, C. S., Schwartz, N. B., and Firlit, M. G. The role of adrenal and ovarian steroids in the control of serum LH and FSH. *Endocrinology,* 1977, *101,* 162–172.

Carter, C. S. Postcopulatory sexual receptivity in the female hamster: The role of the ovary and adrenal. *Hormones and Behavior,* 1972, *3,* 261–265.

Christian, J. J. Hormonal control of population growth. In B. E. Eleftheriou and R. L. Sprott (Eds.), *Hormonal Correlates of Behavior.* New York: Plenum Press, 1975.

Czaja, J. A., and Goy, R. W. Ovarian hormones and food intake in female guinea pigs and rhesus monkeys. *Hormones and Behavior,* 1975, *6,* 329–349.

Dorrington, J. H. Steroidogenesis in vitro. In S. Zuckerman and B. J. Weir (Eds.), *The Ovary* (2nd ed.). Vol. 3. New York: Academic Press, 1977.

Ducker, M. J., Bowman, J. C., and Temple, A. The effect of constant photoperiod on the expression of oestrus in the ewe. *Journal of Reproduction and Fertility Supplement,* 1973, *19,* 143–150.

Duff, R. H., and Bush, L. F. The effect of low environmental temperature on initiation of the breeding season and fertility in sheep. *Journal of Animal Science,* 1955, *14,* 885–896.

Eayrs, J. T., Glass, A., and Swanson, H. H. The ovary and nervous system in relation to behavior. In S. Zuckerman and B. J. Weir (Eds.), *The Ovary* (2nd ed.). Vol. 2. New York: Academic Press, 1977.

Elliott, J. Circadian rhythms and photoperiodic time measurement in mammals. *Federation Proceedings,* 1976, *35,* 2339–2346.

Epple, G. Chemical communication and reproductive processes in non-human primates. In R. L. Doty (Ed.), *Mammalian Olfaction, Reproductive Processes and Behavior.* New York: Academic Press, 1976.

Everett, J. W. The mammalian female reproductive cycle and its controlling mechanisms. In W. C. Young (Ed.), *Sex and Internal Secretions* (3rd ed.). Vol 1. Baltimore: Williams & Wilkins, 1961.

Feder, H. H., and Marrone, B. L. Progesterone: Its role in the central nervous system as a facilitator and inhibitor of sexual behavior and gonadotropin release. *Annals of the New York Academy of Science,* 1977, *286,* 331–354.

Ferin, M., Tempone, A., Zimmering, P. E., and Vande Wiele, R. L. Effects of antibodies to 17B estradiol and progesterone on the estrous cycle of the rat. *Endocrinology*, 1969, *85*, 1070–1078.

Finkelstein, J. S., Baum, F. R., and Campbell, C. S. Entrainment of the female hamster to reversed photoperiod: Role of the pineal. *Physiology and Behavior*, 1978, *21*, 105–111.

Fitzgerald, F. M., and Zucker, I. Circadian organization of the estrous cycle of the golden hamster. *Proceedings of the National Academy of Science, USA,* 1976, *73*, 2923–2927.

Floody, O. R., Pfaff, D. W., and Lewis, C. D. Communication among hamsters by high frequency acoustic signals. II. Determinants of calling by females and males. *Journal of Comparative and Physiological Psychology*, 1977, *91*, 807–819.

Foreman, M. M., and Moss, R. L. Effects of subcutaneous injections and intrahypothalamic infusion of releasing hormones on lordotic response to repetitive coital stimulation. *Hormones and Behavior*, 1977, *8*, 219–234.

Frisch, R. E. Population, food intake and fertility. *Science*, 1978, *199*, 22–30.

Godley, W. C., Wilson, R. L., and Horst, V. Effect of controlled environment on the reproductive performance of ewes. *Journal of Animal Science*, 1966, *25*, 212–216.

Goldfoot, D. A., and Goy, R. W. Abbreviation of behavioral estrus in guinea pigs by coital and vagino-cervical stimulation. *Journal of Comparative and Physiological Psychology*, 1970, *72*, 426–434.

Goldfoot, D. A., Kravetz, M. A., Goy, R. W., and Freeman, S. K. Lack of effect of vaginal lavages and aliphatic acids on ejaculatory responses in rhesus monkeys: Behavioral and chemical analyses. *Hormones and Behavior*, 1976, *7*, 1–27.

Goldman, B. D., Kamberi, I. A., Suteri, P. K., and Porter, J. C. Temporal relationship of progestin secretion, LH release and ovulation in rats. *Endocrinology*, 1969, *85*, 1137–1143.

Goodman, R. L. A quantitative analysis of the physiological role of estradiol and progesterone in the control of tonic and surge secretion of luteinizing hormone in the rat. *Endocrinology*, 1978a, *102*, 142–150.

Goodman, R. L. The site of the positive feedback action of estradiol in the rat. *Endocrinology*, 1978b, *102*, 151–159.

Gorbman, A., and Bern, H. A. *A Textbook of Comparative Endocrinology.* New York: Wiley, 1962.

Grau, G. A. Olfaction and reproduction in ungulates. In R. L. Doty (Ed.), *Mammalian Olfaction, Reproductive Processes, and Behavior.* New York: Academic Press, 1976.

Gray, J. A., and Levine, S. Effect of induced oestrus on emotional behaviour in selected strains of rats. *Nature* (London), 1964, *201*, 1198–1200.

Greenwald, G. S. Exogenous progesterone: Influence on ovulation and hormone levels in the cyclic hamster. *Journal of Endocrinology*, 1977, *73*, 151–155.

Guttman, R., Lieblich, I., and Gross, R. Behavioral correlates of estrous cycle stages in laboratory mice. *Behavioral Biology*, 1975, *13*, 127–132.

Harrison, R. J., and Weir, B. J. Structure of the mammalian ovary. In S. Zuckerman and B. J. Weir (Eds.), *The Ovary* (2nd ed.). Vol. 1. New York: Academic Press, 1977.

Herbert, J. Initial observations on pinealectomized ferrets kept for long periods in either daylight or artificial illumination. *Journal of Endocrinology*, 1972, *55*, 591–597.

Herbert, J. External factors and ovarian activity in mammals. In S. Zuckerman and B. J. Weir (Eds.), *The Ovary* (2nd ed.). Vol. 2. New York: Academic Press, 1977.

Hoffmann, J. C. The influence of photoperiods on reproductive function in female mammals. In R. O. Greep and E. B. Astwood (Eds.), *Handbook of Physiology, Section 7, Endocrinology.* Vol. 2, Part 1. Washington, D.C.: American Physiological Society, 1973.

Howland, B. E. Reduced gonadotropin release in response to progesterone or gonadotropin releasing hormone (GNRH) in old female rats. *Life Sciences*, 1976, *19*, 219–224.

Hyde, J. S., and Sawyer, T. F. Estrous cycle fluctuations in aggressiveness of house mice. *Hormones and Behavior*, 1977, *9*, 290–295.

Johnston, R. E. Sex pheromones in golden hamsters. In D. Müller-Schwarze and M. M. Mozell (Eds.), *Chemical Signals in Vertebrates.* New York: Plenum Press, 1977.

Kent, G. C., Ridgway, D. M., and Strobel, E. F. Continual light and constant estrus in hamsters. *Endocrinology*, 1968, *82*, 699–703.

Lamond, D. R. Seasonal changes in the occurrence of oestrus following progesterone suppression of ovarian function in the Merino ewe. *Journal of Reproduction and Fertility*, 1964, *8*, 101–114.

Lawton, I. E., and Schwartz, N. B. Pituitary–ovarian function in rats exposed to constant light: A chronological study. *Endocrinology*, 1967, *81*, 497–508.

Leatham, J. H. Nutritional effects on endocrine secretions. In W. C. Young (Ed.), *Sex and Internal Secretions* (3rd ed.). Vol. 1. Baltimore: Williams & Wilkins, 1961.

Legan, S. J., and Karsch, F. J. A daily signal for the LH surge in the rat. *Endocrinology*, 1975, *96*, 57–62.

Legan, S. J., and Karsch, F. J. Neuroendocrine regulation of the estrous cycle and seasonal breeding in the ewe. *Biology of Reproduction*, 1979, *20*, 74–85.

Legan, S. J., Karsch, F. J., and Foster, D. L. The endocrine control of seasonal reproductive function in the ewe: A marked change in response to the negative feedback action of estradiol on luteinizing hormone secretion. *Endocrinology*, 1977, *101*, 818–824.

Leikin, M. E., and Campbell, C. S. Reinitiation of estrous cyclicity in underfed rats by constant light. *The Physiologist*, 1978, *21*, 70.

Lipner, H. Mechanism of mammalian ovulation. In R. O. Greep and E. B. Astwood (Eds.), *Handbook of Physiology, Section 7, Endocrinology*. Vol. 2, Part 1. Washington, D.C.: American Physiological Society, 1973.

Lisk, R. O. Hormonal regulation of sexual behavior in polyestrus mammals common to the laboratory. In R. O. Greep and E. B. Astwood (Eds.), *Handbook of Physiology, Section 7, Endocrinology*. Vol. 2, Part 1. Washington D.C.: American Physiological Society, 1973.

Mann, D. R., Korowitz, C. D., MacFarland, L. A., and Cost, M. G. Interaction of the light–dark cycle, adrenal glands and time of steroid administration in determining the temporal sequence of LH and prolactin release in female rats. *Endocrinology*, 1976, *99*, 1252–1262.

McCormack, C. E., and Sridaran, R. Timing of ovulation in rats during exposure to continuous light: Evidence for circadian rhythm of LH secretion. *Journal of Endocrinology*, 1978, *76*, 135–144.

Michael, R. P. The effect of hormones on sexual behavior in female rats and rhesus monkeys. In R. O. Greep and E. B. Astwood (Eds.), *Handbook of Physiology, Section 7, Endocrinology*. Vol. 2, Part 1. Washington, D.C.: American Physiological Society, 1973.

Miller, H. L., and Alliston, C. S. Influence of programmed circadian temperature changes upon levels of luteinizing hormone in the bovine. *Biology of Reproduction*, 1974, *11*, 187–190.

Moore, R. Y., and Eichler, V. B. Central neural mechanisms in diurnal rhythm regulation and neuroendocrine responses to light. *Psychoneuroendocrinology*, 1976, *1*, 265–279.

Moore, R. Y., and Klein, D. C. Visual pathways and the central neural control of a circadian rhythm in pineal serotonin N-acetyltransferase activity. *Brain Research*, 1974, *71*, 17–33.

Morin, L. Progesterone: Inhibition of rodent sexual behavior. *Physiology and Behavior*, 1977, *18*, 701–715.

Morin, L. P., and Fleming, A. S. Variation of food intake and body weight with estrous cycle, ovariectomy and estradiol benzoate treatment in hamsters *(Mesocricetis auratus)*. *Journal of Comparative and Physiological Psychology*, 1978, *92*, 1–6.

Morin, L. P., Fitzgerald, K. M., and Zucker, I. Estradiol shortens the period of hamster circadian rhythms. *Science*, 1977, *196*, 305–307.

Nalbandov, A. V. Control of luteal function in mammals. In R. O. Greep and E. B. Astwood (Eds.), *Handbook of Physiology, Section 7, Endocrinology*. Vol. 2, Part 1. Washington, D.C.: American Physiological Society, 1973.

Negus, N. C., and Berger, P. J. Experimental triggering of reproduction in a natural population of *Microtus montanus*. *Science*, 1977, *191*, 1230–1231.

Norman, R. L., Blake, C. A., and Sawyer, C. H. Estrogen dependent twenty-four hour periodicity in pituitary LH release in the female hamster. *Endocrinology*, 1973, *93*, 965–970.

Oxender, W. D., Noden, P. A., and Hafs, H. D. Estrus, ovulation, and serum progesterone, estradiol and LH concentrations in mares after an increased photoperiod during winter. *American Journal of Veterinary Research*, 1977, *38*, 203–206.

Radford, H. M., and Watson, R. H. Influence of rams on ovarian activity and oestrus in Merino ewes in the spring and early summer. *Australian Journal of Agricultural Research*, 1957, *8*, 460–470.

Raps, D., Barthe, P. L., and Desaulles, P. A. Plasma and adrenal corticosterone levels during the different phases of the sexual cycle in normal female rats. *Experientia*, 1971, *27*, 339–340.

Reiter, R. J. Circannual reproduction rhythms in mammals related to photoperiod and pineal function: A review. *Chronobiologica*, 1974, *1*, 365–395.

Reiter, R. J. Changes in pituitary prolactin levels of female hamsters as a function of age, photoperiod and pinealectomy. *Acta Endocrinologica*, 1975, *79*, 43–50.

Reiter, R. J., Rudeen, P. K., and Vaughan, M. K. Restoration of fertility in light-deprived female hamsters by chronic melatonin treatment. *Journal of Comparative Physiology*, 1976, *111*, 7–13.

Rothchild, I. The nature of the luteotrophic process. *Journal of Reproduction and Fertility Supplement*, 1966, *1*, 49–81.

Rowell, T. E. Female reproduction cycles and social behaviour in primates. In D. S. Lehrman, R. A. Hinde, and E. Shaw (Eds.), *Advances in the Study of Behaviour*. Vol. 4. New York: Academic Press, 1972.

Rowlands, I. W., and Weir, B. J. The ovarian cycle in vertebrates. In S. Zuckerman and B. J. Weir (Eds.), *The Ovary* (2nd ed.). Vol. 2. New York: Academic Press, 1977.

Roy, E. J., and Wade, G. N. Role of food intake in estradiol induced body weight changes in female rats. *Hormones and Behavior*, 1977, *8*, 265–274.

Rusak, B. The role of the suprachiasmatic nuclei in the generation of circadian rhythms in the golden hamster, *Mesocricetus auratus*. *Journal of Comparative and Physiological Psychology*, 1977, *118*, 145–164.

Ryan, K. D. *Estrous Cycles in the Mouse: Influence of Large Group Housing and the Presence of a Male.* Ph.D. dissertation, Northwestern University, 1976.

Ryan, K. D., and Schwartz, N. B. Grouped female mice: Demonstration of pseudopregnancy. *Biology of Reproduction*, 1977, *17*, 578–583.

Sadleir, R. M. F. S. *The Ecology of Reproduction in Wild and Domestic Animals.* London: Methuen, 1969.

Schwartz, N. B. Mechanisms controlling ovulation in small animals. In R. O. Greep and E. B. Astwood (Eds.), *Handbook of Physiology, Section 7, Endocrinology.* Vol. 2, Part 1. Washington, D.C.: American Physiological Society, 1973.

Schwartz, N. B., and Channing, C. P. Evidence for ovarian "inhibin": Suppression of the secondary rise in serum follicle stimulating hormone levels in proestrous rats by injection of porcine follicular fluid. *Proceedings of the National Academy of Science, USA*, 1977, *74*, 5721–5724.

Schwartz, N. B., and Hoffmann, J. C. Ovulation: Basic aspects. In H. Balin and S. Glasser (Eds.), *Reproductive Biology.* Amsterdam: Excerpta Medica, 1972.

Schwartz, N. B., Krone, K., Talley, W. L., and Ely, C. A. Administration of antiserum to ovine FSH in the female rat: Failure to influence immediate events of the cycle. *Endocrinology*, 1973, *92*, 1165–1174.

Signoret, J. P. Chemical communication and reproduction in domestic mammals. In R. L. Doty (Ed.), *Mammalian Olfaction, Reproductive Processes, and Behavior.* New York: Academic Press, 1976.

Smalstig, E. B., and Clemens, J. D. The role of the suprachiasmatic nuclei in reproductive cyclicity. *Neuroscience*, 1975, Abstract 434.

Smith, S. L. Mood and the menstrual cycle. In E. J. Sacher (Ed.), *Topics in Psychoneuroendocrinology.* New York: Raven Press, 1975.

Sridaran, R., and McCormack, C. E. Predicting the time of ovulation in rats by monitoring running activity. *Federation Proceedings*, 1977, *36*, 313.

Steiner, M., and Carroll, B. J. The psychobiology of premenstrual dysphoria: Review of theories and treatment. *Psychoneuroendocrinology*, 1977, *2*, 321–335.

Stetson, M. H., and Watson-Whitmyre, M. Nucleus suprachiasmaticus: The biological clock in the hamster. *Science*, 1976, *191*, 197–199.

Stetson, M. H., Watson-Whitmyre, M., and Matt, K. S. Circadian organization in the regulation of reproduction: Timing of the 4-day estrous cycle of the hamster. *Journal of Interdisciplinary Cycle Research*, 1977, *8*, 350–352.

Swerdloff, R. S., Jacobs, H. S., and Odell, W. D. Synergistic role of progestogens in estrogen induction of LH and FSH surge. *Endocrinology*, 1972, *90*, 1529–1536.

Tamarkin, L., Hollister, C. W., Lefebvre, N. G., and Goldman, B. D. Melatonin induction of gonadal quiescence in pinealectomized Syrian hamsters. *Science*, 1977, *198*, 953–955.

Tartellin, M. D. Cyclic variations in food and water intake of ewes. *Journal of Physiology* (London), 1968, *195*, 29p–31p.

Ter Haar, M. B. Circadian and estrual rhythms in food intake in the rat. *Hormones and Behavior*, 1972, *3*, 213–219.

Turek, F. W., and Campbell, C. S. Photoperiodic regulation of neuroendocrine–gonadal activity. *Biology of Reproduction*, 1979, *20*, 32–50.

Wade, G. M. Sex hormones, regulatory behaviors and body weight. In J. S. Rosenblatt, R. A. Hinde, E. Shaw, and C. Beer. (Eds.), *Advances in the Study of Behavior.* Vol. 6. New York: Academic Press, 1976.

Wang, G. H. The relation between spontaneous activity and oestrous cycle in the white rat. *Comparative Psychology Monographs*, 1923–1925, *2*(6).

Watson, R. H., and Radford, H. M. Influence of rams on the onset of oestrus in Merino ewes in the spring. *Australian Journal of Agricultural Research*, 1960, *11*, 65–71.

Welschen, R., and Dullaart, J. Administration of antiserum against ovine follicle-stimulating hormone or ovine luteinizing hormone at proestrus in the rat: Effects on follicular development during the oncoming cycle. *Journal of Endocrinology*, 1976, *70*, 301–306.

Whitten, W. K., and Champlin, A. K. The role of olfaction in mammalian reproduction. In R. O. Greep and E. B. Astwood (Eds.), *Handbook of Physiology, Section 7, Endocrinology.* Vol. 2, Part 1. Washington, D.C.: American Physiological Society, 1973.

Wise, D. A. Aggression in the female golden hamster: Effects of reproductive state and social isolation. *Hormones and Behavior*, 1977, *5*, 235–250.

Yoshinaga, K. Gonadotropin induced hormone secretion and structural changes in the ovary during the nonpregnant reproductive cycles. In R. O. Greep and E. B. Astwood (Eds.), *Handbook of Physiology, Section 7, Endocrinology*. Vol. 2, Part 1. Washington, D.C.: American Physiological Society, 1973.

Young, W. C., Dempsey, E. W., and Myers, H. I. Cyclic reproductive behavior in the female guinea pig. *Journal of Comparative Physiology*, 1935, *19*, 313–335.

Yuthasastrakosol, P., Palmer, W. M., and Howland, B. E. Luteinizing hormone, oestrogen, and progesterone levels in peripheral serum of anestrous and cyclic ewes as determined by radioimmunoassay. *Journal of Reproduction and Fertility*, 1975, *43*, 57–65.

Zuckerman, S., and Weir, B. J. (Eds.). *The Ovary* (2nd ed., 3 vols.). New York: Academic Press, 1977.

Glossary

Symbols *(For Explanations, see below)*

τ	Period of a biological rhythm (oscillation).
T	Period of a zeitgeber.
$\alpha; \rho$	Activity time; rest time (two fractions of an activity rhythm).
ϕ	Phase angle of biological oscillation.
Φ	Phase angle of zeitgeber.
ψ	Phase-angle difference between zeitgeber and biological oscillation.
LD	Light-dark cycle. A light-dark cycle is composed of light time (L) and dark time (D); the term *photoperiod* is used synonymously with light time.
LL; DD	Continuous illumination; continuous darkness.
c.t.	Circadian time. A time scale covering one full circadian period; the zero point is defined arbitrarily.
z.t.	Zeitgeber time. A time scale covering one full zeitgeber period; the zero point is defined arbitrarily.
PRC	Phase-response curve.

Definitions of Oscillating Systems

1. Classification referring to *internal* features of the oscillating system:

    a. *Active system:* capable of self-sustaining oscillations (endogenous rhythms).
    b. *Passive system:* capable only of forced oscillations (exogenous rhythms) or damped oscillations.

2. Classifications referring to *external* conditions:

    a. *Autonomous system:* not under the influence of a periodic input (self-sustaining and damped oscillations).
    b. *Heteronomous (nonautonomous) system:* under the influence of a periodic input (forced oscillations, whether in an active or in a passive system).

Period: time after which a definite phase of the oscillation recurs.

Frequency: reciprocal of period.

Mean value: arithmetic mean of all instantaneous values of an oscillating variable within one period.

Amplitude: difference between maximum (or minimum) and mean value in a sinusoidal oscillation; often used in a looser sense for other oscillations, too.

Range of oscillation: difference between maximum and minimum value (independent of shape of oscillation).

Phase: instantaneous state of an oscillation within a period, represented by the value of the variable and all its time derivatives.

Phase angle: value of the abscissa corresponding to a phase of the oscillation, given in degree or any other fraction of the whole period with reference to an arbitrarily set zero point. It can be given in units of time, if the length of the period is stated.

EXPLANATION OF FURTHER TERMS

Acrophase: phase angle of the crest (maximal value) of a sine function fitted to the raw data of a rhythm (time series).

Circarhythms: classes of rhythms that are capable of freerunning in constant conditions with periods approximating that of the environmental cycle to which they are normally synchronized, and that are entrainable by zeitgebers (circadian, circatidal, circalunar, circannual rhythms).

Desynchronization: (a) *External:* loss of synchronization between rhythm and zeitgeber. (b) *Internal:* loss of synchronization between two rhythms within one organism.

Entraining agent: synonymous with *zeitgeber.*

Entrainment: synchronization of a self-sustaining oscillation by a forcing oscillation (zeitgeber). During entrainment, the frequencies of the two oscillations are the same or integral multiples (entrainment by frequency demultiplication).

Freerun: state of a nonentrained circarhythm, either in constant conditions or after loss of entrainment by a zeitgeber that is still present but too weak.

Infradian: biological rhythm with a period longer than that of a circadian rhythm.

Pacemaker: localizable functional entity capable of self-sustaining oscillations and of synchronizing other rhythms.

Phase-angle difference: difference between corresponding phase angles in two coupled oscillations, given either in degree or in units of time. Often, "corresponding" phase angles have to be defined arbitrarily.

Phase-response curve: indicates how the amount and the sign of a phase shift, induced by a single stimulus, depends on the phase at which the stimulus is applied.

Phase shift: single displacement of an oscillation along the time axis; may occur instantaneously or after several transients.

Photoperiod: synonymous with light time (*see* symbol LD).

Range of entrainment: range of period (T) within which a self-sustaining oscillation can be entrained by a zeitgeber.

Transients: temporary oscillatory states between two steady states.

Ultradian: biological rhythm with a period shorter than that of a circadian rhythm.

Zeitgeber: the forcing (external) oscillation that entrains a biological (self-sustaining) oscillation.

Index